Culinary Essentials

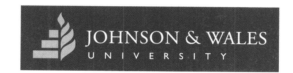

America's Career University®

Second Edition

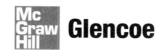 **Glencoe**

New York, New York   Columbus, Ohio   Chicago, Illinois   Woodland Hills, California

Safety Notice

The reader is expressly advised to consider and use all safety precautions described in this textbook or that might also be indicated by undertaking the activities described herein. In addition, common sense should be exercised to help avoid all potential hazards and, in particular, to take relevant safety precautions concerning any known or likely hazards involved in food preparation, or in use of the procedures described in *Culinary Essentials*, such as the risk of knife cuts or burns.

Publisher and Authors assume no responsibility for the activities of the reader or for the subject matter experts who prepared this book. Publisher and Authors make no representation or warranties of any kind, including but not limited to, the warranties of fitness for particular purpose or merchantability, nor for any implied warranties related thereto, or otherwise. Publisher and Authors will not be liable for damages of any type, including any consequential, special or exemplary damages resulting, in whole or in part, from reader's use or reliance upon the information, instructions, warnings or other matter contained in this textbook.

Brand Disclaimer

Publisher does not necessarily recommend or endorse any particular company or brand name product that may be discussed or pictured in this text. Brand name products are used because they are readily available, likely to be known to the reader, and their use may aid in the understanding of the text. Publisher recognizes that other brand name or generic products may be substituted and work as well or better than those featured in the text.

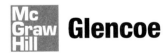

The McGraw-Hill Companies

Copyright ©2006 by The McGraw-Hill Companies, Inc.
All rights reserved. Except as permitted under the United States Copyright Act, no part of this publication may be reproduced or distributed in any form or by any means, or stored in a database or retrieval system, without prior written permission of the publisher, Glencoe/McGraw-Hill.

Send all inquiries to:
Glencoe/McGraw-Hill
21600 Oxnard Street, Suite 500
Woodland Hills, CA 91367

ISBN 0-07-869070-6

Printed in the United States of America

5 6 7 8 9 10 058 08 07

FOREWORD

Johnson & Wales University is known as America's Career University. We are student centered, employment-focused, market-driven, experientially based, and globally oriented. Johnson & Wales University partnered with Glencoe/McGraw-Hill to bring you a unique textbook filled with the essential knowledge and skills needed to become a culinary professional.

Culinary Essentials will show you:

- the value of quality customer service to the dining experience
- the role of foodservice management, standards, regulations, and laws.
- why safety and sanitation must be controlled at all times.
- how to use the equipment found in the professional kitchen
- how culinary nutrition will enable you to create successful menus.
- how to use standardized recipes to control costs.
- the cooking techniques used in quantity food preparation.

Our philosophy is to learn by doing, so we hope you make good use of this learning tool and pursue a rewarding career in culinary arts. We invite you to visit www.jwu.edu to learn more about Johnson & Wales University and culinary arts careers.

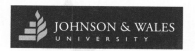

JOHNSON & WALES
UNIVERSITY

America's Career University®

Karl Guggenmos, M.B.A., A.A.C.
University Dean, Culinary Education

Paul J. McVety M.Ed.
Dean, Culinary Academics

Johnson & Wales University Contributors

Dr. Manuel Pimentel, Jr.
Sr. Vice President
University Relations

Robert M. Nograd, C.M.C.
Dean Emeritus
Corporate Executive Chef

Dr. Bradley J. Ware
Professor
Foodservice Academic Studies

John Chiaro, C.E.C., C.C.E., A.A.C
Associate Professor
College of Culinary Arts

Paula Figoni
Associate Professor
College of Culinary Arts

Edward Korry
Department Chair
Beverage and Dining Services
College of Culinary Arts

Johnson & Wales University Contributors (continued)

Martha Crawford
Assistant Dean
International Baking & Pastry Institute

Gary Welling
Department Chair
International Baking & Pastry Institute

Suzanne Vieira
Department Chair
Culinary Nutrition Program

Roger Dwyer
Associate Professor
College of Culinary Arts

Russ Zito
Associate Professor
College of Culinary Arts

William J. Day
Senior Advancement Officer
Johnson & Wales University

Adam Sacks
Associate Instructor
College of Culinary Arts

Louis Serra
Associate Instructor
College of Culinary Arts

Adrian Barber
Associate Instructor
College of Culinary Arts

Debra Bettencourt
Faculty Support
College of Culinary Arts

Special thanks to the students of Johnson & Wales University's Providence Campus for their assistance with photographs throughout this textbook.

Special thanks to the following educators for their important contributions.

Allen B. Asch, Chef-Instructor, C.C.E.
Area Technical Trade Center
North Las Vegas, Nevada

Dorothy M. Gunter,
Retired Culinary Arts Instructor
Elgin U-46 School District
Elgin, IL

Michael Fritch, Vice Principal
The Villages Charter Middle School
The Villages, Florida

Paul Richter, Culinary Arts Instructor
Sea-Tac Occupational Skills Center
Seattle, Washington

Nila Marquard, Career Technical Supervisor
R.G. Drage Career Technical Center
Massillon, Ohio

Denise Brown Johnson, B.A., M.A.
Food Service Instructor
Terrebonne Parish School System
Houma, Louisiana

Reesa Levy, M.S., R.D., Assistant Principal
Cobble Hill School of American Studies
Brooklyn, New York

Shellie A. Fulk Kiedrowski
Hospitality Services & Travel
  Academy Coordinator
Birdville Independent School District
North Richland Hills, Texas

Priscilla Rose Wheeler
Family & Consumer Sciences Instructor
James Island Charter High School
Charleston, South Carolina

Garrett C. Sanborn, C.C.E., C.E.C.
Chef/Instructor
Jefferson County Public Schools
Louisville, Kentucky

Denise Schaefer, C.E.C., C.C.E.
Culinary Arts Chef Instructor
Penta Career Center
Perrysburg, Ohio

Thomas G. Wells Sr.
Culinary/Hospitality Instructor
Herkimer County BOCES
Herkimer, New York

Giorgio Moro, Food Service Coordinator
Miami Dade County Public School System
Miami, Florida

Amy Bergman
Family & Consumer Sciences Instructor
Woodland High School
Cartersville, Georgia

Barbara S. A. Harrison
Culinary Arts Instructor
Copper Hills High School
West Jordan, Utah

Gerald W. Garrett, Culinary Arts Instructor
Pittsylvania Career & Technical Center
Chatham, Virginia

Wealthy Slattery, B.S.
Culinary Arts Instructor
Crenshaw High School
Los Angeles, California

Susan C. Teelin
Family & Consumer Sciences Instructor
Camden Middle School
Camden, New York

Beverly J. Swisher
Family & Consumer Sciences Instructor
Wichita West High School
Wichita, Kansas

Patsy Phelps, Culinary Instructor
Palm Bay High School
Melbourne, Florida

(Continued)

Special thanks to the following educators for their important contributions.

Spankie Lou Basset, Culinary Arts Instructor
Bernalillo High School
Bernalillo, New Mexico

Linda Sader
Family & Consumer Sciences Instructor
Beloit Junior-Senior High School
Beloit, Kansas

Hilde Marschalek
Retired Family & Consumer Sciences
  Instructor
Clifton High School
Clifton, New Jersey

Selene J. Toliver, Chef-Instructor
Breithaupt Career & Technical Center
Detroit, Michigan

Thomas E. Gillen, C.E.C., C.C.E.
Chef-Instructor
Lancaster County Career & Technology Center
Mount Joy, Pennsylvania

Francy M. Johnson
Family & Consumer Sciences Dept. Chair
San Diego High School
San Diego, California

Rev. James E. Laymond, Sr.
Culinary Arts Instructor
Barbara Jordan High School for Careers
Houston, Texas

Contents

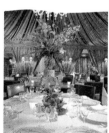

Unit 3: The Professional Kitchen

Unit 4: Culinary Applications

Unit 5: Baking & Pastry Applications

CAREER PATHWAYS...

KEY Math SKILLS

KEY Science SKILLS

Charts

a LINK to the Past

Recipes

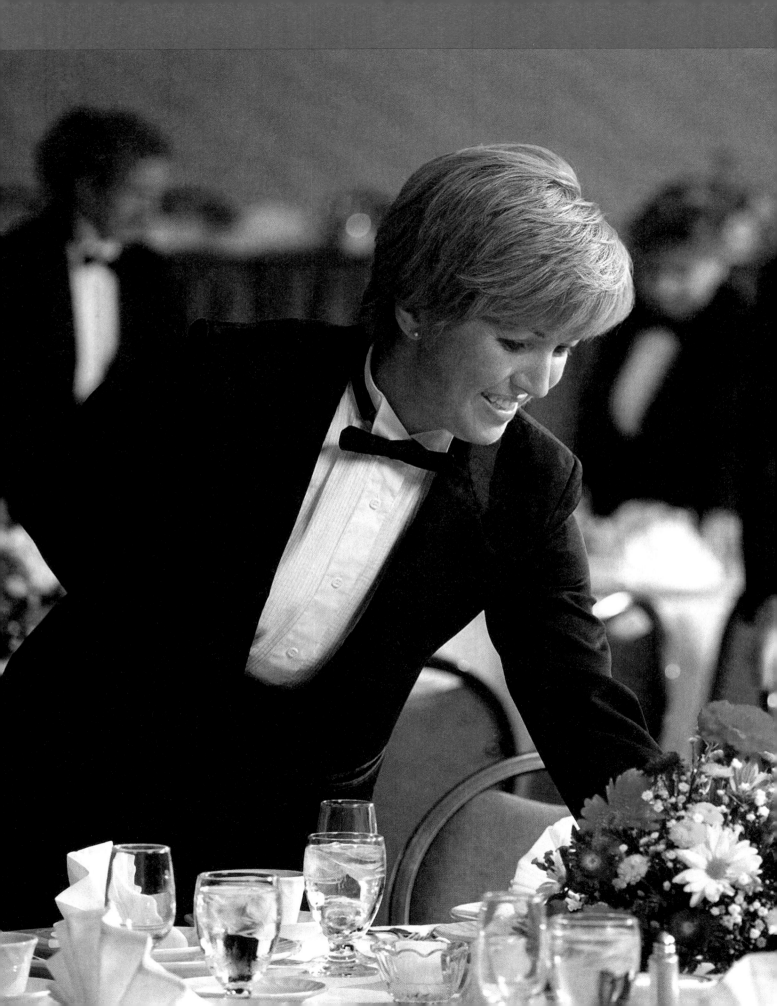

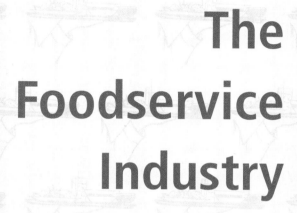

UNIT 1

The Foodservice Industry

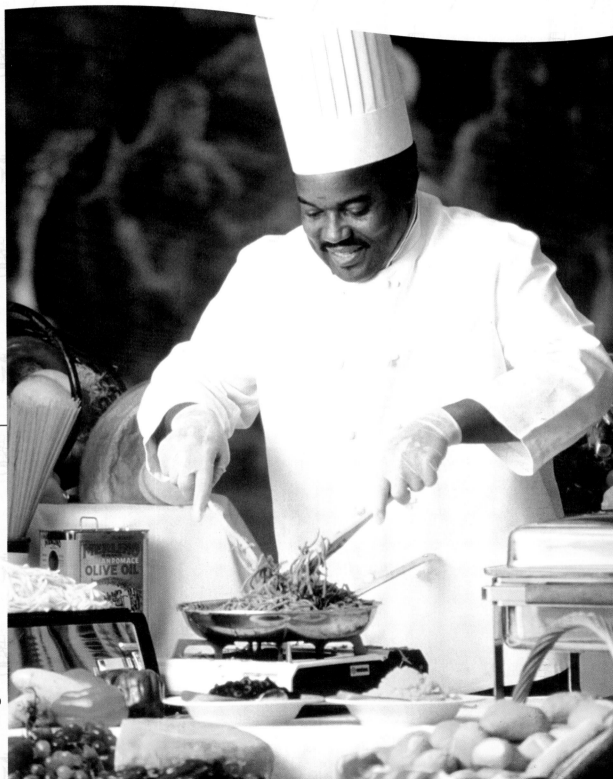

Foodservice Career Opportunities

1

CHAPTER

16

Careers in Foodservice

KEY TERMS

- **brigade**
- **cross-train**
- **sous chef**
- **garde manger**
- **vendor**

OBJECTIVES

After reading this section, you will be able to:

- Describe different food production and service opportunities.
- Describe career opportunities related to food production and service.

THE foodservice industry is about people—the people it serves and the people it employs. Foodservice continues to change, grow, and expand to meet the ever-changing needs of its customers. This growth creates exciting job opportunities. Before starting on your career path, explore the variety of job opportunities available to you.

⊠ FOODSERVICE AT A GLANCE

The foodservice industry employs over 11 million people in the United States ranging from street vendors to fine-dining restaurants. This makes it one of the largest employment segments in the country. Many people are drawn to foodservice careers because of job availability, advancement opportunities, and the creative environment. Others have an interest, a natural ability, or personal experience that draws them into this field of work. The growing interest in global foods, cooking shows, cookbooks, and star chefs has created an increased interest in the food industry.

Employment in foodservice continues to increase as the industry grows and expands. The majority of foodservice positions depend upon providing a service, such as cooking food or waiting on customers. Customers are willing to spend time and money for a pleasant dining experience.

You can choose from an array of foodservice career options. Advancement is also possible if you are willing to work hard and obtain the required training and education.

Employees who take pride in their work and treat customers with courtesy and respect will find many rewarding opportunities in foodservice. The industry welcomes dependable team players that have positive attitudes and a willingness to learn. See Fig. 1-1.

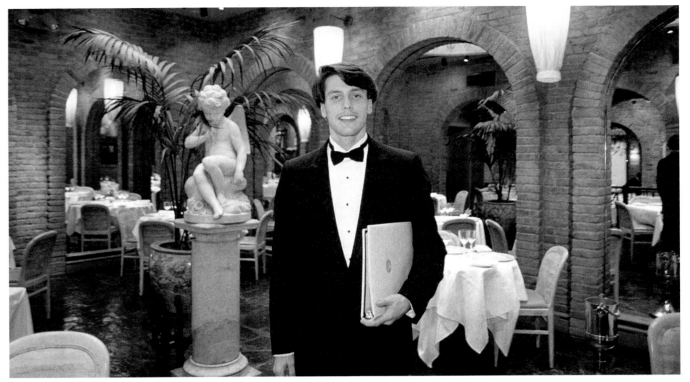

Fig. 1-1. The host must remain calm especially during peak dining times. What other service staff opportunities are available in foodservice?

SERVICE OPPORTUNITIES

Foodservice jobs generally fall into two categories: those that require working directly with customers and those that involve actual food preparation. Individuals who are part of the service staff need to be able to relate to all kinds of customers. Working directly with the public is emotionally and physically demanding. No matter what the situation, the service staff must maintain a pleasant and helpful attitude that promotes good customer service. Four general categories of service staff are: host, cashier, server, and busser. These positions and the duties required are described in Chapter 3.

PRODUCTION OPPORTUNITIES

Historically, foodservice operations have used a kitchen brigade system to divide food production responsibilities. In a kitchen **brigade**, special tasks are assigned to each member of the kitchen staff. These assignments are in line with the person's title. See Fig. 1-2.

Today, most restaurants **cross-train**, or provide work experience in a variety of tasks. Cross-training reduces the cost of labor and results in fast service. The line cooks/station cooks, sous chef, pastry chef, prep cook, and garde manger usually have fairly separate functions in the kitchen, yet by being trained in more than one of these positions, an employee can provide more than one service to the foodservice operation.

■ **Line cooks/station cooks.** Line cooks and station cooks work the production line. They have experience preparing meals quickly. Work is usually divided into stations such as the grill station and the fry station.

■ **Sous chef.** The "under" chef, or **sous** (soo) **chef**, reports to the executive chef. Sous chefs supervise and sometime assist other chefs in the kitchen. They may also fill in for the executive chef when necessary.

■ **Pastry chef.** Pastry chefs are responsible for making baked items, such as breads, desserts, and pastries. Pastry chefs must be skilled in a variety

Fig. 1-2.
Traditional Kitchen Brigade

FRENCH TERM	ENGLISH TERM
Sous Chef (soo)	"Under" Chef
Chefs de Partie (chef-duh-par-TEE)	Line or Station Chefs
Saucier (saw-see-YAY)	Sauce Cook
Poissonier (pwah-sawng-YAY)	Fish Cook
Grillardin (gree-yar-DAHN)	Grill Cook
Friturier (free-too-ree-YAY)	Fry Cook
Rotisseur (roh-tess-UHR)	Roast Cook
Entremetier (ehn-tray-mee-tee-YAY)	Vegetable Cook
Potager (poh-tah-ZHAY)	Soup Cook
Tournant (toor-NAHN)	Swing Cook
Garde Manger (gahrd-mohn-ZHAY)	Pantry Chef
Patissier (pah-tees-ee-YAY)	Pastry Chef
Boucher (boo-CHER)	Butcher

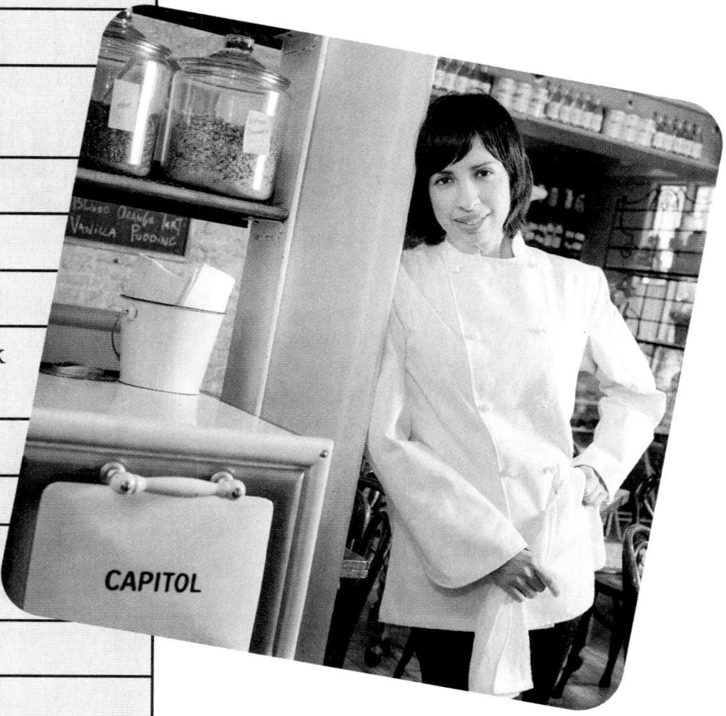

of bread and pastry techniques. They produce muffins, biscuits, cakes, pies, and other baked goods.

■ **Prep cook.** Prep cooks prepare ingredients to be used on the food line. For example, they might wash and peel fruits and vegetables or cut and trim meats. Prep cooks then properly store these items to maintain freshness and allow for easy access.

■ **Garde manger.** The pantry chef, or **garde manger** (gahrd-mohn-ZHAY), is responsible for preparing cold food items. These items may include salads, cold meats and cheeses, and cold sauces.

✗ MANAGEMENT OPPORTUNITIES

Management opportunities in the foodservice industry are offered to individuals with appropriate work experience, training, and education. Careful selection of managers is critical for a foodservice operation to run efficiently and smoothly.

■ **Executive chef.** The executive chef manages all kitchen operations. Depending on the size of the operation, the executive chef works with the restaurant manager and the dining room supervisor as part of the management team. Executive chefs order supplies, organize work schedules, and supervise food preparation and service. They

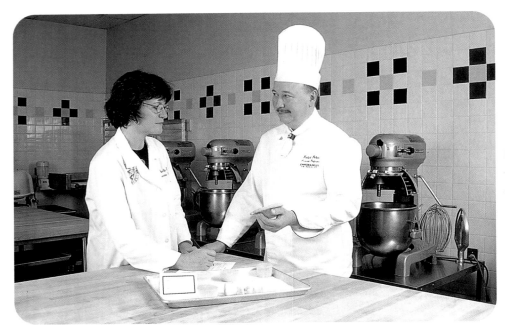

Fig. 1-3. Research chefs help turn recipes into prepackaged foods.

also work with management to develop menus. Executive chefs keep up with the latest developments in the industry by continuing their education and attending conferences and seminars.

■ **Research chef.** Large food manufacturers, such as Pillsbury® and Kraft®, have experienced research chefs working in their labs or test kitchens. Many restaurant chains also employ research chefs. Research chefs work closely with food scientists to produce new food products. Research chefs can also turn favorite recipes into packaged food products and develop nutrition labels. See Fig. 1-3.

■ **Culinary scientist.** The field of culinary science integrates two disciplines—culinary arts and food science. This occupation sets new standards in the food technology industry. Knowledge of culinary arts, nutrition, food science, and technology are required for this career.

■ **Foodservice director.** Foodservice directors oversee the banquet operations of hotels, banquet facilities, hospitals, and universities. They coordinate events that require food and servers. In a large operation, the foodservice director is in charge of all self-service or full-service dining operations. The foodservice director works closely with the executive chef to ensure quality foodservice.

■ **Catering director.** The catering director reports to the foodservice director or general manager. In large operations, there can be numerous functions going on at once. The catering director coordinates the menus for each function. Each event requires careful planning and coordination.

■ **Kitchen manager.** The kitchen manager takes the place of the executive chef in most chain restaurants. The kitchen manager orders ingredients and makes sure that they are prepared correctly. Kitchen managers also supervise non-production kitchen staff, such as employees involved in purchasing. Unlike an executive chef, a kitchen manager might not have the authority to determine the culinary direction of the operation.

■ **Dining room supervisor.** Depending on the size and budget of the restaurant, there may or may not be a dining room supervisor. The dining room supervisor coordinates the hosts, servers, and bussers and also assigns responsibilities to each of these positions. The supervisor's goal is to make each customer's dining experience pleasant.

■ **Restaurant manager.** The kitchen manager and dining room supervisor report to the restaurant manager. The restaurant manager oversees the entire restaurant. This includes the day-to-day operations, such as record keeping, payroll, advertising, and hiring. The restaurant manager may perform other roles, especially if staffing or the budget is limited.

RELATED OPPORTUNITIES

As you can see, the foodservice industry has many opportunities for motivated, hard-working, experienced, and educated people. Other positions, such as purchaser and sales representative, also help an operation run smoothly.

■ **Purchaser.** A purchaser buys goods according to his or her restaurant clients' current needs. This involves shopping around for the best prices and ordering the amount of each ingredient needed to meet the demands of the menu.

■ **Sales representative.** A sales representative often represents a **vendor**, or a company that sells products to the foodservice industry. Sales representatives assist chefs in selecting food and equipment that will best fit their needs and budgets. A successful salesperson will also allow customers to test new products and equipment.

REWARDS AND DEMANDS

The food industry has many rewards and demands. The area of the industry or level of employment will determine what those demands and rewards will be. For example, an executive chef has more responsibility, liability, and demands than a line cook. The rewards are also greater. The executive chef makes a much larger income than someone who works on the line.

The foodservice industry does operate on a schedule of long hours and oftentimes, little regard for the holidays. This is a committed business with many exciting and creative opportunities.

The following job opportunities also offer bright futures in the foodservice industry:

- Food researchers.
- Food writers.
- Food scientists.
- Food processors.
- Food stylists.
- Food marketers.
- Menu developers.
- Recipe developers.
- Foodservice trainers.

After years of experience in the culinary field, chefs can choose to take a teaching position at a culinary school or university. See Fig. 1-4.

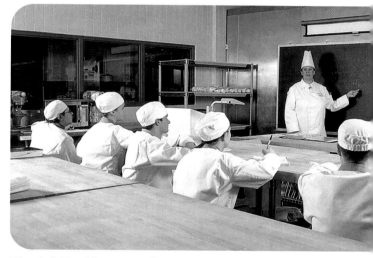

Fig. 1-4. Teaching at a culinary school or university is an excellent option for an experienced chef.

SECTION 1-1   Knowledge Check

1. What are the differences between the service staff and food preparation positions?
2. Describe two types of management job opportunities.
3. Compare the rewards and demands in the foodservice industry.

MINI LAB

Choose three foodservice job opportunities that interest you. Use print and Internet resources to explore them further. Make a list of the education and training, work experience, and key skills needed for each. Discuss your findings with the class.

Foodservice Trends

KEY TERMS

- trends
- entry-level
- noncommercial operations
- commercial operations
- quick-service
- full-service
- fine-dining

OBJECTIVES

After reading this section, you will be able to:

- Analyze how foodservice trends affect foodservice and food production operations.

- Identify job opportunities in various commercial and noncommercial foodservice and food production operations.

TO be successful, the foodservice industry must reflect the changing needs of the people and communities it serves. One way to determine how foodservice and food production operations can do this is to track and analyze industry trends. **Trends** are general developments or movements in a certain direction within an industry. These trends may be societal, cultural, ethnic, demographic, or economic in nature. As the needs and expectations of customers have changed, so has the industry. Understanding how trends affect the foodservice and food production industry will help you be a successful employee.

⊠ THE HOSPITALITY INDUSTRY

The hospitality industry includes businesses such as restaurants and hotels. As long ago as 3000 B.C., grain traders traveled to different regions selling their products. They needed food, beverages, and shelter on their journeys. When people began offering these services, the hospitality industry was born. Today the hospitality industry is a large, complex network of businesses that stretch around the world. It employs millions of people and services billions.

Food service is a critical part of the hospitality industry. People who are away from home depend on food service for snacks, meals, and beverages. Whether people are on vacation, too busy to cook, or meeting friends for dinner, eating out has become routine. Institutions such as schools and hospitals also provide food service to large numbers of people. With the continued growth of these establishments, job opportunities will also increase. See Fig. 1-5.

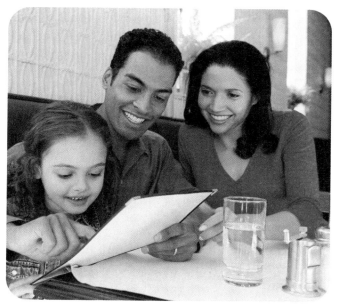

Fig. 1-5. When parents work outside the home, little time may be left for meal preparation. How does a variety of foodservice options benefit families?

TRACKING TRENDS

To understand how foodservice and food production operations can best meet customers' needs, industry experts analyze societal, cultural, demographic, and economic foodservice trends. For example, as the aging population increases, additional workers will be needed at places such as retirement centers and nursing homes. In addition to growing older, the workforce in the United States is more equally divided between men and women. It is also more ethnically and culturally diverse.

Foodservice managers must understand these trends so they can develop methods to attract and keep employees. Trends in foodservice and food production include:

- An increase in the number of theme and chain restaurants.
- A family-friendly atmosphere is easily found.
- Ethnic foods are served at many restaurants.
- Foodservice operations are expanding in sports facilities.
- Special events and private parties center their events around food.
- Supermarkets are carrying prepared and packaged RTE (ready-to-eat) meals.

Industry experts also analyze trends in customer needs. Three societal factors influencing customer needs are family structure, work, and preferences.

- **Family structure.** Family structure is changing as the number of single and single-parent households increases. Another trend in family structure is the increased amount of money children spend on food away from home. See Fig. 1-6.
- **Work.** The number of people who work and the hours they spend working is another important economic trend. Men and women are both working more hours. This leaves them with little time to prepare meals. Restaurants and supermarkets that offer take-out and delivery services have helped fill this need by offering food quickly and conveniently.
- **Preferences.** Customer tastes and preferences also are changing. Customers are more knowledgeable about food choices and also are more concerned with eating healthful foods. As the population becomes more ethnically and culturally diverse, people desire a larger number of cuisines. Customers also expect to get value for the money they spend on food.

Fig. 1-6. The customer's desire for attractive, healthful, and flavorful food greatly impacts foodservice trends.

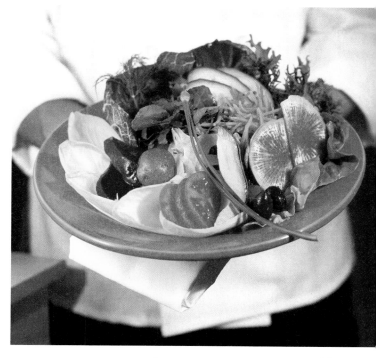

WHAT DOES THE FUTURE HOLD?

The customers it serves will determine the future of the foodservice industry. As customer needs change, foodservice operations will have to find ways to meet those needs.

Technology will also impact the future of food service. Computers and improved commercial equipment will continue to make food preparation and service faster and more efficient. However, technology cannot replace the smile of a helpful server or the artistic skill of a chef. The foodservice industry will always rely on people to provide personal service to customers.

WHERE ARE THE OPPORTUNITIES?

The foodservice industry offers hundreds of jobs in many different settings. These range from **entry-level**, or beginning jobs that require little or no experience, to jobs that require years of work experience and education. Moving up from an entry-level position takes hard work and the proper training and education. See Fig. 1-7.

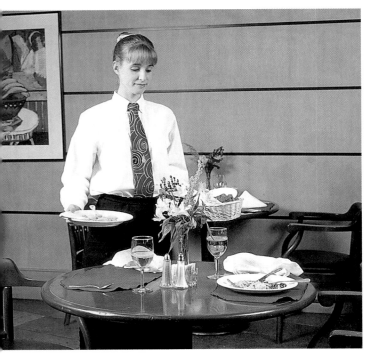

There are two settings in which food service takes place: noncommercial and commercial. **Noncommercial operations**, such as government facilities, schools, and hospitals, aim to cover daily expenses, such as wages and food costs. **Commercial operations**, such as fast-food chains and fine-dining restaurants, earn more than enough to cover daily expenses, resulting in a profit.

Restaurants

Job opportunities at restaurants are available across the country. See Fig. 1-8. More people are eating out than ever before and restaurants are multiplying to meet this demand. Customers choose a restaurant based on different needs and expectations. For example, to celebrate a special occasion, they may choose a fine-dining restaurant. To quickly feed a family before a baseball game, customers may choose a quick-service restaurant.

- **Quick-service restaurants.** Establishments that quickly provide a limited selection of food at low prices are called **quick-service** restaurants. Customers order their food at the counter and then carry it home or to a table to eat. Many quick-service restaurants, such as fast-food chains, also offer take-out and delivery services. Entry-level opportunities, such as a cook or cashier, are common at quick-service restaurants. Many of these facilities hire high school students on a part-time basis.

- **Full-service restaurants.** Servers take customer orders and then bring the food to the table in **full-service** restaurants. Customers seeking a relaxed foodservice operation that offers full service without high prices will choose a casual restaurant. Casual, full-service restaurants range from themed facilities to family restaurants that offer child-friendly menus.

- **Fine-dining restaurants.** A **fine-dining** restaurant offers an upscale atmosphere, excellent food

Fig. 1-7. Entry-level jobs are a great way to get a taste of the foodservice industry.

Fig. 1-8.

RESTAURANT	JOB OPPORTUNITIES
Quick-Service	Manager, Assistant Manager, Cashier, Prep Cook, Line Cook.
Full-Service	Dining Room Manager, Host, Cashier, Server, Busser, Dishwasher, Kitchen Manager, Line Cook, Prep Cook, Sauté Cook, Pantry Chef.
Fine-Dining	Dining Room Manager, Maitre d', Head Server, Server, Captain, Busser, Dishwasher, Executive Chef, Sous Chef, Sauté Cook, Pastry Chef, Pantry Chef.

and service, and higher menu prices. Staff members at a fine-dining restaurant are exceptionally skilled in their positions, whether as a server or executive chef. Most job opportunities in fine-dining restaurants require both work experience and training.

Hotels & Resorts

Providing customers with food and beverages is an essential service in a lodging facility. Many lodging facilities have a combination of foodservice operations from which customers can choose. This range of food service provides a wide array of jobs.

Health spas are one way hotels and resorts offer customers services that calm and relax customers. They are often known for their healthful food and personal service. Job opportunities include a team of chefs, dietitians, and service staff.

Banquet Facilities

It is not uncommon for banquet facilities to be booked months in advance for weddings and other special occasions. Most banquet facilities are open only for catered events or meetings. They usually offer both full and part-time employment. Job opportunities include banquet manager, banquet captain, server, executive chef, sous chef, sauté cook, pantry chef, and catering manager.

Government Facilities

In addition to traditional food service, many military bases feature food from quick-service restaurants, such as Pizza Hut®. Bases also use a lot of vending machines. Job opportunities include cooks, entry-level counter help, and fast food preparation. See Fig. 1-9.

On-Site Catering

Chefs, cooks, servers, bussers, and managers can all be employed by on-site catering operations. To increase their income, many schools, hospitals, nursing homes, and government facilities offer catering services. Many restaurants also cater on-site. They have also developed frozen food products that are now available in super-

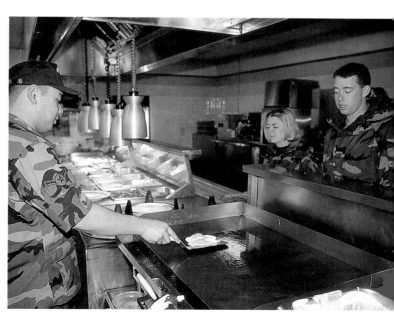

Fig. 1-9. Foodservice opportunities also exist on military bases.

markets. For example, food products from Marie Callender® and Bob Evans® restaurants can be found in many supermarkets.

Off-Site Catering

With off-site catering, a caterer or catering company prepares and delivers food from a centralized kitchen to different locations. Catering companies have an advantage over restaurants because they know in advance how many guests will attend and the amount of food required. If the function is canceled, the client must still pay the original amount. This decreases food waste and allows the caterer to staff the appropriate number of servers. Job opportunities are available for chefs, cooks, and servers.

Bakeries & Pastry Shops

Commercial kitchens often purchase baked goods from bakeries and pastry shops. This method is often less costly than making the food in house. There has also been a recent increase in customers wanting homestyle baked goods. As a result, employment at bakeries and pastry shops is increasing. See Fig. 1-10.

Other Opportunities

Ready-to-eat (RTE) food products from various restaurants and manufacturers are now available at supermarkets and specialty food stores. Many supermarkets include an on-site deli, bakery, and butcher shop. Some supermarkets also offer catering services. The following settings also offer great foodservice job opportunities: cruise ships, airlines, resorts, athletic clubs, and corporate headquarters.

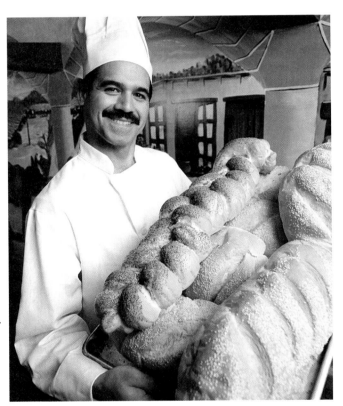

Fig. 1-10. Bakeries and pastry shops offer many opportunities for pastry chefs and bakers. Investigate the skills needed to become a pastry chef.

SECTION 1-2 Knowledge Check

1. Analyze how trends impact foodservice and food production operations.
2. Define the two categories of foodservice operations.
3. List several foodservice and food production job opportunities.

MINI LAB

Using print and Internet resources, analyze the societal, cultural, ethnic, demographic, and economic factors that affect the foodservice industry. Discuss your findings with the class.

Education & Training

OBJECTIVES

After reading this section, you will be able to:

- Describe educational and training programs that can prepare you for a foodservice career.

- List ways you can prepare while still in high school for a foodservice career.

YOU can begin preparing for a career in the foodservice industry while you're still in high school. This section discusses how you can get foodservice experience now. It also describes different educational and training programs that you can enter after high school graduation. These programs will help you gain the skills and experience necessary for a successful foodservice career.

✕ PREPARING FOR FOODSERVICE CAREERS

There are many different ways you can prepare for a career in foodservice. You can begin in high school by taking culinary arts or foodservice courses and trying to get part-time work at a foodservice operation. After high school, you can enroll in an apprenticeship program, a certificate program, or an associate or bachelor degree program. Corporate training programs are another way to gain valuable skills and experience.

Remember that it is possible to work your way up in the foodservice industry. However, the more education and training you have, the faster you will advance. Choose an education or training program that will best fit your goals.

A high school education is a solid foundation on which to build your foodservice career. Learning excellent communication skills—reading, writing, listening, and speaking—is critical. Classes in English and mathematics will teach you the basic skills you'll need for any foodservice job. Special programs in foodservice production and the culinary arts are offered at many high schools, career centers, and vocational-technical schools. See Fig. 1-11.

Another way to learn about the industry is through a part-time, entry-level job in a foodservice operation. Entry-level positions, such as dishwasher and counter worker, require little or no

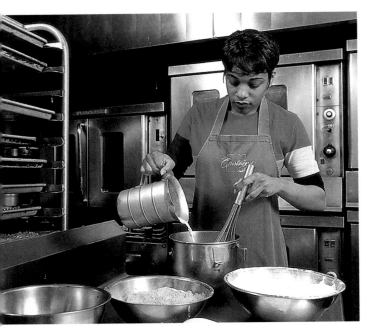

Fig. 1-11. Taking a class such as this will help jump-start your foodservice career.

training or experience. Instead, you learn on the job. Entry-level positions are readily available in quick-service or full-service restaurants. Most operations offer flexible hours, so you can build your work schedule around school. An entry-level job will show you what it's really like to work in the foodservice industry.

✖ CERTIFICATE PROGRAMS

Many culinary schools, community colleges, and foodservice operations offer certificate programs. These programs often involve work experience, coursework, and a certification test. **Certification**, or proof of expertise, is available in different areas, such as culinary, baking, and pastry. Obtaining certification in any area of the culinary arts will make you more marketable.

Before enrolling in a certificate program, carefully evaluate the program and the reputation of the school or operation. Find out what job opportunities are available for individuals with that particular certification. Remember, certification programs usually focus on particular skills. Advancement opportunities may require that you attain more formal education.

a LINK to the Past

The Emperor of Chefs

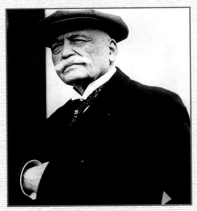

Auguste Escoffier is one of the most famous and innovative chefs in history. His accomplishments serve as an inspiration to culinary professionals today.

Born in France in 1846, Escoffier began his career at the age of 13 working in his uncle's restaurant in Nice. For the next 30 years, he worked in cities throughout Europe gaining fame for his culinary skills.

In 1890, Escoffier was hired by César Ritz as head chef of the elegant Savoy Hotel in London. In 1898, he moved on to the famous Carlton Hotel. During this time, Escoffier defined French cuisine and dining among the rich and famous. Escoffier's culinary innovations include eliminating elaborate food displays and garnishes, reducing the number of courses served at a formal meal, making sauces less heavy, and serving seasonal foods. He respected and preserved the basic principles of classical cuisine, but simplified the process. Escoffier also restructured the kitchen so that it operated as a single unit—the brigade system, which is still in use today.

APPRENTICESHIPS

An **apprentice** works under the guidance of a skilled worker in order to learn a particular trade or art. In the foodservice industry, an apprentice would learn under an experienced chef or manager. An apprenticeship involves a combination of hands-on training and classroom learning.

Professional organizations and industry associations often operate apprenticeship programs. The American Culinary Federation sponsors apprenticeships across the U.S. The amount of time spent in an apprenticeship program varies greatly.

ASSOCIATE DEGREE PROGRAMS

Many colleges and universities offer two-year, or associate, degrees in the culinary field. Good associate degree programs offer more than just classroom learning. They provide hands-on experience so you can apply the techniques you've learned in class. Selecting a program that meets your needs is important. Evaluate the program, the college or university credentials, and the employment rate for graduates.

BACHELOR DEGREE PROGRAMS

Four-year, or bachelor, degrees prepare students for supervisory and management positions in the foodservice industry. They provide in-depth training in one or more areas. For example, Johnson & Wales University offers several bachelor degree programs. These include Culinary Arts, Baking and Pastry Arts, Culinary Nutrition, and Foodservice Management. See Fig. 1-12.

Two types of bachelor degrees are common in the foodservice industry. Foodservice-related bachelor degrees provide students with hands-on learning and industry-specific information. General bachelor degrees in subjects such as marketing, business, and management provide the basis of a wide array of skills and information.

While pursuing bachelor degrees, students may have the opportunity to participate in a cooperative education or work experience program. These programs match students with a company whose business is related to their interests. This is an excellent way to gain work experience while getting an education.

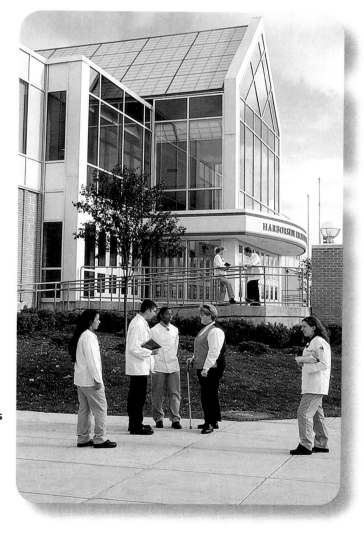

Fig. 1-12. Bachelor degrees are offered at many colleges and universities, such as the Providence, Rhode Island campus of Johnson & Wales University.

CORPORATE TRAINING PROGRAMS

Some corporations, such as large hotels and restaurants, offer specialized training programs. For example, McDonald's® trains its management staff at Hamburger University®, a worldwide training center in Oak Brook, Illinois. This training promotes a consistent style of management in all McDonald's® locations. Large hotels, such as Marriott® and Hilton®, also provide corporate training programs.

Employees do not pay for corporate training programs. These programs provide employees with the opportunity for advancement within the corporation that sponsors them. To get involved in corporate training programs, you usually interview with a company before you graduate from college. See Fig. 1-13.

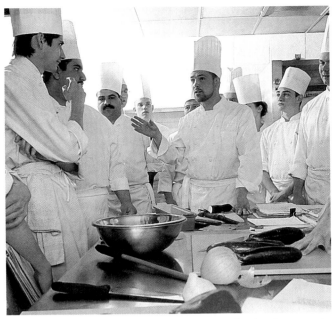
Fig. 1-13. Corporate training programs also lead to excellent job opportunities.

MILITARY TRAINING PROGRAMS

Many opportunities exist for foodservice training in all branches of the military. Entry-level foodservice positions through management positions are available in this military occupational specialty. Most military foodservice personnel leave the military with effective job skills. This allows them to find employment once out of the military.

ON-THE-JOB TRAINING PROGRAMS

On-the-job training is an option for many people. When training employees, some foodservice managers use a training method called job rotation. In this method, entry-level employees are rotated through a series of jobs, which allows them to learn a variety of skills.

Internships are another form of on-the-job training. Classroom instruction and job training are combined in internship programs.

SECTION 1-3 Knowledge Check

1. Name three valuable foodservice skills that you can develop while in high school.
2. Contrast apprenticeships and certificate programs.
3. What are two advantages of corporate training programs?

MINI LAB

Using print and Internet resources, locate information on certificate and apprenticeship programs in your area. Also locate information on the associate and bachelor degree programs available in your state. How many opportunities are there?

Entrepreneurship Opportunities

OBJECTIVES

After reading this section, you will be able to:

- Identify small business opportunities available in foodservice.

- Explain the governmental requirements for starting and running a food business.

- Describe the function of a business plan.

IMAGINE being the boss. An **entrepreneur** (ahn-truh-pruh-NYOOR) is a self-motivated person who creates and runs a business. Entrepreneurs are willing to take personal and financial risks in search of personal satisfaction and financial rewards. Although it may be risky, the rewards of entrepreneurship can be high. Entrepreneurs in the foodservice industry usually begin by opening a small business such as a deli, bakery, or small restaurant.

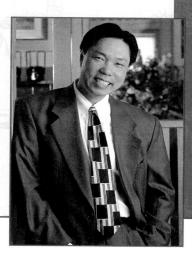

SMALL BUSINESS OPPORTUNITIES

A small business starts with a person's dream. Through hard work and dedication, an entrepreneur turns that dream into a reality. Small businesses, those with fewer than 100 employees, are a vital part of our economy. These businesses produce a wide range of goods and services and employ many people. In fact, more than 53% of the U.S. workforce is made up of people working for small businesses.

Food Production

The fast-paced world creates a strong need for food products that are quick and easy to prepare. Many food entrepreneurs share the dream of creating a new taste sensation. Imagine, for example, taking the family's secret recipe and mass-producing it. Does this appeal to you? Would the rewards of entrepreneurship outweigh the costs? Being an entrepreneur in the food-production business offers the following advantages:

PARTNERSHIP IN PROPORTION

Although you may have a wonderful idea for a new restaurant, you may not have enough money to actually put your ideas into motion. Instead, you may need to form a partnership. A partnership involves splitting profits and losses. Profits and losses are distributed in proportion to each partner's investment.

For instance, two brothers decide to open a new diner. The oldest brother invests $40,000 into the business and the youngest brother invests $60,000. At the end of the first year, this diner makes a 10% net profit of $82,000. The remaining $738,000 covers the operating expenses for the diner. The partnership agreement states that the profits be split in proportion to the amount of money each person invested. To calculate this amount, you would write each amount invested as a fractional part of the total investment. You know that the total investment for the diner was $40,000 + $60,000 = $100,000.

$$\text{Oldest Brother's Share} = \frac{\$40,000}{\$100,000} = \frac{4}{10} = \frac{2}{5}$$

$$\frac{2}{5} \times \$82,000 = \frac{\$164,000}{5} = \$32,800$$

Youngest Brother's Share =

$$\frac{\$60,000}{\$100,000} = \frac{6}{10} = \frac{3}{5}$$

$$\frac{3}{5} \times \$82,000 = \frac{\$246,000}{5} = \$49,200$$

Based on the proportion invested, the younger brother receives $49,200 and the older brother receives $32,800 of the $82,000 net profit of the diner.

TRY IT!

In each of the following, the partnership agreement states that the partners shall distribute the net profit or loss in proportion to their investments.

1. Michele invested $15,000 and Alonzo invested $25,000 in their new deli. Their net profit above operating expenses for the first year was $30,000. What is each partner's share of the profit?

2. Carlos invested $20,000 and Amber invested $5,000 in their new restaurant. Their net loss for the first year was $10,000. What is each partner's share of the loss?

- **Ownership.** You decide what to produce and how to produce it.
- **Job satisfaction.** With the help of food-processing facilities, your secret recipe can make its way to supermarket shelves.
- **Earning potential.** If you've got what it takes, you could be the next Mrs. Fields®!

Entrepreneurship in the food-production business also offers these disadvantages:

- **Financial risk.** Taking a product all the way from an idea to the market involves a lot of money. You could lose all the money you invest, or even more.
- **Competition.** You're not the only one trying to create a new food product.

- **No guarantees.** New products have a high rate of failure. Your food product must also meet strict government regulations.

Food Service

Restaurant ownership often follows one of three patterns: independent, chain, or franchise.

1. An **independent restaurant** has one or more owners and is not affiliated with a national name or brand. The concept, theme , or style is a personal choice.

2. A **chain restaurant** such as Pizza Hut® has many individual restaurants that all have the same atmosphere, service, menu, and quality of food. These restaurants are consistent in appearance and procedures.

3. A **franchise** is a common form of ownership used by chain restaurants. A franchise company sells the business owner the rights to its name, logo, concept, and products. In return, the business owner agrees to run the business as outlined by the franchise company. While certain guidelines are set there is some room for individualizing.

Entrepreneurship in the restaurant business has the following advantages:

- **Ownership.** You can decide what type of restaurant to open.
- **Job satisfaction.** Imagine the creativity and flexibility involved in running your own restaurant.
- **Earning potential.** Some restaurant owners discover financial independence as their business grows.

As with other forms of entrepreneurship, restaurant ownership also has its disadvantages:

- **Financial risk.** Most restaurants have annual sales of less than $500,000. **Overhead costs**— all costs outside food and labor—and expenses consume much of the sales, leaving little profit.
- **Competition.** The restaurant business is a very competitive segment of the retail world.
- **No guarantees.** Nearly half of all individually owned restaurants fail within 12 months. About 85% close within the first five years.

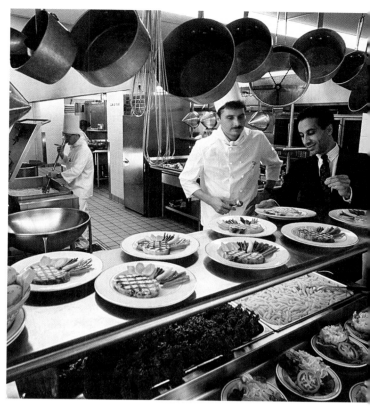

Fig. 1-14. Some food corporations rely on an experienced chef to help them with product development.

Foodservice Management

Foodservice management offers several routes for entrepreneurs. A foodservice consultant is one possible career. For example, an experienced chef might be quite useful to restaurant owners or a corporation opening a new chain of restaurants. Such a chef-consultant might be hired just long enough to oversee the opening of the restaurant(s) to ensure initial success. See Fig. 1-14. Large corporations might hire a culinary expert to work with the marketing team to develop a new food product or service.

Another avenue an entrepreneur might take in foodservice management is that of an employee recruiter. With a tight labor market, many companies hire outside agencies to locate and staff their foodservice operations. To find the right person for the job, an employee recruiter must have a knowledge of the different jobs and skill levels.

DEVELOPING BUSINESS PLANS

One of the primary reasons start-up businesses fail is that a business plan was not followed. A **business plan** is a document that gives specific information about the future of a business. All business plans should include a vision, goals, strategies, and an action plan.

- **Vision.** A business plan starts with an entrepreneur's vision. This vision may include the goods and services the business will offer, how much it will cost to start and run the business, and the business location. It must also include the targeted customer base and an estimate of the profits.
- **Goals.** Once the vision is stated, goals must be put in place. These goals must be specific, concrete, and measurable. The plan must also give a timetable for meeting these goals.
- **Strategies.** A business plan should include strategies for meeting goals. These strategies may include the type of marketing the business will use to attract customers. **Marketing** is the process of promoting and supplying goods and services to customers. It includes a sales and marketing strategy, packaging, advertising, selling, and in some cases, shipping or distribution.
- **Action plan.** An action plan is another part of any business plan. It helps a business reach its goals by giving a specific course of action.

Types of Business Ownership

Once you decide to open a business, you must choose the form of ownership. There are three common types of legal business ownership. Each must be carefully evaluated when developing a business.

- **Sole proprietorship** (proh-PRI-uh-tor-ship). When a business has only one owner, it is called a **sole proprietorship**. Most U.S. businesses—about 75%—are sole proprietorships.
- **Partnership.** The second type of business ownership is a **partnership**, or a legal association of two or more people who share the ownership of the business. Control and profits of the business are divided among partners according to a partnership agreement.
- **Corporation.** The third type of ownership, a **corporation**, is created when a state grants an individual or a group of people a charter with

Fig. 1-15.

BUSINESS OWNERSHIP	ADVANTAGES	DISADVANTAGES
Sole Proprietorship	• Owner makes all decisions. • Easiest form of business to set up. • Least regulated of three forms of business.	• Limited by the skills, abilities, and financial resources of one person. • Difficult to raise funds to finance business. • Owner has sole financial responsibility for company; personal assets sometimes at risk.
Partnership	• Can draw on the skills, abilities, and financial resources of more than one person. • Easier to raise funds than in sole proprietorship.	• More complicated than sole proprietorship. • Tensions and conflicts may develop among partners. • Owners liable for all business losses; personal property sometimes in jeopardy.
Corporation	• Easier to finance than other forms of business. • Financial liability of shareholders limited.	• Expensive to set up. • Record keeping often time-consuming and costly. • Often pays more taxes than other forms of business.

legal rights. The owners buy shares, or parts of the company. If the business fails, the owners lose only the amount of money that they have invested in the business. These owners are called shareholders and earn a profit based on the number of shares they own. See Fig. 1-15.

Government Requirements

The U.S. economic system is known as the free enterprise system. **Free enterprise** means that businesses or individuals may buy, sell, and set prices with little government control. A business decides how many goods and services to provide.

Businesses in a free enterprise system, however, are subject to some government controls. The government passes important laws that set workplace safety standards, prices, and wages. These laws are meant to protect everyone who buys and uses goods and services. You'll learn more about these laws in Chapter 6.

Zoning & Licensing

Although the United States has a free enterprise system, government still has a voice in how businesses are run. Health codes, regulations, and zoning requirements must be met if you're preparing food for sale. **Zoning** divides land into sections used for different purposes. These purposes include residential, business, and manufacturing. Zoning laws help city planners regulate the growth of an area. Only certain activities are permitted within these defined zones.

Before you set up a foodservice business, you must investigate the laws in the area where the product will be produced. For example, you will need to obtain a license that grants you permission to open a business. Special liability insurance is also necessary for food products and some services. You will need to check the licensing and insurance requirements in your city and state.

✖ RECORD KEEPING

You must maintain accurate financial records to run a successful business. These records will include a detailed account of all income and spending. The records are normally updated and maintained by the business owner or an accountant. Many people prefer to use record keeping software. This software helps you set up your records and store this important information on disk as well as on paper. See Fig. 1-16.

Fig. 1-16. Accurate record keeping is an important part of running a successful business.

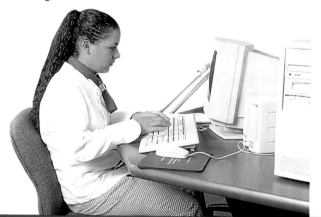

SECTION 1-4   Knowledge Check

1. Contrast various ownership structures in the food production and service industry.
2. What is the function of a business plan?
3. Describe the governmental requirements for starting and running a foodservice business.

MINI LAB

Working in teams, plan to open a new restaurant. Determine the following: the potential customers and their foodservice needs, the staff positions needed, and the location desired. Share your team's decisions with the class.

SECTION SUMMARIES

1-1 Foodservice careers can be divided into two categories: service opportunities and food production or cooking opportunities.

1-1 Management opportunities include positions as research chef, culinary scientist, catering director, kitchen manager, and executive chef.

1-2 Workforce changes and customer needs are two trends tracked by industry experts.

1-2 Cashiers, cooks, servers, sous chefs, and hosts are some of the jobs in commercial and noncommercial foodservice operations.

1-3 Foodservice professionals begin their careers with a solid high school education that may include foodservice courses.

1-3 Working a part-time, entry-level foodservice position while in high school is one way to prepare for a foodservice career.

1-4 Food production, restaurant ownership, and management are three small business opportunities for entrepreneurs.

1-4 A business plan helps you envision the future of your business.

1-4 Businesses operate in a system of free enterprise.

CHECK YOUR KNOWLEDGE

1. Identify three positions in foodservice that require working directly with customers.
2. List the members of a traditional kitchen brigade system.
3. What do trends in foodservice tell experts?
4. What is the difference between a commercial and noncommercial foodservice operation?
5. Name three ways to prepare for a foodservice career.
6. How does an independent restaurant differ from a chain?
7. What information should be included in a business plan?
8. Name three types of business ownership?

CRITICAL-THINKING ACTIVITIES

1. Debate the pros and cons of food production and management opportunities. Why are positions in management more demanding?
2. After studying foodservice in high school, you decide to continue your education in the field. Explain which would be a better choice—an apprenticeship program or a college degree.

WORKPLACE KNOW-HOW

Decision making. Imagine that you currently work as a part-time server in a local restaurant. You take foodservice courses in school and are interested in management. Two positions become available where you work: one for a host, the other for a prep cook. Which position would you apply for? Why?

LAB-BASED ACTIVITY:

Foodservice Careers

STEP 1 Identify at least five different job titles from the chart on this page that are of interest to you.

STEP 2 Use print and Internet resources to research the job titles you selected. Your research should include:

- A thorough description of the job title. This should include the duties to be performed, the required job skills, the responsibilities, the career path, the career opportunities, job outlook, and rewards. Discover how far the position will take you in foodservice, and where you can move for a career change.
- A complete list of other job titles that the job may be known as.
- Key skills needed.
- Education and training requirements.
- National average salary ranges.
- A list of the resources you used for your research.
- A list of the demands and rewards of different jobs in the foodservice industry.

STEP 3 If possible, interview someone who holds each position. Ask what role personal priorities and family responsibilities played in his or her career choice.

STEP 4 Once you have completed your research, organize the job title information into a report.

STEP 5 Present your report to the class. When you're done, explain why you would or would not want to pursue a career in the five job areas you researched.

Service Jobs	Production Jobs
• Assistant Manager	• Assistant Pastry Chef
• Banquet Captain	• Baker
• Banquet Manager	• Caterer
• Cafeteria Manager	• Chef
• Chef Instructor	• Dietician
• Culinary Educator	• Director of Research
• Dining Room Captain	• Executive Chef
• Dining Room Manager	• Federal Food Inspector
• Director of Foodservice Marketing	• Garde Manger
• District Manager	• Kitchen Manager
• Food Service Director	• Line Cook
• General Manager	• Menu Planner
• Host	• Nutritionist
• Maitre d'	• Pantry Worker
• Purchasing Agent	• Pastry Chef
• Quality Assurance Specialist	• Pastry Cook
• Research Development Specialist	• Prep Cook
• Sales Manager	• Production Manager
• Sales Representative	• Sanitation Supervisor
	• Sauce Cook
	• Seafood Cook
	• Soup Cook
	• Storeroom Supervisor
	• Swing Cook
	• Vegetable Cook

Becoming a Culinary Professional

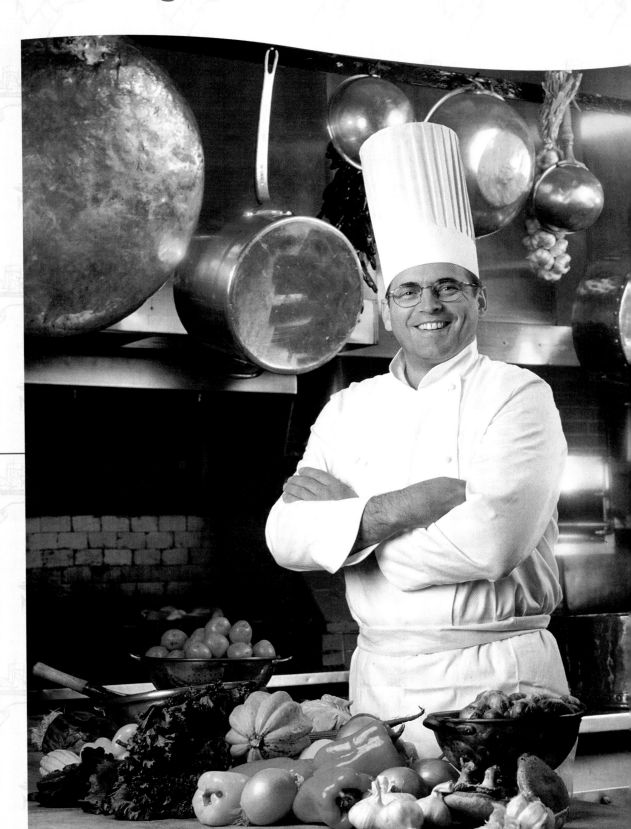

Employability Skills

KEY TERMS

- calculate
- active listening
- distractions
- work ethic
- flexibility
- leadership
- prioritize

OBJECTIVES

After reading this section, you will be able to:

- Apply basic employability skills in foodservice.
- Demonstrate a positive work ethic.
- Practice leadership skills in foodservice.

CONGRATULATIONS! You've decided to pursue a career in food service. Whether you see yourself as a pastry chef or a restaurant manager, your next step is to make your goal a reality. The first skills you will need to become employed in food service are the same skills you will draw on to find and keep a job in any other field. You may already have many of these basic skills. This section will help you polish the abilities you have and develop the skills you need. You'll also learn how employment skills are applied in the foodservice industry.

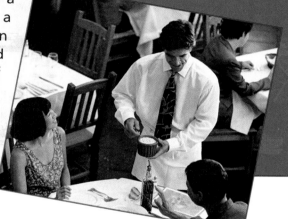

✕ SHARPENING YOUR BASIC SKILLS

Imagine you are a foodservice employer looking to fill an opening. What would you look for in a potential new employee? Depending on the position, you might look for someone with a particular type of education, training, and work experience. For example, you would want a dining-room manager to have supervisory experience.

Beyond this specialized knowledge and experience, however, every employer expects you to have certain basic skills. One of the best moves you can make toward a career in foodservice is to sharpen your basic skills. The ability to calculate, communicate, think, negotiate, and work as a member of a team is critical. These skills will help you acquire the knowledge and experience you'll need to pursue your career goal. These skills will also help you pursue a culinary degree after high school. Basic skills provide you with a strong foundation for finding and keeping employment and advancing on the job.

Math Skills

The ability to **calculate**, or work with numbers, is a fundamental part of every food service job. See Fig. 2-1. You'll add, subtract, multiply, and divide in countless ways. For example:

• Cooks must use math skills to adjust recipe yields, weigh ingredients, and adjust cooking times and temperatures.

• Servers use math skills to total customers' bills, calculate tax, make change, and keep track of tips.

• Foodservice managers use math skills to order supplies, schedule deliveries, set up employee work rosters, complete payroll and tax forms, determine portion sizes, and estimate profits.

• All employees use basic math skills to keep track of their work hours and pay rates.

Here are three situations in which sharpening your basic math skills will improve your chances of employment in food service.

■ **Working with percentages.** Foodservice workers often encounter percentages in recipes. For example, "The fat should make up 40% of the dough." Percentages are also used to calculate the tax on the cost of a food item or a meal. A tax of 8%, for example, means adding 8¢ for every dollar to the total. Converting the percent to a decimal may help.

■ **Making change.** Servers, cashiers, and hosts need to know how to make change for customers. Fig. 2-2 shows the organization of a typical cash

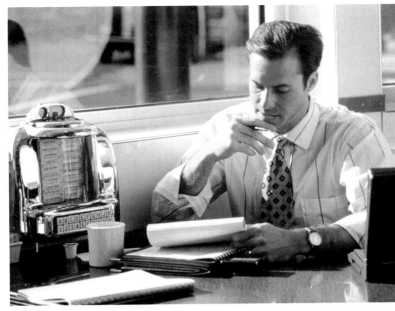

Fig. 2-1. Math skills are important on the job. In what ways will you use math skills in food service?

drawer. When making change at a table or at a cash register that doesn't calculate the change, count up from the amount of the bill to the amount of money the customer gave you. Begin with the smallest coin and count up to the largest bill.

When using a point-of-sales system that indicates the amount of change due the customer, count out the change from the largest bill to the smallest coin. For example, two dollars and forty-two cents.

■ **Weighing and measuring.** Recipes require accurate weighing and measuring of ingredients to ensure product quality and consistency. You'll also need to understand simple fractions to read and follow most recipes. Fractions may need to be multiplied or divided for recipe conversions as well. They may also need to be converted to percents like these:

• ¼ = .25 = 25%
• ⅓ = .33 = 33%
• ½ = .50 = 50%
• ⅔ = .66 = 66%
• ¾ = .75 = 75%

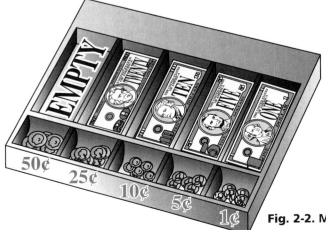

Fig. 2-2. Most cash drawers are organized this way. How does an organized cash drawer help you make correct change?

Listening Skills

You'll be listening and speaking almost constantly while at work. The kinds of listening and speaking skills you need on the job are aimed at promoting understanding.

Listening isn't just appearing to hear what's being said. It is hearing the message and responding to it. To listen you need to avoid distractions. Whether you're taking a customer's order in a restaurant or carrying out the instructions of a chef, you'll need to practice **active listening**, the skill of paying attention and interacting with the speaker. Fig. 2-3 lists key steps in the active listening process.

Try to avoid **distractions** or turning your attention to something else. Focus on what is being said. Even if you disagree with the speaker, listen carefully. Don't let your feelings about the speaker get in the way of your understanding of the message. Wait until the speaker has finished before speaking.

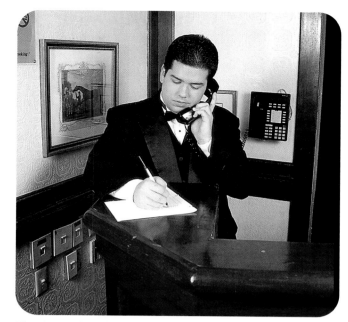

Fig. 2-4. Using the telephone correctly is an important communication skill.

Fig. 2-3.

Be an Active Listener

1. Think about the purpose of the message. Why are you listening?
2. Signal your level of understanding with eye contact and body language, such as nodding your head.
3. Ask questions to help clarify points you do not understand.
4. Listen for the speaker's inflections—the rising and falling tones of voice that communicate emotional content.
5. Look at the speaker's body language. What is he or she saying with posture, gestures, and facial expressions?
6. Select the most important points of the message.
7. Take notes on the message.
8. Listen for the conclusion of the message.

Speaking Skills

How well you are understood depends on how clearly you speak. Pay attention to the following qualities of speech:

- **Pronounce words clearly and correctly.** If you're unsure how to pronounce a word or a name, check a dictionary or ask someone.
- **Don't use slang on the job.** Slang is not appropriate for use in the workplace.
- **Speak each syllable of a word.** Don't slur your words together or drop the endings of words.
- **Try to speak at a medium pace.** Your message will be missed if you speak too quickly, and your listener may become distracted if you speak too slowly.
- **Regulate your volume.** If you speak too softly, people will not hear you. If you speak too loudly, you will annoy your listeners.

When using the telephone, speak clearly at a moderate volume. Even though you can't be seen, smile while you speak on the telephone. The person on the other end of the phone can sense when you're smiling. Your voice on the telephone may be a customer's first or only impression of your business. See Fig. 2-4.

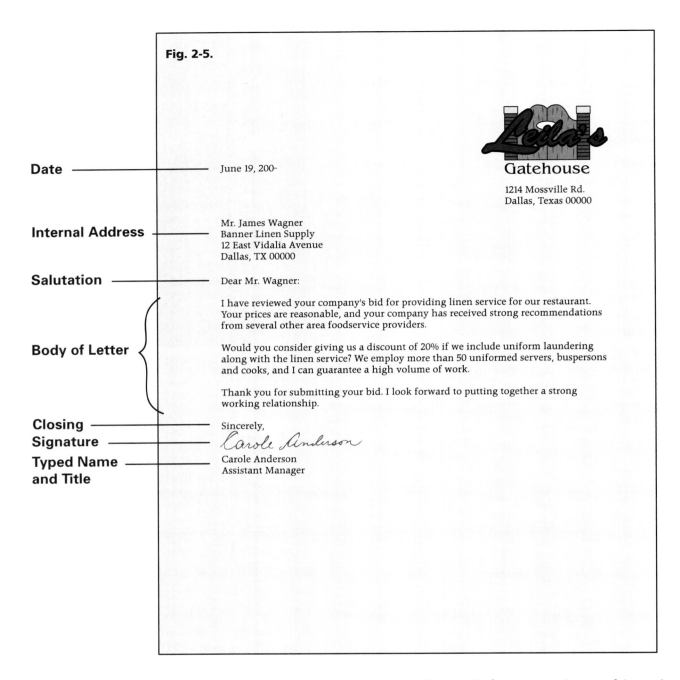

Fig. 2-5.

Date — June 19, 200-

Leila's
Gatehouse
1214 Mossville Rd.
Dallas, Texas 00000

Internal Address —
Mr. James Wagner
Banner Linen Supply
12 East Vidalia Avenue
Dallas, TX 00000

Salutation — Dear Mr. Wagner:

Body of Letter —
I have reviewed your company's bid for providing linen service for our restaurant. Your prices are reasonable, and your company has received strong recommendations from several other area foodservice providers.

Would you consider giving us a discount of 20% if we include uniform laundering along with the linen service? We employ more than 50 uniformed servers, buspersons and cooks, and I can guarantee a high volume of work.

Thank you for submitting your bid. I look forward to putting together a strong working relationship.

Closing — Sincerely,

Signature — *Carole Anderson*

Typed Name and Title —
Carole Anderson
Assistant Manager

■ **Body language.** You also speak without saying a word. Body language, or how you physically respond, also "speaks" for you. The way you sit, stand, move your hands, look, and smile or frown sends a clear message to the listener(s).

Writing Skills

Your ability to communicate in writing will help you find a job and perform well on the job. From business letters to work orders to menus, your writing will improve if you pay attention to the following points.

■ **Your audience.** Before you write anything, picture the person or group who will be reading it. Tailor what you write to the reader's needs.

■ **Your purpose.** Choose language that suits the purpose of your writing. Read what you have written and decide if your writing fulfills its purpose. Most business communications are intended to carry out one of the following purposes:

• To inform or give information or instructions.

• To request or ask for information, seek a decision, or call for action.

• To persuade or convince the reader to agree or to pursue a course of action.

• To complain or to protest.

- **The right style.** The style of your communication involves your choice of language and tone. Business communications are written in a direct style with a professional tone.
- **The correct form.** The two most common forms of business writing are memos and business letters. See Fig. 2-5. Follow basic grammar and punctuation rules when you write. Be sure to use the spell check and grammar check features on the computer to check your writing. It is also a good idea to have someone else proofread your letters before sending them.

Reading Skills

Reading is an important skill both on and off the job. Much of the information you receive from the world around you comes through reading. In foodservice you'll use reading skills to:

- Prepare food by reading ingredient labels and recipes or formulas.
- Operate foodservice equipment by reading instruction manuals and safety precautions.
- Serve customers by reading menus.
- Carry out general job responsibilities by reading workplace policies and communications.

In order to read well, you'll need to develop good reading skills. Here are some basic reading skills you will use on the job.

- **Previewing.** Before you read anything, read the headlines and subheads to get an overview.
- **Skimming.** When reading you should always look for key points. This is called skimming.
- **Focusing.** After you've previewed or skimmed material, give what you're reading your full attention. Think about what you're reading.
- **Visualizing.** If the text is not illustrated, imagine a set of pictures or charts that would accompany what you read.
- **Checking.** Ask yourself how well you're comprehending what you read. If there are words you don't understand, look them up in a dictionary.

Thinking Skills

In addition to basic math and communication skills, you also need to think critically, make decisions, and solve problems.

- **Think critically.** An employee who can think critically can respond to a variety of situations.
- **Make decisions.** When you consistently make good decisions, you will demonstrate the responsibility needed to succeed in the workplace.
- **Solve problems.** Your ability to find quick, practical solutions will make the difference between success and failure.

✖ WORK ETHIC

In addition to basic skills, employers look for certain key qualities in their employees. Demonstrating these qualities shows a strong **work ethic**—a personal commitment to doing your very best as part of the team. The qualities that mark a strong work ethic can be developed with practice. See Fig. 2-6.

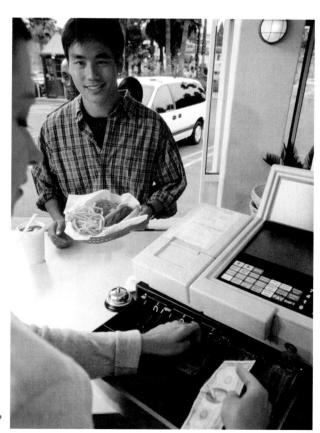

Fig. 2-6. Responsibility is part of a strong work ethic. In what ways can you show responsibility on the job?

Responsibility

Being responsible is one of the most important qualifications for success in any job. Think of responsibility as your ability to respond—to be aware of what a particular situation demands of you. Being responsible means showing up for work on time, even when you'd rather sleep in or go to the beach. It means becoming familiar with the tasks that make up your job and carrying them out correctly. When you are responsible, you accept the consequences of your choices and actions instead of blaming others.

Flexibility

In today's rapidly changing work environment, **flexibility**—the ability to adapt willingly to changing circumstances—is very important. Being flexible on the job means being willing and able to adjust to changes without complaining. The more confident you are in your skills, the easier you'll find it to be flexible when circumstances demand it.

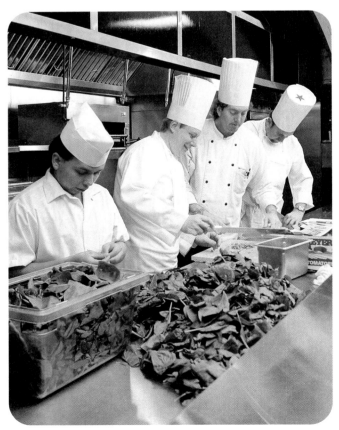

Honesty

Honesty is another important part of a strong work ethic. You practice honesty on the job when you're truthful and loyal in your words and actions. For example, if you make a mistake on the job, don't cover it up or blame someone else. Instead, admit to your mistake and find out how to prevent making the same error in the future. This quality is always appreciated by employers.

Reliability

Reliability (ree-lie-ah-BILL-lah-tee) is an extension of responsibility. When you demonstrate reliability on the job, you contribute to the success of the business. Reliable people are more likely to advance on the job than employees who can't be counted on. A reliable employee is someone who:

- Arrives at work on time.
- Works a full shift.
- Carries out a variety of assigned tasks without constant prompting.
- Takes on extra work when necessary.
- Gets enough rest to work effectively.
- Maintains good physical and mental health.

Teamwork

As a foodservice worker, you will often find yourself part of a large team. A winning team, however, is more than just a collection of talented individuals. If you've ever played a team sport or served as a committee member, you know how important it is that every member participates. Learning to effectively communicate, resolve conflicts, and develop negotiation skills makes for good team members. Just as a star player must support his or her teammates throughout the game, you'll practice teamwork on the job by supporting the efforts of your coworkers. See Fig. 2-7.

Fig. 2-7. Teamwork is part of every job.

How can you demonstrate teamwork?

Commitment

Commitment is the quality that supports all your abilities and skills to build a strong work ethic. The level of commitment you demonstrate on the job will set you apart as a valuable employee. By displaying good business etiquette and always doing your best, you show a commitment to quality and excellence.

■ **Quality.** A commitment to quality means doing work you can be proud of. In food service, a commitment to quality involves using quality ingredients and preparing and serving them in the most pleasing way. When you're committed to quality, you strive to meet the highest standards.

■ **Excellence.** Employees committed to excellence strive to do their very best at all times. They make the most of opportunities to improve their abilities and learn new skills. People who are committed to excellence aren't willing to settle for work that's "just good enough."

LEADERSHIP SKILLS

Beyond basic skills and a strong work ethic, employers look for employees with leadership skills. **Leadership** is the ability to motivate others to cooperate in accomplishing a common task. It is a quality every employee should practice.

You don't need to wait until you're employed to develop leadership skills. Many organizations and programs have been designed to help students develop leadership skills. Two organizations that develop leadership skills are FCCLA and SkillsUSA. See Fig. 2-8 below.

■ **Family, Career and Community Leaders of America (FCCLA).** FCCLA is a national organization of middle and high school students enrolled in family and consumer sciences courses. FCCLA activities and skill events provide opportunities for leadership development. One FCCLA program, Leaders at Work, offers opportunities for students working in food production and services or hospitality and tourism to create projects to strengthen their communication, interpersonal, management, and entrepreneurship skills.

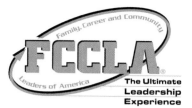

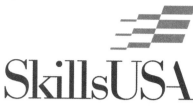

Students also can participate in challenging competitions such as the STAR (Students Taking Action with Recognition) events. Members may compete in such areas as culinary arts, entrepreneurship, and interpersonal communications.

■ **SkillsUSA.** SkillsUSA is a national organization of high school and college students enrolled in training programs for technical, skilled, and service occupations. SkillsUSA programs partner students with industry professionals to provide the SkillsUSA Championships.

Foodservice students can participate in contests for culinary arts and commercial baking. Students are judged on technical skills, sanitation and food safety practices, the quality of prepared items, and their creative presentation. Students can also compete in the area of food and beverage service, demonstrating skills in table setting, greeting guests, taking reservations, menu presentations, and meal service.

Using Resources Effectively

Resources are the raw materials with which you do your work. It's up to you to make the best use of these resources and to avoid wasting them. These key resources are:

• **Time.** You can use time effectively by performing activities quickly and carefully. You can also learn to **prioritize**, or put things in order of importance. Because the world of food service is fast-paced, time is your most limited resource. That's all the more reason to use your time well.

- **Energy.** Use personal energy resources effectively by getting the right amount of rest, nutrition, and health care to do your job well.
- **Money.** Whenever you perform a job transaction that costs or earns money for your employer, you have an opportunity to practice leadership. If you're responsible for making purchases, look for good value for the money. If you're receiving money in payment, be careful and honest.
- **Things.** The materials, equipment, and tools associated with your job are resources. Use supplies properly and carefully. Immediately report any problems with or damage to equipment and supplies. Always take care of your uniform, tools, supplies, and work area.
- **People.** The foodservice industry has busy, almost rushed, service times preceded by slower preparation periods. You waste people resources when you perform your job so poorly that someone else has to redo the job.

Using Information Effectively

Information is coming at you from countless sources. On the job, you will need to acquire, use, and share information.

■ **Acquiring information.** From newspaper headlines to radio and TV news bulletins, information is everywhere. Learn the difference between useful information and idle chatter, false statements, and misleading opinions. Be careful when retrieving information from the Internet. Some Web sites contain false information. Reliable information comes from known sources, such as government agencies or businesses. See Fig. 2-9.

■ **Using information.** Information is worthless until you use it. You show leadership when you can acquire, understand, and use information appropriately.

■ **Sharing information.** Don't keep important information to yourself. The whole team benefits from shared knowledge. Effective leaders share the information they acquire. They also recognize the difference between sharing useful job information and negative conversation, such as gossip.

Fig. 2-9. Leaders acquire, use, and share reliable information. What are some reliable information sources?

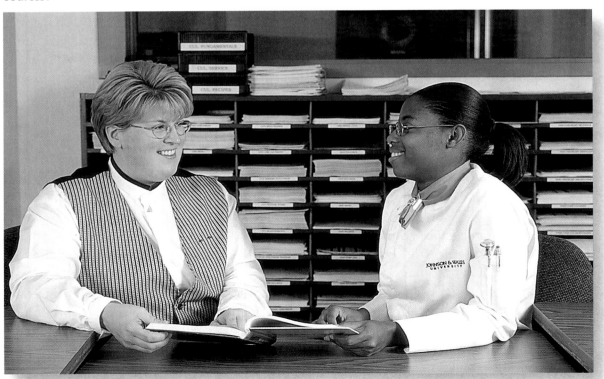

Using Technology Effectively

Technology is a resource, not a replacement for a skilled employee. You can learn to use technology as effectively as you use any other resource. Depending on your job, this can mean knowing how to operate anything from a point-of-sales system to an entire automated production line. Kitchen equipment has also become high-tech. Today there are instant-read thermometers, convection ovens, and ovens that use light waves to cook food. No matter what your role in the foodservice industry, you'll encounter and use computer technology. Here are some tips to keep in mind:

- **Apply your basic computer skills.** Once you know how to work with standard computer software, you can adapt your knowledge and abilities to a variety of uses. These range from entering restaurant orders and tracking inventory to running automated food production equipment, converting recipes, and conducting nutritional analyses (uh-NAL-uh-sees).
- **Respect computer resources on the job.** If your employer provides you with access to a computer, remember to use it for business purposes only. Personal e-mail, Web-surfing, on-line chatting, and computer games are inappropriate uses of work equipment.
- **Don't expect computers to do your job.** Computer technology can assist you enormously, but a computer can't think or solve

problems. Be sure your basic skills are strong enough to compensate when the computer system goes down. Commit yourself to learning and maintaining the technological processes that apply to your job. See Fig. 2-10.

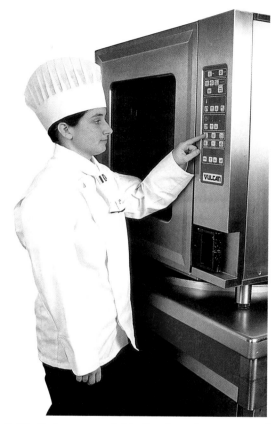

Fig. 2-10. To be successful in food service, you need to know how to use technology effectively. How might you use this *combi-oven* (a combination of convection and steam) in a foodservice kitchen.

SECTION 2-1   Knowledge Check

1. What kinds of basic skills will you need to practice in any job? Give an example of each.
2. What qualities contribute to developing a strong work ethic?
3. List the kinds of resources leaders are expected to use effectively on the job.

MINI LAB

Imagine that you have been asked to lead a team that will prepare and serve refreshments for an upcoming school event. Write a short "help wanted" ad, listing the qualities you want in team members to help you carry out your task.

Seeking Employment

OBJECTIVES

After reading this section, you will be able to:

- Analyze the employment outlook in food production, management, and services.

- Use practical job-search skills.

- Prepare a résumé.

- Complete a job application.

YOUR culinary career begins with your first foodservice job. Whether you enter food service as a server in a restaurant or a counter worker in a bakery, obtaining your first foodservice job will involve sorting through options. This section will familiarize you with the process of seeking and applying for employment.

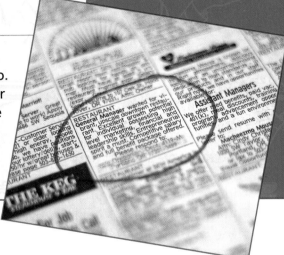

✖ FOODSERVICE EMPLOYMENT

Foodservice offers a positive employment picture. The foodservice industry employs more people than any other segment of the sales and service world. According to the National Restaurant Association, more than 11 million people in the United States are involved in preparing and serving food. Total U.S. sales in foodservice exceed $376 billion annually. The industry continues to grow at a steady rate. New employment opportunities are constantly opening. The popularity of dining out and the steady growth of the restaurant industry make food service an ideal career choice. Entry-level jobs are plentiful and opportunities for advancement are almost unlimited.

✖ EMPLOYMENT RESOURCES

Where can you find out about foodservice job openings? Many first-time job seekers mistakenly believe that classified ads are the only place to search for a job. While it's true that foodservice jobs are frequently listed in the newspaper, there are many resources that can bring a job opportunity to your attention.

Networking

If you've ever followed up on a job tip you received from a family member or friend, you have practiced networking. **Networking** means

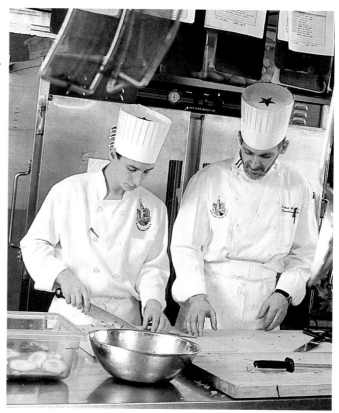

Fig. 2-11. Mentors are always there to give advice and support as you learn new things.

making use of all your personal connections to achieve your career goals. When you seek job information from people you know, you have a good chance of going into the job application process informed and confident. Networking is the most direct way of finding a job. In addition to networking with your family members and relatives, you can also network with:

- **Friends and classmates.** Others who are interested in culinary arts will also be doing job research. They may be willing to share information with you.
- **Teachers and mentors.** These are adults who know you. They are familiar with your strengths and how you could make use of those strengths on the job. See Fig. 2-11.
- **Employers and coworkers.** If you are already employed, your workplace may also be a source of information about job openings. Many companies list internal job postings and opportunities for advancement before telling the general public. Your coworkers may also know about upcoming job openings within or outside of your present workplace.
- **Organizations.** School organizations, such as FCCLA and SkillsUSA, are often willing to help put you in contact with other members. Community organizations can also provide networking information. Collect business cards for future contacts.

When you network, be courteous. Don't pressure people for information. Every reference you receive through networking is a personal gift. Treat it with respect. If you are given a job lead by someone you know, follow up in a responsible manner. Be on time for interviews. Return phone calls and always present yourself professionally. Your dress, communication skills, and behavior reflect not only on you, but on the person who recommended you. And remember to return the favor—when you become aware of job information, share it with the members of your network.

Professional Organizations

Another source of job postings is through professional organizations. These organizations are made up of people already employed in a field. They network on a state, national, or international level. Professional culinary organizations focus on the industry in general or specialized areas such as baking. Here are a few for you to investigate:

- National Restaurant Association (NRA)
- Council of Hotel, Restaurant and Institutional Educators (CHRIE)
- American Culinary Federation (ACF)
- Society for Foodservice Management (SFM)
- Research Chefs Association (RCA)

Although you must pay a membership fee to join professional organizations, the membership benefits almost always outweigh the investment. The services they offer include employment listings, job placement services, scholarships, and network opportunities. Foodservice jobs listed with professional organizations are usually higher paying jobs that require more skill than those listed in the local newspaper.

a LINK to the Past

Being an Apprentice

Today, many foodservice workers get valuable on-the-job training as apprentices via the American Culinary Federation. This concept is not new. In fact, European craftsmen from about 1000–1600 A.D. had apprentices in many professions, including baking.

Apprenticeship was also popular in colonial America, since only the wealthiest families could afford formal schooling for their children. Typically, a boy of 11 or 12 would go to live with a master who would agree to teach him a craft and provide for his food, clothing, and shelter. Some agreements also included a promise to teach the apprentice reading and writing.

The apprentice would agree to work for the master for a certain period of time. At the end of this time, he would become a journeyman and could be paid for jobs, even under another employer.

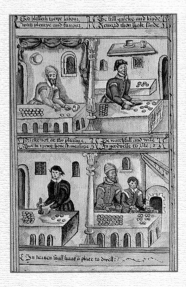

Trade Publications

You can extend your job search resources by reading culinary **trade publications**. These professional magazines and newsletters are produced by and for members of the foodservice industry. They contain helpful articles on all aspects of the industry. Most of them also list job opportunities. Fig. 2-12 lists some prominent foodservice trade publications. Subscriptions to many of these publications are included as part of membership in professional organizations. Some of these trade publications can also be found in public libraries or on the Internet. Many trade publications list job banks that offer a wide and varied range of career opportunities.

Employment Agencies

There may be times when it's best to use an employment agency to assist in your job search. Employment agencies are businesses that put employers in touch with potential employees. Employment agencies maintain lists of job openings and information given to them by people seeking jobs. Most employment agencies charge fees for their services.

The Internet

Thousands of employment resources are available to you in one place. By using the Internet, you can:

- Network with others.
- Contact professional organizations.
- Check out on-line versions of trade publications.
- Register with on-line employment agencies.

You can make the best use of job-search resources by keeping a job file. Use a computer file or a set of index cards to record and review job information you receive from each source. An entry in your job file is a **job lead** or possible employment opportunity. Fig. 2-13 shows a sample job lead card.

Fig. 2-12.

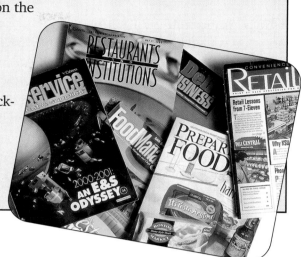

⬛ APPLYING FOR A JOB

If you have identified several good job leads, rank the possible jobs in order of your preference. Apply for the job you want most first.

The first step is usually to request, complete, and return a job application. Some job leads may require you to begin the application process with a telephone call. Other job leads will ask you to contact the employer by mail, sending a letter of application and a résumé (REH-zuh-may). A **résumé** is a summary of your career objectives, work experience, job qualifications, education, and training. The second step in responding to a job lead will be one or more job interviews. **Job interviews** are formal meetings between you and your potential employer. It is important to perform each step of the job application process in a professional manner.

Filling Out an Application

Remember to make a good professional impression from the beginning. Don't walk into a potential workplace, even to ask for an application, unless your clothing is neat and appropriate and you're clean and well-groomed. A job posting won't disappear in the time it takes you to clean up and change clothes.

Even if an application form is not your first step, you'll be asked to complete one at some point during the job application process. That's why you need to know how to fill out the form correctly and completely.

Job application forms vary, but they all ask for the same kinds of information. Keep these tips in mind when completing an application:

- Print neatly, using blue or black ink. Use cursive handwriting for your signature only.

Fig. 2-13.

> ## Job Lead
>
> **Job:** *Kitchen Worker*
>
> **Key Details:** *35 hours per week, mostly evenings and weekends, on-the-job training provided*
>
> **Employer:** *The Limberlost Restaurant*
>
> **Contact Person:** *Maria Smith, Kitchen Manager*
>
> **Source of Lead:** *Mike Smith, neighbor*
>
> **Next Steps:** *Complete and return job application by October 25*

- Read the instructions for completing each blank before responding. Try not to make errors. If you need to correct something you have written, draw a line through what you need to correct.
- Carry important information with you. This includes your Social Security number; driver's license number; and the names, addresses, and phone numbers of previous employers.
- Don't leave any part of the application form blank unless you're asked to do so. If a question doesn't apply, put NA—or not applicable—in the space provided.
- Always tell the truth on an application. Submitting false information is illegal.

Responding by Telephone

Your job leads may come from listings that give phone numbers and ask you to call for more information. When making a phone call, follow these guidelines:

1. Call the number you've been given.

2. Tell the person who answers the phone that you are calling in response to a job opening. He or she will direct your call to the contact person.

3. When you're connected to the contact person, give your name and which job opening you are interested in. If you were referred by someone, mention that person's name.

4. The contact person will tell you what the next steps will be in the application process. These may include asking you to send a letter of application and a résumé. The contact person may offer to send you a job application or set up an appointment for an interview.

5. Write down everything you are told to do. Repeat it back to the contact person to make sure you understood the next steps.

6. Ask any questions you may have about the application process. Answer any questions the contact person asks you.

7. Thank the contact person for his or her time.

Responding in Writing

Responding to a job lead in writing means composing an effective letter of request or a cover letter to accompany your résumé.

■ **Letter of request.** Write a letter of request when you need to ask for an application form or request an interview. Include a brief summary of your education, experience, and qualifications in the letter.

■ **Cover letter.** Write a cover letter when a job lead asks you to send a written response. Your cover letter should introduce you to your prospective employer without repeating your résumé. Fig. 2-14 shows an example of a cover letter accompanying a résumé.

Preparing Your Résumé

Your résumé is a very important job-seeking tool. It gives a prospective employer the information he or she needs to help determine if you are suitable for a position. Choose your work experience, skills, and education or training that will convince an employer that you're the best candidate for the job. Always be truthful and accurate. Here are some guidelines for preparing a résumé:

- Keep your résumé brief.
- Stress relevant education, training, work experience, and key skills. If you have foodservice experience of any kind, include it.
- Include your career objective.
- Use correct spelling and grammar.
- Present your résumé on quality paper.
- Avoid using decorative graphics and pictures.
- Include accurate contact information.
- Use keywords to describe your work experience. **Keywords** are significant words that make it easier for employers to search for relevant information. If your résumé contains keywords such as foodservice, restaurant, or baking, employers with foodservice opportunities will be more likely to call up your résumé in an electronic search.

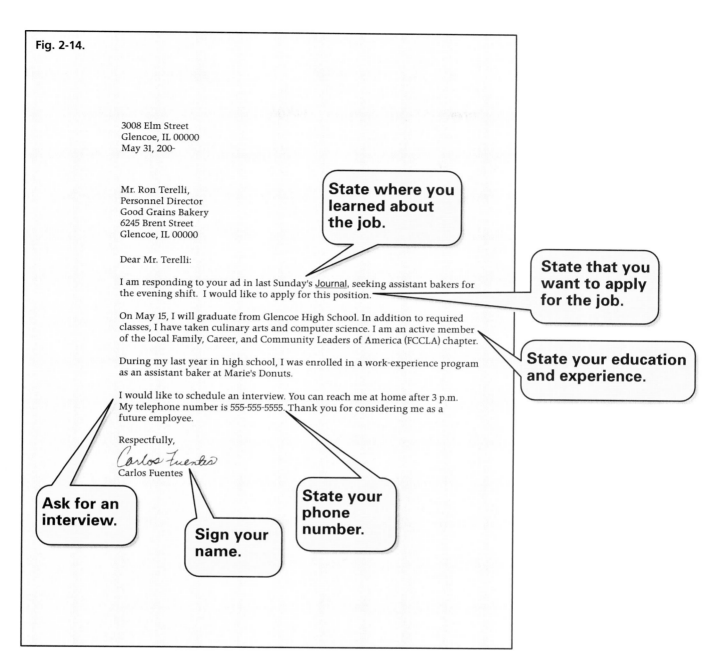

Fig. 2-14.

3008 Elm Street
Glencoe, IL 00000
May 31, 200-

Mr. Ron Terelli,
Personnel Director
Good Grains Bakery
6245 Brent Street
Glencoe, IL 00000

Dear Mr. Terelli:

I am responding to your ad in last Sunday's Journal, seeking assistant bakers for the evening shift. I would like to apply for this position.

On May 15, I will graduate from Glencoe High School. In addition to required classes, I have taken culinary arts and computer science. I am an active member of the local Family, Career, and Community Leaders of America (FCCLA) chapter.

During my last year in high school, I was enrolled in a work-experience program as an assistant baker at Marie's Donuts.

I would like to schedule an interview. You can reach me at home after 3 p.m. My telephone number is 555-555-5555. Thank you for considering me as a future employee.

Respectfully,

Carlos Fuentes
Carlos Fuentes

State where you learned about the job.

State that you want to apply for the job.

State your education and experience.

Ask for an interview.

Sign your name.

State your phone number.

THE INTERVIEW PROCESS

Once you've completed the application process, you'll need to prepare for your job interview. At an interview, you'll have the chance to convince an employer that you're the right person for the job. You will be evaluated by your appearance, attitude, and answers to the employer's questions. Sometimes the interview also includes having a meal with the employer or supervisor. Remember to demonstrate good table manners. How you present yourself indicates how you will conduct yourself in different situations.

Before the Interview

The interview process begins when an employer sets an appointment for your interview. Write down the date, time, and place of the interview.

■ **Do your homework.** The more you know about your prospective employer and the job you're seeking, the better you'll do in the interview. Check resources, such as community business publications, local newspapers, Internet directories, or professional organizations. You will want to learn how large the business is, how profitable it has been, and what its plans for future growth may be. Make notes about what you learn.

■ **Choose appropriate clothing.** Your employer's first impression of you will be based on your appearance. Choose appropriate clothing that fits properly and is clean, pressed, and in good condition. Your grooming habits can make or break a job interview. You should be clean, your hair well trimmed and conservatively styled, and your fingernails clean and neatly trimmed.

■ **Be prompt and courteous.** On the day of the interview, allow plenty of time to locate your destination. It is best to arrive a few minutes early. As you introduce yourself to a receptionist, guard, or other person before meeting with the interviewer, be polite and respectful. The interviewer may check with these people later.

During the Interview

The interview is very important. You'll do well if you are prepared, positive, and relaxed. Remember, business etiquette is not unlike the good manners that should be used at home. Keep the following points in mind.

■ **Shake hands.** The interviewer will introduce himself or herself to you. Introduce yourself in return, and offer your hand for a firm, confident handshake. Remain standing until the interviewer asks you to be seated. He or she will probably begin with a few simple questions or comments to help you feel more at ease. Smiling never hurts.

■ **Make eye contact.** Throughout the interview, and when talking directly to anyone, maintaining eye contact is important. Eye contact with the interviewer helps show that you are listening and are interested in what the interviewer is saying.

■ **Speak clearly.** Use correct grammar and speak clearly. The interviewer will ask you questions designed to determine if you are the person they need for the job.

■ **Use good office manners.** Sit up straight, with both feet on the floor. Avoid nervous gestures such as tapping. Never chew gum during an interview.

■ **Answer thoughtfully and completely.** Do not interrupt the interviewer or become sidetracked. If you don't understand a question or don't know the answer, say so politely and ask for clarification. See Fig. 2-15.

■ **Ask questions.** The interview process is meant to help you gain information, too. Don't hesitate to ask the interviewer about the nature of the job,

Fig. 2-15.

Questions Often Asked in a Job Interview

1. Why would you like to work for this company?
2. What do you want to be doing in five years?
3. What are your qualifications for this job?
4. What are your strengths and weaknesses?
5. Why did you leave your last job?
6. Tell me about a challenge you met or a problem you solved in school or on the job.
7. What do you enjoy doing in your spare time?
8. Have you ever been part of a team or a club? What did you like best and least about that experience?
9. What questions do you have about the job or this company?
10. Why should we hire you?

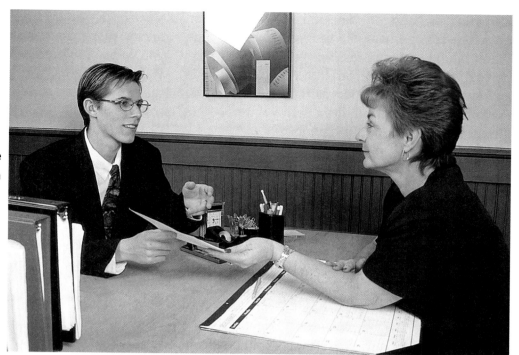

Fig. 2-16A. The job interview is your chance to make a good impression. How can your manners affect an employer's decision to hire you?

your responsibilities, and the working environment. Save questions about the rate of pay and employee benefits, such as vacation time, for the end of the interview.

■ **Leave gracefully.** Regardless of how the interview ends, thank the interviewer for his or her time. A professional attitude accompanied by good manners will always be remembered. Shake hands as you leave. The interviewer will signal the end of the interview in one of the following ways:

• The interviewer may tell you that you will be contacted later. If the interviewer does not specify a time period, politely ask, "When may I expect to hear from you?"

• You may be asked to contact the employer later. Note the telephone number, the preferred time to call, and the contact person.

• You may be offered the job. You may be asked to decide right away whether you'll take the job. If you are unsure, ask the interviewer if you may think about the offer. If this option is offered, be sure to follow up by responding promptly.

• You may not be offered the job. Don't be discouraged by being turned down for a job. You may not have the necessary qualifications, or

the employer may have found another applicant more suited to the job. The interviewer is under no obligation to tell you why you are not being offered the job. Accept the decision gracefully. See Fig. 2-16A.

After the Interview

The interview process does not end when the interview is over. After each job interview, you have the following responsibilities.

■ **Send a thank-you letter.** The day after the interview, send the interviewer a letter thanking him or her for the interview. Do this even if you have been turned down for the job. Be sure the employer's correct address and the right amount of postage are on the envelope. This is good business etiquette.

■ **Follow up.** If you have been asked to contact the employer, do so at the specified time. Send or deliver any materials or information, such as references, you have agreed to supply. If the employer has promised to contact you, wait the specified amount of time. If this time passes, telephone the employer and politely request information about the status of your application. You may be asked to go through a second interview.

■ **Review the session.** As soon as possible after the interview, go over the session in your mind. Think about the impression you made. Make notes on anything you could do to improve. Note any key information, such as employer expectations and job responsibilities. List any unanswered questions you have about the job.

Responding to a Job Offer

When you receive an offer of employment, you have three options.

■ **Accept the offer.** The employer will give you information on when you can begin work. You may be asked to participate in employee orientation or a training session before formally beginning your job. The employer will usually set up another interview during which you will be given specific details on pay, benefits, schedules, and other job expectations.

■ **Ask for time to consider the offer.** This is the time to bring up any unanswered questions that might affect your decision. With the employer, come to an agreement on when you will notify him or her of your decision. Do not put off responding to the employer.

■ **Turn down the job offer.** Perhaps you will decide that the job is not right for you. Or, maybe you've been offered a better job in the meantime. Whatever the case, if you do not intend to take the position, say so. You don't need to supply reasons for turning down a job offer. Simply say, "Thank you for considering me, but I am not interested in taking the position." See Fig. 2-16B.

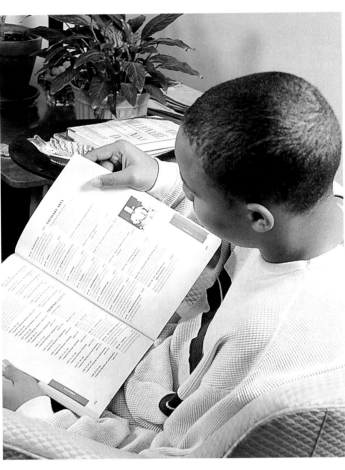

Fig. 2-16B. After you turn down a job offer, be sure to check out additional sources, such as the *Occupational Outlook Handbook*.

SECTION 2-2   Knowledge Check

1. Why is the employment outlook for the food-service industry so positive?
2. List five sources for job leads.
3. What is the purpose of a résumé?

MINI LAB

Write a résumé, cover letter, and thank-you letter in response to a job ad from the newspaper or the Internet.

On the Job

KEY TERMS

- **workers' compensation**
- **repetitive stress injuries**
- **minimum wage**
- **compensatory time**
- **labor union**
- **discrimination**
- **sexual harassment**
- **probation**
- **deductions**
- **empathy**
- **ethics**

OBJECTIVES

After reading this section, you will be able to:

- Summarize the rights and responsibilities of employees and employers.
- Perform calculations related to wages and benefits.
- Practice workplace etiquette.
- Identify opportunities and qualifications for advancement in foodservice.

WHETHER a job makes you part of a large workforce or of a small business, it really comes down to the relationship between you and your employer. When you accept a job, you enter into a relationship in which both parties have rights and responsibilities. The specific expectations and regulations will be explained to you by your employer when you begin your job. In this section, you will learn about your rights as an employee and your responsibilities to your employer. You will become familiar with wages, taxes, and benefits. You will practice skills for getting along with others on the job. You'll also identify some of the qualities required for advancement in the foodservice industry.

✖ EMPLOYEE RESPONSIBILITIES

As an employee, your main responsibility is to do the very best job possible for your employer. This means being responsible, reliable, flexible, and honest. It means using job resources appropriately and effectively. Here are some general ways to carry out your responsibilities:

- **Use time responsibly.** Be on time for work. Return promptly from designated breaks and meal periods. Stay at work for your full shift, or specified hours of employment. Keep busy on the job. Don't waste time chatting with coworkers and never use company time or resources to do personal business.

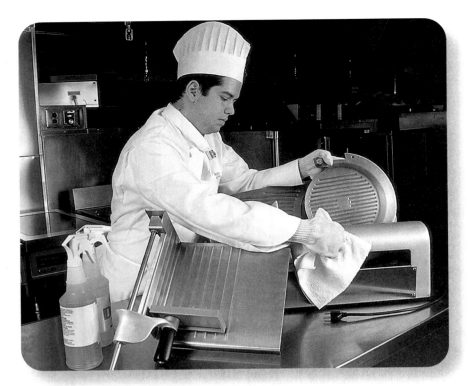

Fig. 2-17. Performing your work safely protects you and your employer.

- **Respect the rules.** Learn and follow your employer's rules, regulations, and policies. You'll probably be given an employee handbook. If you are in doubt about a company policy, ask your employer.
- **Work safely.** Familiarize yourself with the safety requirements of your job. Learn how to operate and maintain equipment safely. Report any unsafe conditions or practices to your supervisor immediately. See Fig. 2-17.
- **Earn your pay.** Complete each task you are assigned. Keep your work area neat and well organized. Use company resources responsibly.

✖ EMPLOYER RESPONSIBILITIES

The employer-employee relationship goes both ways. Your employer has responsibilities to you, too. Your employer's chief responsibility is to make sure that you are compensated fairly for the work you do. Other employer responsibilities include supplying what you need to do your job, providing safe working conditions, and making sure you're treated fairly on the job.

■ **Employee support.** Your employer has the responsibility to supply what you need to do your job well. Your employer will outline your job responsibilities and expectations clearly. You also may be offered on-the-job training.

■ **Safe working conditions.** Federal, state, and local regulations require your employer to provide you with safe working conditions. This responsibility includes:

- Eliminating any recognized health and safety hazards.
- Providing equipment and materials necessary to do the job safely.
- Informing employees when conditions or materials pose dangers to health and safety.
- Maintaining records of job-related illnesses and injuries.
- Complying with environmental protection policies for safely disposing of waste materials.

■ **Workers' compensation.** If you're injured on the job and can't work, your employer has a legal responsibility to provide financial help—called **workers' compensation**—to cover medical expenses and lost wages. Injury prevention is another important part of your employer's safety responsibility. For example, employers have supported research into **repetitive stress injuries**, the potentially disabling ailments that develop among workers who must perform the same motions repeatedly. These conditions can affect a person's employability.

Fair Labor Practices

Your employer has a legal responsibility to protect you from unfair treatment on the job. U.S. labor laws are meant to protect the following rights of employees:

- To have an equal opportunity to obtain and keep employment.
- To be paid a fair wage.
- To be considered fairly for promotion.
- To be protected in times of personal and economic change.

Among other legally mandated responsibilities, employers must pay their employees at least the federal **minimum wage**, the lowest hourly amount a worker can earn. See Fig. 2-18. Some locations pay employees a higher minimum wage than the federal government requires. Employers must compensate employees who work overtime with extra pay or time off, called **compensatory time**.

American workers are guaranteed the right to join a **labor union**, an organization of workers in a similar field. Labor unions act as the voice of their members in collective bargaining, the process of negotiating working conditions, contracts, and other job benefits. About 15% of American workers are represented by labor unions.

Employers must also protect their employees from **discrimination**—unfair treatment based on age, gender, race, ethnicity, religion, physical appearance, disability, or other factors. For exam-

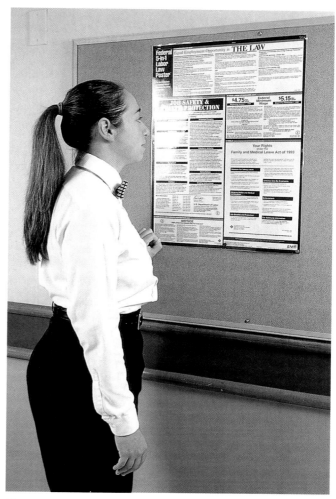

Fig. 2-18. Employers post information updates that affect employees.

ple, **sexual harassment**, any unwelcome behavior of a sexual nature, is prohibited in the workplace. If you think you have been sexually harassed, report the incident to your supervisor immediately so action can be taken.

Performance Evaluations

Your employer is also responsible for providing feedback on your job performance. Some employers consider the first few months of your time on a new job to be a **probation** (pro-BAY-shun) period. This time period gives your employer a chance to monitor your job performance closely to confirm you can do the job.

✖ WAGES AND BENEFITS

When you agree to take a job, you trade your skills and efforts for pay. Your pay is determined by a number of factors, including your level of experience, the difficulty of the work, and the number of people competing for the same job. Pay periods differ from employer to employer. Some employers pay weekly, others every two weeks, still others once a month.

Your employer will pay you in one of two ways. If you are paid an hourly wage, your employer will pay you a certain amount for each hour you work. With an hourly wage, your pay will vary depending on how many hours you work. If you receive a salary, your employer will pay you a set amount of money regardless of the hours worked.

■ **Deductions.** The amount of money you actually receive is called your net pay or take-home pay. **Deductions** are the money withheld from your gross pay for taxes, insurance, and other fees. Ask your employer to explain the type and amount of deductions that will be taken from your pay. Fig. 2-19 lists some common deductions.

■ **Benefits.** In addition to your salary, your employer may offer benefits. Among the benefits your employer may offer are:

• Health and accident insurance.
• Paid vacation days.
• Discounts on meals or company products.
• Life insurance.
• Disability insurance, a policy that helps pay your expenses if you become disabled and can no longer work.
• Tuition reimbursement, or full or partial repayment of tuition and fees you pay for education courses that are directly related to your career.
• Savings and investment plans, such as a 401K, to help you earn money for retirement.

Be sure to figure in any benefits when you are calculating your job compensation. A high wage may make up for few benefits. A good range of benefits, on the other hand, can compensate for a lower wage.

KEY Math SKILLS

OVERTIME PAY

Some employers would rather have an employee work overtime than hire additional help. The costs related to hiring and training new employees and the added cost of employee benefits outweigh the amount paid in overtime. Overtime pay may be paid at time-and-a-half or two times your hourly wage.

To calculate time-and-a-half pay, multiply your hourly rate by 1.5. If your hourly rate is $8.30, your overtime pay will be $12.45 per hour:

$$\begin{array}{r} \$8.30 \\ \times\,1.5 \\ \hline \$12.45 \end{array}$$

If your employer pays you double time, your hourly overtime rate is calculated as 2 times your regular rate:

$$\begin{array}{r} \$8.30 \\ \times\,2 \\ \hline \$16.60 \end{array}$$

So, if you worked 6 overtime hours based on time-and-a-half pay and 2 hours based on double time, your overtime pay for the week is calculated as follows:

$$\begin{array}{r} \$12.45 \\ \times\,6 \text{ hours} \\ \hline \$74.70 \end{array} \qquad \begin{array}{r} \$16.60 \\ \times\,2 \text{ hours} \\ \hline \$33.20 \end{array}$$

$$\begin{array}{r} \$74.70 \\ +\,\$33.20 \\ \hline \$107.90 \end{array}$$

Your overtime pay is $107.90

TRY IT!

Garrett Jones is paid time-and-a-half overtime for any time he works over 40 hours at Mason's Cafeteria. Last week Garrett worked 44 hours. If Garrett's hourly rate is $10.40, how much did he make last week?

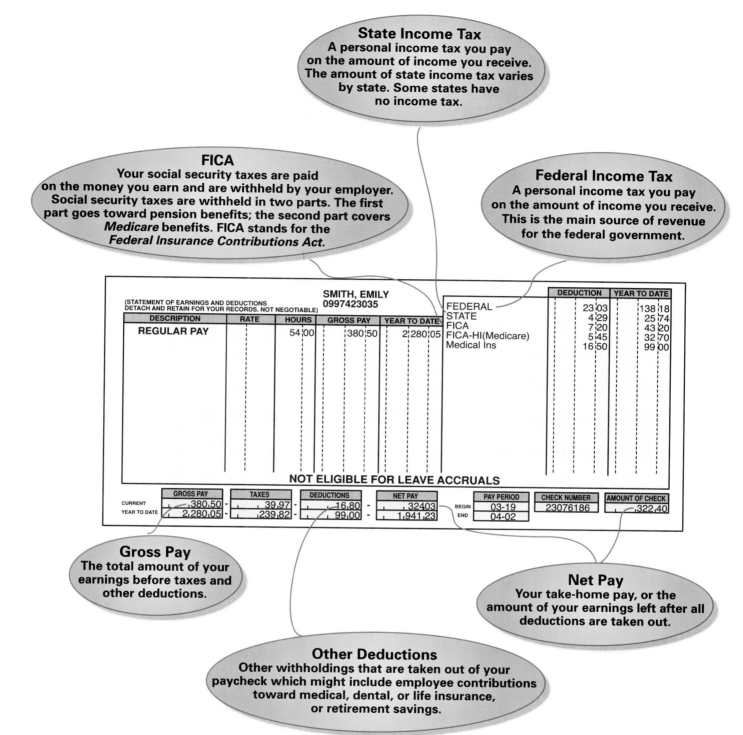

State Income Tax
A personal income tax you pay on the amount of income you receive. The amount of state income tax varies by state. Some states have no income tax.

FICA
Your social security taxes are paid on the money you earn and are withheld by your employer. Social security taxes are withheld in two parts. The first part goes toward pension benefits; the second part covers *Medicare* benefits. FICA stands for the *Federal Insurance Contributions Act.*

Federal Income Tax
A personal income tax you pay on the amount of income you receive. This is the main source of revenue for the federal government.

				DEDUCTION	YEAR TO DATE
FEDERAL				23 03	138 18
STATE				4 29	25 74
FICA				7 20	43 20
FICA-HI(Medicare)				5 45	32 70
Medical Ins				16 50	99 00

SMITH, EMILY
0997423035

(STATEMENT OF EARNINGS AND DEDUCTIONS
DETACH AND RETAIN FOR YOUR RECORDS. NOT NEGOTIABLE)

DESCRIPTION	RATE	HOURS	GROSS PAY	YEAR TO DATE
REGULAR PAY		54 00	380 50	2 280 05

NOT ELIGIBLE FOR LEAVE ACCRUALS

	GROSS PAY	TAXES	DEDUCTIONS	NET PAY	PAY PERIOD	CHECK NUMBER	AMOUNT OF CHECK
CURRENT	380,50 -	39,97 -	16,80 -	32403	BEGIN 03-19	23076186	322,40
YEAR TO DATE	2,280,05 -	239,82 -	99,00 -	1,941,23	END 04-02		

Gross Pay
The total amount of your earnings before taxes and other deductions.

Net Pay
Your take-home pay, or the amount of your earnings left after all deductions are taken out.

Other Deductions
Other withholdings that are taken out of your paycheck which might include employee contributions toward medical, dental, or life insurance, or retirement savings.

Fig. 2-19. A pay stub shows you the amount of each deduction taken from your paycheck. What types of deductions may be withheld from your gross pay?

■ **Tips.** Some foodservice workers earn tips amounting to between 10% and 20% of the customer's check. Because employers are entitled to count tips as part of the minimum wage, foodservice workers may actually earn more in tips than they do in wages. If you earn tips as part of your job, it is your responsibility to keep a record of the money you earn. You will need to report your tips as income when you file a tax return.

✖ TEAMWORK

In addition to the employer-employee relationship, you also enter into a relationship with your coworkers when you take a job. Every worker is an individual, with his or her own personality traits, strengths, and weaknesses. In order to bring individuals together into an effective team, each employee must practice good teamwork.

■ **Keep a positive attitude.** An upbeat, positive outlook contributes to the team spirit of the group. Complaining can bring the whole team down and affect your job performance.

Fig. 2-20. Your coworkers may represent different backgrounds, and opinions. How can you demonstrate positive interpersonal skills with coworkers?

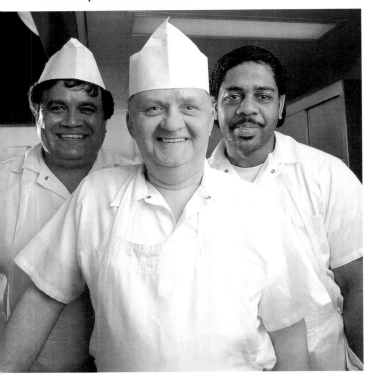

■ **Respect yourself.** You demonstrate self-respect when you accept responsibility for your actions, learn from your mistakes, and take care of your appearance.

■ **Respect others.** Disrespectful actions can result in unemployment. Learn to practice **empathy** (EHM-pah-thee), the skill of putting yourself in another's place. Empathy will help you understand the people you work with.

Resolving Conflicts

No matter how well you and your coworkers get along, you will not always agree. Disputes and conflicts are an inevitable part of team interaction. While conflict can be unpleasant, you can learn something from the process of working to resolve conflicts respectfully. There must be give and take. Learn to negotiate. See Fig. 2-20.

You may encounter conflicts that can't be resolved. Remember to focus on the problem, not the personalities involved.

Ethical Behavior

Your **ethics** (EH-thicks) are your internal guidelines for distinguishing right from wrong. Ethical behavior consists of doing what is right. Much of the time, it's easy to recognize the ethical course of action. Some choices, however, are more difficult. When two choices appear equally right or equally wrong, ask yourself the following questions:

• Does the choice comply with the law?
• Is the choice fair to those involved?
• Does the choice harm anyone?
• Has the choice been communicated honestly?
• Can I live with the choice without embarrassment or guilt?

Behaving ethically also means taking responsibility. If you make a mistake, you should admit it. Responsible employees learn from their mistakes and adapt their behavior to make better choices.

ADVANCING ON THE JOB

Food service offers many advancement opportunities. Advancement may involve a promotion or be at the same job level. Advancement may also involve leaving for a better job elsewhere, or beginning your own business. See Fig. 2-21.

Here are some qualities that will help you advance in your career:

- **Show initiative.** The willingness to take on new tasks and levels of responsibility shows initiative (ih-NIH-shuh-tihv). Workers with initiative don't wait to be told what to do next.
- **The desire to learn.** Continuing your education or training through formal classes, workshops, or independent study.

TERMINATING EMPLOYMENT

Terminating employment can be an uncomfortable situation. Always leave on good terms. You may want to return or obtain a letter of recommendation. Always give at least two weeks notice prior to leaving your job. Work these final weeks as hard as you would if you were keeping the job.

Fig. 2-21.

Advancement Opportunities

FROM:	TO:
Server	Head server
Busser	Server
Dishwasher	Kitchen helper
Counter worker	Assistant manager
Host	Server
Dining room supervisor	Banquet captain
Cafeteria attendant	Cafeteria supervisor
Short-order cook	Line cook
Kitchen worker	Pantry supervisor
Baker's assistant	Baker
Cook	Sous chef
Caterer or chef	Restaurant owner
Prep cook	Line cook
Garde manger	Caterer
Pastry cook	Pastry chef
Line cook	Sous chef
Sous chef	Executive chef
Executive chef	Corporate chef

SECTION 2-3   Knowledge Check

1. What are the main responsibilities of an employee and an employer?
2. What steps can you take to practice good workplace etiquette?
3. How much notice should you give an employer prior to terminating your employment?

MINI LAB

Working with another student, role-play an employer and an employee in different work-place scenarios. Then switch roles. How did you act as an employee? How did you act differently as an employer?

SECTION SUMMARIES

2-1 The basic skills for employment in the foodservice industry include math, reading and writing, speaking, and listening skills.

2-1 A positive work ethic equates to a personal commitment of doing the best job possible.

2-1 Future foodservice employees can begin to develop leadership skills in organizations such as FCCLA and SkillsUSA.

2-2 The employment outlook in food service is positive with unlimited growth and opportunities.

2-2 Job searching includes networking, joining professional organizations, and reading trade publications.

2-2 When preparing a résumé, be brief and positive, and stress relevant education and experience.

2-2 Completing a job application is typically the first step in applying for a job.

2-3 Employers and employees have different rights and responsibilities in the workplace, but each has the right to a safe workplace.

2-3 When calculating your job compensation, you should consider benefits in addition to wages.

2-3 Working in teams means coworkers have a common goal.

2-3 Advancement opportunities in foodservice include those from server to head server, cook to chef, and chef to owner.

CHECK YOUR KNOWLEDGE

1. What specific thinking skills are expected from employees?
2. Name five traits you can demonstrate to show a positive work ethic.
3. What is leadership?
4. Name the key resources leaders use effectively.
5. What sources can be used for networking?
6. How should you prepare for a job interview?
7. List two employee and two employer responsibilities in the workplace.
8. What deductions may be taken from your pay?
9. How can you practice workplace etiquette?
10. What qualities help people advance in the workplace?

CRITICAL-THINKING ACTIVITIES

1. As an employee in a bakery, you are responsible for preparing everything in the shop prior to opening. Today you overslept and are running late. You call a coworker and ask if he or she can fill in for you until you arrive. Why is this important to do?

2. You have recently graduated from community college with a degree in culinary arts. You haven't been able to get a job. How might you alter the situation?

WORKPLACE KNOW-HOW

Networking. Imagine you've recently talked to a friend about a job opening at another foodservice establishment, but know very little about the company or the position. How can you find out more before applying for the job?

LAB-BASED ACTIVITY: Interview Practice

STEP 1 Invite three or more local chefs and restaurant managers to conduct mock interviews with all students in your class.

STEP 2 Research background information about the foodservice operations for which the guest interviewers work. You should be prepared to answer questions as well as ask questions of the interviewers. For example, what foodservice organizations are you a member of? What are the goals of that organization?

STEP 3 Write your résumé and complete a sample employment application.

STEP 4 Participate in mock interviews with the guest interviewers. Include an interview done during lunch. Videotape each interview to share later with the class.

STEP 5 Create evaluation charts like the sample below. Use the following rating scale:

Poor=1; Fair=2; Good=3; Great=4

STEP 6 Evaluate the videotaped interviews using the evaluation charts. Have the class evaluate each interview and offer suggestions for improvement.

Sample Interview Evaluation Chart

	Rating	Comments:
Appearance (initial impression)	3	I dressed appropriately.
Communication Skills	2	The interviewer corrected my speech twice. I also said "I guess" too much.
Enthusiasm Level	3	I expressed my sincere interest in this job.
Preparation for Interview	1	I should have done more research about this foodservice operation.

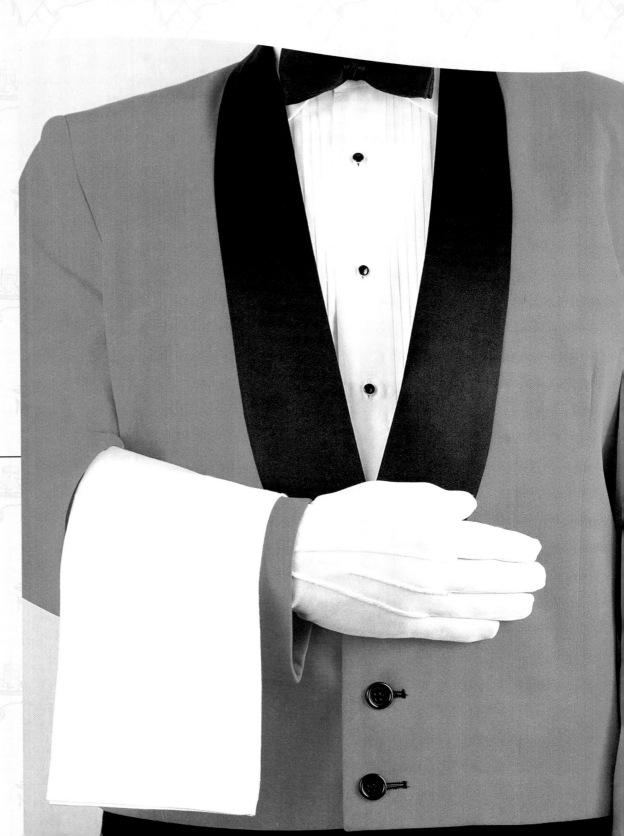

Service Basics

KEY TERMS

• patronage

• body language

• section

• station

OBJECTIVES

After reading this section, you will be able to:

• Identify the role and duties of each member of the service staff.

• Demonstrate service skills that provide exceptional customer service.

PROVIDING quality customer service is one of the most important ways a foodservice operation can draw repeat business from satisfied customers. Well-prepared meals and a charming atmosphere will not offset slow or inefficient service. It is important to know how to provide quality customer service.

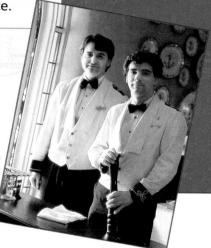

☒ THE SERVICE STAFF

Customers expect competent and friendly service, consistency in the food served, and a clean, comfortable environment. Each member of the service staff plays a key role in ensuring the success of the foodservice operation. Customers who are greeted with a smile feel welcome. If they can make eye contact with you, they will feel more relaxed. Going beyond customers' expectations gives a facility a good reputation, and it improves the chance of repeat business.

No employee can afford to be rude or unskilled in serving customers or resolving their complaints. By treating all customers with warmth and courtesy, the service staff helps make the dining experience pleasant. If there is a problem with an order, the food, or the service, the server should bring it to the manager's attention. The manager should then acknowledge the issue and resolve the complaint quickly and positively.

Every member of the service staff contributes to a customer's impressions of a foodservice operation. The host, server, busser, and cashier are all members of the service team.

Host

Initially, the host greets the customers by smiling warmly and welcoming them. If the foodservice operation uses a reservation system, customers should be asked if they have made a reservation and in what name. Keeping track of reservations and waiting lists is another responsibility of the host. Hosts often track empty and occupied tables on a printed or computerized chart. See Fig. 3-1.

In case of a waiting list, the host tells customers how long their wait will be. Many restaurants use pagers to alert customers that their seats are available.

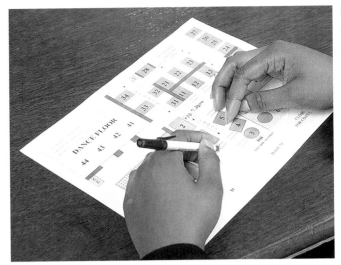

Fig. 3-1. One important responsibility of the host is to chart empty and filled tables. What are some other duties of a host?

The host also leads the way to the table, walking slowly in order not to lose the customers. The host then seats the customers and presents them with the menus. If there are special needs, such as a child's booster chair, the host will either provide the chair or inform a server of the need. None of the services provided by the host should be rushed. A sense of being hurried will make customers feel uncomfortable.

Server

The server has the most contact with the customers. Servers perform four tasks: They represent the foodservice operation, sell the menu, serve menu items skillfully, and receive correct payment from the customer.

Servers must have good communication and interpersonal skills. They help set the tone of the dining experience. Servers are the sales staff of every foodservice operation. They also help customers make beverage and food decisions by recommending menu items. A server must know the ingredients and preparation methods of all beverage and food items.

Busser

The busser helps maintain an inviting table and keeps the service station stocked with supplies. Bussers sometimes serve water and bread to customers as soon as they are seated. Then, as cus-

tomers finish eating, the busser clears the table. The busser also cleans and resets the table prior to seating the next customer.

In some restaurants, the server or busser will clear the table between courses of a meal. Remember, dishes should not be removed until all the customers have finished. When in doubt, you should ask the customers whether you may clear their dishes. Bussers also keep the dining room tidy.

Cashier

Some busy, informal, or family-style restaurants employ a cashier. A cashier is responsible for correctly reading the amount of the bill, processing the payment, and making change. See Fig. 3-2. Other restaurants have servers process payments.

The cashier should always thank customers for their support, or **patronage** (PAY-truh-nij). Some establishments also offer additional items for sale at the cash register. These may include such items as cakes, pies, bottled dressings, sauces, or syrups.

Fig. 3-2. During training chefs also learn basic cashier skills.

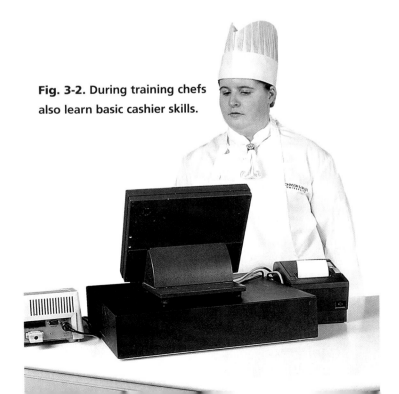

SERVICE SKILLS

All foodservice employees, especially those who interact with customers, must possess the following qualities. Each of these qualities is important to a successful career.

- A positive attitude.
- A neat and clean appearance.
- Good communication and teamwork skills.
- Thorough job knowledge and the ability to use time wisely.
- An ability to resolve customer complaints by positive means.

Positive Attitude

It is critical to have a positive attitude at all times when dealing with customers. You can't allow one difficult customer to affect your attitude. For example, a server who has just dealt with a difficult customer must be able to serve other customers without being visibly upset.

The proper attitude is a willingness to please the customer. Without this willingness, you can't succeed, despite any other skills you may have. This is also a way to build and maintain a client base. The following list of behaviors shows a willingness to please customers:

- Take pride in your work, regardless of your job assignment.
- Be cheerful. Friendliness matters to everyone around you. See Fig. 3-3.
- Try to resolve complaints in a positive manner.
- Show courtesy to customers and coworkers alike. This includes helping your coworkers if they need it.
- Never argue with customers. People prefer a relaxed, pleasant setting when dining out. Remember that the customer is never "wrong." Your role is to find solutions that will keep customers happy.
- Don't hold conversations with coworkers in the dining area. Customers need to know that they are your only priority.

Fig. 3-3. A positive attitude is vital to providing customers with excellent service.

Personal Attire

The service staff's appearance is key to giving customers a good first impression of both the staff members and the foodservice operation. Most foodservice operations have their own policies regarding proper attire or dress. However, here are some general guidelines.

- Be sure your uniform fits properly and that it is clean and pressed.
- Keep your work shoes clean and polished.
- Remove nail polish before going to work.
- For safety and sanitation reasons, keep jewelry to a minimum.

Personal Hygiene

When you are working directly with the public, personal hygiene is very important. Follow these guidelines for personal hygiene:

- Keep your hair pulled back and out of the way.
- Keep your hands clean by washing them frequently, including after handling food, clearing tables, coughing, or sneezing. Washing your hands after using the restroom is required.
- Keep your fingernails trimmed and clean.
- Be sure that your teeth are clean and your breath is fresh.
- Use body deodorant daily.
- Don't wear heavy colognes or perfumes.

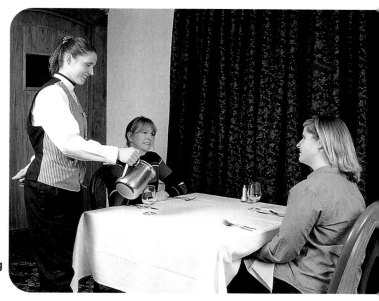

Personal Health

The energy and skills demanded in food service can be best achieved when you are in good physical and mental health.

■ **Rest.** Foodservice careers often involve long hours on your feet. Getting enough sleep is key. Too little sleep weakens the body's immune system and puts the body at risk for illness. A lack of sleep does not promote good physical or mental health.

■ **Fitness.** Foodservice careers often require lifting heavy objects, such as loaded serving trays. Exercising regularly increases your strength and will help you handle stress, making you more successful at your job. See Fig. 3-4.

■ **Illness.** In the foodservice industry, disease can spread easily to coworkers and customers. If you have a fever or are vomiting, don't go to work. Call your supervisor and see a doctor, rather than trying to "wait and see." Return to work only when you are completely well.

Communication & Teamwork

Service staff members must be able to communicate well with customers and coworkers. They also must be able to work as a team member. Teamwork is shown through verbal and nonverbal communication.

■ **Verbal communication.** Verbal communication involves speaking to another person. It is important to speak clearly and loudly enough to be heard when talking with others. Don't speak so rapidly that your words run together. Otherwise, customers may have to ask you to repeat information. Your tone of voice should be professional, pleasant, and friendly.

■ **Nonverbal communication.** One form of nonverbal communication includes **body language**, or expressing your thoughts through physical action. For example, standing attentively when taking orders shows customers you are listening carefully. Here are some general guidelines:

• Don't chew gum, eat, or drink while serving customers.

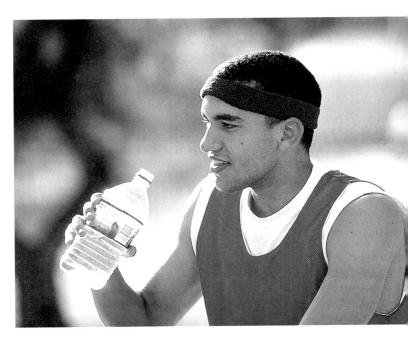

Fig. 3-4. A healthful lifestyle will help you meet the demands of a foodservice career. List ways that physical and mental health issues can affect your success at work.

• Don't lean, slouch, or stand around with your hands in your pockets.
• Don't touch your mouth, nose, or hair while serving customers.

When you write out an order, you are also using nonverbal communication. See Fig. 3-5. It is always important to write clearly and concisely so that your message is understood. For example, you may need to leave a note for a coworker or write out an accident report.

Required Job Knowledge

Service staff members must have a thorough understanding of the following:

• How to interact with customers.
• Dining room equipment.
• Menu selections and the ingredients used.
• How to take a customer's order.
• Beverage service techniques.
• Proper serving and clearing techniques.
• How to write and compute a customer check.
• Presenting a check and collecting payment.
• How to manage time wisely.

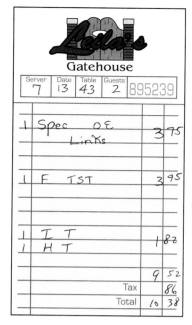

Fig. 3-5. Servers must be able to communicate clearly when writing out orders. What does the shorthand used here tell you about this order?

Other ways to save time and motion include setting more than one table at a time, delivering food items for more than one table at a time, and clearing more than one table at a time. Being constantly aware of customers at all the tables in a station allows the server to be more effective and efficient. See Fig. 3-6.

USE OF TIME & MOTION

Service staff members are often responsible for serving a group of tables, called a **section** or **station**. The server should always be looking for ways to save time and energy. Servers must be well organized and know how to set priorities, using as few steps as possible. For example, avoiding empty-handed trips to and from the kitchen increases efficiency. In addition, when pouring water at a table, the server should check his or her other tables to see if anyone else needs water.

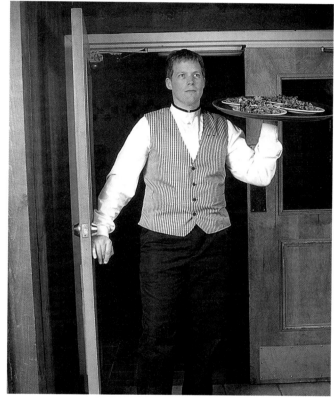

Fig. 3-6. Looking for ways to save time, energy, and motion are important for every server.

| SECTION 3-1 | Knowledge Check |

1. Describe the duties of a host and a busser.
2. How do servers function as the sales staff of a foodservice operation?
3. Give one example of how an employee could use time or motion effectively.

MINI LAB

Observe the service staff at a restaurant. How were you greeted? Was the server knowledgeable about the menu? Were the dishes cleared quickly? How was your bill processed? How could your dining experience have been more enjoyable?

Serving Customers

KEY TERMS

- **highlighting**
- **upselling**
- **preset**
- **appetizers**
- **underliner**
- **cover**

OBJECTIVES

After reading this section, you will be able to:

- Describe the role and duties of the server.

- Use selling techniques to increase sales.

- Serve food and beverages properly.

- Calculate customer checks.

CUSTOMERS have the most contact with servers when dining out. From taking orders to presenting checks, the server plays a key role in how the customer rates his or her dining experience. In this section you will learn about the role of servers and how their duties should be performed.

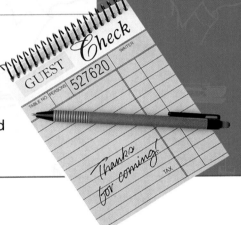

⊠ THE SERVER'S ROLE

The host or busser may serve bread and water before the server arrives at the table. However, the server is the main caretaker of customers' needs throughout the meal. The server is responsible for greeting customers, taking the order, serving the meal, and presenting the check. The server should do everything possible to make the total dining experience enjoyable and relaxing.

Greeting Customers

As a server, you should give the customer a moment to adjust to his or her surroundings before approaching the table. Be sure to smile and maintain good eye contact with each customer. If your customers are gathering to celebrate a spe-

cial event, try to determine who is the guest of honor. Your objective is to make customers comfortable by letting them know that you are a caring and attentive server.

Taking the Beverage Order

Taking the beverage order is the first point of service. Confirm the beverage order by repeating it to the customer. As illustrated in Fig. 3-7, you can use position numbers to make sure the right beverage is served to each customer. This can be done by taking the order in a clockwise direction. It can also be done by numbering each customer at a table by seat position.

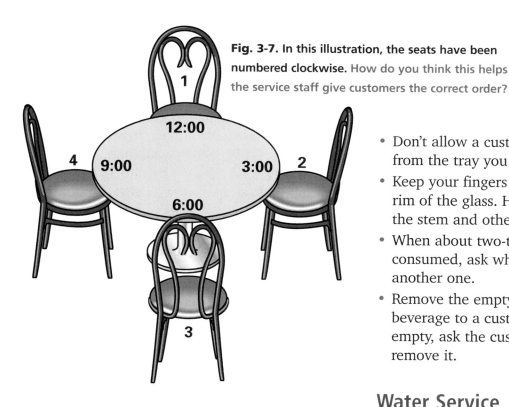

Fig. 3-7. In this illustration, the seats have been numbered clockwise. How do you think this helps the service staff give customers the correct order?

Serving Cold Beverages

Beverages are either cold or hot. They are served on a small, handheld tray called a beverage tray. Cold beverages include milk, iced tea, soft drinks, juice, and water. Serve cold beverages by following these guidelines:

- Be sure that the tray is clean and dry before using it at a table.
- Use beverage napkins for each beverage if the table surface is not covered with a cloth.
- Try arranging the glasses so that the beverage being served first is closest to the rim of the tray. However, be sure to place the tallest and heaviest glasses in the center of the tray to help maintain balance. Adjust the positions of the glasses on the tray as they are served.
- Carry trays at waist level and with your left hand under the center of the tray. Use your right hand to place the beverage on the customer's right.
- When possible, beverages should be served from the right side. Don't reach across the customer.
- Don't hold the tray between you and the customer or you and the table.

- Don't allow a customer to remove beverages from the tray you are holding.
- Keep your fingers as far as possible from the rim of the glass. Handle a stemmed glass by the stem and other glasses at the base.
- When about two-thirds of a beverage has been consumed, ask whether the customer wants another one.
- Remove the empty glass before serving a fresh beverage to a customer. Unless the glass is empty, ask the customer whether you may remove it.

Water Service

Some foodservice operations serve customers water as soon as they are seated. Many customers will want only water with their meals or water in addition to another beverage. Follow these guidelines when serving water:

- Place water glasses above the entrée knife and in line with its tip. See Figure 3-8.

Fig. 3-8. Beverage service is important because it is the first point of service. In what order do you serve beverages to customers?

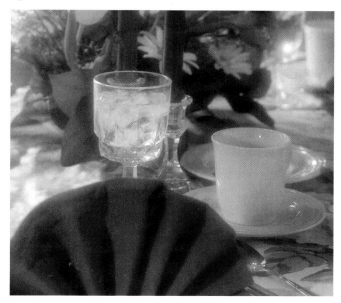

- Don't allow a serving pitcher to touch the rim of a customer's glass.
- Don't fill a glass more than one-half inch from the rim. Overfilling is a sign of sloppy service and causes spilling.
- Refill water glasses whenever needed during the meal. Don't allow customers' glasses to be less than one-third full.

Serving Hot Beverages

Many customers have coffee or hot tea with their meals. A hot beverage may be the customer's last impression of the meal and the service. To ensure quality service, warm the cups or mugs before presetting the table or placing them in front of the customer. A customer who receives hot coffee in a cold cup or mug will have lukewarm coffee especially if he or she adds milk.

The setup for coffee or hot tea must be completed before the beverage is served. The setup for coffee consists of cream, sugar, cup and saucer or mug, and a teaspoon. Coffee is poured from the customer's right side with your right hand. Hot tea is often served as a separate container of hot water, a tea bag and slice of lemon, and a teaspoon along with a cup and saucer or a mug. You should offer to bring more hot water as needed. See Fig. 3-9.

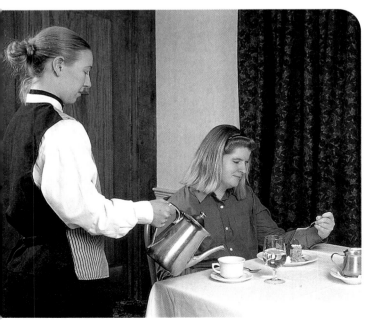

Selling the Menu

Servers represent the menu to customers. A thorough knowledge of the menu items and their preparation is critical to a server's success. Servers must know the descriptions, ingredients, and prices of all regular and special menu items. An effective server encourages customers to try different items. To suggest menu items comfortably, you can use several sales techniques, which include highlighting, open-ended questions, and upselling.

- **Highlighting.** Emphasizing a particular menu item, or **highlighting**, can be used to promote specials of the day or regular menu items. Servers use this technique to draw attention to a certain menu item. It is important for servers to have favorite items on the menu. It is easier to recommend items that you personally like. The enthusiasm showed by a server for a food item will be evident through his or her description.

- **Open-ended questions.** Ask questions that require a specific answer. Open-ended questions can't be answered with "yes" or "no." For example, rather than asking, "Would you like something to start with?" you might ask, "What would you like to start with?" This suggests that the customer is expected to order something right away.

- **Upselling.** A technique for suggesting a larger size or better quality than the customer's original order is called **upselling**. For example, if the prime rib is offered in 10-oz. and 16-oz. servings, ask the customer, "Would you like the 16-oz. size?"

When servers use these selling techniques, customers may be more inclined to try something new or order more items. Increasing sales and enhancing the customer's dining experience are also part of the server's role.

Fig. 3-9. Many customers choose to have a hot beverage with or at the end of their meals.

Taking the Order

When taking food orders, servers use the same position numbers that were used for taking beverage orders. Servers should follow these guidelines:

- Smile, maintain eye contact, and use a pleasant tone of voice.
- Listen carefully to each customer. See Fig. 3-10.
- Take the order in its entirety and confirm the order before moving to the next customer.
- Take the menu from each customer after you have taken his or her order.

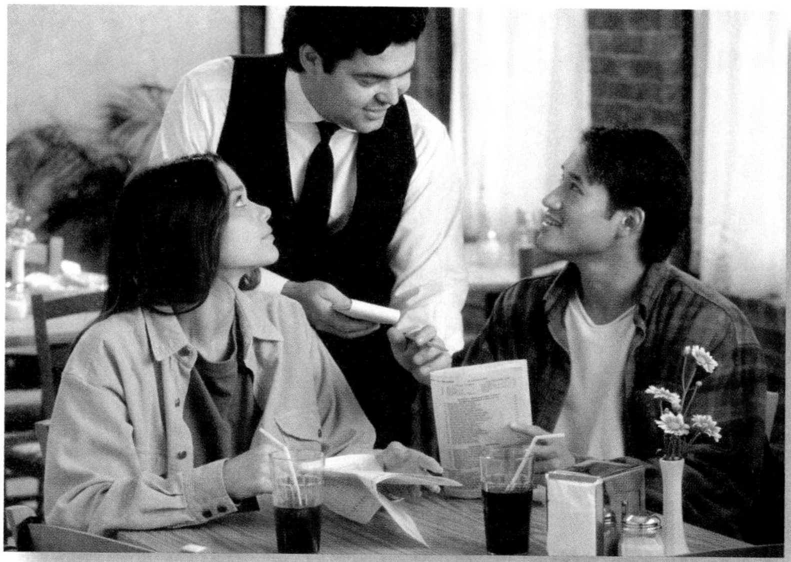

Fig. 3-10. When taking food orders, listen carefully to each customer.

Writing the Order

In most foodservice operations, the server takes orders on a customer check or transfers it directly into a computerized point-of-sales system. You need to write quickly and clearly when taking an order. Be sure to learn the abbreviations (uh-BREE-vee-A-shunz) that are understood by the kitchen staff.

When using an order pad, write down the table number. You might also want to write the customer's position number next to each item ordered. If a customer orders the same item as another customer, add the second customer's seat number next to the item. Be sure to place the quantity of each item in front of it. This technique will make it easier for the kitchen to fill the order. It will also help you serve the items ordered to the right customer. You may also need to write down additional information about the order. For example, the degree of doneness for red meat or "dressing on the side."

Transmitting the Order

The three ways to place an order in the kitchen are by writing out a customer check, reciting the order from memory, or using a computerized point-of-sales system. Using a point-of-sales system involves a computer that has either a number or a button code for each item on the menu. By simply pressing a button or entering a code, the order is sent to the kitchen.

A verbal ordering system is sometimes used in very elegant restaurants. Most foodservice operations use a computerized point-of-sales system, but a handwritten system of customer checks is used if the computer system breaks down. Servers must be able to clearly write an order in an organized way. Each course should be listed in the correct order.

Electronic Ordering

Point-of-sales computer technology is becoming more common in the foodservice industry. Nearly every foodservice establishment uses a computer to help communication and service flow smoothly. Just a touch makes transferring orders to the kitchen faster, easier, and more accurate. The benefits of point-of-sales computer technology include:

- The computer sends orders to a printer in the proper workstations. For example, cold food orders are sent to the pantry and hot food orders are sent to the hot line. See Fig. 3-11.
- Using a touch pad computer to send orders cuts down on steps for the server and increases efficiency and accuracy in ordering.

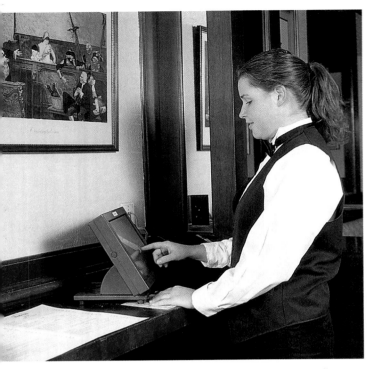

Fig. 3-11. Computerized point-of-sales systems make transferring orders to the kitchen faster and easier.

- Orders are organized and easy to read.
- The system prints accurate customer checks.
- Customers receive itemized checks with clearly marked totals. Management can also add messages to checks, such as "Make Your Reservations Early."
- Requiring a printout of every item ordered helps reduce employee theft.
- The computer keeps detailed, accurate sales records. Each server's sales output is available for the manager to check during the server's shift.
- The computer tracks each menu item and may be programmed to tell the server how many portions are available to sell.

To prevent misuse of the computer, each server receives an identity code or key. The computer prompts the server to enter information such as the check number, the number of customers, and the table number. After this information is displayed or entered, the server enters the order into the computer.

SERVING THE ORDER

The technical aspects of service refer to the way items are physically placed before a customer. More important to customers, however, is the manner in which they are served. The areas of most concern to customers are the following:

- When delivering dishes, did the server keep his or her fingers on the edge of the plate, away from the food?
- Was the plate placed in front of the customer according to the chef's wishes?
- Did the server use his or her left hand to serve the food from the customer's left side?
- Did the server anticipate customer needs instead of waiting to be asked?

Hand Service

Many restaurants use hand service instead of tray service. Hand service is effective if the distance from the service line in the kitchen to all points of the dining room is short. Hand service requires more skill to be performed effectively. See Fig. 3-12.

A server should be able to carry three soup cups or soup plates on the left arm and hand and the fourth in the right hand. The server should be able to carry plates on the right arm with the last plate in the left hand when serving the appetizer, salad, dinner, or dessert courses. It is essential that servers develop the skill to carry plates, cups, or bowls without tipping or angling them to ruin the presentation or have soup or sauces run onto the rim.

Hand service often requires a greater degree of teamwork because the size of a party may prevent one server from carrying all the plates to a table at one time. No matter what type of service is used, everyone at a table should be served at approximately the same time.

Tray Service

Tray service has the advantage of allowing the server to carry more cups, bowls, and plates without worrying as much about affecting the presentation. If soup spills along the rim of the bowl, the server should wipe it clean using a server napkin or towel.

Tray service is almost universally used in banquet service. A single server can carry a course for 10–12 guests at a time. Dinner plates will be covered with plate covers to allow dinners to be stacked one on top of another.

Service Trays & Stands

Tray stands have metal, wood, or plastic leg frames that will fold. They are usually connected by two fiber or cloth support straps that hold the legs steady when the tray stand is set up. Some frames include a low-level shelf to use as a small side stand. Tray stands are also referred to as tray jacks. Follow these guidelines when using service trays and tray stands.

Fig. 3-12. When performing hand service, the server must be careful not to ruin the presentation of the food on the plate.

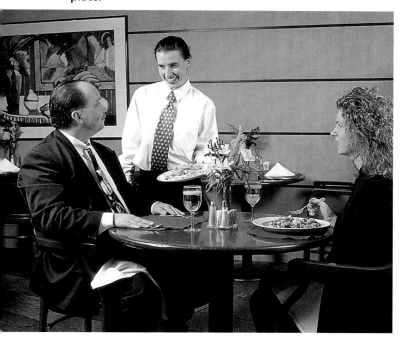

1. To prevent plate slippage and accidents, service trays are usually lined with rubber or cork. If the service tray is not already lined, use a wet service napkin to line the tray.
2. Arrange items on the tray so it is as evenly balanced as possible.
3. Pick up and carry the heaviest part of the tray closest to your body.
4. Always carry a service tray in the left hand, above the shoulder. This allows you to go through a doorway without the door swinging back and hitting the tray.
5. Carry the tray on your fingertips or palm, depending on the tray's weight.
6. Use your left shoulder to help balance the tray if necessary.
7. Carry the folded tray stand on your right while walking in the dining room.
8. Try not to place the tray stand right next to the customer's table when setting it up.
9. Extend the right arm holding the tray stand and flick your wrist. The support legs will separate, bringing the tray stand to an open position. Place the tray stand so that one set of legs is facing your right side. This will ensure that as you place the tray on the stand, the top cross bar will not obstruct your movements. The frame legs should be parallel to your body.
10. Turn to the right, bend your knees, and lower the tray horizontally until it sits on the tray stand.
11. Slide the tray across the top of the tray stand to distribute the tray weight evenly.
12. Keep your back straight, and bend and lift with your knees and legs when picking up or putting down a loaded tray.
13. Reverse the process when removing the tray. While holding the tray level, collapse the tray stand against your right hip.
14. After clearing a customer's table, use a service napkin to cover the tray before carrying it from the dining room.
15. Remove the tray and tray stand as soon as the table is cleared. See Fig. 3-13.

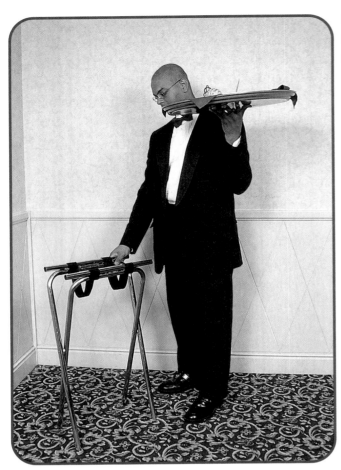

In addition to following procedures for using trays and stands, servers must follow procedures for serving each course. There are separate guidelines for serving bread, appetizers, soup, salad, entrées, and desserts. Food is always served from the customer's left with your left hand. Dishes are cleared from the customer's right with your right hand whenever possible.

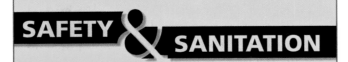

SAFETY & SANITATION

PREVENTING ACCIDENTS—To prevent accidents, tray stands should always be folded and placed out of busy traffic lanes when they are not being used.

Serving Bread

Many foodservice operations require that bread be served once the beverage order has been taken and served. Use the following guidelines for serving bread:

- Preset butter or olive oil. To **preset** items means to set them on the table before food is served.
- Place bread or rolls in the center of the table.
- Don't touch the bread or rolls with your hands.
- Serve enough bread or rolls initially for each customer to have one-and-a-half servings.

Serving Appetizers

Appetizers are frequently offered on a menu. **Appetizers** are small portions of hot or cold food meant to stimulate the appetite that are served as the first course of a meal.

If a customer orders a cold and a hot appetizer, serve the cold appetizer first, unless otherwise requested. If two or more customers are sharing an appetizer, divide and plate equal, attractive portions. An alternative would be to place it between the customers with serving utensils and a clean plate for each customer who is sharing the appetizer.

Serving Soup

If the customer orders a cup or bowl of soup or chowder, you will serve it from the customer's left in a cup or bowl placed on a saucer or an underliner. An **underliner** is a dish placed under another dish to protect the table from spills. If the underliner doesn't have an insert for the bowl to sit in, use a paper doily to keep the dishes from slipping. When clearing soup cups or bowls and saucers or underliners, place the soup spoon on the saucer or underliner before clearing the soup to prevent accidents and spills.

Serving Salad

The salad can be presented before or after the entrée. In the United States, the salad is usually served before the entrée. In other countries, a salad is often served after the entrée.

Serve cold salads from the customer's left on chilled plates. Preset a salad fork and knife. Salad forks are generally smaller than dinner forks.

Serving Entrées

The correct rotation of the plate is important to the presentation of the entrée. When hand-carrying plates or using food trays, be sure the plates stay level. Sauces can flow together if a plate is tipped. When placing the plate in front of the customer, allow about an inch between the edge of the plate and the table edge. Use your left hand to place the plate from the customer's left side.

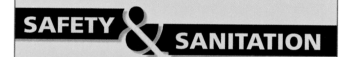

SAFETY & SANITATION

SERVING HOT PLATES—Present hot entrées on hot plates. Always use a clean, folded service towel when handling hot plates. This will prevent hot plates from burning or hurting you or the customer. Be sure to warn customers when plates are hot.

Serving Dessert

Dessert is usually the final chance to impress customers. Showing desserts is a very effective way of selling them. Many foodservice operations display their desserts on trays or on rolling carts. See Fig. 3-14. When presetting the dessert course, be sure to set the appropriate utensil at the customer's place before serving dessert. A dessert fork should be placed to the left for cake and pie. A dessert spoon is placed to the right for ice cream and pudding. Serve all desserts from the customer's left.

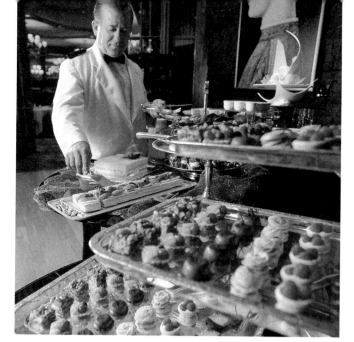

Fig. 3-14. Dessert trays or carts are often used to display the desserts offered.

Adjusting Flatware

Flatware should be adjusted to suit the food order. For example, the customer may need specialty flatware, such as a seafood fork, or may have used a preset utensil intended for another course. If the customer used a piece of flatware before its intended use, clear it with that course and preset the correct flatware for the next course. Always make sure that customers have the necessary flatware for the food you are about to serve.

Checking Back with the Customer

Servers should check back with their customers during the meal to see whether they are satisfied. However, be careful not to interrupt the customer too often. You can check back with customers by sight as well as sound. Make yourself available to the customer. Check back with the customers once they have been given a minute or two to taste the food. Watch their reactions as they taste the food. If they appear content, no further action is required on your part. If the customer's facial expression shows disappointment or displeasure, however, return to the table and ask whether the dish is prepared to his or her liking.

Clearing the Table

Using a tray makes clearing and carrying soiled dishes and service items safer, easier, and more efficient. Observe tables regularly to decide whether all customers have finished eating before clearing any dish. Customers might push the dish away, place their napkins on the table, or lay the flatware side by side across the dish to show that they have finished with a course.

Clearing an individual customer's dish before all of the customers are finished will make them feel rushed. Once the customers have finished eating, clear the dishes from the table as follows.

- Using your right hand, clear the dishes from the right side. Don't reach across the table or in front of customers unless absolutely necessary.
- Keep cleared plates in your left hand away from the customer and table, and move around the table clockwise.
- Don't overstack dishes on your arm or on the tray, and don't stack dishes on top of food.
- Don't scrape leftover food from one plate onto another plate when stacking dishes.
- Clear the table quietly and quickly.

Although many foodservice operations are smoke-free, some have separate smoking areas. Ashtrays should be changed by placing a clean ashtray over the dirty one. Remove both from the table and then place the clean one back on the table.

CULINARY TIP

CRUMBING THE TABLE—When clearing the table between the entrée and dessert courses, it is desirable to "crumb" the table. Crumbing is the process of removing crumbs that may have accumulated during the meal. The proper way to crumb a table is to fold a service towel into a small square and brush the particles onto a small plate or use a crumbing set. Do not brush the crumbs into your hand or onto the floor.

✕ CALCULATING CUSTOMER CHECKS

Every foodservice operation has its own policy about customer checks. In some places, the server or cashier figures the check, while in other operations, a computer is used. Regardless of the method, accurately listing charges is a must. For example, some foodservice operations charge for beverage refills or a second bread serving. Any extra charges must be clearly listed on the check.

Because the costs of operating a foodservice operation are so high, profit margins are very important. If servers do not accurately charge customers, profit will be lost. Managers generally double-check the accuracy of customer checks at the end of each business day.

Hand-Calculated Checks

There are still a few foodservice operations where servers need to figure the check by hand. Do this away from the table and use a calculator. To prepare the check, list all of the charges and double-check that prices are correct. Next, add the prices of all the food and beverage items. This is the subtotal. Then add the sales tax to the subtotal, which gives you the grand total.

Computer-Calculated Checks

Most foodservice operations use computers to create checks. In these operations, the server puts the order into the computer. That information then appears on the computerized check. Computer-calculated checks are convenient and reliable. Totals are accurately figured, and each item's price, the subtotal, the tax, and the grand total all appear on the check. See Fig. 3-15.

Handling Check Errors

Errors are always possible when you calculate a customer check. Errors are fairly simple to correct if you catch them before you give the check to the customer. If you make an error, simply draw a line through the error and begin again. Most foodser-

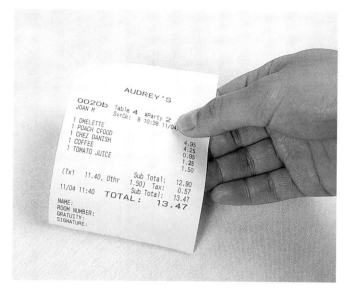

Fig. 3-15. Many foodservice operations use computer-generated checks.

vice operations use numbered checks. If a computerized check is printed before the error is noticed, or if a written check is beyond fixing, ask your supervisor what to do.

✖ PRESENTING THE CHECK

Prepare the customer check once you are certain the customer has finished ordering. A good server anticipates the request for the check. Make sure that all items and the check total are accurate. The check should be legible and clean.

Before presenting the check, all unnecessary serviceware should have been cleared from the table. Give the check to the host of the party, or place it in the center of the table. When the server is to collect the money, the check is placed on a check tray, a small plate, or in a check folder. The server then returns the change or credit card receipt to the customer in the same manner.

If the customer has paid with cash, be sure that the correct payment is received. Never ask customers if they want change. Always give them the change and thank them for their business.

a LINK to the Past

History of Tipping

The history of tipping—an acronym for "to ensure promptness"—is anything but clear. One theory states that tipping has its roots in the coffeehouses of sixteenth-century England. Still another theory says tipping has its roots in the Roman Empire. Tipping didn't become widespread in America until the middle of the nineteenth century.

Regardless of its origin, there have always been opponents of the practice. In fact, a group called the Anti-Tipping Society of America, an alliance of 100,000 traveling salesmen, had tipping abolished in seven states between 1905 and 1919.

For many years, the standard tip in America was 10%. This rose to 15% in the 1970s. Today, many foodservice workers are receiving a tip of 20% or more for a job well done.

Internationally, tipping practices are varied. In much of Europe, the tip is automatically added to the bill or included in the price of the menu items. In many Asian countries, tipping is considered rude.

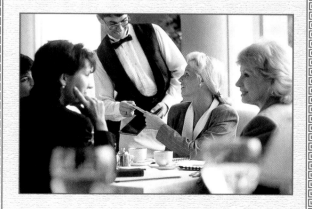

Handling Money

In many foodservice operations, the customers pay the server directly. Be sensitive to whether customers seem to want to sit and talk or pay the bill immediately. After presenting the check, return to the table within five minutes, or when you see the customer has placed money or a credit card with the bill. Take the money directly to the cash register. Either give the money and the check to the cashier or ring up the bill yourself. Be sure the change is correct before returning it to the table. Place the money to the left of the person who paid the bill. Thank your customers for coming in and invite them to return.

Handling Credit Cards

Many customers pay by credit card. These cards are easier to carry than cash, and they provide customers with an accurate expense record.

Most restaurants today use an electronic credit card machine which may be part of a point-of-sales computer. The card will need to be swiped correctly and the amount entered into the computer. It should be double-checked prior to transmission.

1. Check the card for the customer's signature.
2. Check the card's expiration date.
3. Make sure the customer signs the credit slip.
4. Compare the signatures to see that they match.
5. Return the credit card to the correct customer. Never leave credit cards laying around.

Handling Tips

Customers show their appreciation for good service by tipping. A tip is usually based on a percentage of the check, depending on the type of establishment. A good guide is a minimum of 15% of the total check, although outstanding service might warrant a tip of 20–30%.

Although the federal government sets a minimum wage, servers are often paid less than the minimum wage because tips are expected to make up the difference.

✖ RESETTING TABLES

To prepare for the next customer, you will need to reset the cover. A **cover** is an individual place setting that includes flatware, glassware, and dishes. First, thoroughly wipe and dry the tabletop. If a tablecloth is used, replace it if it is soiled. Then gather all of the flatware, glassware, and dishes on a tray or cart. Carry the flatware to the table on a service napkin or serviette. Carry the glassware on a beverage tray, making sure that the glasses are right side up. Place them in the correct position. Next, set any required dishes, such as bread plates. Finally, place the folded napkins in the desired location. See Chapter 4 for more information on setting tables.

SECTION 3-2   Knowledge Check

1. Describe three selling techniques a server can use to enhance sales.
2. What are three guidelines you should follow when using service trays or tray stands?
3. Describe the types of checks used in foodservice operations.

MINI LAB

In teams of three, role-play serving customers. Two students will be the customers, and the other student will act as the server. Rotate roles until each person has been the server. Discuss what you learned with the class.

Serving Beverages

OBJECTIVES

After reading this section, you will be able to:

- Operate and maintain hot and cold beverage equipment.

- Explain how to prepare beverages.

PROVIDING good customer service includes offering a full range of well-prepared beverages. Whether it is juice, milk, coffee, tea, or soft drinks, customers expect a refreshing beverage that is safe to drink. To accomplish this, each member of the service staff must know how to operate cold and hot beverage equipment.

✖ COLD BEVERAGE EQUIPMENT

Cold beverages range from bottled water to soft drinks, milk, iced tea, and juice. Each is dispensed from a special machine. Dispensers for tea, milk, or juice should be taken apart, cleaned, and sanitized daily. The Food and Drug Administration (FDA) recommends this practice to keep harmful bacteria from multiplying in the tubing.

Ice Makers

Since ice can be contaminated easily, always use a plastic or metal scoop. Never use your hands or a glass to scoop ice. See Fig. 3-16. After removing ice from the ice maker, place the scoop on a hook or in a holder on the outside of the ice maker. The ice maker should not be used for chilling any other food or objects. Always close the ice maker and put away the ice scoop when it is not in use.

SAFETY & SANITATION

ICE SAFETY—Never scoop ice with a glass. It is too fragile and could easily be broken by the ice. Keep the floor around the ice machine dry to prevent slips and falls.

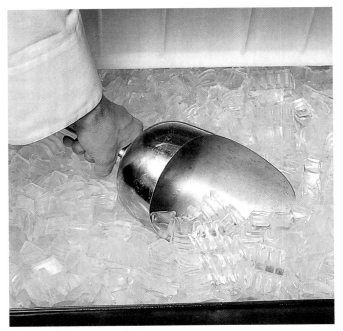

Fig. 3-16. Ice makers should be used only for ice. What do you do with the scoop after you are finished using it?

Soft Drink Machines

Soft drinks are often dispensed from a system that consists of a container of concentrated soda syrup, a tank of carbon dioxide (CO_2), and a soda gun dispenser. Two popular types of systems are the "bag in the box" and the tank system. The "bag in the box" is a cardboard box with a bag of concentrated soda syrup inside.

In the tank system, two plastic lines are connected to each tank. One leads to the CO_2 tank and allows it to pressurize the soda syrup. The other line permits the soda to pass to the dispensing gun.

You must clean the nozzle and rubber holster on a daily basis. Place the nozzle in a pitcher of warm water with a sanitizer for 15 minutes and then allow it to air dry. The soda lines should be maintained by the soda purveyor according to state sanitation laws.

SOFT DRINKS—FLAT OR FIZZY?

Have you ever wondered what makes a soft drink fizz, or what makes a soft drink go flat? The fizz in soft drinks is caused by carbonization. Carbon dioxide (CO_2), a clear, colorless gas, is dissolved in the soda mixture under pressure. In a container of soda, there is CO_2 in the soda and in the space between the soda and the top of the container. When the CO_2 in that space is lower than the CO_2 in the soda, more of the CO_2 comes out of the soda than returns to the soda. In other words, the CO_2 moves from the soda to the empty space. This causes the soda to become flat.

APPLY IT!

To see how CO_2 affects soft drinks, obtain a soft drink bottle with a replaceable lid. Let the bottle sit open at room temperature, without its cap, overnight. The next day, replace the cap tightly and shake the container. Remove the cap and pour about half of the liquid into a glass and taste it. Pour the remaining liquid into the sink. Record your observations.

When the soda bottle was left open, the CO_2 could only come into balance by using some of the CO_2 from the liquid. The larger the space above the liquid, the more CO_2 will be required to reach a balance. With the cap off, the CO_2 level will come to balance with the CO_2 levels in the air, causing the soda to go flat. In this experiment, you tasted for yourself how important it is to serve customers fresh soft drinks.

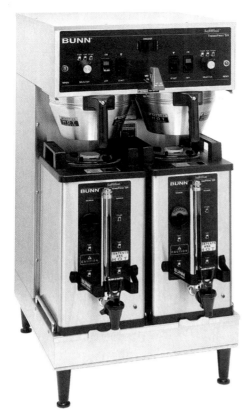

Fig. 3-17. A foodservice coffee maker.

⊠ HOT BEVERAGE EQUIPMENT

Many customers order hot beverages with or following their meals. With the exception of water, tea, in the form of loose tea leaves or tea bags, is the most popular beverage in the world. Coffee, prepared in a variety of ways, has long been a favorite beverage as well.

Coffee Makers

Most restaurants lease coffee makers from the same company that supplies the coffee. See Fig. 3-17. This procedure reduces expense and provides regular maintenance of the machines. Some coffee machines make regular grind coffee only, while others make only espresso and cappuccino. **Espresso** (ess-PRESS-oh) is a beverage made by forcing hot water and steam through finely ground, dark-roasted coffee beans. **Cappuccino** (kahp-uh-CHEE-noh) is a beverage made from espresso and steamed and foamed milk. Here are some general guidelines for using foodservice coffee makers:

- Turn on the hot plates and set the adjustable plates to "high" so that water will boil for tea.
- Don't place empty or near-empty glass pots on warming plates. They may break.
- Always ensure that the brewing cycle has finished completely before removing the pot. Interrupting the brew cycle by removing a pot too early will result in the first pot being too strong and incorrectly balanced while the second pot will be too weak and bitter.
- Be sure to use coffee within 15 minutes if it is kept on a direct heat source such as a warming plate. After one hour coffee will begin to lose flavor.
- If the coffee is kept in a vacuum or insulated container, it will maintain its quality and temperature for over an hour.

■ **Proportion of coffee to water.** The proportion of coffee to water affects the strength of coffee, a preference that varies with customers. In general, the recommended proportion is 1 lb. of coffee to 1¾–2½ gallons of water. Don't try to brew more coffee than the machine can make at one time. For the best flavor, use good quality water.

Many commercial coffee makers use premeasured vacuum-sealed packets of coffee. They are available in a wide variety of sizes to make small and large quantities of coffee. Follow the manufacturer's instructions to use this type of coffee. Some restaurants use fresh coffee beans. A coffee filter is placed under the bean hopper to catch the coffee as the beans are ground.

■ **Brew cycles.** Always match the grind of coffee to the coffee machine's brew cycle. Coffee beans can be ground from coarse to fine. A coarser grind takes longer to brew than a fine grind.

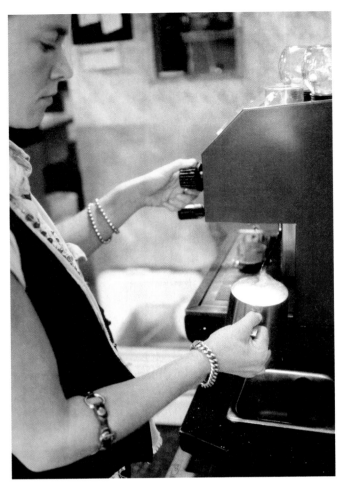

Fig. 3-18. Espresso is the basis for hot beverages such as this. In what kind of cup do you serve a single espresso?

■ **Using foodservice coffee makers.** To make coffee, first put the coffee pot on the burner. Check the filter basket to make sure it is clean. Then line the filter basket with a coffee filter and add the correct amount of coffee. Note that the amount of coffee used will vary depending on the type of coffee maker. Return the filter basket to the coffee maker. Press the "on" switch and then the "start" switch.

Espresso Machines

Espresso and espresso-based coffee drinks are becoming the fastest growing segment of this market. Espresso machines produce only one or two cups at a time, but each ounce of espresso takes only 17–23 seconds to run through the machine. Most machines require a grinder to finely grind the espresso coffee beans. This is done immediately prior to dispensing a designated por-

tion into the portafilter. For convenience and freshness, vacuum-packed single and double doses of espresso, called pods, are available.

Traditionally, espresso is served in a half-size cup, called a **demitasse** (DEHM-ee-tahss) cup, rather than the standard coffee cup. The cup should be filled about ⅓ full. Double espressos may be served in regular coffee cups. A shot of espresso is the basis for other beverages, as shown in Fig. 3-18. A quality serving of espresso should be covered with an amber-colored thin layer of froth called a "crema" (KRAI-mah). This reflects that the coffee beans are fresh, the grind is correct, the water temperature was sufficiently hot and pressurized, the brewing cycle was correct, and the equipment was clean. Always leave the machine turned on.

Tea-Making Equipment

Tea can be made in a wide variety of equipment. Pottery, china, stoneware, porcelain, and glass are all used to make strainers, kettles, teapots, and teacups. These may be simple or decorative in design. Like coffee, tea made in metallic equipment will give the liquid a metallic taste. Humidity, temperature, oxygen, and light all have an impact on tea leaves. Store tea in a sealed container in a cool, dry place.

■ **Proportion of tea to water.** The final taste of tea is determined by the proportion of tea to water. Depending on the type and quality of tea leaves, use 6 ounces of water with 1 rounded teaspoon of loose tea or one tea bag.

■ **Infusing tea.** When infusing tea in fresh water, consider the water temperature and the length of time that the leaves and water are in contact. To **infuse** a substance means to extract its flavors by placing it in a hot liquid. Infusion usually lasts from 2–4 minutes. The water should be at or near boiling to release the flavors and aromas of most teas. Color shouldn't be used to determine how long to infuse tea, since a good cup of tea depends on its flavor and aroma.

Cleaning Hot Beverage Equipment

To provide flavorful and sanitary hot beverages, you must clean hot beverage equipment, such as coffee makers, espresso machines, and tea containers, frequently and thoroughly.

■ **Coffee makers.** Turn off or unplug the coffee machine, and remove the used filter and grounds from the filter basket. Remove the water spray fixture and clean it. Be sure to clean and replace the filter basket. Clean coffeepots at the end of each shift with a brush and commercial cleaner.

■ **Espresso machines.** The portafilter should be removed immediately after serving the beverage. After each use, knock the spent grounds out into a special "knock box." Rinse the portafilter by running a cycle of hot water through it without coffee grounds. Place the portafilter upside down on top of the machine to air dry. To clean the machine, use an approved cleaner. Dispense the recommended amount into a portafilter which has a "blind" screen, or a screen with no holes.

Turn on the brewing cycle up to eight times once the blind portafilter has been inserted into the machine's group or housing. Leave the cleaner in the system for 15 minutes or according to the manufacturer's instructions. Remove the blind portafilter. Flush out by running at least two brewing cycles.

■ **Tea containers.** Tea-making equipment must be kept free of mineral deposits that build up from water and tea. This buildup gives tea an unpleasant flavor. Boil equipment with a solution of diluted white vinegar to remove deposits. See Fig. 3-19.

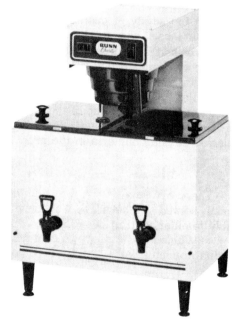

Fig. 3-19. Tea equipment must be cleaned and sanitized regularly.

SECTION 3-3 Knowledge Check

1. What are two guidelines to follow when using an ice maker?
2. List three guidelines for using a coffee maker.
3. What steps should you take to clean an espresso machine?

MINI LAB

In teams, learn how to safely operate and clean each piece of beverage equipment in your lab. Practice serving the beverages you make while learning to operate each machine. Rotate stations until each team has mastered using all of the equipment.

CHAPTER ③ Review & Activities

SECTION SUMMARIES

3-1 The host, server, busser, and cashier each have a role in making the customer's experience enjoyable.

3-1 Qualities that service employees should possess include a positive attitude, a neat and clean appearance, good communication and teamwork skills, job knowledge, and the ability to use time wisely.

3-1 Because foodservice jobs often require long hours, maintaining good health with rest and exercise will help the foodservice employee thrive in his or her job.

3-2 Server's duties include greeting customers; taking the beverage order; serving hot and cold beverages; selling the menu; taking, writing, transmitting, and serving the order; and presenting the check.

3-2 Thorough knowledge of the menu helps servers sell items by highlighting menu choices, asking open-ended questions, and upselling larger sizes.

3-2 Serving food and beverages and clearing tableware and glassware require physical strength and constant consideration for customers and coworkers.

3-2 Servers are responsible for accurately calculating customers' checks or, if using a computerized point-of-sales system, ensuring that each item ordered is listed.

3-3 The types of machines used to make beverages include an ice maker, a soft drink machine, milk and juice dispensers, coffee and espresso makers, and tea-making equipment.

3-3 Quality ingredients, correct portions, and attention to detail are important when preparing coffee, tea, and espresso.

CHECK YOUR KNOWLEDGE

1. List three skills that show a proper attitude in the foodservice business.
2. Contrast verbal and nonverbal communication.
3. How does asking customers open-ended questions help sell menu items?
4. How does a computerized point-of-sales system make service easier and faster?
5. What concerns do customers have with how their food is served?
6. When should the server clear dishes from the table?
7. What should be cleared from the table before the server presents the check to the customer?
8. How do you check the taste and color of a new tank or bag of soda?
9. Contrast the process of making coffee with that of making tea.

CRITICAL-THINKING ACTIVITIES

1. Analyze various companies' practices regarding customer satisfaction. How can this help you improve your service to customers?
2. How do the host, server, busser, and cashier work together as a team? Describe how good teamwork benefits the customer.

WORKPLACE KNOW-HOW

Decision making. Suppose you are a restaurant manager hiring for server positions. What qualities would you look for in potential employees? Why might these qualities be beneficial for a server to have?

LAB-BASED ACTIVITY: Practicing Table Service

STEP 1 **Divide into teams of four.** Each student will take turns being a server to a table set for three people.

STEP 2 **Gather the following supplies:**
- Linen.
- Beverage tray.
- Serving tray and tray stand.
- Glasses, cups, and saucers.
- Bread plates.
- Salad plates.
- Soup bowls.
- Dinner plates.
- Dessert plates.
- Flatware for each course.
- Blank customer check and a pencil or pen.
- Check tray or folder.

STEP 3 **Determine the role each person will play.**
- Greet the customers and offer them beverages.
- Serve beverages.
- Offer appetizers to start the meal.
- Serve appetizers.
- Clear appetizer tableware and flatware.
- Take an order for a meal.
- Serve a salad.
- Clear salad plates and flatware.
- Serve the main course.
- Clear the main course.
- Take the dessert and coffee order.
- Serve the dessert and coffee.
- Clear the table.
- Present the check.
- Make correct change and present it to the customer.

STEP 4 **Number a sheet of paper for as many students as will be servers.** After each participant serves, write down what you thought of his or her service.

STEP 5 **Watch and listen closely as each server takes his or her turn:**
- How does the server talk to the customer? What does the server's posture and eye contact convey?
- How does the server move around the table while serving and clearing dishes?
- Does the server place and clear from the correct positions?
- Does the server place the tableware and glassware appropriately?
- What does the server do with tableware and glassware when clearing them from the table?

STEP 6 **After everyone has had a turn, discuss what you observed with the rest of the class.**

STEP 7 **Make a list of the areas with which people had the most problems.**
- How does each area affect customer service?
- How can these problems be resolved?

The Dining Experience

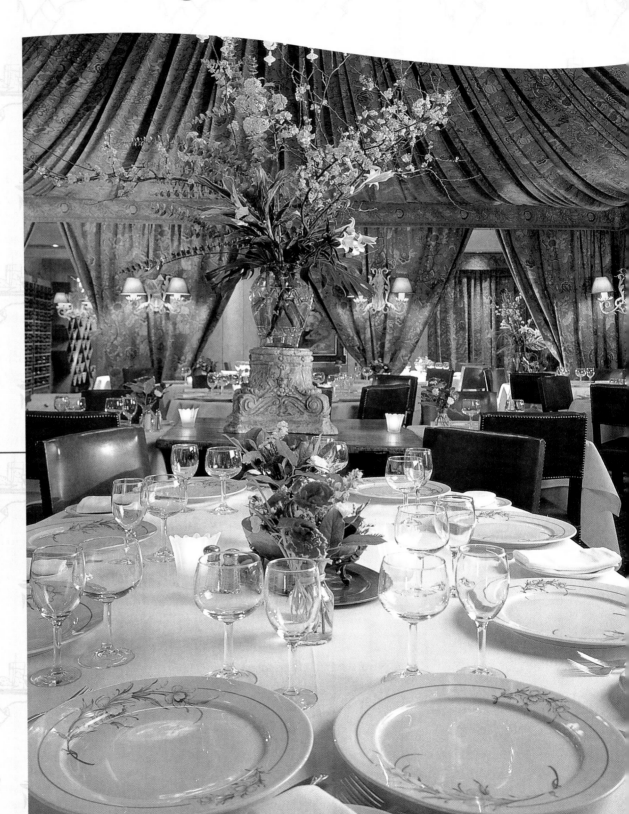

Dining Today

KEY TERMS

- food court
- focal point
- banquette
- tableside
- flambé
- hors d'oeuvre
- chafing dish

OBJECTIVES

After reading this section, you will be able to:

- Describe the five different types of dining environments.
- Explain the characteristics of the various types of meal service.
- Demonstrate different styles of meal service.

E A C H type of dining environment presents unique challenges to the foodservice professional. The type of establishment and its meal service strongly influence a customer's dining experience. Learning about these factors will help you better serve customers and build a rewarding foodservice career.

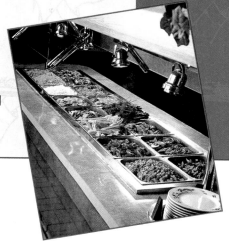

✕ TYPES OF DINING

Different types of dining appeal to different customers and situations. The five most common types of dining are fine-dining restaurants, theme restaurants, casual-dining establishments, quick-service restaurants, and catering services. These types differ in menu prices, decor, the type of food served, and the way food is served.

Some restaurants promote themes and special events, such as special birthday dinners, holiday buffets, or seasonal specialties. Marketing these themes and events can bring in a strong customer base.

Fine-Dining Restaurants

Fine-dining restaurants provide an environment featuring excellent food, elegant decor, and superior service. Customers are willing to pay top prices for a meal in fine-dining establishements. Some of these restaurants are known for their chef's exceptional culinary skills and some for their specific location.

Theme Restaurants

Theme restaurants often try to recreate another place or time. Customers enjoy seeing sports memorabilia or an indoor waterfall in the middle of a simulated rain forest. They are attracted to the fun and unique atmosphere. The food can often be secondary or the food related to the theme becomes the focus, as in a table top grill restaurant. Most theme restaurants have a moderate priced menu.

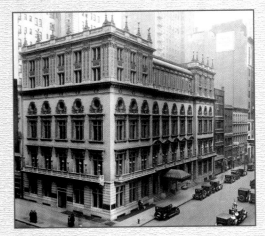
Casual-Dining Establishments

Casual-dining establishments attract people who like to eat out, but are not interested in a formal atmosphere or high prices. Instead, they enjoy the relaxed environment and mid-range prices of casual dining.

Sometimes casual-dining restaurants also have a theme, such as the music theme of the Hard Rock Café®. Steak houses with a theme of "grill your own dinner" have become very popular for those who crave food and adventure. Other common casual-dining establishments include family-style restaurants, neighborhood establishments, grills and buffets, and vending machines. See Fig. 4-1.

■ **Family-style restaurants.** The menu is more limited in a casual, family-style restaurant. Traditional, child-friendly favorites, such as fried chicken, macaroni and cheese, and mashed potatoes, are often served.

Fig. 4-1. Theme restaurants offer customers the chance to dine in a unique dining environment.

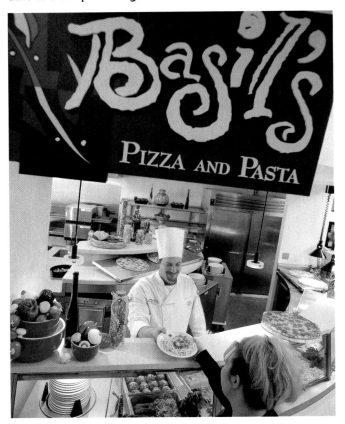

- **Neighborhood establishments.** Two popular types of casual neighborhood establishments are lunch counters and coffee shops. The food is usually simple, inexpensive, and generously portioned. Coffee houses, for example, are increasing in number. Neighborhood establishments attract customers with their convenient location and friendly atmosphere.

- **Grills and buffets.** Casual grill and buffet restaurants offer self-service meals at budget prices. Buffet restaurants also offer all-you-can-eat specials that appeal to families and senior citizens.

- **Vending machines.** Casual dining wouldn't be complete without vending machines. Vending machines offer a wide variety of foods and beverages. Because vending machines operate 24 hours a day, they are popular with college students and factory workers. Many companies have saved money by using vending machines rather than running a full-service dining room or cafeteria.

Quick-Service Restaurants

This category of restaurants, also known as fast food, is the largest section of the foodservice industry. Quick-service restaurants offer limited menus, low prices, and speedy service. Food is prepared according to exact standards through factory-like production, such as Kentucky Fried Chicken® and Pizza Hut®.

Malls and shopping centers often place several quick-service restaurants into a single area, called a **food court**. This allows shoppers quick and convenient access to a variety of meals. Small food courts, offering three or four options, are found in many hospitals, colleges, and supermarkets.

Catering Services

Catering is a growing segment of the foodservice industry. It often involves purchasing, receiving, storing, preparing, cooking, delivering, and serving food to a client in another location. Catered meals range from beverages and doughnuts for a breakfast meeting to a six-course dinner for an awards banquet.

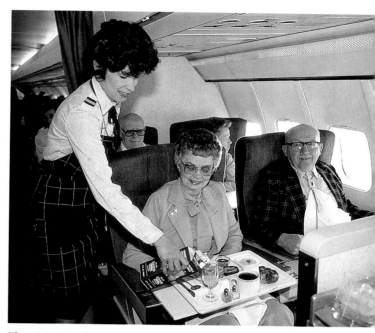

Fig. 4-2. Food service on airlines is limited by storage needs, flight length, and transportation.

In an attempt to increase sales, many institutions have begun providing catering services. For example, some supermarkets, restaurants, schools, and hospitals use their kitchens to cater outside the institution. Because caterers generally know how many portions to make, waste is kept to a minimum.

- **Contract foodservice.** For a management fee, a foodservice contractor will provide cost-effective food and beverage service for organizations such as schools, businesses, hospitals, and nursing homes. For example, an organization such as a hospital may decide to move from a self-operated facility to a contract facility in order to save money. Meals may still be prepared on-site; however, management of the foodservice is not run by the hospital.

- **Airline meals.** Food catered for airlines is limited by storage needs and transportation. Depending on the flight length, customers may be served one or more full meals or just snacks and beverages. See Fig. 4-2. Meals for travelers are prepared in a commissary (CAH-muh-sair-ee), where food is purchased, prepared, and loaded onto airplanes for people to eat. Special meals, such as vegetarian or low-fat requests, are made available when ordered in advance.

■ **Hotel and motel restaurants.** Hotel and motel restaurants offer customers longer service hours. Most of these restaurants serve three meals a day, seven days a week. Labor costs are high, with room service being the most labor-intensive service. Prices vary, depending on the hotel or motel in which the restaurant is located.

■ **Cruise ship dining.** For many people, one of the highlights of taking a cruise is the excellent food. There is no limit on the amount of food eaten, and the cost is included in the price of the cruise. Food on a cruise ship is often offered in different settings, such as a poolside snack shop or a fine-dining restaurant. Special dietary needs can also be met with advance notice.

⊠ TYPES OF MEAL SERVICE

From buffet service to classical French service, there is a style of meal service to match every dining establishment's customers and goals. Different elements of each style can also be mixed. The following types of meal service are commonly found in commercial foodservice operations: modern American plated, booth, banquette (bang-KEHT), family style, classical French, Russian, butler, and buffet service.

Modern American Plated Service

Modern American plated service originated in the United States, but is now used worldwide. It is popular because it requires fewer and less extensively-trained service staff members than other types of meal service. It is also appreciated

by many restaurant chefs. It gives the chef complete control over the preparation, portioning, and presentation of the food. This is not always the case with other styles of service.

In modern American plated service, the food is completely prepared, portioned, plated, and garnished in the kitchen. The servers carry the plated food from the kitchen and place the prepared dishes in front of the customer. In order to follow modern American plated service guidelines, the server must be able to serve from both the left and right side of each customer.

Follow these general guidelines for modern American plated service:

• Serve beverages and soup from the customer's right side, with your right hand and right foot forward. Move clockwise to the next customer.

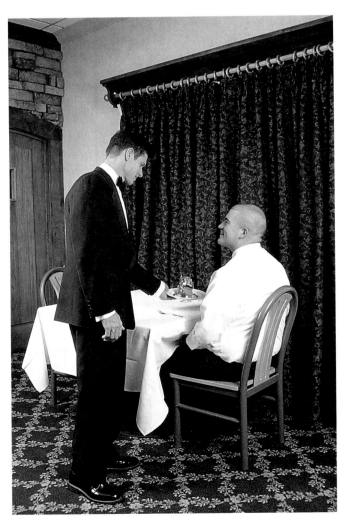

Fig. 4-3. American plated service is popular around the world. Name two reasons for its popularity.

- Serve solid foods from the customer's left side, with your left hand and left foot forward. Move counterclockwise to the next customer. See Fig. 4-3.
- Clear from the right with your right hand and right foot forward, except when clearing items on the customer's left, such as forks or bread plates.
- Completely serve and clear one guest before moving onto the next.
- Never break the order of service.

This type of service is more efficient than many other styles of service. The savings can be passed on to the customer through reasonable menu prices. It can also be helpful in boosting profits.

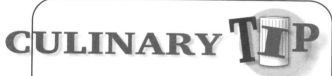

USING THE CORRECT HAND—Notice that whenever a server performs a function from the guest's left, the left hand is used. When working from the customer's right, the right hand is used. This is true regardless of the type of table being served or the type of service being performed.

Booth Service

Booth and banquette service have different service guidelines because the server can't go to the customer's left or right side. A booth table rests against, or is attached to, a wall. Since the server can't walk to each customer, all customers must be served from a single **focal point**, or service point. The customers on the right side of the booth will be served from the left with the server's left hand. The customers on the left side will be served from the right with the server's right hand. See Fig. 4-4.

Use the following guidelines when serving at a booth:

- Serve customers in the back of the booth first. Then serve the customers in the front of the booth.
- Using the same hand procedures, clear soiled tableware first from the customers seated closest to the back.
- For beverage service, however, don't switch hands. Keep the tray in your left hand and serve beverages with the right. Try not to get in the way of the guest. To ensure safety, you could say, "pardon me" as you serve.
- To maintain proper etiquette, always keep your hands as close to table level as possible.
- Avoid handing items to customers whenever possible. Instead, place the item on the table.

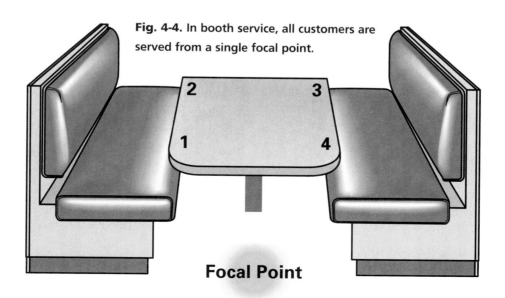

Fig. 4-4. In booth service, all customers are served from a single focal point.

Focal Point

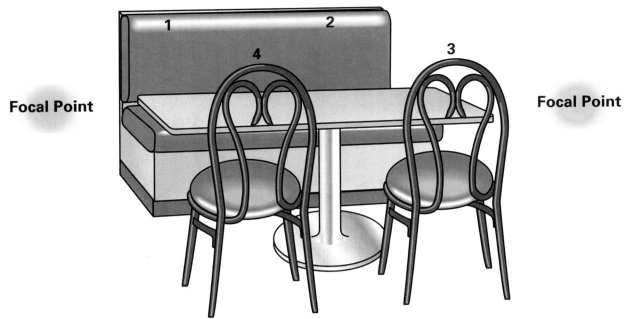

Focal Point

Focal Point

Fig. 4-5. In banquette service, both ends of the banquette are focal points.

Banquette Service

Banquette (bang-KEHT) is a type of seating arrangement in which customers are seated facing the server with their backs against the wall. See Fig. 4-5. Use the following guidelines when serving at a banquette:

- Treat both ends of the banquette as focal points. Serve one side of the table at a time; then proceed to the other side of the table and serve those guests.
- When serving a banquette with more than four people, serve each end of the table as you would a booth.
- Hold the beverage tray in your left hand. Serve with the right hand. Stand with your right hip close to the table and your left arm farthest away.

Family-Style Service

Family-style service is used in a casual-dining atmosphere. Customers serve themselves and pass the food around the table. This type of service creates an atmosphere of eating dinner at home. Foods are prepared completely in the kitchen and placed on platters or in casseroles. Then they are placed in the center of the customers' table with the correct serving utensils and a service plate for each customer. After serving themselves, customers pass each dish to the person on their right.

One advantage of family-style service is that it allows customers to choose their own portion sizes. On the other hand, this service style can result in a large amount of food waste. It also lacks personalized service.

Classical French Service

The most elegant and elaborate style of service is classical French service. It is used internationally when a formal style of service is desired. An important element of classical French service is that some foods are fully or partially prepared **tableside**, or at the table, in full view of the customer. For this reason, this service is more time-consuming and labor-intensive than modern American plated service.

Servers of this style must be highly skilled, with a thorough knowledge of food preparation and fine-dining service. Successful classical French service uses a team system. The typical French brigade consists of a four-member team—a captain, a front waiter, a back waiter or runner, and a busser. Each member of the service staff has a specific duty as follows:

- **Captain.** The captain is responsible for supervising and organizing all aspects of classical French service in his or her station.
- **Front waiter.** The front waiter assists the captain when serving food and should be able to perform the duties of the captain in his or her absence.
- **Back waiter or runner.** The back waiter or runner brings all of the food from the kitchen area to the service area.
- **Busser.** The busser serves bread, butter, and water. He or she also clears the table and cleans the table when customers leave.

■ **Tableside preparation.** Tableside food preparation is an important part of classical French service, but it also can be used with other services. Tableside preparations are made on a cart called a guéridon (gha-ree-dawn) using a cooking unit called a réchaud (ray-choh). These preparations are classified into four categories:

1. **Assembling.** This includes salads or dishes such as Caesar salad that require the simple assembly of ingredients.
2. **Saucing and garnishing.** This category includes dishes precooked in the kitchen that need finishing touches, such as sauces and garnishes.
3. **Sautéing or flambéing.** Items in this category are sautéed or flambéed quickly in the dining room. To **flambé** (flahm-BAY) an item is to "flame" it tableside as part of the preparation. See Fig. 4-6. Examples include shrimp with garlic or bananas foster.
4. **Carving and deboning.** Fish, game, meat, and poultry dishes are often carved or deboned tableside for the customer's enjoy-

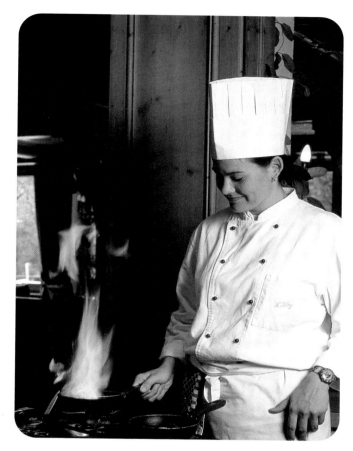

Fig. 4-6. Flambéing food tableside.

ment and convenience. This category also includes the slicing of cheese and the peeling of fruit. Peeling, coring, pitting, and slicing fruit allows customers to eat fruit easily without using their fingers.

Russian Service

Russian service is another elegant, formal service that is used internationally. Russian service is ideal for banquets where everyone is eating the same meal. Each course is completely prepared, cooked, portioned, and garnished in the kitchen and then placed on a service plate or platters. Each customer is served a portion of the product from large platters. The portion is placed on service plates that have been previously set on the table. It is served from the left, using a serving set that is held in the server's right hand. Two different

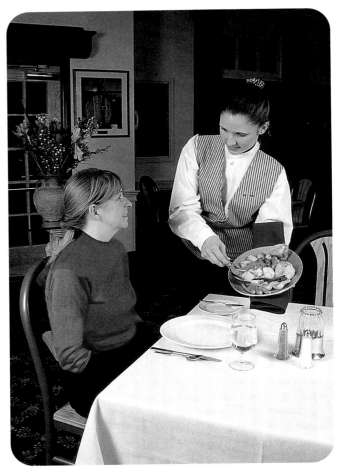

Fig. 4-7. Russian service is often used at formal banquets where everyone is eating the same meal.

servers usually perform Russian service. One server delivers the entrée. The other server brings the rest of the meal. See Fig. 4-7. Some general guidelines of Russian service include:

- Servers have a clean service napkin or towel draped over their left forearm. Platters are held in the left hand.
- Service always moves counterclockwise.
- Empty plates and soup bowls are placed in front of the customer from the right side.
- Items are served with the right hand from the customer's left side. The server is standing with his or her left foot forward.
- A serving set is used to transfer food from the platter to the customer's plate.
- All items are removed with the server's right hand from the customer's right side.

Butler Service

In butler service, the server carries the prepared food on a silver tray to standing or seated customers. Customers serve themselves from the trays. This is an efficient and cost-effective way to serve bite-size foods such as an **hors d'oeuvre** (ohr-DURV), or very small portions of food served before a meal to a large number of people. You will learn more about hors d'oeuvres in Chapters 18 and 21.

At a butler-served meal, each course is presented on a platter from the left side of each customer. Customers serve themselves while the server or butler holds the platter. Customers choose how much or how little they want of each food. Butler service is cost-effective; however, there is no control over how much food is eaten or how it is presented on the customer's plate.

Buffet Service

A buffet is a style of service in which all the food is attractively displayed on a table for the customers to see. Customers go to the buffet, choose what they want, and serve themselves. Customers must get a clean plate each time they return to the buffet line.

Buffet service can range from customers helping themselves to all food and beverages, to customers being served certain foods. Since buffets are mostly self-service, servers can attend to a greater number of customers. Three types of buffet service include:

- **Self-service**—Customers serve themselves.
- **Staff-service**—Customers indicate their choice, but are served by a member of the service staff. Some items are prepared to order.
- **Mixed service**—Different stations along the buffet offer self-service and other stations offer staff-service.

Advantages of buffet service include its low labor costs and its wide selection of food. Disadvantages include the possibility of large amounts of wasted food. If servers are inattentive, tables may not be properly cleared and guests may not receive timely beverage service.

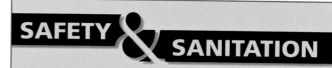

SAFETY & SANITATION

KEEPING BUFFET FOODS SAFE—Buffets can include both hot and cold foods. All foods must be held at the proper temperatures. Maintain the temperature of hot foods by placing them in chafing (CHAYF-ing) dishes. A **chafing dish** is a device that holds a large pan of food over a canned heat source. The temperature of cold food is maintained by setting the platters of food in beds of ice. See Fig. 4-8.

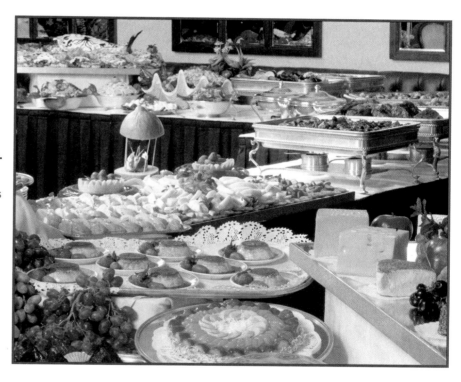

Fig. 4-8. Buffet service offers customers a wide variety of food choices. How can you make sure hot and cold foods stay at the proper temperatures on a buffet table?

SECTION 4-1 Knowledge Check

1. Name three types of catering services.
2. What does it mean to serve a meal family style?
3. Describe two categories of tableside service.

MINI LAB

Working in teams, choose a style of service. Practice that style of service until each team member has been the server. Rotate styles until each team has practiced all styles of service.

The Dining Room Environment

KEY TERMS

- side work
- condiments
- perishable
- nonperishable
- heat treated
- flatware
- serviette
- preset menu
- centerpieces
- candelabra

OBJECTIVES

After reading this section, you will be able to:

- Restock side station items.
- Set glassware, tableware, and flatware appropriately.
- Fold napkins into various decorative shapes.
- Use appropriate table settings and centerpieces.

MAKING sure that customers dine in an inviting atmosphere is the task of every member of the service staff. In this section, you will learn about some of the elements that help contribute to a pleasant dining experience. From folding napkins to choosing centerpieces, there are many things you can do to make customers feel welcome.

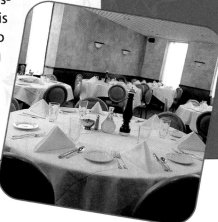

⊠ CREATING A DINING ENVIRONMENT

The atmosphere of a restaurant refers to the textures, colors, aromas, lighting, and sounds that create a dining environment. From the type of tableware used to the background music played, all elements work together to create a pleasing environment. This atmosphere helps determine the type of service and menu used.

Service is another important factor in creating the dining environment. To be able to provide quality service, the service staff must understand and properly use all dining room equipment.

Side Work

Preparing and placing all necessary equipment is the first step in providing quality service. Every service member has clearly defined duties to perform, called **side work**, before opening the dining room to the public. Side work generally includes:

- Cleaning and refilling salt and pepper shakers.
- Cleaning and refilling sugar containers.
- Cleaning and refilling glass and metal containers used to hold condiments.

Fig. 4-9. Learning to set tables properly is an important skill.

- Stocking side stations with all the materials needed for service.
- Cleaning the seats, table, table base, and floor.
- Folding napkins.
- Setting tables. See Fig. 4-9.

Refilling Salt & Pepper Shakers

Refill salt and pepper shakers before each shift begins. Be sure they are clean and not greasy or sticky. Empty and clean them regularly. Here are some guidelines for cleaning and refilling salt and pepper shakers:

1. Use a tray to collect the salt and pepper shakers. Take them to the kitchen and empty them.

2. Wash both the inside and outside of each shaker. To clean the inside, use a bottle brush.

3. Wash the shaker tops, unplugging the holes.

4. Be sure the tops and shakers are completely dry before refilling. Otherwise, the salt and pepper will not flow properly.

5. Fill the shakers. Be sure to use the right-sized grain of salt and pepper. If the grains are too fine or too coarse, customers may become frustrated when shaking too much or too little salt and pepper onto their food.

6. After filling the shakers with fresh salt and pepper, tap them to clear out air pockets. Place the shakers on a tray and return them to the tables.

Refilling Sugar Bowls

Some state laws do not permit the use of sugar bowls because loose sugar is not sanitary. Instead, restaurants use individual sugar packets. If sugar bowls are used, however, clean the bowls daily. Check for lumps, and remove them with a dry spoon. Always check and refill sugar containers before they become empty.

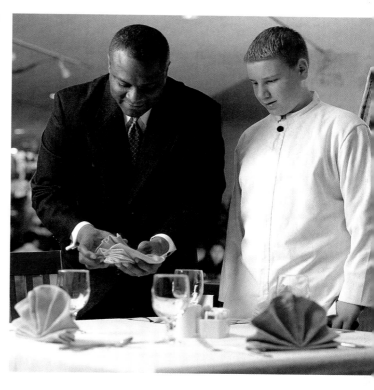

Refilling Condiments

Condiments, such as mustard, pickle relish, and ketchup, are traditionally served as accompaniments to food. Be sure to clean condiment containers daily. When refilling the containers, check that no condiments have gotten into the grooves around the cap. Never use a paper towel when drying or wiping off a condiment container. Original condiment containers, such as a ketchup bottle, should not be refilled due to safety and sanitation regulations. Containers of condiments, such as vinegar and oil, can be grouped into a caddy and placed on the table.

■ **Perishable condiments.** Some sauces and most salad dressings are perishable (PEHR-ih-shuh-bul). **Perishable** products can spoil quickly, even when stored correctly. Refrigerate these items when they are not being served to customers.

■ **Nonperishable condiments.** Nearly all condiments served in individual packets are **nonperishable**, meaning they will not spoil quickly when stored correctly. Nonperishable condiments include ketchup and steak sauces, mustard, syrups, jams, and preserves.

Fig. 4-10.

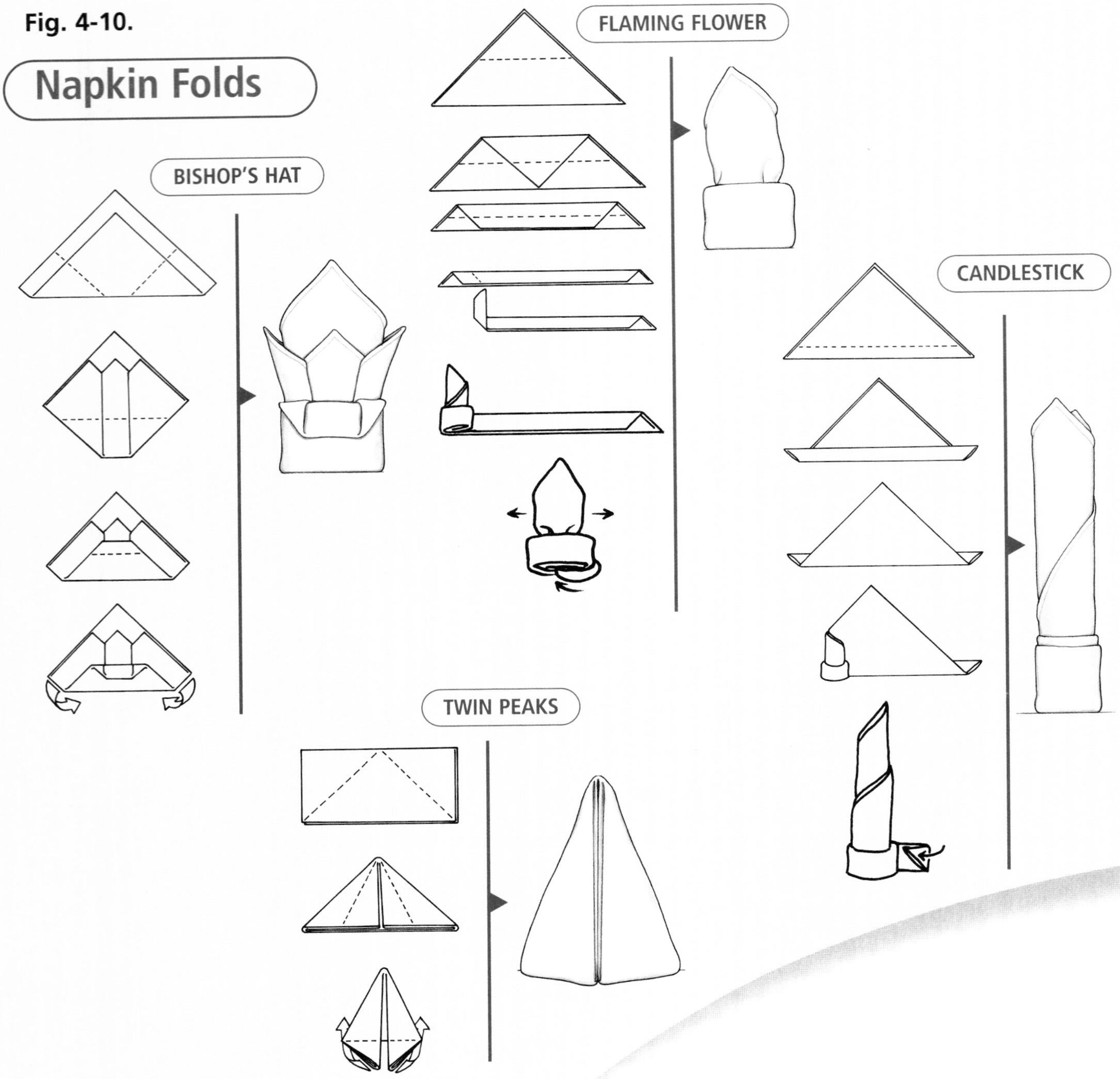

Napkin Folds

BISHOP'S HAT

FLAMING FLOWER

CANDLESTICK

TWIN PEAKS

Folding Napkins for Service

The restaurant owner or manager decides how napkins are to be folded. Fig. 4-10 shows a few ways to fold napkins. Use the following guidelines when folding napkins:

• Place linen on a clean surface.
• Be sure that your hands are clean before handling linen.
• Handle customer napkins as little as possible.

GEOMETRY & NAPKIN FOLDING

As you fold napkins into a water lily design as shown here, you will notice some familiar geometric shapes. To begin with, your napkin is probably in the shape of a square. A square has four right angles (90°) and four equal sides. In Step 1, you create a smaller square when you fold the corners of the napkin into the center.

If you look closely, you will notice that the square is made up of two large congruent triangles. For triangles to be congruent, all of the corresponding angles and sides must be the same. In this case, the two large congruent triangles are classified as isosceles triangles. Isosceles triangles have at least two congruent sides. These two isosceles triangles can also be classified as right triangles because each triangle contains a 90° angle.

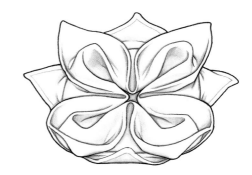

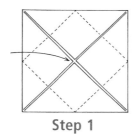

Step 1

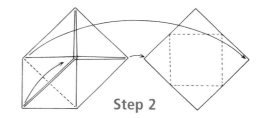

Step 2

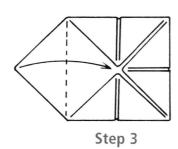

Step 3

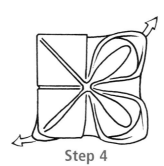

Step 4

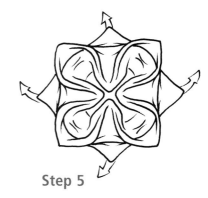

Step 5

TRY IT!

1. Look at the napkin in Step 1. How many total triangles do you see? Classify each triangle.

2. Classify each triangle that you see in Steps 2 and 3. What pattern do you notice?

3. The sum of the angle measures in a triangle has to equal 180°. What are the angle measures in a right isosceles triangle?

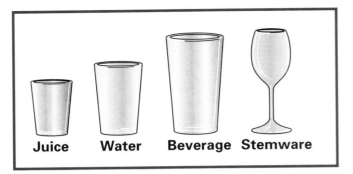

Fig. 4-11. The two categories of glassware are lead crystal and heat treated. How do these two types differ?

GLASSWARE

Restaurants use glassware for beverages such as juice, water, and iced tea. Although there are many styles and patterns to choose from, glassware can be divided into two categories: lead crystal and heat-treated glass. See Fig. 4-11.

■ **Lead crystal.** Lead crystal glassware is very hard, clear, and bright. Because this glassware is expensive and easily chipped, it is not practical for busy, casual restaurants. It is generally used in formal, fine-dining restaurants.

■ **Heat treated.** Glass that is heated and then cooled rapidly is called **heat treated**. It is strong and resists breaking and chipping. Most foodservice operations use heat-treated glassware.

Use the following guidelines for handling all types of glassware.

• Store glassware upside down in a glass rack or on air mats on a shelf.

• Always hold glassware by the base or stem.

• Never use chipped or cracked glassware.

• Always use a beverage tray to carry glassware in the dining room.

TABLEWARE

Restaurants use a variety of tableware, from dinner plates to soup bowls to coffee cups. Setting a visually pleasing table includes choosing the correct tableware. For a formal presentation, you might use porcelain or fine china. For a more casual look, you might use ceramic tableware. Fig. 4-12 shows tableware commonly used in food service.

FLATWARE

Flatware refers to dining utensils, such as spoons, forks, and knives. See Fig. 4-12. Flatware can also be referred to as cutlery. Flatware can be made of different quality grades of stainless steel or of silver. Like glassware and tableware, flatware is available in many different styles.

Flatware is carried through a dining room on a **serviette**, or napkin-lined plate. Handle flatware by the "waist," or midsection of the handle. This keeps fingers from coming into contact with the end of the utensil that will go into the customer's mouth. It also prevents fingerprints from being left on the handles.

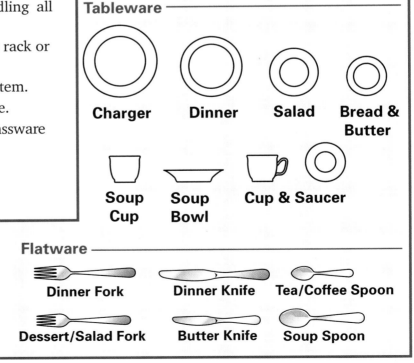

Fig. 4-12. Foodservice operations use many types of tableware and flatware.

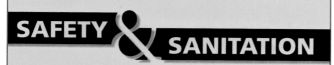
✖ TABLE SETTING

Restaurant management determines the type and style of table setting that is used. The setting will depend on the menu offered and the type of dining environment. See Fig. 4-13. Customer comfort, cleanliness, and uniformity are important factors to remember when setting tables. Here are some general guidelines for setting tables.

1. Place chairs around the table to establish the location of each place setting.

2. Place centerpieces, salt and pepper shakers, and condiment holders at the same location on each table.

3. To center each place setting, first place the napkin. If a placemat is used, center it in the place setting about 1 in. from the edge of the table. Place a napkin to the left side of the placemat or in the center.

4. Set forks on the left side of each place setting and knives and spoons on the right side of the place setting.

5. Always set knives with the cutting edge toward the center of the place setting.

6. Flatware should not hang over the edge of the placemat or table. Place flatware 1 in. from the edge of the placemat or table.

7. Place all flatware from the outside in, following the order of use. Make sure there is room for the dinner plate in the center of the place setting.

8. If presetting dessert spoons or forks, place them at the top of the place setting, perpendicular (purh-puhn-DIH-kyuh-luhr) to the other flatware. If both are used, the spoon is placed above the fork. Point the spoon's handle to the right and the fork's handle to the left.

9. Place the bread-and-butter plate on the left, above the fork(s).

10. If a butter knife is used, it should be placed on the top of the bread-and-butter plate with the cutting edge facing down.

11. Place the water glass above the tip of the dinner knife.

12. Preset coffee cups to the right of the knives and spoons, with handles at the 4 o'clock position.

Fig. 4-13.

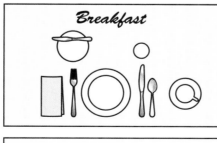

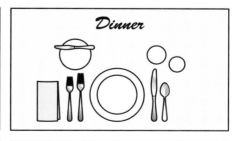

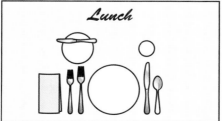

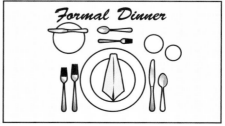

Table Preparation

Regardless of the table setting used, the server must be sure that the tabletop, benches, chairs, and the floor area around the table are clean. Check the underside of tabletops for any chewing gum that may have been placed there by a customer. Be sure the chairs and booth seats are wiped clean. Constantly inspect tables and the floor below them, especially when the tables are being reset.

■ **Table linens.** Linen napkins and tablecloths can dramatically enhance a room's appearance. Using linen, however, is expensive. Many foodservice establishments use place mats, paper or vinyl tablecloths, or glass tabletops instead. Restaurants that do use linen usually rent it from companies that specialize in linen rental. There are many different styles, types, and colors of linen. Servers must set each tablecloth with the seam toward the table and make sure it is even on all sides. Use the following guidelines for changing a tablecloth. See Fig 4-14.

1. Remove all glassware and dishes from the table.

2. Place standard accessories, such as candles or flowers, on a tray. Never use a chair to hold such items.

3. Fold the soiled cloth back about one fourth of its length. Fold it onto the table, but don't show any of the surface underneath.

4. Bring out the clean tablecloth and place it over the folded portion of the soiled cloth.

5. With the seam down, drop the end of the new cloth so that it is opened one fold and hangs over the end of the table.

6. Using both hands, hold the two corners of both the clean and soiled cloths. Pull them toward the other end of the table.

7. When you reach the other end of the table, let go of the cloth corners.

8. Grasp the hanging corners of the soiled cloth and bring them to the other corners of the folded cloth.

9. Hold all corners and drop the top edge of the new cloth over the table. Do not let go of the corners of the soiled cloth.

10. Neatly fold the soiled cloth again, making sure that the trapped crumbs don't fall onto the floor.

11. Place the cloth on the tray.

12. Before placing the soiled linen in a linen bag, empty the crumbs in a lined trash can in the back of the foodservice operation.

Table Setting for Preset Menus

A **preset menu** is a meal served to a group of customers who have decided in advance on the menu and the time of service. A banquet often uses a preset menu. The particular menu determines how the table will be set.

An à la carte (ah lah KART) table setting is placed on the table in advance. The appropriate flatware is brought to the table, using a serviette, after customers place their orders.

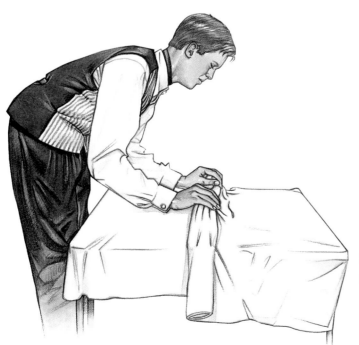

Fig. 4-14. When properly changing a tablecloth, you should never expose the surface of the table.

CENTERPIECES

Centerpieces are decorative objects placed on tables to add beauty and interest. Place centerpieces on the table so they do not get in the way of the customer's view. Properly maintaining centerpieces and keeping them clean will ensure customer safety. There are four types of centerpieces.

■ **Lighting centerpieces.** Lighting provides the most common centerpieces used in the industry. Generally, lighting centerpieces are used during the evening hours to create a soothing environment. Lights may range from a simple votive candleholder to an elaborate **candelabra** (can-duh-LAH-brah), or branched candlestick. Candlesticks and candelabras must be polished. Votive or glass-enclosed candles are used most frequently. Electrical or battery-powered lights may also be used.

■ **Floral centerpieces.** This type of centerpiece can be made from fresh, dried, or artificial flowers, leaves, and branches. Fresh flowers require extra care and are not always available. If they are properly cared for, dried and artificial flowers can be reused for a long period of time.

■ **Edible centerpieces.** Edible (EH-duh-bul) centerpieces are made from items that can be eaten, such as fruit or carved vegetables. Centerpieces can also be sugar-based creations, which showcase the artistic skills of the chef. Handle sugar-based centerpieces carefully, since they are very delicate and will break easily.

■ **Sculpted centerpieces.** Ice, butter, chocolate, and beeswax can all be carved into sculpted centerpieces. Large ice sculptures are often used to adorn buffet tables. Ice sculptures are not practical as regular table centerpieces. Butter, chocolate, or beeswax are better choices for regular tabletops if a sculpture is desired. See Fig. 4-15.

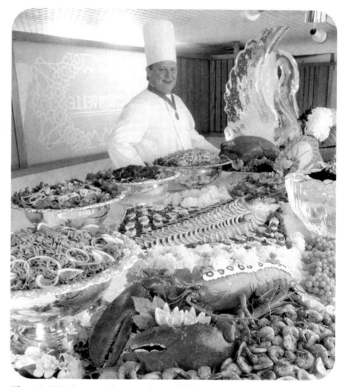

Fig. 4-15. Centerpieces also add beauty and interest to a buffet.

SECTION 4-2 Knowledge Check

1. What are three duties involved in side work?
2. List two guidelines for using or caring for glassware.
3. Name at least three types of centerpieces.

MINI LAB

Practice folding napkins like those shown on page 102. You should be able to make each of these napkin folds easily.

SECTION SUMMARIES

4-1 The five different types of dining environments include: fine-dining restaurants, theme restaurants, casual-dining establishments, quick-service restaurants, and catering services.

4-1 While dining establishments with limited menus include airlines and family-style and quick-service restaurants, more varied menus are offered at buffets and on cruise ships.

4-1 The different types of meal service include: modern American plated, booth, banquette, family style, classical French, Russian, butler, and buffet service.

4-1 A variety of similar service methods are used at the different types of dining establishments, while a few procedures are exclusive to one type of establishment.

4-2 Restock side stations regularly with needed supplies.

4-2 Store glassware upside down in a glass rack or on an air mat. Hold glassware by the base or stem and never use chipped or cracked glassware.

4-2 Handle flatware appropriately at all times in order to keep it clean and prevent soiling the end from which customers eat.

4-2 Cleanliness, uniformity, and customer comfort should always be stressed when preparing table settings.

CHECK YOUR KNOWLEDGE

1. Contrast fine-dining restaurants and casual-dining establishments.

2. Name three types of foodservice operations that provide an inexpensive dining experience.

3. How do people with special dietary needs eat on airlines or cruise ships?

4. Why is modern American plated service considered more efficient than some other types of service?

5. Name five side work tasks.

6. Why do some states prohibit foodservice establishments from using sugar bowls at tables?

7. Why should cracked or chipped glassware and tableware never be used?

8. What do you do to prepare a table between customers?

CRITICAL-THINKING ACTIVITIES

1. How might the tableware, glassware, and flatware used in a fine-dining restaurant differ from those used in a quick-service restaurant? Why?

2. Why is side work an important part of providing good customer service?

WORKPLACE KNOW-HOW

Decision making. One of your friends is starting a family-style restaurant that will use modern American plated service. He is debating what type of table covering to use—linen tablecloths, place mats, paper tablecloths, vinyl tablecloths, or glass tabletops. Which would you advise, and why?

LAB-BASED ACTIVITY: Planning a New Restaurant

STEP ① Working in teams, plan a new restaurant for your area.

STEP ② To begin, think of all the restaurants already in your area. Try to find a location that isn't already flooded with the same type of establishments.

STEP ③ Use the chart below to help you decide on the type of restaurant and meal service for your plan.

STEP ④ While considering the market, research the following situations that could make or break even the best of ideas:

- What is the general income level of the people in the area? If you live in an area where most people work in factory jobs, then a fine-dining restaurant may not prosper.
- Does your restaurant need to be accessible by car, by bus, or by foot? Do you need to consider parking for your customers? Is there a parking garage or parking lot close by?
- What kind of area will your restaurant be in—suburb, city, small town, tourist center, or another type of location?

STEP ⑤ After selecting the type of operation and meal service for your restaurant, answer the following questions about your restaurant:

- What will be the per-person price range of your menu?
- Why did you choose this price range?
- What sort of environment will you create in your restaurant? If you chose to start a catering business, environments are usually determined by the occasion—but be prepared to fit in with a variety of needs.
- Why do you think this choice will work well with the type of restaurant and service style that you have chosen?
- Will you have centerpieces? If so, which type?

STEP ⑥ Create a poster showing the location, type, and meal service of your restaurant.

STEP ⑦ Share your team's plans for a new restaurant with the class. When listening to other teams describe their restaurant, think about why their plan sounds like it could succeed.

Basic Restaurant Planning Decisions

Type of Restaurant
- Theme
- Family Style
- Lunch Counter
- Coffee Shop
- Grill
- Bistro
- Quick-Service
- Fine-Dining

Type of Meal Service
- Modern American Plated
- Booth
- Banquette
- Family Style
- Classical French
- Russian
- Butler
- Buffet

Management & Supervision

People in foodservice management and supervision have a strong background in business math, accounting, and food safety, as well as accurate record-keeping skills and basic computer skills. Their ability to organize and communicate effectively with diverse groups of people ensures a smooth and consistent operation. In some settings, several languages may be spoken in one foodservice operation. Being multilingual is an asset for managers and supervisors.

Along with staff training and managing budgets, foodservice managers and supervisors are also responsible for maintaining a safe and sanitary work environment.

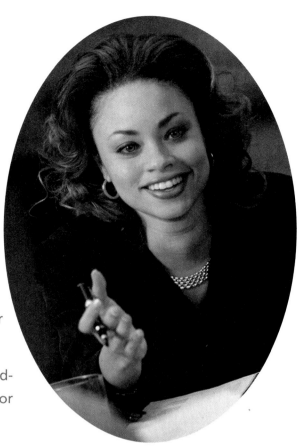

Food and beverage managers are responsible for a foodservice operation's entire food and beverage department. They coordinate the daily operation of all kitchen services, and are also responsible for tracking costs, profits, and losses.

Assistant managers oversee the dining room or the kitchen staff under the guidance of the manager.

Dining room managers are responsible for supervising and scheduling staff, as well as managing the dining room during meal service. Dining room managers must be outgoing and customer focused. A dining room manager may sometimes be called a mâitre d´ (may-truh-DEE).

Executive chefs have many years of experience. They are responsible for menu development, food orders, and supervising the cooking staff.

Production managers are responsible for supervising the kitchen staff and all food preparation. Knowledge of cost control and quality food preparation is essential.

Purchasing agents are in charge of buying all the food and equipment necessary for food production. Effective communication and negotiation skills are important.

Storeroom supervisors are responsible for receiving, issuing, and properly storing all food products. Attention to detail and accurate record-keeping skills help them maintain inventory control.

Working in the Real World...

CAREER RESEARCH ACTIVITY

1. Select one of the careers on page 110. Use print and Internet resources to research all aspects of this career, including education, training, skills, salary range, and working conditions. Summarize your findings in a written report.

2. Interview two people in foodservice management or supervisory positions. Ask them to describe their career pathways. Share your findings in an oral presentation.

FOOD & BEVERAGE MANAGER

My name is Herman Schumacher. I am a food and beverage manager with Wyndam Hotels™. After high school graduation in my home country of the Netherlands, I worked in many restaurants trying to gain as much knowledge and experience as I could. Like other food and beverage managers, I also started in the business by attending culinary school.

After completing culinary school, I went to work on a cruise ship to see the world and hone my culinary skills. Working aboard ship taught me speed and dexterity with my cooking. However, to achieve a successful career, I needed to return to school and earn another degree. I chose Johnson & Wales University, where I received a degree in Hospitality Management.

I believe that a successful chef is one who constantly approaches each day as an opportunity to learn and improve his or her skills. Each job experience builds on the next, which prepares you for your long-term goals. I feel that the sum total of my life experiences has prepared me for my future success. My goal is to become the general manager of a hotel.

For young culinarians starting in the foodservice industry, my advice would be to focus on the fundamentals. Communication and strong interpersonal skills are valuable assets in becoming a food and beverage manager.

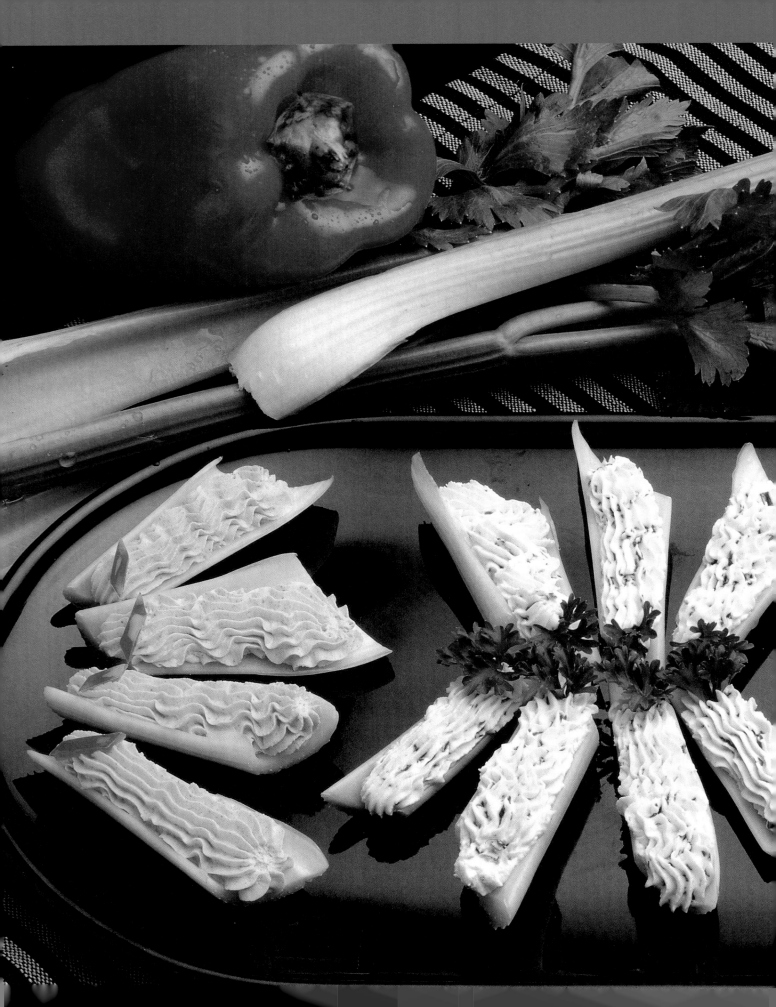

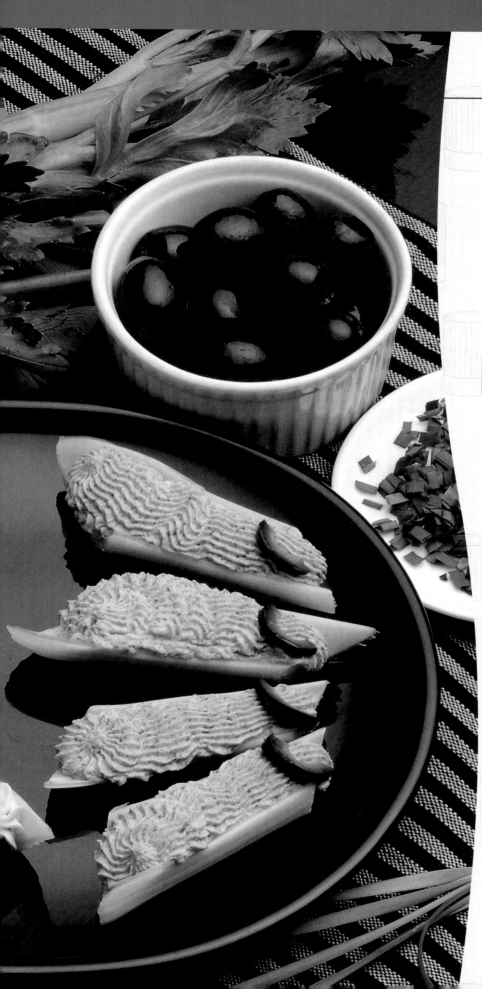

UNIT 2

Quality Foodservice Practices

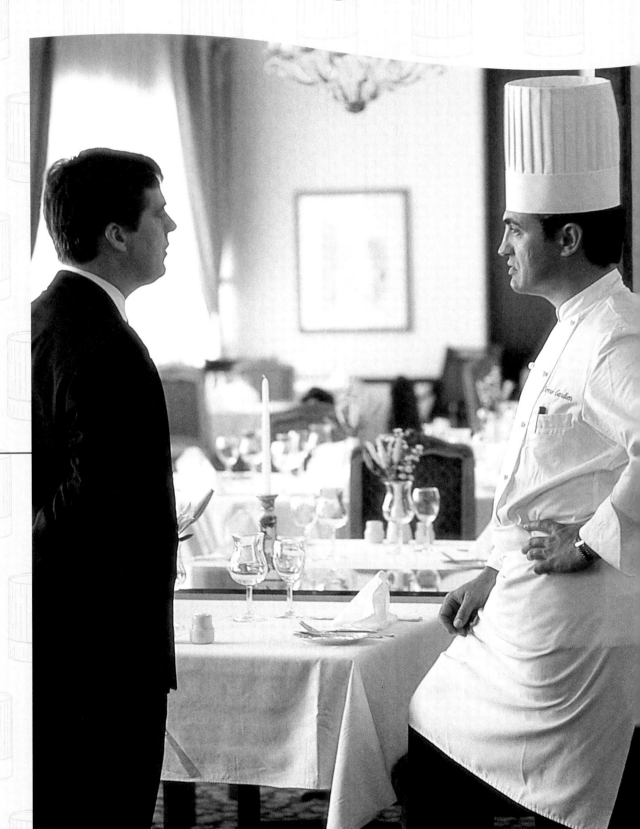

Foodservice Management

Management Basics

OBJECTIVES

After reading this section, you will be able to:

- List the qualities of an effective manager.

- Describe how to manage time and human resources within a foodservice operation.

- Describe how management is structured in a foodservice organization.

- Explain the foodservice manager's role in implementing cost control techniques.

KEY TERMS

- overstaffing
- human resources
- direct labor
- indirect labor
- profit and loss statement
- forecast
- break even

MANAGING a foodservice operation has never been more challenging than it is today. The success of a foodservice operation often depends on the manager's ability to do his or her job well. Good managers are sensitive to business and facility needs as well as the needs of their staff. To be an effective manager, you must understand how a business operates and how to lead people. If you are in your first foodservice job, being a manager may seem a long way off. However, closely observing how managers operate and learning their responsibilities will help you be a better employee.

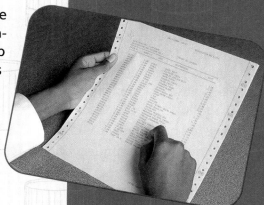

✖ EFFECTIVE MANAGEMENT

You may want to be a foodservice manager someday. If so, you'll need to know how to manage people and facilities. You'll also need to advertise and market your foodservice operation to the public. Maybe you have an idea for a restaurant and want to start a new business. To accomplish any of these goals, you'll need to become an effective manager. Effective managers are skilled in communication, time management, resource management, and leadership.

Communication

Managers need to encourage good on-the-job communication, whether it is communicating with customers or with other staff members. No matter where communication lapses occur, poor communication can severely affect a foodservice operation's success. Good managers also follow an "open-door policy," meaning that they always make time for employees to talk about ideas and problems. See Fig. 5-1.

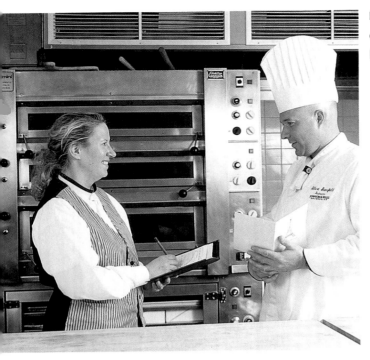

Fig. 5-1. Open and clear communication between employees is essential to the success of a foodservice business.

many people are scheduled, employees will be bored. **Overstaffing**, or scheduling too many people to work on a given shift, can quickly result in lost money.

Effective time management also involves looking for ways employees can save time. In other words, good managers determine how time is wasted and how work can be done more efficiently. Managers who look for ways to improve time management often cause changes that make a business more profitable. These changes include:

- Changes in the way a task is done.
- Reorganizing storage space. See Fig. 5-2.
- Changing staff or schedules.
- Adding employee training.

Foodservice operations often establish their own guidelines for dealing with customer complaints. Many policies require the manager to handle customer complaints. Good interpersonal skills are very important in these situations. Keep the following guidelines in mind:

- Listen attentively to the customer's concerns.
- Show that you understand the customer's frustrations.
- Address the customer's concern as quickly as possible and offer compensation if necessary. For example, you might not charge a customer for an unsatisfactory meal.
- Reassure the customer that the problem will not happen again.
- Determine the cause of the problem and the steps that need to be taken to prevent it from happening again.

Time Management

Managers must be skilled in how to balance time schedules so that each shift is covered by an adequate number of staff. For example, enough people need to be working to keep the business running smoothly and efficiently. However, if too

Fig. 5-2. Reorganizing storage space to be more effective saves time for everyone who uses the supplies.

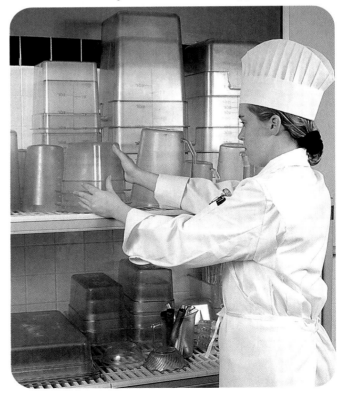

Resource Management

The success of a foodservice operation always depends on how its resources are managed. Hiring the right people for the job is challenging and important. Managing staff, or **human resources**, involves knowing the strengths and weaknesses of each employee.

In addition to managing human resources, a good foodservice manager also manages the facility. This means making sure the facility is safe, clean, and properly equipped.

Leadership

One of the most important qualities of a successful manager or supervisor is leadership style. Successful managers must be able to lead people. Their staff must look to them for guidance and answers. The staff should also feel confident that their manager's decisions are best for the business, its employees, and its customers. The best managers are those who make employees feel that they are part of a team. The best foodservice managers coach, delegate, direct, and support their staff. When employees feel that they have a stake in the success of a foodservice operation, everyone wins—including the customer. See Fig. 5-3.

Some managers use an *autocratic leadership* style. Everything moves from the top down. Other managers are *democratic leaders*. They involve everyone in the decision-making process.

Many foodservice employers prefer to hire managers who hold the Foodservice Management Professional (FMP) credential. Managers who hold this National Restaurant Association credential stand out. They have achieved a certain level of professionalism, knowledge, experience, and leadership. To obtain the FMP credential, candidates have to meet the following requirements:

• Three years of supervisory experience in a restaurant or foodservice operation. Only two years of supervisory experience are required if a candidate has an associate, or higher, degree in business or hospitality.

• Candidates must receive food protection manager certification within five years of applying for the FMP credential.

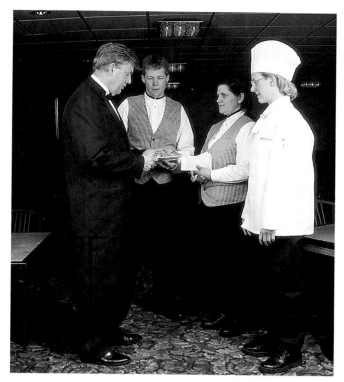

Fig. 5-3. Being part of a team helps employees feel that they have a stake in the success of the foodservice operation.

✕ MANAGEMENT STRUCTURES

Each foodservice facility has its own organizational structure. Some smaller operations may have an owner who also acts as the restaurant manager and supervisor. In most foodservice operations, there are several managers who are responsible for people and other resources. In larger operations, there may be many "layers" of organization. Several managers or supervisors may oversee different segments of food production and service.

■ **Employees.** These people work in positions such as cook, server, and cleaning staff. Employees make up the largest group of people in a foodservice organizational structure.

■ **First-line managers.** Sometimes called "supervisors," first-line managers are directly responsible for the day-to-day supervision of employees. Some facilities might have different first-line managers who oversee food production, service, and cleaning.

- **Middle managers.** These managers usually direct the activities of the first-line managers rather than the employees. They coordinate activities and make sure policies are followed. These managers help facilitate communication between first-line and top managers.

- **Top managers.** The top managers, or administrators, control the organization. Top managers establish policies and procedures for the organization, and make the major decisions about sales, personnel matters, and finance.

⊠ MAINTAINING PROFITABILITY

If a commercial foodservice operation doesn't make money, it won't survive. Maintaining profitability is not just a concern for managers. The actions of every foodservice employee affect an operation's profitability. For example, if a busser is careless in clearing a table and breaks dishes, he or she has caused the operation to lose money. In contrast, if a chef is so skilled that customers return just to sample more of his or her creations, then that chef has helped the operation make money.

Managing time as profitably and efficiently as possible is essential to success. Here are some guidelines managers use to manage time:

- Prepare daily and weekly plans. What needs to be accomplished that day or that week? Make lists and mark off tasks as they are accomplished.
- Delegate responsibility. Let employees have the opportunity to prove themselves as good workers.
- Limit meetings. Invite only the employees that need to be involved in a meeting. Keep meetings to a specific time limit.
- Take time to plan for emergencies. Prepare a plan of action for concerns such as employee illness and overdue food deliveries.

Effective Record-Keeping Systems

In a growing number of facilities, records are kept on a computerized point-of-sales system. These systems track every menu item ordered, so managers can see what foods are most and least popular. See Fig. 5-4.

Specialized computer software can also help managers track the following information:

- Expenses, profits, marketing, and advertising expenses.
- Purchases, price lists, and inventory expenses.
- Reservations.
- Recipes and expenses involved in recipe development.
- Work schedules and employee hours and wages.

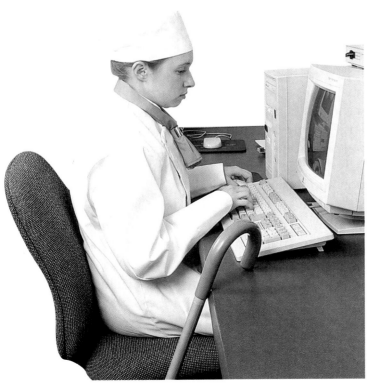

Fig. 5-4. Many foodservice operations track their records with computer software.

Food, Beverage & Labor Costs

Computerized systems also allow managers to analyze the three elements that make up most of an operation's cost: food, beverages, and labor. A facility's food cost percentage is the ratio of the cost of food served to the sales of food served. For example, the cost of food served during the month of June was $14,800. The income received from sales of food in June was $37,000. To find the food cost percentage, divide the food cost by the food sales cost.

$$\begin{array}{r} .40 \\ \$37,000\,\overline{)\$14,800.00} \\ \underline{14,800.0} \\ 0 \end{array}$$

.40 = 40% (food cost percentage)

A 40% food cost percentage means that for every dollar received in sales, 40 cents were spent toward payment for the food.

An operation's third major cost is labor. This involves the direct and indirect labor costs of running a facility. Wages paid to employees are **direct labor**. An operation's costs for employee health insurance, taxes, and vacations are considered **indirect labor**. The more food processing done in-house, the higher the direct labor costs.

The amount of money going "out" (expenses) cannot exceed the amount of money coming "in" (income). Income generally includes food and beverage sales. Expenses include:

• Food costs.
• Beverage costs.
• Nonedible supplies, such as paper napkins.
• Rent and insurance.
• Employee salaries and wages.
• Benefits.
• Marketing and advertising.
• Operating expenses, such as uniforms.
• Utility costs, such as water, gas, electricity, and waste removal.

Profit & Loss Statements

As a manager, you'll want to know where the money is going and how much profit is being made. A **profit and loss statement**, sometimes called an income statement, shows exactly how money flows in a business. Statements such as these usually cover a limited time span, such as a one-month period. For that period, the statement lists all the expenses incurred and shows a total of those expenses. The profit and loss statement also lists the income for that time period and a total income. To find the total income after expenses, or the facility's profit during a particular month, you would subtract the total expenses from the total income.

Managers are often asked to "look into the future" and **forecast**, or anticipate what things will cost, how much money will be needed, what staffing needs there will be, and what profits will be expected. When projected cost equals projected income, an operation is said to **break even**. If your facility is in business to make money, you'll need to do better than break even to stay in business. You'll need to make a profit.

Purchasing Procedures

Making wise purchasing decisions is an important first step toward making a business profitable. Purchasing more food than the restaurant uses produces waste. Not purchasing enough food will result in the restaurant running out of items. Both scenarios quickly lead to lost profits. Good managers will always ask questions when making purchasing decisions. Knowing the answers to the following questions will lessen the chances that money and food will be wasted:

• How much food do we need to prepare the items on our menu?
• How long will the food products last?
• How much food do we already have in stock?
• How far ahead of time does the food need to be ordered so that it will be on-hand?

KEY Math SKILLS

PROFIT AND LOSS

Businesses use profit and loss statements to analyze how well or how poorly they are doing. By using both the percentage analysis method and comparing dollar figures, a manager can more effectively compare the income patterns of the business.

For instance, in March a coffee shop had a total income of $36,000 and expenses of $30,000. In April, the same coffee shop had a total income of $44,800 and expenses of $38,600. When you calculate the net profit for each month, it appears that both months were equally profitable.

Total Income − Total Expenses = Net Profit

March: $36,000
       − $30,000
        $6,000

April: $44,800
       − $38,600
        $6,200

However, when you compare the net profit percent to the total income for both months, you will see that the coffee shop actually operated more efficiently in the month of March. Use the following formula for the percentage analysis method:

$$\frac{\text{Net Profit}}{\text{Total Income}} \times 100 = \text{Percentage Analysis}$$

March: $\frac{\$6,000}{\$36,000} \times 100 = 16.7\%$

April: $\frac{\$6,200}{\$44,800} \times 100 = 13.8\%$

Although both months showed the same profit in dollars, April clearly has a reduced net profit percent. In the month of March, for every dollar earned, 16.7¢ went to net profit. In the month of April, for every dollar earned, only 13.8¢ went to net profit. This difference in net profit percent is a signal to the manager to investigate what happened to cause this difference. Perhaps there was more employee waste, or there was a rise in the cost of food.

TRY IT!

In May, the manager of a chain restaurant recorded an income of $25,000 with expenses of $21,000. In June, the same restaurant made $30,000 and had expenses of $27,000. Use the percentage analysis method to calculate which month had the highest percent of net profit to total income.

Inspecting Food

When food is received, it must be inspected closely to make sure that:

- The product's quality matches the specification, or description, for the product.
- The product is what was ordered, in the correct quantity. Check the amount received against the purchase order and invoice.
- The product's unit size is what was ordered.
- The product price on the invoice matches the product price on the purchase order.
- The product was not damaged during shipment.
- The product was shipped under the proper conditions. For example, check frozen food items for evidence of thawing.
- The product shows no sign of insect or pest damage. See Fig. 5-5.

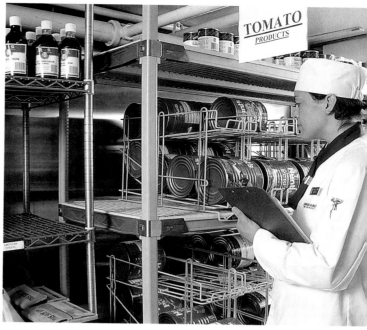

Fig. 5-6. An important step in inventory is tracking product use.

Fig. 5-5. Food must be closely inspected upon delivery.

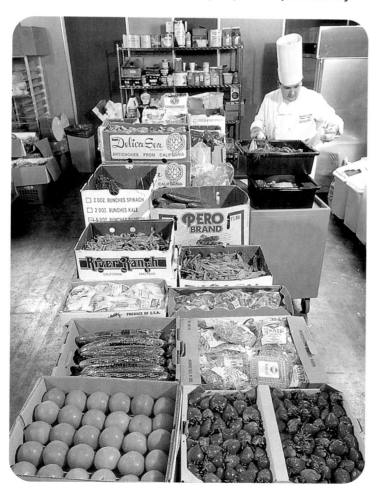

Inventory Control

Following standard inventory procedures will help ensure that food is stored correctly and that you will never run out of important items. Food that is ordered but has not yet arrived at the facility is not considered part of the inventory.

Food and supplies are usually purchased in large quantities, which can bring down the per-item cost. For example, if a manager bought a dozen eggs, it might cost $1.00. However, buying 30 dozen, or a case of, eggs might bring down the cost per dozen to 67 cents.

Most facilities have established an inventory tracking system to keep track of how much of a product is in inventory. It's important that managers make sure their employees know how to use these procedures effectively. See Fig. 5-6.

Properly storing food and supplies helps maintain an adequate inventory. For example, food products should be labeled with the date of storage. In addition to food products, facilities must track the use of nonedible supplies, such as cleaning products. These should be kept in their assigned storage area away from food.

Portion Control

If two customers order the same menu item, such as a slice of pie, they expect both slices to be approximately the same size. To control costs and keep customers happy, foodservice operations should follow strict portion control guidelines. See Fig. 5-7. Recipes specify how many servings or portions will be created from each batch. By following portion control guidelines:

- No one has to guess about serving sizes.
- The right amount of each menu item will be prepared.
- Food waste is minimized and cost is kept in line.
- Customers will be satisfied.

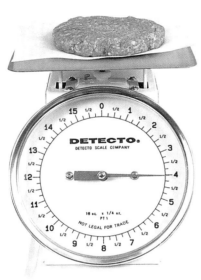

Fig. 5-7. Portion control techniques minimize waste by standardizing food item quantities.

Waste Control

Here are several techniques managers and employees can use to minimize waste:

- Follow strict inventory procedures to identify product needs.
- Follow good purchasing procedures and order only what's needed.
- Minimize waste during production.
- Train employees on proper food preparation methods.
- Train employees in the proper use of nonedible supplies.

COMPLYING WITH LAWS

Foodservice managers need to adhere to many laws and regulations. Chapter 6 covers these items in detail. Rules apply to different areas of the operation, from hiring and firing, to the safety of the food that is served to customers. It is the manager's responsibility to know and follow rules and regulations and to make sure that employees understand and follow them as well.

Public policy also affects the food production and service industry. These policies are usually posted and relate to: no smoking, wearing shoes and shirts, and the ability to refuse service.

SECTION 5-1

Knowledge Check

1. Contrast the leadership styles used by foodservice managers and supervisors.
2. What are the four levels in a foodservice organizational structure?
3. Name two advantages of following portion control guidelines.

MINI LAB

After finishing his meal, a customer complains that the food was unsatisfactory. Describe two possible ways that you could deal with this customer. Identify the advantages and disadvantages of each possible solution.

Managing People

KEY TERMS

* orientation

* positive reinforcement

* mentors

OBJECTIVES

After reading this section, you will be able to:

* Summarize the importance of decision making and problem solving as management skills.

* Explain the process of employee selection and evaluation.

* Describe effective training techniques and mentoring programs.

* Explain the duties involved in employee supervision.

I T can be exciting to be in charge, but a management position also means a lot of responsibility. People who oversee employees are usually called managers or supervisors. Managers make sure that all employees are properly trained and that they complete tasks efficiently. To do this, managers must be good problem-solvers and decision-makers. Managers are often promoted to their positions after working in lower level positions. Most companies recognize outstanding work and promote those who have experience in the jobs they will be supervising. Managers interview and hire new employees and evaluate their work performance.

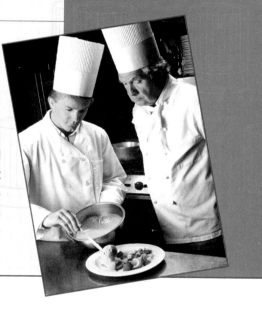

✖ THE MANAGER'S ROLE

Successful managers are respected by the employees they supervise. They encourage and train employees in how to get a job done, to work as a team, and to meet challenges with a positive attitude. In addition, managers must master two important skills: problem solving and decision making. Employees can begin learning these skills by observing how their supervisors manage difficult situations and negotiate resolutions.

■ **Problem solving.** One of the most important responsibilities of every manager is to solve problems. A problem-solver can spot problems and take swift action to resolve them. Unfortunately, businesses often have scheduling conflicts, delayed orders, and equipment breakdowns. Managers who are the best problem-solvers understand their business from top to bottom. See Fig. 5-8.

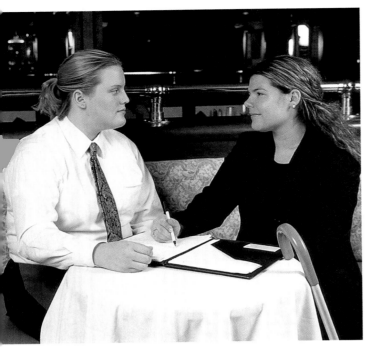

Fig. 5-8. Good managers spot problems in the workplace and then act swiftly to solve them.

■ **Decision making.** Managers must make good decisions about how the business will operate. They weigh the possible outcomes of a decision before making it. Foodservice managers must make frequent decisions about:

• Staffing.
• Purchasing.
• Menus.
• Pricing.
• Production and sales goals.
• Customer complaints.
• Rules and standards.
• Facility safety and appearance.

✖ SELECTING EMPLOYEES

What should managers look for when they interview prospective employees? All the qualities an interviewer looks for are not obvious. Most managers look for qualities such as honesty and the ability to work well with others. They also look for an employee whose past education and work experience best fits the job description.

Job Descriptions

Each job has its own unique set of duties and responsibilities. These duties are listed in the job description. Many job descriptions also list the skills and tasks involved in a particular position.

A job description has several different uses. First, it can be shared with prospective employees during an interview. By using the job description, the manager can explain what the job will entail. In addition, job descriptions can be used to evaluate job performance. Employees who don't meet a job description requirement may need more training to improve their skills.

Job Applications

Choosing the right employee for the job can be difficult. The first step a manager takes is to review job applications to make sure they are neat and completely filled out. See Fig. 5-9. The following items signal a warning to managers reviewing job applications:

• Reasons for leaving a job, such as "problems with coworkers," may indicate poor interpersonal skills.
• Reasons for time spent between jobs may indicate serious conflicts with a former employer. On the other hand, the person may have taken time off to have children or to go to college.

Interviewing Skills

The next and perhaps most important step in the hiring process is the interview. During an interview, the manager looks for a person who is:

• Clean and well groomed.
• A good communicator.
• Self-confident.
• A team player.
• Honest.
• Organized.
• Willing to learn new things.

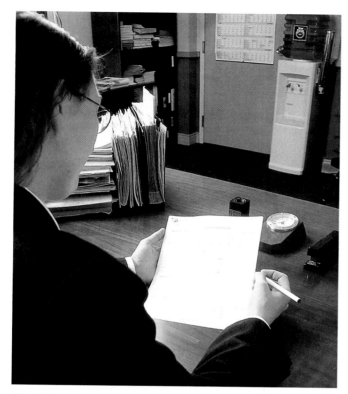

Fig. 5-9. Reviewing job applications is the first step in hiring an employee. **What should a manager look for when reviewing applications?**

Effective managers ask interview questions that require more than a one- or two-word answer. For example, instead of asking, "When did you leave your last job?" they will ask, "Why did you leave your last job?" They also listen carefully to a person's answers and note his or her body language. Thus, it is important to be positive and answer questions thoroughly and clearly.

During an interview, the manager needs to get an idea of whether or not the potential employee is right for the job. The best way to do this is to ask questions that often reveal a person's work ethic and attitude.

• What were the customers like in the last place you worked?
• If you could have changed anything about your last job, what would it have been?
• Describe a difficult challenge you had on the job and how you overcame it.
• Why should we hire you?

✖ TRAINING EMPLOYEES

Employees may show up the first day on the job eager and ready to work. However, most new employees need to be trained to do their jobs. Managers are usually responsible for training new employees. **Orientation** is the process of making a new employee familiar with a foodservice organization, its policies and procedures, and specific job duties. The orientation period can last several hours to several weeks, depending on the position. See Fig. 5-10.

Positive Reinforcement

People learn better when they believe they are capable of doing a job correctly. People also act in ways that they feel will be rewarded. Because of this, it's important for managers to build an employee's confidence during training. Managers use a technique called **positive reinforcement**, or praising an employee when a job or task is done correctly.

Fig. 5-10. During orientation, the manager may take the new employee on a tour of the facility.

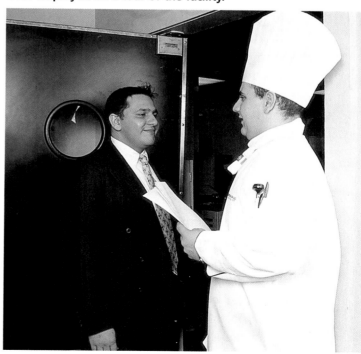

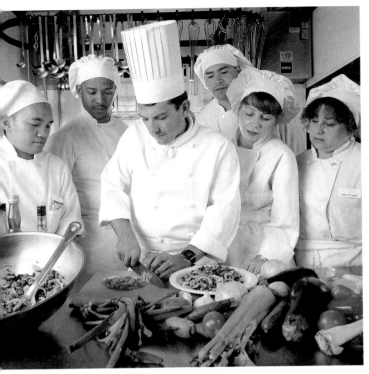

Fig. 5-11. Mentors introduce new employees to the procedures they will follow and the equipment they will use on the job.

Mentorship

When a new employee is hired at a foodservice establishment, the manager may assign him or her to work with another employee. **Mentors** are employees who have a solid understanding of their jobs. Employees can ask their mentors questions and receive immediate feedback.

Mentoring is an excellent way to bring new employees up to speed on the procedures of a foodservice facility. It's also a quick way to train existing employees who have changed jobs or been given new responsibilities. See Fig. 5-11.

⊠ SUPERVISING EMPLOYEES

Managers need to make sure employees understand and follow policies. These policies relate to standards of conduct, customer relations, drugs and alcohol, and work schedules.

■ **Standards of conduct.** Most employees want to do a good job. Having established standards of conduct can help guide employees in a variety of situations. Each foodservice operation usually has its own standards of conduct. They may include information such as:

- The customer is always right. Never argue with a customer. Assume that you made the error and continue offering service with a smile.
- Suggest alternatives. If a customer is dissatisfied with a food item, suggest an alternative menu choice.
- Avoid public arguments. Never argue with other employees in front of customers.
- Help out without being asked. If your workload is slow and a coworker is extremely busy, offer to help if you have been trained in that task.
- Take appropriate breaks. Never take a break during peak hours without permission.

■ **Customer relations.** Returning customers keep foodservice operations in business. An unsatisfied customer may tell friends about the experience. Good customer service keeps customers coming back.

■ **Drugs and alcohol.** There are strict rules that prohibit drug and alcohol use. The manager is responsible for ensuring a safe facility for employees and customers. An employee who arrives at work under the influence of drugs or alcohol could lose his or her job.

■ **Work schedules.** Most foodservice operations have established policies regarding schedules and work assignments. The manager must juggle each employee's availability with the master work schedule. See Fig. 5-12.

Managers consider several things when determining the work schedule:

- Managers must figure out how many employees will be needed to prepare, serve, and bus each menu item. Managers rely on their past experience to tell them how many employees will be needed.
- Managers must consider who is available to work at different times.
- Managers should have a balance of new and experienced workers on each shift.

Fig. 5-12.
Tuesday's Production Schedule

LUNCH 11:30 A.M.–1:00 P.M.			
Employee	**Item/Activity**	**Portions**	**Station**
LH and FZ	Country Fried Steak with Gravy	25	Fry Station
TG	New Potatoes	25	Hot Station
CS	Green Beans	25	Hot Station
AP	Cloverleaf Rolls	50	Bake Station
JH	Strawberry Shortcake	25	Bake Station
CI and LM	Mixed Greens with Ranch Dressing	25	Garde Manger Station
PS and CF	Coffee & Iced Tea	50	Beverage Station & Servers
BW and RN	Kitchen Clean-up		Dishwashing Station
MD	Floater		As Needed

Fig. 5-12. Developing an employee work schedule is an important part of a manager's job. What are some factors managers should consider when scheduling employees? For example, in what ways can managers help employees in managing multiple family, community, and wage-earner roles?

✖ EVALUATING EMPLOYEES

Foodservice employees are evaluated on their work performance. Typically, the manager conducts the performance evaluation, and focuses on how well the employee is performing assigned tasks, overall work attendance and attitude, and teamwork skills.

During the evaluation, the manager identifies the employee's strengths and weaknesses, and provides an opportunity for the employee to ask questions. The results of the performance appraisal are often used to determine promotions and raises.

SECTION 5-2 Knowledge Check

1. Why is problem solving a valuable skill for managers to have?
2. What are two warning signs a manager should look for on job applications?
3. Name two advantages of mentorship.

MINI LAB

Imagine that you're interviewing potential employees for these positions: server, cashier, busser, and host. Choose a position and make a list of 5–10 questions that you would ask in the interview. Exchange lists and discuss the questions.

Managing Facilities

OBJECTIVES

After reading this section, you will be able to:

- Describe how workplace design impacts employee performance and the success of a foodservice operation.
- Identify management's responsibility for implementing loss prevention factors.
- Explain the importance of effective equipment handling, maintenance, and repair.

Y O U might be surprised at the amount of work that goes into managing a foodservice facility. The design of a facility can affect how productive and successful it is. Equally important is how a facility and its contents are maintained. A dirty or neglected operation will drive off customers. Learning about the factors that can prevent a foodservice facility from losing money will help you manage and maintain any type of foodservice operation.

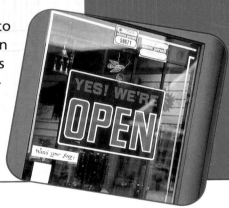

✖ FACILITIES DESIGN

The design of a foodservice operation is important to customers. As a foodservice employee, you will also be affected by the design of the workplace—the space in which you will perform your job. A foodservice operation must be designed so that employees can complete tasks efficiently and customers can enjoy their dining experience.

■ **Balance.** Dividing space to meet customer and preparation staff needs is called **balance**. For example, suppose a manager squeezes the maximum number of customers into the dining area as allowed by law. The remaining space is where the kitchen is built. While more customers can dine at

the facility, the kitchen may not be able to handle large numbers of orders efficiently. This demonstrates the need to balance space allotments between the dining room and kitchen area.

■ **Menu.** One of the most important factors in foodservice facility design is the menu. The equipment, storage space, and work surfaces needed to make the menu items all affect facility design.

■ **Turnover rate.** Another factor in facility design is the desired **turnover rate**, or the average number of times a seat will be occupied during a given block of time. For example, if customers stay an average of 20 minutes for breakfast, the potential turnover rate is 2½ times per hour. A facility's design can help achieve a certain turnover rate. If a high turnover rate is desired, for example, the tables can be placed closer together and more staff can be hired to provide quick and efficient service.

■ **Traffic paths.** The movements of people and materials within the foodservice operation follow certain traffic paths. Managers must determine the easiest way to allow movement along traffic paths, while keeping the space they require to a minimum. For example, if carts or containers will be pushed or carried down a traffic path, the path must be wide enough for the cart to pass behind someone working in that area.

■ **Bypassing.** Facilities should be designed so that work stations are laid out in a logical sequence. This keeps bypassing to a minimum. **Bypassing** happens when people or materials must walk or be moved past unrelated stations during the food-service process. For example, after vegetables have been cleaned and cut for grilling, they must be passed from the pantry station to the grill station. If the baking station is in between the two areas, this unneeded motion interrupts the smooth and efficient flow of business.

■ **Production space.** The total amount of production space to allow for a foodservice operation depends upon the type and size of the facility. Managers must divide this space by all of the work areas, such as storage, food preparation, and dishwashing as shown in Fig. 5-13.

Layout of Work Areas

When laying out work areas, managers will try to keep the movement of people and goods to a minimum. The first step of layout is to arrange the individual pieces of equipment into a work area. Secondly, the work area must be fitted into the entire facility. An effective work area layout will:

• Allow for easy maintenance and inventory access.
• Provide a safe and productive environment for employees.
• Make the work process flexible.
• Protect equipment from damage.

Fig. 5-13.

WORK AREA	SPACE
Receiving and storage	25%
Food preparation	42%
Dishwashing	8%
Traffic paths	15%
Employee facilities	10%
Total	**100%**

☒ LOSS PREVENTION FACTORS

A foodservice operation must focus on loss prevention factors to stay profitable. Taking steps to ensure that each factor is handled appropriately will save a foodservice operation time and money. Factors to consider include:

• Safety.
• Sanitation.
• Food handling.
• Equipment handling.
• Maintenance and repairs.
• Insurance.

Safety

Having a safe workplace is a must for all food-service facilities. Unfortunately, foodservice employees are particularly at risk for on-the-job injuries. The most common injuries include slips and falls, burns, and cuts. Chapter 7 addresses specific safety issues.

Managers can improve the safety of their facilities by properly training employees. This is especially important when employees first learn about their job duties. This training should be taken seriously. No matter how long you've been an employee, safety precautions must always be followed. See Fig. 5-14 for some of the standards inspectors look for in a facility.

Depending on the size of the operation, a risk management coordinator may be responsible for implementing and overseeing safety procedures. Smaller foodservice operations with smaller budgets often contact insurance companies regarding risk management. Some insurance companies provide free or low-cost advice on keeping employees and customers safe. Organizations such as the American Red Cross and some local fire departments also provide free or inexpensive risk management training programs. For example, all employees should be trained in basic first aid, CPR, and how to extinguish fires.

Sanitation

Foodborne illness is a major health concern. In food service, there are many different kinds of food and many different people handling it. If a facility is not kept clean, the chances of contamination are high. Managers must properly train employees about sanitation practices. In particular, employees must follow strict rules about personal hygiene. Chapters 7 and 8 address sanitation and how it should be applied on the job.

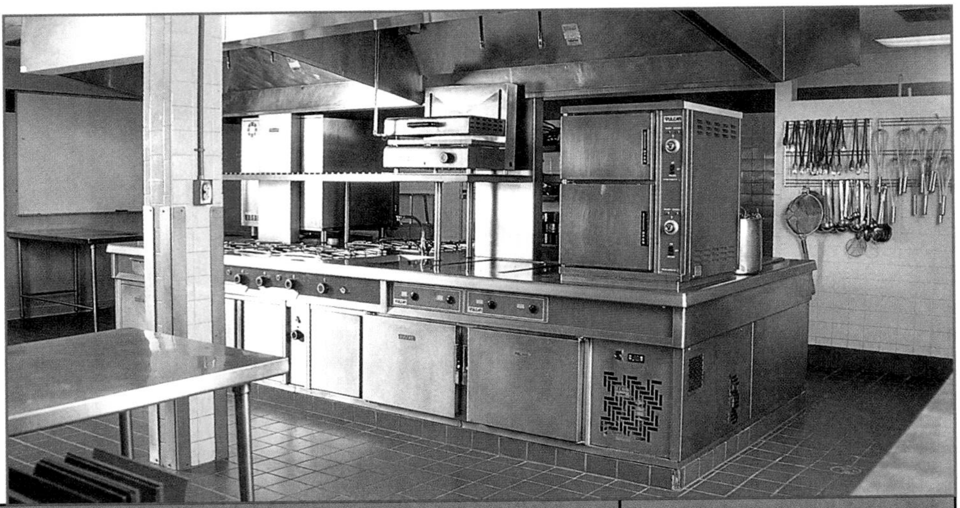

Fig. 5-14.

AREA	✔	SAMPLE INSPECTION POINTS	FREQUENCY
Hot Station	✔	Clean the surfaces of all cooking and baking equipment according to the manufacturer's directions.	• Daily
Work Surfaces	✔	Clean and sanitize all work surfaces.	• Every 4 hours or before use of each raw food or when changing from raw to ready-to-eat food
Ice Machine	✔	Top clean and free of objects; rim of door free of mold; ice scoop available.	• Daily
	✔	Floor is clean under machine; vent hood is clean; side and back wall next to the machine also clean.	• Daily
Dishwashing	✔	Spray hose is leak-free; prevents backflow.	• Daily
	✔	Glass-rack shelf is neat and clean.	• Monthly
	✔	Walls next to the dish machine are clean.	• Monthly
	✔	Dish machine is lime- and crust-free.	• Daily

Food Handling

Federal, state, and local governments regulate the safe handling of food. In addition, many trade associations, such as the National Turkey Federation, publish their own standards and guidelines for safe food handling and storage. Improper food handling can result in contamination. Chapter 8 addresses safe food handling.

Foodservice operations are periodically inspected to make sure they are following government regulations for food handling. Health and safety inspectors will examine such things as:

• The cleanliness of the facility.
• Food preparation processes.
• Food storage areas.
• Worker sanitation practices.

Equipment Handling

Foodservice operations spend thousands of dollars on the equipment needed to prepare and serve food. Incorrectly handling or operating a piece of equipment can damage it.

Managers are responsible for training employees in the correct use of equipment. Mishandling equipment is costly and dangerous. Managers must make sure employees are properly trained to operate each piece of equipment they'll use on the job. Do not hesitate to ask questions if you are unsure of these procedures. See Fig. 5-15.

Maintenance & Repairs

Although employees may carefully follow safety, sanitation, and handling guidelines, equipment must be constantly maintained. This will ensure top operating condition. If equipment needs to be fixed, repairs must be made promptly to keep the foodservice operation running smoothly.

Whether you are using a deep fat fryer or a manual can opener, it is important to follow proper maintenance procedures. Management will usually establish an equipment maintenance and cleaning schedule.

a LINK to the Past

Protecting Workers

Determined to do something about the high number of job-related deaths and injuries to workers in the 1970s, the Occupational Safety and Health Act was signed on December 29, 1970. The Act created the Occupational Safety and Health Administration (OSHA), which formally came into being on April 28, 1971.

Before 1970, no comprehensive programs existed to protect against workplace safety and health hazards. Since it started, OSHA's job has been to protect American workers. OSHA's main goal is to make sure every worker is safe on the job.

Since 1970, OSHA has cut the work-related fatality rate in half and reduced overall injury and illness rates in targeted industries. Foodservice workers are particularly at risk for injuries. Burns, cuts, falls, and back strain are all hazards of the trade. OSHA strives to protect workers by making frequent inspections.

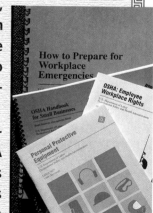

In addition to enforcing safety rules, OSHA tries to prevent accidents by educating employers and employees. Posters and handouts about on-the-job safety are available free of charge. OSHA encourages voluntary safety and health programs in the workplace.

Insurance

Owners of foodservice operations purchase insurance to cover their business operations, facility, employees, and customers. Insurance is costly. It is purchased to cover:

- Fire damage.
- Injury to customers.
- Equipment.
- Employee disability.
- Employee health.
- Loss of life.
- Theft.
- Loss of the business.

✕ FACILITY MAINTENANCE

Many foodservice operations sign contracts with repair companies for their maintenance needs. Under these contracts, repair companies routinely visit the facility and perform routine maintenance. Everything from the roof to floor tiles to doors and windows needs to be kept in good working order. Routine maintenance often prevents large repair bills.

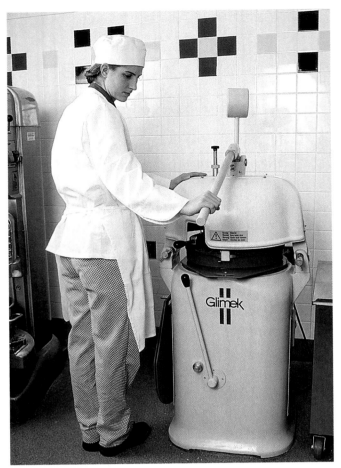

Fig. 5-15. Managers must enforce safety precautions for using equipment to prevent injury. What could happen if an employee incorrectly operates the dough divider in the above photo?

SECTION 5-3 Knowledge Check

1. Name two elements of an effective work area.
2. Why is it important for managers to train employees about sanitation practices?
3. What are two things that can be done to prevent high equipment repair costs for a foodservice facility?

MINI LAB

Imagine that a large piece of foodservice equipment breaks down during the dinner shift. Explain how a manager could keep the business running smoothly while the equipment is being repaired?

Foodservice Marketing

OBJECTIVES

After reading this section, you will be able to:

- Explain the purpose of marketing.

- Analyze location, customer base, competition, and trends to develop a marketing strategy.

- Describe how positioning, atmosphere, and customer needs influence marketing.

- Summarize the elements involved in public relations.

TO survive in today's foodservice industry, a business must do more than provide quality food and service. Competition has made marketing a top priority. Marketing involves planning and researching locations, menus, customers, competitors, and trends. Different marketing strategies help managers maintain their customer base and attract new customers. In successful foodservice operations, the management has spent hours planning and marketing the facility—even before the doors opened to its first customers. This section will tell you how this is done.

☒ TYPES OF BUSINESS OWNERSHIP

When deciding upon the type of operation you would like to have, there are several options for business ownership. These options include independent ownership, chain ownership, and franchise ownership.

■ **Independent ownership.** With independent ownership, the owner is in control of the business operation. The independent owner sets company policies and establishes product prices. The owner makes the profit, but also bears the burden of all the expenses.

■ **Chain ownership.** When a restaurant operation has two or more locations that sell the same products and are operated by the same company, it is known as a **chain**. Unlike independent ownership, chain operations are run by a manager-employee. The manager-employee does not make policy decisions. This individual reports to the person or "parent" company that owns the operation. Chain operations usually have lower expenses due to centralized buying of food and equipment by the parent company.

■ **Franchise ownership.** When a parent company grants an individual the right to sell the company's products, a **franchise** is formed. The franchise is given the trademark and logo of the company along with a complete operational system for dealing with day-to-day business. Many quick-service restaurants are franchise businesses.

A large amount of money is needed to purchase a franchise operation. In addition, the franchise owner generally pays an ongoing fee to the parent company every year for use of the company name, logo, and products. The franchisee gets a well-developed business package and the marketing power of the parent company.

✖ ANALYZING THE MARKETPLACE

The first step in creating a new business is to analyze the marketplace. The **marketplace** includes the physical location, the people, and the atmosphere of a particular geographic area. New business owners must thoroughly research these factors to determine whether a new business will succeed in a certain location. See Fig. 5-16.

For example, suppose that you wanted to open a pastry shop. To analyze the marketplace you would investigate several different areas where you think the shop could be located. When checking these areas, you might ask yourself:

• How busy is this location at mealtimes?
• Is this location convenient and accessible to a large number of people?
• Does this area have a need for this type of foodservice facility? Or is this service already being provided by a nearby operation?
• How much does it cost to rent or purchase space at this location versus other locations?
• Is this area showing signs of growth?
• Does this area draw from a multicultural population?

Fig. 5-16. An important step for new business owners is to investigate the marketplace.

Marketing Strategies

Marketing affects the location of the foodservice operation, what food products are offered, how items are promoted, and who presents the product. The reality is that a large percentage of foodservice operations go out of business within one to five years because many fail to take all of these strategies with serious consideration.

Several basic marketing strategies can be used to provide key information to give an operation the best possible start toward profitability. These strategies include:
• Analyzing the location.
• Analyzing the customer base and the diversity of those customers.
• Analyzing the competition.
• Analyzing trends.

■ **Location.** Suppose you have an idea for a new foodservice facility. The location you choose for your new business is one of the most important decisions you'll make. Whether it is an existing building that you plan to renovate or simply an empty lot, the location should be carefully analyzed before any construction or renovation begins.

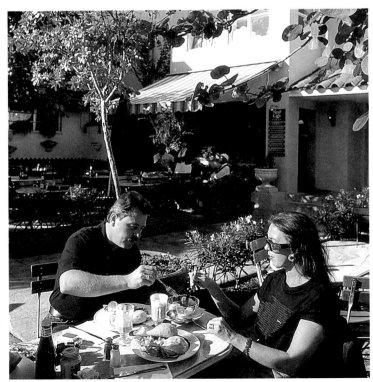

Many businesses fail because they don't consider traffic patterns, such as a new highway or an existing one that has been closed or rerouted. Customers want easy, convenient access to their food choices. If it's difficult to get to a location, chances are customers will find another foodservice facility. Business owners can start by asking questions about the location, such as:

- What physical locations or structures are affordable?
- How much money must be spent on the physical structure? Consider the lot and the building construction or the rental space.
- Should a new structure be built, or should an existing structure be renovated?
- Why did the last owner leave?

■ **Customer Base.** Next, business owners must analyze the clientele, or the people who will be their main customers. This strategy involves examining what type of people you want to attract as customers. Are they, for example, business people, young, health-conscious, ethnic food lovers, or families? Perhaps they are looking for familiar foods and flavors from their cultural heritage. Knowing your customer base is important when presenting and promoting a foodservice operation. See Fig. 5-17.

This information is also important when pricing menu items. For example, if you know your average customer rarely spends more than $10 for a meal, you would price your menu accordingly. Too many menu items over $10 could turn away your customers.

■ **Competition.** It's not enough to find the perfect location and create an attractive, inviting foodservice facility. If there are several other facilities in an area that offer similar foods at similar prices, you may have a hard time winning over new customers.

Business owners are always very conscious of who their competitors are. **Competitors** are businesses that offer similar products or services. When deciding how to market a business and where it will be located, business owners always investigate the competition. Answers should be sought for the following questions:

- Will my business have competition, or is it a one-of-a-kind operation?
- If competition exists, how close is it to my location?
- In what ways will my operation be different and more attractive than what's offered by the competition?

■ **Trends.** Just because a business idea seems perfect now doesn't necessarily mean it will be a great idea next year or ten years from now. Business owners always need to keep the future in mind. For example, you might have a great idea for a hot dog stand. You've investigated a location, and it seems just right. There are lots of potential customers and no current competition. However, did you know that plans were being drawn up for a new baseball field one block away from your chosen location? How will the new ballpark affect your business a year from now?

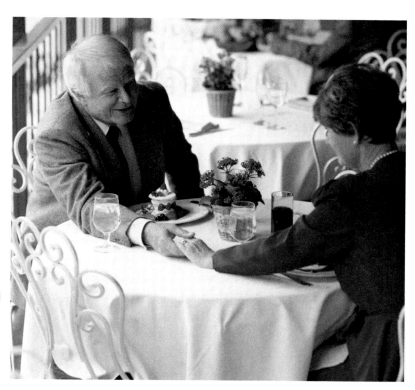

Fig. 5-17. These customers are celebrating a special event. What type of menu items would appeal to them?

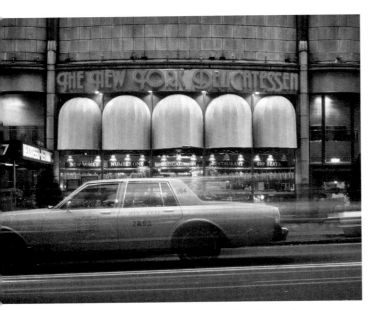

Fig. 5-18. Customers expect to find restaurants near shopping, work, and entertainment areas.

To investigate trends in the marketplace, business owners should ask:

- Is the location in an established area with other thriving businesses? See Fig. 5-18.
- Will customers have easy access to my facility?
- Is there adequate parking?
- Are other businesses nearby that might offer a steady supply of hungry customers?
- What is planned for the future of my chosen location?

✖ POSITIONING

Strong and accurate positioning can attract new customers and keep existing customers coming back again and again. **Positioning** is the way a foodservice operation presents itself to the community. Many foodservice operations develop a position statement that helps guide their decision-making and marketing efforts. This statement explains what the business stands for and its main goals. A brief position statement might read: "The Healthy Alternative Café emphasizes healthful food choices at affordable prices."

Atmosphere

Have you ever noticed how every foodservice facility has its own atmosphere? A facility's **atmosphere** is the "feeling" or "sense" that customers receive from the interior and exterior of the facility. The way a facility is designed, from its carpet and wall coverings to its music and staff uniforms, helps shape its atmosphere. Great care should be taken to create an atmosphere that fits your foodservice operation.

Business owners must thoroughly investigate their customer's needs and wants before establishing "atmosphere." Keep in mind that defining customer needs isn't something that happens only before a business opens its doors. It's an ongoing process. Foodservice operations often use customer comment cards to gather information. This feedback is used to determine whether the business is on track, or if management should alter the food choices, hours, or atmosphere to better meet customer needs. See Fig. 5-19.

Fig. 5-19. Operations that take specific customer needs into account are more likely to be successful. What methods can an operation use to monitor customer needs?

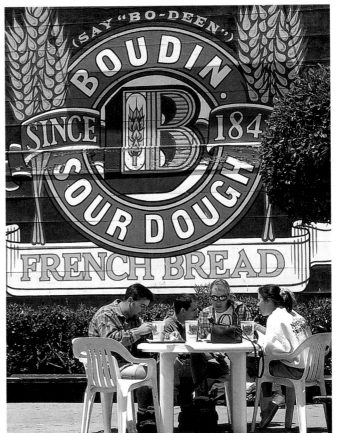

PUBLIC RELATIONS

Having good public relations is critical to the success of a foodservice facility. **Public relations** includes publicity and advertising that a foodservice operation uses to enhance its image. **Publicity** includes the free or low-cost efforts of a facility to improve its image. Keep in mind that publicity can be both negative and positive. Negative publicity, such as news of an outbreak of foodborne illness, may take months or even years to overcome. Positive publicity can include the use of special events and promotions. Charity events, fundraisers, and educational food seminars can produce great customer interest.

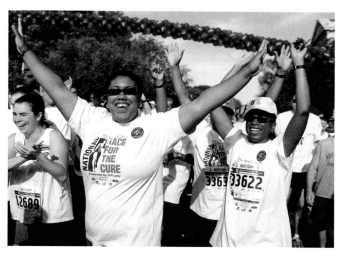

Fig. 5-20. Restaurants get positive publicity by sponsoring charitable events in the community.

Advertising

To become and remain successful in today's marketplace, foodservice facilities must advertise. **Advertising** is a paid form of promotion that persuades and informs the public about what a facility has to offer. Newspapers, television, radio, and the Internet are some of the options facilities can use to advertise.

Businesses can also improve their image and standing in the community by sponsoring events their customers care about. Let's say you work at a pizza parlor. Your managers might improve public relations by donating pizzas to a charity bike-a-thon. Sponsorships and donations like this enhance a business's community standing. See Fig. 5-20.

Direct Marketing

Direct marketing is a form of advertising in which materials, such as letters and advertisements, are mailed directly to customers. Direct marketing over the Internet allows an operation's message to reach its desired audience. However, direct marketing has its disadvantages. People often don't read every piece of mail they receive. It is also expensive to write, design, print, and mail direct marketing materials. To enhance your understanding of direct marketing, try researching technological innovations used in foodservice to market products on the Internet. How do these innovations help to enhance sales and marketing strategies?

SECTION 5-4   Knowledge Check

1. How can a position statement help a foodservice operation?
2. Contrast advertising and publicity.
3. Name one advantage and one disadvantage of direct marketing.

MINI LAB

Briefly analyze the location, customer base, competition, and trends affecting a recognized restaurant in your area. Explain to the class why you think this restaurant will or will not continue to be successful.

SECTION SUMMARIES

5-1 An effective manager is skilled in the areas of communication, time management, resource management, and leadership.

5-1 Managers must be able to balance time and know the strengths and weaknesses of each staff member to effectively manage human resources.

5-1 With the help of effective record-keeping systems, managers can keep an operation's costs under control.

5-2 Problem solving and decision making are two skills that managers must have to keep their operations running smoothly.

5-2 Managers can successfully train employees during orientation by using positive reinforcement and mentoring programs.

5-2 Managers must make sure employees understand all of the operation's policies.

5-3 The design of a facility, such as its traffic paths, turnover rates, and balance, affects the performance of employees.

5-3 To protect the operation and employees, managers consider loss prevention factors.

5-3 Correctly handling, maintaining, and repairing equipment will save a foodservice operation time and money.

5-4 Marketing helps a foodservice operation maintain its current customer base and attract new customers.

5-4 Analyzing the location, customer base, competition, and trends of a business helps direct its marketing efforts.

5-4 Public relations includes the methods through which a foodservice operation enhances its image.

CHECK YOUR KNOWLEDGE

1. What are two guidelines managers can use to handle dissatisfied customers?
2. Why isn't profitability a concern just for managers?
3. What three elements make up most of a foodservice operation's costs?
4. Name one use for a job description.
5. What are three standards of conduct?
6. Name two factors a supervisor might consider when planning a work schedule.
7. How does the menu influence the design of a foodservice operation?
8. List five elements for which a foodservice operation can purchase insurance coverage.
9. Why is it important to analyze the marketplace when creating a new business?

CRITICAL-THINKING ACTIVITIES

1. A quick-service restaurant has just hired a new manager. The employees are part-time college students. What style of leadership would you recommend the manager use? Why?
2. You are a new foodservice employee. Your manager has asked you to analyze your family, community, and wage-earner roles to help him in determining your work schedule. How can this help you balance your life?

WORKPLACE KNOW-HOW

Problem solving. In examining a recent profit and loss statement, a foodservice manager notices that labor costs are higher than usual. What might be the cause of the increase? How might the manager keep labor costs down?

LAB-BASED ACTIVITY: Marketing a Foodservice Operation

STEP 1 Suppose you have an idea for a new restaurant. You've already analyzed the marketplace, location, customer base, competition, and trends. Now you need to develop a marketing plan for your new restaurant.

STEP 2 Develop a position statement for your restaurant.

- Your position statement should explain what your business stands for and its main goals.
- You must also determine how you will set your facility apart from the competition.

STEP 3 Describe the atmosphere of your facility. Think of the design of the interior and exterior.

- What "feel" or "sense" do you want to communicate to customers?
- How can you convey these emotions through the design of the facility?

STEP 4 Describe your customers.

STEP 5 Design an ad for your restaurant. Incorporate the look and feel of the restaurant's atmosphere into the design of the ad.

STEP 6 Share your restaurant ad with the class.

- What do they expect your restaurant to be like based on your ad?
- Are their impressions correct? If not, how could you change your advertisement to convey the correct information?

STEP 7 Develop a customer comment card to place on tables in your restaurant. See the example below as a guide.

- Think about what you want to know about your customers. Write questions that will help you get this information.
- How might customers' answers to these questions affect your restaurant?

STEP 8 Name three other ways you could advertise your restaurant. Consider the cost of each method and what types of customers it might reach.

Sample Customer Comment Card

	Poor			Excellent	
1. How was your overall dining experience?	1	2	3	4	5
2. Was your greeting friendly?	1	2	3	4	5
3. Did your server attend to your needs?	1	2	3	4	5
4. Was your order taken promptly?	1	2	3	4	5
5. Was your food served in a reasonable amount of time?	1	2	3	4	5
6. Was your food flavorful?	1	2	3	4	5
7. Was the diner clean?	1	2	3	4	5
8. Would you visit us again?	1	2	3	4	5

Comments:_____

Standards, Regulations & Laws

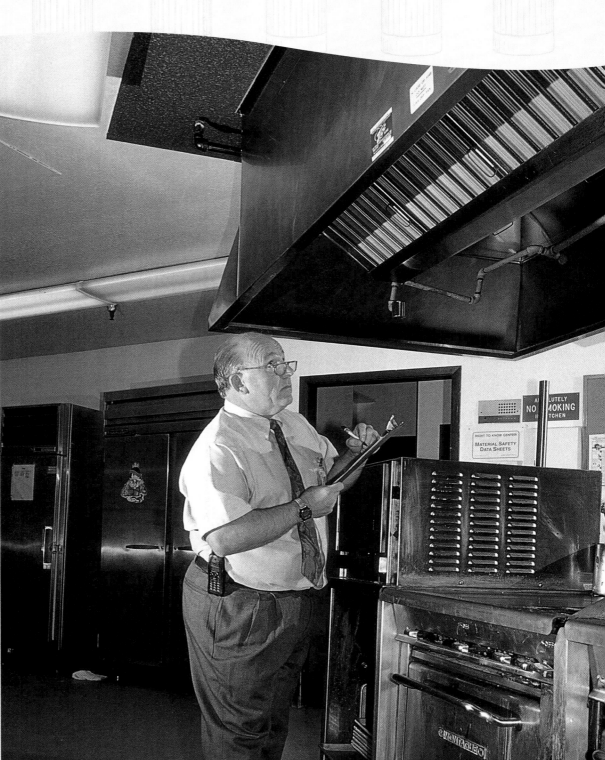

Foodservice Standards & Regulations

KEY TERMS

- standards
- regulations
- grading
- genetically engineered
- irradiated food
- solid waste
- material safety data sheets (MSDS)

OBJECTIVES

After reading this section, you will be able to:

- List the standards of quality used to evaluate food.
- Explain the role of various government agencies in the foodservice industry.
- Describe food gradings and inspections.
- Identify industry standards for handling food safely.

IMAGINE that you've just received a shipment of eggs from a supplier. Would you know if the eggs met industry standards? Would you know if the eggs were safe? Foodservice industry standards take away much of the guesswork. Government laws and regulations increase the safety level of food products. They also regulate safety in the workplace. As a foodservice professional, you need to be familiar with industry standards and government laws and regulations.

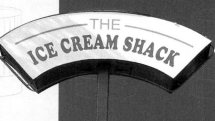

✖ INDUSTRY STANDARDS

Quality goes hand in hand with standards. **Standards** are established models or examples used to compare quality. These standards are the result of planning and state expectations. With standards in place, managers and food safety professionals can judge the performance of a foodservice operation. If a standard isn't met, the foodservice operation is written up as "in violation." Action must then be taken to correct the problem.

The main goal of the foodservice industry is to provide quality food and service to customers. To achieve this, all of the following quality standards must be considered:

- Safety.
- Nutritional value.
- Appearance.
- Consistency.
- Flavor.
- Texture.
- Convenience.
- Ease of handling.
- Packaging.
- Storage.

USDA REGULATIONS

In addition to standards, the foodservice industry is governed by regulations. **Regulations** are rules by which government agencies enforce minimum standards of quality. Federal, state, and local governments oversee these regulations, each with a different responsibility. For example, the U.S. Department of Agriculture (USDA) grades and inspects poultry and poultry products, eggs and egg products, and meat and meat products. The USDA also supervises food grading, processing plant inspections, and the use of pesticides, preservatives, and food additives.

Food Grading

When the USDA inspects food and food products, they apply grades to them. **Grading** food products involves applying specific standards of quality to those products. Grading helps the foodservice manager decide what to buy. Some products must be graded. Others are graded on a voluntary basis, and the manufacturer pays for the service.

A product receives a grade based on its quality when it is packaged. The package is then stamped with the grading seal. Changes in the product may occur during handling and storing that can affect the food's quality. Different grades exist for different kinds of products. For example, there are three grades of chicken and eight grades of beef. See Fig. 6-1 below.

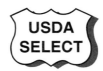

Food Inspections

Inspections are conducted to ensure that food is sanitary and labeled correctly. These inspections are conducted by the Food Safety and Inspection Service (FSIS). The FSIS is a public health agency that is part of the USDA. The FSIS checks that egg, poultry, and meat products are wholesome, safe, and correctly packaged and labeled. Inspected food is stamped to let you know that the food meets safety standards. See Fig. 6-2.

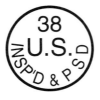

Fig. 6-2. FSIS stamps.

FDA REGULATIONS

The Food and Drug Administration (FDA) is part of the U.S. Department of Health and Human Services. The FDA enforces the Food, Drug, and Cosmetic Act of 1938. This law covers food and the packaging of foods other than fish, poultry, and meat.

In 1992, the FDA stated that food would be judged by its characteristics, not by the process used to make it. This also applies to genetically engineered and irradiated foods.

Genetically (juh-NET-i-kuh-lee) **engineered** foods are those foods made by recombining genes. Genes can be omitted or held back, or new genes can be spliced into a food. These foods may become new varieties, such as the combination of broccoli and cauliflower to create broccoflower. Genes may also be combined to improve foods, packing them with nutrients.

Irradiated (ih-RAY-dee-ay-tuhd) **food** has been exposed to radiation to kill harmful bacteria. Beef, lamb, and pork are the three foods most commonly exposed to radiation. Other food products that may be irradiated include spices and some fruits and vegetables. The FDA regulates the irradiation process to ensure that the foods are safe and do not contain radioactive particles. They also require these foods carry a label to indicate they've been irradiated. See Fig. 6-3.

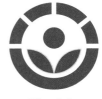

Fig. 6-3.

■ **Labels.** The FDA also requires nutrition labels to be placed on food packages, as a result of the 1990 Nutrition Labeling and Education Act. The nutrition label shows the percent of daily dietary value

The 1906 Food & Drug Act

The United States was slow to recognize the need for a national food and drug law. In 1883, Dr. Harvey W. Wiley was appointed chief of the U.S. Department of Chemistry. This government agency was a predecessor to the Food and Drug Administration. Dr. Wiley, sometimes called the "Crusading Chemist," set out to put a stop to inferior food products and quack remedies. He and his staff performed countless investigations and made their findings public.

In 1903, Dr. Wiley captured the attention of the country by establishing a "poison squad." These young men volunteered to eat foods treated with measured amounts of chemical preservatives. The objective was to determine whether these ingredients were dangerous.

Dr. Wiley's determination led to the passage of the original Food and Drug Act on June 30, 1906. The Meat Inspection Act was passed the same day.

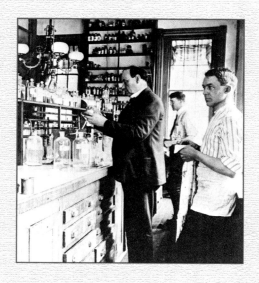

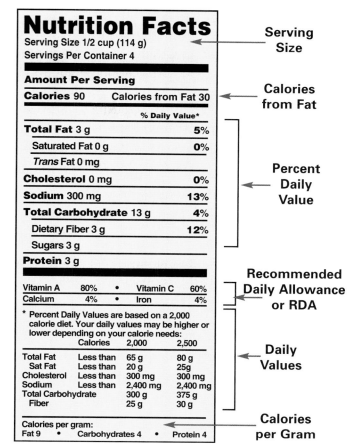

Fig. 6-4. Nutrition labels provide valuable information.

in the food, usually based on a daily 2,000- or 2,500-calorie intake. The nutrition label also shows the number of calories per serving, the total calories, as well as the amount of vitamins and minerals, fat, cholesterol, sodium, carbohydrates, and protein in the food. See Fig. 6-4.

■ **Menus.** Since 1997, the FDA has regulated health claims made by restaurants, such as low-fat menu items. These claims must meet FDA standards as listed in the Nutrition Labeling and Education Act. For example, the FDA standard for "low fat" is 3 grams or less per serving. A food-service establishment must be able to provide nutritional information to any customer who asks for it. If the menu does not make any special claims, nutritional information is not required.

■ **Food Code.** The FDA also recommends food-service standards in the Food Code. The Food Code provides states with specific guidelines for safe food handling. It is updated every two years. Since the code isn't a law, states may choose to adopt the Food Code or write their own code, using the Food Code as a guide.

SAFE FOOD HANDLING

Most states require that foodservice managers take special training and certification in safe food handling. You can contact your local health department for information regarding certification requirements for safe food handling and environmental considerations for safe food production. Chapters 7 and 8 address safe food handling.

FACILITIES MAINTENANCE

Standards and regulations also apply to how a facility is maintained. Foodservice operations must have sanitary facilities designed and equipped in a way that permits thorough cleaning. Any facility that cannot be thoroughly cleaned isn't sanitary and would not provide a safe environment for food supplies or food production. These main areas must meet industry standards:

- Floors, walls, and ceilings.
- Equipment.
- Facility design.

Floors, Walls & Ceilings

Industry standards state that floors, walls, and ceilings should be constructed for durability. They must also meet health and safety regulations. The FDA Food Code recommends that floors be slip resistant, nonporous, and nonabsorbent.

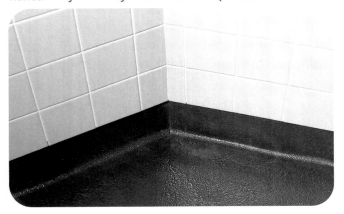

Fig. 6-5. Foodservice standards extend to facility maintenance. Why is facility maintenance important?

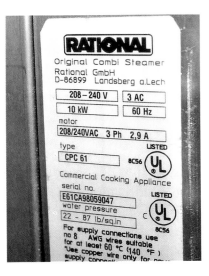

Fig. 6-6. The NSF International and UL certification marks help ensure that foodservice equipment is safe.

Common materials used for floors include rubber tile, vinyl tile, and quarry tile. See Fig. 6-5.

Walls and ceilings should be light in color. This is especially true in food preparation areas. Light-colored walls and ceilings allow soil to be easily seen. All floors, walls, and ceilings should be kept in good condition. They should not have any holes, cracks, or peeling paint. They should be kept clean and sanitized at all times.

Equipment

The National Sanitation Foundation (NSF) International issues sanitation standards for equipment. In addition, the Underwriter's Laboratories (UL) classifies electrical equipment that meets NSF International standards. The equipment used in commercial kitchens must bear the NSF International and UL sanitation classification marks. See Fig. 6-6.

When equipment is purchased, it should:

- Be easy to clean.
- Have smooth, nontoxic, nonabsorbent food-contact surfaces.
- Have corrosion-resistant surfaces that are nontoxic and chip resistant.
- Be free of surface pits and crevices. Bolts and rivets should be flush with the surface of the equipment—not sticking out.
- Have rounded off corners or edges.
- Be easy to take apart for cleaning.
- Be for commercial use only.

Facility Design

Industry standards for kitchen design include effective workflow, minimized risk of contamination, and easy access to equipment. Facility maintenance standards also apply to restrooms, sinks, hand-washing stations, ventilation, lighting, and waste management systems. See Fig. 6-7. Facilities should be designed in a way that allows easy access to all equipment. This is so the equipment can be thoroughly cleaned and the disposal of grease can be accomplished in a safe, environment-friendly way. Areas that can't be cleaned well may become breeding grounds for bacteria and pests.

ENVIRONMENTAL REGULATIONS

The Environmental Protection Agency (EPA) determines how solid waste is managed. **Solid waste** includes packaging material, containers, and recyclables. The EPA recommends reducing solid waste by eliminating packaging where possible. It also recommends that reusable food containers be cleaned and sanitized before reusing. Dispose of containers that hold chemicals—never reuse for food products. In addition, make sure chemicals are not stored near food.

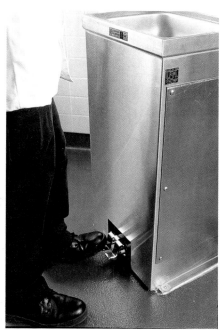

Fig. 6-7. Built-in sanitation features include the foot control on this hand-washing station.

THE pH SCALE

The food industry has very strict specifications for raw materials. One of those specifications is pH. The pH scale measures the acidity or alkalinity of a solution on a scale ranging from 0–14. A pH of 7 means the substance is neutral. Pure water has a pH of 7. Tomatoes have a 1.8–2.4 pH. A pH of less than 7 means the solution is an acid. A pH of more than 7 means the solution is a base. With a few exceptions, such as E. coli, most bacteria grow between 4.6 and 7.5 on the pH scale.

Indicators, such as litmus (LIT-muhs) paper, can be used to determine whether a substance is an acid or a base. If the litmus paper changes to red, the solution is considered an acid. If it changes to blue, the solution is considered a base.

APPLY IT!

1. Break off three or four red cabbage leaves.
2. Cut them into small pieces and add them to 1 cup of boiling water.
3. Boil them for 25 minutes.
4. Remove the red cabbage leaves from the water using tongs.
5. Pour the juice into a small pitcher.
6. Add 2-3 drops of red cabbage juice to one ounce of each of the following substances: vinegar, baking soda in water, milk, orange juice, dish detergent mixed in water, and pickle juice. If the substance turns a pinkish red, it is an acid. If it turns blue, it is a base.
7. Record your observations.

The National Environmental Policy Act (NEPA) of 1969 protects the environment from damage caused by building development. Whenever a new restaurant is proposed, an Environmental Impact Statement (EIS) must be completed. An EIS describes the impact of the proposed facility and any negative effects to the environment.

OSHA REGULATIONS

The Occupational Safety and Health Administration (OSHA) has two main responsibilities: to set standards and to inspect workplaces to ensure that employers provide safe and healthful environments. Standards, such as the three that follow, are the same in all workplaces:

• Employers must provide personal protective equipment, such as gloves. Refer to Chapter 7 for more information on protective clothing.

• Manufacturers of hazardous materials must evaluate their products for danger. If products are hazardous, they must be labeled. OSHA also requires that employers have **material safety data sheets** (MSDS) that identify any hazardous chemicals and their components. Employers must inform employees where these sheets are located.

• Employers must allow employees access to any records of exposure to toxic materials.

OSHA also regulates record keeping of job-related illness and injury. One required form is an accident report log. See Fig. 6-8. If an accident causes three or more employees to be hospitalized, or one or more people to die, that accident must be reported to a local OSHA representative within eight hours. OSHA will then investigate to determine whether any standards were violated.

STATE & LOCAL REGULATIONS

Many of the health regulations affecting foodservice operations are written at the state level. Local health departments then enforce state regulations. A large city may also have its own health department that enforces regulations within city limits. The county health department enforces regulations in rural areas and small cities. Likewise, most national and statewide companies also have standards maintained by their own inspectors.

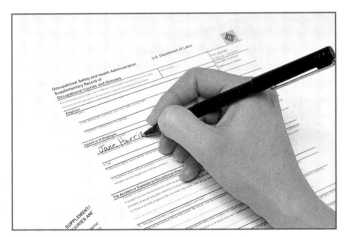

Fig. 6-8. OSHA accident and injury forms are available in cases of employee injury. When should this form be completed? By whom?

SECTION 6-1   Knowledge Check

1. List five standards of quality used to evaluate food.

2. Contrast food gradings and food inspections.

3. What government agency oversees workplace safety?

MINI LAB

Research a foodservice standard, law, or regulation on the Web site of a government agency, such as the USDA. Present a summary of your research to the class.

Employment Laws

KEY TERMS

- laws
- discrimination
- sexual harassment
- disability
- musculoskeletal disorders
- ergonomics

OBJECTIVES

After reading this section, you will be able to:

- Identify laws related to workers' rights and safety.
- Identify laws that protect certain groups of people.

INDUSTRY standards and government regulations address the rights of employees and employers in the workplace. **Laws**, or established rules, protect various groups of people from discrimination and ensure that workers are treated fairly. These include right-to-know laws. These laws require that employers tell employees about their rights in the workplace. Foodservice professionals should know the laws that protect them on the job and follow them responsibly.

EQUAL EMPLOYMENT OPPORTUNITIES

The United States federal government has passed a number of laws to ensure that everyone has a chance for equal employment. The Equal Employment Opportunities Act, passed in 1972, expanded some of the laws in the 1964 Civil Rights Act. It requires businesses to have affirmative action programs. The goal of affirmative action is to keep discrimination from occurring. **Discrimination** (dis-krih-mah-NAE-shun) is the unfair treatment of people based on age, gender, race, or religion.

This applies to all public and private employers involved in interstate commerce. This includes restaurants with at least 15 employees who work at least 20 weeks per year. State and local governments also have laws to protect employees from discrimination. See Fig. 6-9.

Affirmative Action

Following the 1964 Civil Rights Act, employers put in place programs to locate, hire, train, and promote women and people of color. The goal of these programs is to prevent discriminatory practices that would prevent qualified people from getting jobs because of their age, race, or gender.

Affirmative action programs are also required of employers with federal contracts of more than $50,000. This might include, for example, a foodservice company that supplies meals to a U.S. military base.

Fig. 6-9.

EMPLOYMENT LAWS	PROVISIONS
Civil Rights Act	Employers may not discriminate based on race, color, national origin, sex, or religion; protects U.S. citizens working for U.S. companies overseas.
Equal Employment Opportunities Act	Requires businesses to have affirmative action programs. This includes restaurants with at least 15 employees who work at least 20 weeks per year.
Age Discrimination in Employment Act	Protects people 40 years of age and older from being discriminated against in any aspect of employment.
Americans with Disabilities Act	Prevents employers from refusing to hire or promote disabled persons, and ensures that all employees are treated equally. This law also requires public facilities make "reasonable accommodations" for the disabled.
Immigration Reform and Control Act	Only U.S. citizens and people who are authorized to work in the U.S. may be legally hired.
Immigration and Nationality Act	Prevents employers from hiring illegal immigrants for low-skill, low-paying jobs without providing them with pension or insurance benefits.
Federal Employment Compensation Act	Protects employees who are injured or disabled due to work-related accidents.

Age Discrimination

The Age Discrimination in Employment Act of 1967 protects people 40 years of age and older from being discriminated against in any aspect of employment. This applies to hiring, promotion, and wages. This law helps prevent people from not being hired based on their age. Hiring should focus on ability. This law has been amended several times. In 1974, it was extended to state, local, and federal positions. See Fig. 6-10.

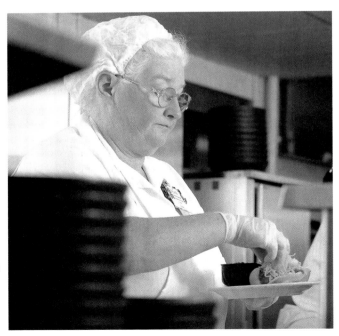

Fig. 6-10. Workers over the age of 60 can make a positive impact in the workplace.

In 1987, the age limit, which originally applied only to those between the ages of 40–65, was amended to remove all upper age limits. Experts predict that by 2010, one in four persons in the United States will be age 55 or older, and that by 2030, one in three persons will be that age. Working beyond a standard retirement age is becoming common, since better health care allows people to be active and mentally alert longer.

Sexual Harassment

"Unwelcome advances, requests for sexual favors, and other verbal or physical conduct of a sexual nature" are defined as **sexual harassment** by the Equal Employment Opportunity Commission. When such behavior affects an employee's job performance or leads to an unfriendly workplace, it violates Title VII of the Civil Rights Act of 1964. Sexual harassment incidents affect an employee's chance for a promotion or pay raise. They can also get you fired.

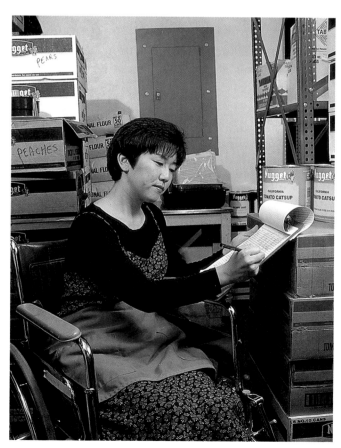

Employees need to know what type of behavior is considered sexual harassment. An employer is responsible for the harassment if he or she does not take action to either prevent the harassment or discipline the person causing the problem. Every workplace has a policy for dealing with sexual harassment. Sexual harassment policies should cover the following items:

- Communication of the policy to all employees.
- Supervisor training in the legal aspects of harassment cases.
- A formal system for complaints and how they will be investigated and solved.
- A plan for action on any complaints received, being careful to protect the person who brought the complaint.
- Disciplinary action for any person guilty of harassment.
- Follow up on all harassment cases.

Americans with Disabilities

The Americans with Disabilities Act (ADA) became law in 1990 to protect the civil rights of the disabled. This law makes it illegal to put disabled people in lower-paying jobs just because of their disabilities. It also makes it illegal to offer different pay to a disabled person doing the same job as an able-bodied person. The ADA also prevents employers from refusing to hire or promote disabled persons, and ensures that all employees are treated equally. See Fig. 6-11.

The ADA defines **disability** as "a physical or mental impairment that substantially limits one or more major life activities." The law requires public facilities make "reasonable accommodation" for the disabled, whether they are employees or customers. This might mean adding access ramps near stairs, providing adaptive equipment for an employee to use, or adapting customer bathrooms to accommodate wheelchairs, and provide special handles on sinks.

Fig. 6-11. Certain accommodations need to be met for those with disabilities.

WAGE & LABOR LAWS

The hourly minimum wage that employers can pay employees is determined by the federal government. The U.S. Department of Labor does issue certificates for a lower rate for some employees, such as apprentices, student learners, and full-time college students.

IMMIGRATION LAWS

In times of economic uncertainty, war, or political troubles, some people choose to leave their native countries looking for a better life. The United States limits the number of immigrants permitted to enter the country each year. Before immigrants can be hired, they must receive special work permits. It is against the law to hire illegal immigrants for low-skill, low-paying jobs, without giving them pension or insurance benefits.

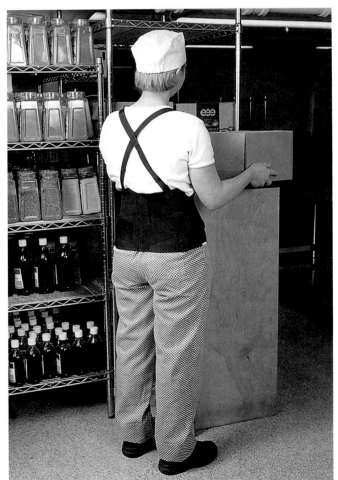

The Immigration Reform and Control Act (IRCA) of 1986 states that only U.S. citizens and others who are authorized to work in the United States may be legally hired. All employers are also subject to the Immigration and Nationality Act (INA) of 1952. This law states that employers must fill out an Employment Eligibility Verification Form, also called an I-9, for each person hired. These forms may be checked by the Immigration and Naturalization Service (INS) to determine an employee's immigration status. The I-9 form must be kept on file for at least three years, or for one year after the person is no longer employed, whichever is longer. The IRCA and the INA were designed to protect people from being discriminated against because of their national origin.

WORKERS' COMPENSATION

No matter how careful employees are, sometimes accidents occur. Workers' compensation laws make sure that injured or disabled workers have an income while they are unable to work. One goal of this policy is to cut down on the number of lawsuits filed against employers.

Federal employees are covered under the Federal Employment Compensation Act, passed in 1993. Money is awarded in cases of death or disability that occur while on the job. Injured or disabled employees may be required to retrain for another job. If an employee is killed on the job, benefits are paid to the surviving family. The protections of this law have been extended to state and local employees, too. Employers purchase workers' compensation insurance to cover the possibility of accidents. This insurance is part of the employee benefits package. See Fig. 6-12.

Fig. 6-12. By wearing safety equipment, workers may be able to prevent injuries caused by repetitive motion.

WORKPLACE INJURIES & DEATHS

Since the establishment of the Occupational Safety and Health Administration (OSHA) in 1971, workplace injury and illness rates have dropped 40% and fatalities have dropped 50%. One of the largest injury categories is **musculoskeletal** (muhs-kyoo-loh-SKEH-luh-tahl) **disorders**, such as carpal (car-PUHL) tunnel syndrome, lower back pain, and tendinitis (ten-dah-NY-tahs). These conditions are caused by repeated trauma to muscles or bones.

In light of the high rate of musculoskeletal disorders, OSHA is taking a closer look at the area of ergonomics. **Ergonomics** (URH-guh-nah-mihks) is the science concerned with the efficient and safe interaction between people and the things in their environment. In the workplace, ergonomics involves arranging and using equipment and your work space safely and efficiently.

WHO IS RESPONSIBLE?

Each of the laws discussed in this section affects a foodservice worker every day of his or her career. Knowing the law helps both employees and employers understand their rights as well as their responsibilities under the law. Following laws means a safer workplace. The role of federal, state, and local government agencies in protecting workers is important to everyone.

- **Employee responsibilities.** All employees need to be aware of their rights under the law. You must follow the laws and provide correct information about yourself and your job. See Fig. 6-13.
- **Managerial responsibilities.** Managers are required to post certain notices, such as the minimum wage laws and annual injury/accident reports. Managers must keep accurate records. They are responsible for knowing the law and enforcing it.

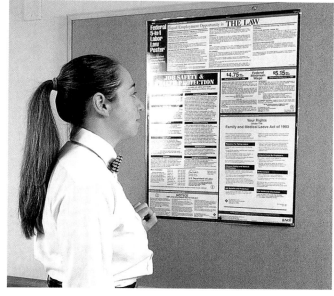

Fig. 6-13. As a foodservice employee, it is important to read all legal notices that are posted by your employer.

SECTION 6-2 Knowledge Check

1. What role does OSHA play in changing the workplace?
2. What law governs the hiring of older people?
3. Name three laws all foodservice workers should be aware of and the rights that each law protects.

MINI LAB

Choose one of the laws presented in this section and research how that law affects foodservice operations in your county. For example, did passage of the Americans with Disabilities Act require any construction changes? Report your findings.

CHAPTER 6 Review & Activities

SECTION SUMMARIES

6-1 Foodservice professionals evaluate the quality of foods and food products. Standards such as appearance, flavor, texture, and safety are followed.

6-1 The USDA and the FDA are government agencies that recommend regulations for the foodservice industry.

6-1 Foods inspected by the USDA receive either a grading seal or an FSIS stamp that informs the buyer that the product meets the standards of safety.

6-1 The foodservice industry follows strict standards concerning safe food handling. These standards include good personal hygiene and sanitation practices.

6-2 The Equal Employment Opportunities Act and the Civil Rights Act ensure that all workers are treated fairly. They also protect people from discrimination.

6-2 Laws also protect workers from discrimination based on age, disability, or national origin.

6-2 The employee's right to work in a safe and healthful environment is protected by OSHA regulations and worker compensation laws.

CHECK YOUR KNOWLEDGE

1. What foods and food products does the USDA regulate?
2. What is the grading system for food based on?
3. What government agency inspects nutrition labels?
4. What is irradiated food? What government agency regulates irradiated food?
5. List three industry standards involving good personal hygiene.
6. What industry standard should be followed when cooling food?
7. What are the benefits of affirmative action?
8. Define sexual harassment.
9. How can a restaurant make reasonable accommodations for disabled employees?
10. What are your legal responsibilities as a foodservice employee?

CRITICAL-THINKING ACTIVITIES

1. Debate the pros and cons of genetically engineered or irradiated foods. How can these processes impact the foodservice industry?
2. The foodservice industry has strict standards concerning the temperature of foods. Why do you think this is important? What are the potential consequences of not following these standards?

WORKPLACE KNOW-HOW

Communication. As manager for a restaurant, you are hiring several new employees. What government standards, laws, and regulations do you need to follow?

LAB-BASED ACTIVITY:

Knowing the Law

STEP ❶ Working in teams, make a chart of the various laws and regulations presented in this chapter. Use the chart below as a guide.

STEP ❷ Use print and Internet resources to research the items on your team's chart. Your chart should list each law or regulation by name and explain how each one impacts employees in the workplace.

STEP ❸ Select one law or regulation from the chart and create an educational poster that would inform foodservice employees about this law or regulation. Display the posters in class.

Laws & Regulations

Law or Regulation	Its Impact
Right-to-Know Law	Prevents employers from taking advantage of employees. Empowers employees in the workplace. Keeps employees safe.
Equal Employment Opportunities Act	
Civil Rights Act	
Food, Drug, and Cosmetic Act	
Meat Inspection Act	
Nutrition Labeling and Education Act	
Vietnam Era Veterans Readjustment Act	
Pregnancy Discrimination Act	
Americans with Disabilities Act	
Federal Employment Compensation Act	
Immigration and Nationality Act	
Immigration Reform and Control Act	
Age Discrimination and Employment Act	

7 Safety & Sanitation Principles

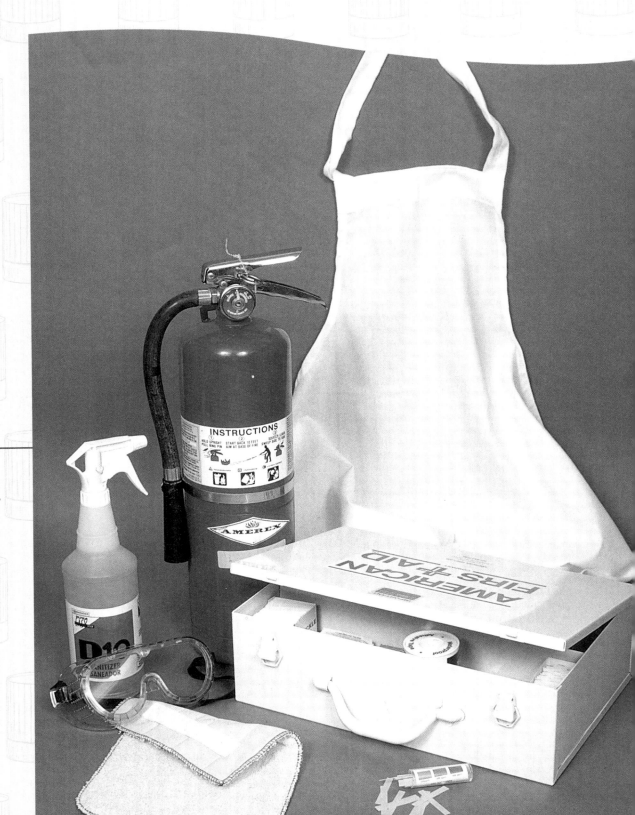

Safety Know-How

OBJECTIVES

After reading this section, you will be able to:

- Identify workplace safety guidelines and equipment.

- Explain fire safety measures.

- Describe first aid measures for burns, wounds, and choking.

- Explain cardiopulmonary resuscitation.

ACCIDENTS can easily happen in a busy kitchen. Burns, bruises, cuts, and even broken bones are all possible injuries that can occur. The government has established legislation to help protect workers on the job. However, it's the personal responsibility of each worker to practice safety at all times.

⊠ WORKING SAFELY

Workplace accidents cost the foodservice industry over $48 billion per year. Foodservice workers are particularly at risk for injuries. Fatigue, poor kitchen design, and minimal training all contribute to these accidents.

Despite the frequency of workplace accidents, they can be controlled. The Occupational Safety and Health Administration (OSHA) plays a large role in keeping the workplace safe. OSHA accomplishes this task by enforcing workplace standards. These standards are outlined in the Occupational Safety and Health Act. Employers are required to post OSHA safety and health information in their facilities. Employees are required to follow OSHA regulations.

The Environmental Protection Agency (EPA) also plays a role in workplace safety. The EPA requires foodservice operations to track how they handle and dispose of hazardous materials such as cleaning products and pesticides. This is very important since hazardous materials pose a danger to all forms of life.

Following OSHA and EPA regulations is an important part of being a foodservice professional. By practicing safety every day, you can help prevent accidents in the workplace. See Fig. 7-1.

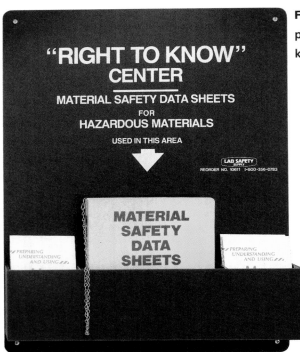

Fig. 7-1. Foodservice workers are responsible for properly using hazardous materials. It is important to know how to use a material safety data sheet.

Always wash your hands thoroughly with soap and water before putting on gloves. Follow proper hand-washing procedures to ensure cleanliness. See Chapter 8 for more details.

The type of gloves worn depends on the task you are doing. For example, you should use heavy-duty plastic gloves when cleaning pots. You would use wire-mesh gloves when cleaning a slicer. Other types of gloves include:

• Uniseal gloves.
• Powder-free gloves.
• Nitrile (NY-truhl) powder-free gloves.
• Plastic disposable gloves.
• Vinyl gloves.

Personal Protective Clothing

Wearing personal protective clothing correctly, such as uniforms, aprons, and gloves, is one way to practice safety in the workplace. Foodservice operations often provide protective clothing to help to control contamination. See Fig. 7-2. When putting on an apron, make sure it is clean. Dirty aprons are an ideal place for bacteria to grow. Change aprons when yours gets dirty on the job. You should always remove your apron if you leave the food preparation area to go into the dining area or the restroom. You also should remove it to take garbage out.

■ **Gloves.** Gloves should be worn to protect your hands from injury. Gloves also serve as a precaution against food contamination. However, you should always wash your hands—even when wearing gloves.

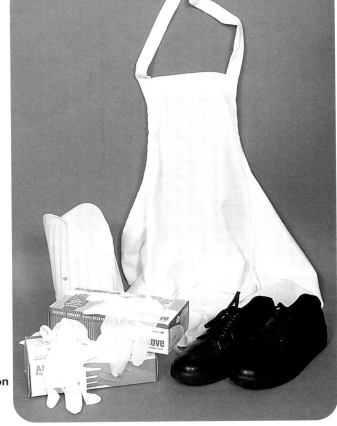

Fig. 7-2. Protective clothing helps keep you safe on the job.

Foodservice gloves are for single use only. For example, the gloves you wear to crack and mix eggs shouldn't be re-used to make a sandwich. You should change your gloves:

• When they become soiled or torn.
• At least every four hours of single-use.
• After handling any raw food.

■ **Shoes.** Shoes are also considered protective clothing. The type of shoes worn in the foodservice industry varies. Shoes should be sturdy and slip resistant for safety. All shoes must be closed-toe shoes.

■ **Back braces.** When lifting heavy items, foodservice workers may wear a back brace. A back brace is designed to support the lower back.

Personal Injuries

Foodservice workers are responsible for helping prevent slips and falls, cuts, burns and scalds, and other personal injuries in the kitchen. For example, when transporting large containers full of hot liquids, call out "Hot cart coming through!" This will warn others in the kitchen and help prevent accidents. The following guidelines can help you minimize injuries while at work. See Fig. 7-3.

Fig. 7-3. Caution signs should be placed on the floor to warn coworkers of potential danger. Why do you think this is important?

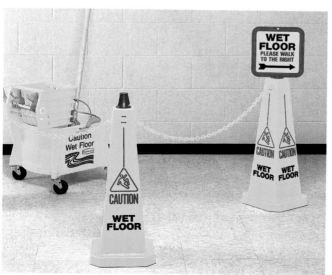

■ **Slips and falls.** Slips and falls are a common work-related injury. Yet most falls can be avoided. Perform your tasks carefully. Don't rush. Keep the walking area uncluttered and free of spills, especially around exits, aisles, and stairs. You can help prevent falls in the kitchen by:

• Walking. Never run in the kitchen.
• Wiping up spills immediately.
• Using slip-resistant floor mats and making sure floors are in good repair.
• Wearing shoes that are slip resistant.
• Using safe ladders or stools for climbing. Never use a chair or box for climbing.
• Always closing drawers and doors when you're through with them.
• Asking for help or using a cart when moving heavy objects.
• Keeping traffic paths open at all times.

Keeping floors clean is important in the foodservice industry. However, floors still wet from cleaning are dangerous. Many falls occur on wet floors because they are slick with water and cleaning products. When cleaning floors, always follow the cleaning fluid directions carefully.

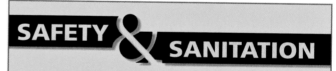

CAUTION SIGNS—Always place caution or wet floor signs after mopping or cleaning up spills. This will warn people to be careful.

■ **Cuts.** With so many sharp tools in a commercial kitchen, the risk of being cut is high. You can minimize this risk by following these safety guidelines while working with sharp tools:

• Always use knives for their intended purpose only. Never use them to open plastic overwrap or boxes, for example.
• Always cut away from your body, not toward your body.
• Always carry a knife down at your side with the blade tip pointed toward the floor and the sharp edge facing behind you.

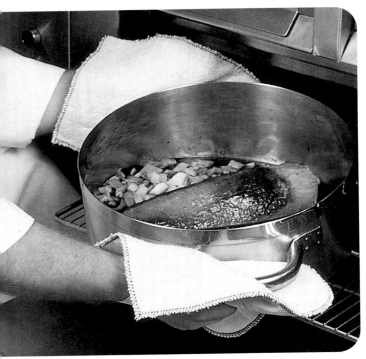

Fig. 7-4. Always use dry pot holders or oven mitts when handling hot items.

- Look where you are placing your hands when reaching for a knife.
- Never wave your hands while holding a knife.
- If you drop a knife, don't try to grab for it. Pick the knife up after it falls to the table or floor.
- Hold knives with a firm grip on the handle.
- Never leave a knife handle hanging over the edge of the work surface.
- Keep knife handles and hands dry when using knives.
- Keep knives sharp. Dull knives require you to apply more pressure, possibly causing slipping.
- Use a cutting board.
- When cleaning slicers, wear protective gloves and cuff guards.
- Always unplug appliances before cleaning them.
- Wash sharp tools separately from other utensils. Never leave knives in the sink.
- Throw away broken knives or knives with loose blades.
- Store knives in a knife kit or a rack for safety.

■ **Burns and scalds.** Commercial kitchens also provide many occasions to get burned. Follow these safety tips to prevent burns and scalds:

- Remove lids by tilting them away from your body to let the steam escape.
- Use dry pot holders or oven mitts. Wet cloth forms steam when it touches hot pots and pans. See Fig. 7-4.
- Turn the handles of pots and pans away from the front of the range.
- Step aside, while opening oven doors, to avoid the rush of heat.
- Ask for help to move hot containers.
- Follow manufacturer's directions when operating hot beverage machines.
- Be careful when filtering or changing shortening in fryers. Always wear gloves and aprons for protection.
- Keep all cooking surfaces, vent hoods, and other surfaces free of grease.
- Keep oven doors closed.
- Don't clean an oven until it has cooled.
- Always keep papers, plastic, and other **flammable**, or quick-to-burn, materials away from hot cooking areas.

■ **Back injuries and strains.** Back injuries from improper lifting and bending are one of the most common workplace injuries. They account for 20-25% of all workers' compensation claims. Many could have been prevented if employees had taken the proper precautions.

Fig. 7-5. If you decide to lift an object by yourself, follow the steps on page 159 to avoid unnecessary back strain. How might a back brace be helpful?

For example, pushing and pulling puts less strain on your back than lifting. Use rollers under the object if they are available. Ask for help if needed.

Before lifting a heavy object, first ask yourself these questions:

- Can I lift this object by myself?
- Is the object too heavy or too awkward?
- Do I need help moving or lifting the object?
- Is the path that I need to take free of clutter?

When lifting heavy objects follow these steps:

1. Bend at your knees.
2. Keep your back straight.
3. Keep your feet close to the object.
4. Center your body over the load. See Fig. 7-5.
5. Lift straight up without jerking.
6. Don't twist your body as you pick up or move the object.
7. Set the load down slowly, keeping your back straight.

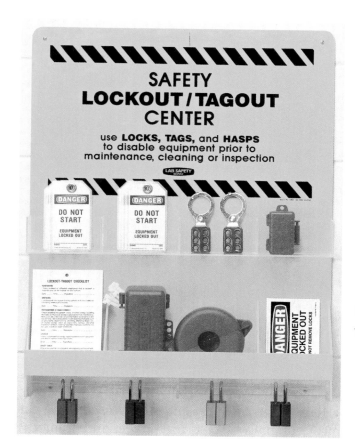

SAFETY & SANITATION

LOCKOUT/TAGOUT—To protect workers from faulty equipment, OSHA implemented a lockout/tagout procedure. **Lockout/tagout** requires all necessary switches on electrical equipment to be locked out and tagged when they are malfunctioning. This prevents the equipment from being used while it is being repaired.

Cleaning Kitchen Equipment

Each kitchen is different in its design and the equipment used. If you're unsure about how a piece of equipment works or how to clean it, ask. You should be familiar with each piece of equipment before you operate it.

You also should be familiar with equipment safety features, such as guards and safety devices. For example, a slicer is equipped with a hand guard that must be in place to operate the machine. Make sure you know how to use all the safety features on equipment. See Fig. 7-6.

In addition to operating equipment to prepare and cook food, you will also need to clean and maintain it. To clean kitchen equipment safely, always follow these precautionary measures:

- Turn switches to the "off" position.
- Unplug the machine from its power source.
- Follow the manufacturer's instruction manual and the food establishment's directions for cleaning.

Fig. 7-6. Lockout/tagout is an essential guideline for worker safety.

CLASS OF FIRE		TYPE OF FLAMMABLE MATERIAL	TYPE OF FIRE EXTINGUISHER TO USE	
Class A		Wood, paper, cloth, plastic	Class A Class A:B	
Class B		Grease, oil, chemicals	Class A:B Class A:B:C	
Class C		Electrical cords, switches, wiring	Class A:C Class B:C	
Class D		Combustible switches, wiring, metals, iron	Class D	
Class K		Fires in cooking appliances involving combustible vegetable or animal oils and fats	Class K	

Fig. 7-7. The universal picture symbols above not only identify types of fires, but are also found on fire extinguisher labels. When located on a fire extinguisher label, these symbols indicate the types of fires on which the fire extinguisher can and cannot be used.

FIRE SAFETY

Each year, fires in the workplace cause substantial property and equipment damage. They also cause injuries, and even death. The flames and high heat sources associated with the foodservice industry increase the probability of fires. Fires are classified according to the type of material that catches fire. See Fig. 7-7.

Fire Prevention

Keeping the workplace clean, especially of built-up grease, is an important first step in fire prevention. Practicing good work habits and being prepared are your best weapons for preventing and controlling fires. Here are some other tips to help keep your work environment safe:

• In facilities where smoking is permitted, be sure the contents are extinguished before emptying ashtrays.

• Use precautions around gas appliances. Built-up gasses can explode if a match is lit nearby.
• Store oily rags in proper metal containers.
• Make sure all smoke alarms are working.
• Store flammable or combustible materials away from heat sources.
• Keep water away from electrical outlets.
• Clean range and oven hoods and filters regularly.
• Keep all exits unlocked and accessible from the inside. Never block an exit.

Fire Protection Equipment

Precaution is your best course of action when it comes to fire, even then fires can happen. Having the proper fire protection equipment, and knowing how to use it, is essential. See Fig. 7-8.

■ **Fire extinguishers.** Fire extinguishers are the most common type of fire protection equipment

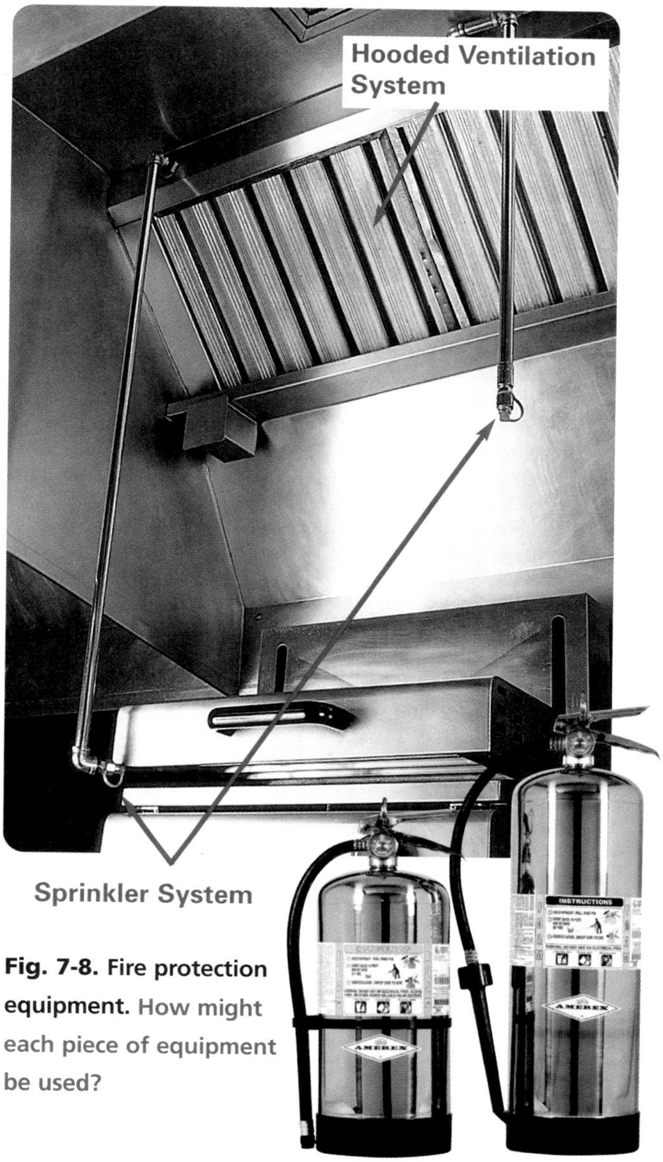

Hooded Ventilation System

Sprinkler System

Fig. 7-8. Fire protection equipment. How might each piece of equipment be used?

upright and remove the safety pin. Direct the nozzle at the bottom of the fire and push the handle down. This will release the contents that will extinguish the fire.

■ **Hood and sprinkler systems.** In addition to fire extinguishers, foodservice operations should have hood and sprinkler systems. A properly ventilated hood system can help remove excess smoke, heat, and vapors. Make sure hoods are cleaned regularly and are working properly. If your establishment has a sprinkler system, be sure products and supplies are kept the regulated distance away from the sprinkler equipment.

used in foodservice operations. The type, number, and location of fire extinguishers needed in a commercial kitchen varies by location. However, a working fire extinguisher should be located within each work area.

Fire extinguishers use several types of chemicals to fight different kinds of fires. To fight a fire properly, you must use the appropriate type, or class, of extinguisher.

Fire extinguishers are inspected and tagged on a regular basis. The fire department or a state-certified fire protection company can do this. To use a fire extinguisher properly, hold the extinguisher

KEY Science SKILLS

EXTINGUISHING A GREASE FIRE

The best way to extinguish an oil or grease fire is to use sodium bicarbonate, $NaHCO_3$, or in simpler terms, baking soda. When heated, baking soda breaks down and forms carbon dioxide gas, CO_2. Unlike oxygen, carbon dioxide is not readily combustible, which means it does not ignite. Carbon dioxide gas also has an atomic weight greater than that of nitrogen, N_2, and oxygen, O_2, the other gases that make up the atmosphere. Basically this means that CO_2 is heavier than N_2 and O_2. So when baking soda is spread over a grease or oil fire, the carbon dioxide gas that is formed fills up the space around the fire and actually suffocates or smothers the flames.

APPLY IT!

Contact your local fire department. Ask if a firefighter can come to your class to demonstrate operating fire extinguishers. Summarize the instructions on the different classes of fire extinguishers.

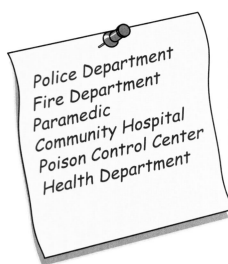

Police Department
Fire Department
Paramedic
Community Hospital
Poison Control Center
Health Department

Fig. 7-9. Keep emergency numbers near the phone. **What other emergency numbers might be on such a list?**

⊠ PREPARING FOR EMERGENCIES

In addition to fires, other emergencies sometimes happen. An emergency is a potentially life-threatening situation that usually occurs suddenly and unexpectedly. It's important to be prepared so you will know how to respond. When an emergency happens, how you react may make all the difference.

Always post telephone numbers of emergency services, such as the fire department, poison control, and the health department, near the phone. See Fig. 7-9. You should also learn basic first aid and CPR. It is your responsibility to be familiar with your employer's policies regarding emergencies. You must trigger the Emergency Response System if there is an emergency. Waiting for management to arrive could cost a person his or her life.

Fire Emergency Procedures

Every foodservice establishment has fire emergency procedures. It's the employees responsibility to be familiar with them. Employers must have fire exit signs posted in plain view above exits. Employees should know where they are to meet outside the establishment for a head count in case of a fire. Employees should also know how to direct customers out of the building.

The foodservice staff is responsible for keeping customers calm during emergencies. If you discover a fire, call the fire department regardless of the size of the fire. Fires can grow large very quickly. Then help customers and coworkers leave the building as quickly and calmly as possible.

First Aid

The immediate response to an emergency often involves first aid. First aid involves assisting an injured person until professional medical help can be provided. The American Red Cross offers courses that teach hands-on practical information about first aid in the workplace. You can contact your local chapter of the American Red Cross for additional information.

Fig. 7-10. An accident report is designed to help medical staff in an emergency.

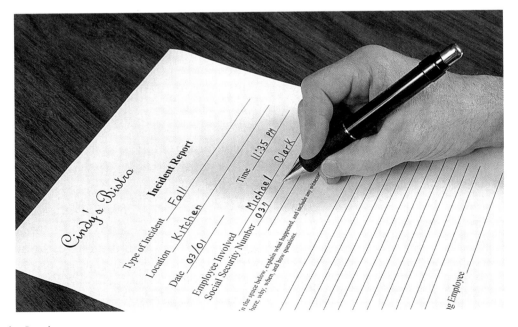

Fig. 7-11.

TYPES OF BURNS	CHARACTERISTICS OF BURNS
First-degree burns 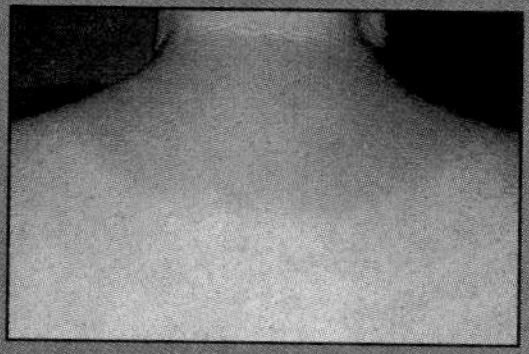	The skin becomes red, sensitive, and sometimes swollen. These are the least severe of all burns.
Second-degree burns 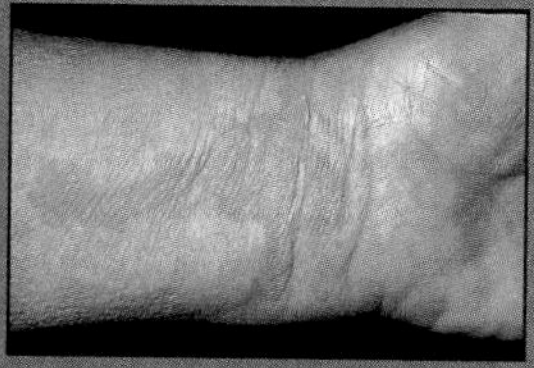	These burns cause deeper, painful damage, and blisters form on the skin. The blisters ooze and they are painful.
Third-degree burns 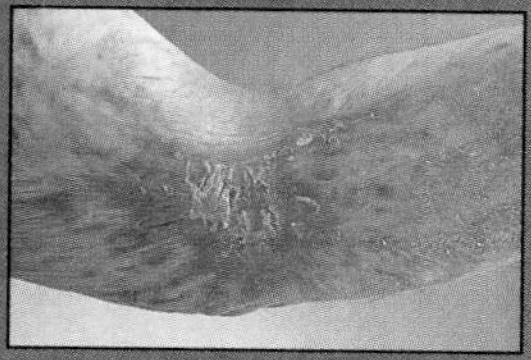	The skin may be white and soft or black, charred, and leathery. The burned area has no feeling. Sometimes third-degree burns aren't painful because the nerves in the skin have been destroyed. These are the worst kinds of burns. Third-degree burns require immediate medical attention, at a hospital.

The general emergency action tips in the list below should be followed in an emergency. They do not replace the need to be trained in first aid.

- Check the scene and stay calm.
- Check the victim. Keep him or her comfortable and calm.
- Call the local emergency number for professional medical help.
- Care for the victim by administering first aid according to the first aid manual.
- Keep people who are not needed away from the victim.
- Complete an accident report. See Fig. 7-10. Write the victim's name, the date and time of the accident, the type of injury or illness, the treatment, and how long it took for assistance to arrive.

■ **First aid for burns.** Any degree of burn requires immediate treatment. See Fig. 7-11. In the event you or someone in the workplace is burned, call your local emergency number for medical assistance. Until help arrives, follow these general guidelines:

- Remove the person from the source of the heat.
- Cool the burned skin to stop the burning. Do this by applying cold water over the affected area. You can use water from a faucet or soaked towels. Do not use ice or ice water.
- Never apply ointments, sprays, antiseptics, or remedies unless instructed to do so by a medical professional.
- Bandage the burn as directed in your first aid manual.
- Minimize the risk of shock. Keep the victim from getting chilled or overheated. Have the victim rest.

■ **First aid for wounds.** There are four types of open wounds, or cuts: abrasions, lacerations, avulsions, and punctures.

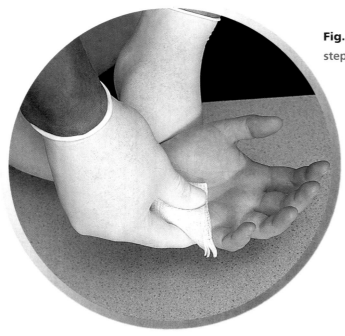

- An **abrasion** is a scrape, and is considered a minor cut. A rug burn is an abrasion.
- **Lacerations** (LASS-uh-ray-shuns) are cuts or tears in the skin that can be quite deep. A knife wound is a type of laceration.
- An **avulsion** (auh-VUHL-shun) occurs when a portion of the skin is partially or completely torn off. A severed finger is an avulsion.
- **Puncture** wounds occur when the skin is pierced with a pointed object, such as an ice pick, making a deep hole in the skin. Puncture wounds can be deep.

Cuts often require immediate attention. If a cut is severe, call for emergency help immediately.

For a minor cut, you can follow these guidelines for treating the injured person:

- Put on disposable gloves to protect against infection.
- Clean the cut with soap and rinse it under water.
- Place a bandage over the cut. Use sterile gauze if possible.
- Apply direct pressure over the sterile gauze or bandage to stop any bleeding from the cut. See Fig. 7-12.

- If bleeding doesn't stop, elevate the limb above the heart to reduce the amount of blood going to the cut area.
- Follow instructions in the first aid manual.

As you wait for medical help for an injured person with a laceration, avulsion, or puncture wound, follow these guidelines:

- Put on disposable gloves.
- Control the bleeding by applying pressure using sterile gauze or a clean cloth towel. Do not waste time washing the wound first. Elevate the area while applying pressure.
- Cover the wound with clean bandages. Continue to apply pressure.
- Wash your hands thoroughly after treating the wound.

■ **First aid for choking.** One of the most frightening on-the-job emergencies you may encounter is someone choking. Choking is often caused by food blocking a person's airway. If the object is stuck in the airway, the person will have difficulty speaking and breathing.

You may be able to save the life of someone who is choking by using the **Heimlich maneuver**. See Fig. 7-13. Use this maneuver only on someone who is conscious and choking. If the person can cough or speak, or is unconscious, do not perform this maneuver. Doing so can cause physical injury. Also, never perform the Heimlich maneuver on someone who is pregnant.

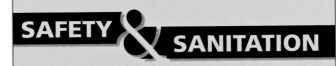

SAFETY & SANITATION

PREGNANT VICTIM—The Heimlich maneuver should never be performed on a pregnant woman. Doing so could harm the baby.

Here are the basic guidelines for performing the Heimlich maneuver:

1. Stand behind the victim. Wrap your arms around the victim's waist.

2. Locate the victim's navel.

3. Make a fist with one hand. Place the thumb side of your fist against the middle of the abdomen. Position your hand just above the navel and below the bottom of the breast bone.

4. Place your other hand on top of your fist.

5. Press your hands into the victim's abdomen. Use quick, inward and upward thrusts. Each thrust should be a separate and distinct action.

6. Repeat this motion as many times as it takes to dislodge the object or food from the victim's throat. Note that a conscious victim can become unconscious during this maneuver if the object is not dislodged.

Cardiopulmonary Resuscitation (CPR)

Cardiopulmonary resuscitation (CAR-dee-oh-PALL-mun-air-eeree-CESS-ah-tay-shun) is emergency care that is performed on people who are unresponsive. Unresponsive victims include those who are unconscious because of choking, cardiac arrest, stroke, or heart attack.

The sooner CPR is performed, the greater the victim's chance of survival. CPR helps keep oxygen flowing to the brain and heart. This is done until advanced care can restore normal heart function.

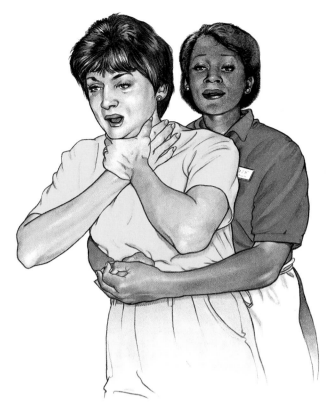

Fig. 7-13. The Heimlich maneuver can be performed on a choking, conscious adult. When would you not perform the Heimlich maneuver?

In many communities, an emergency services operator will give you directions to follow over the phone. However, you may be in a situation where you have to perform CPR on a customer or coworker without help. You can contact your local chapter of the American Heart Association or the American Red Cross for additional information.

SECTION 7-1   Knowledge Check

1. What equipment is used to keep you safe at work?

2. Name three general first aid guidelines you should follow in an emergency.

3. What is CPR?

MINI LAB

Using the information from this section, create a safety procedures checklist that would help new employees know how to prevent accidents, and what to do when one occurs.

Sanitation Challenges

- **sanitary**
- **contaminated**
- **direct contamination**
- **toxins**
- **cross-contamination**
- **sanitation**
- **hazard**
- **bacteria**
- **parasites**
- **fungi**
- **sanitizing**

OBJECTIVES

After reading this section, you will be able to:

- Describe the sources of direct contamination and cross-contamination.
- Identify biological, chemical, and physical hazards.
- Explain how to respond to an outbreak of foodborne illness.

FOODBORNE illnesses kill thousands of people each year and make many more people sick. For this reason, foodservice professionals need to know how to create a clean, disease-free environment for food preparation. They also need to know how to prevent and respond to foodborne illnesses.

☒ WHAT IS CONTAMINATION?

When consumers eat out, they expect the food to be prepared and served in a **sanitary**, or clean, environment. When harmful microorganisms or substances are present in food, the food is **contaminated**. Contaminated food is food that is unfit to be eaten. Eating contaminated food can make you sick and may even cause death. See Fig. 7-14.

Contamination can happen in one of two ways. **Direct contamination** occurs when raw foods, or the plants or animals from which they come, are exposed to **toxins**, or harmful organisms or substances. For example, toxins in soil used to grow grains could contaminate the grain and any products produced from the grain.

The other way foods become tainted is by cross-contamination. **Cross-contamination** is the movement of chemicals or microorganisms from one place to another. The most common mode of cross-contamination is people. For example, food handlers can transfer biological, chemical, and physical organisms or substances simply by preparing or serving foods.

Foodservice professionals need to be concerned about both types of contamination. You'll want to take precautions to minimize direct contamination of foods. You also need to prevent cross-contamination when you prepare and serve foods. Sanitation measures can help foodservice professionals achieve this.

Fig. 7-14.

Foodborne Illnesses

ILLNESS & CAUSE	SYMPTOMS	FOODS INVOLVED
Salmonellosis—Bacteria	Cramps, nausea, headache, fever, diarrhea, vomiting.	Poultry and poultry products, meat and meat products, fish, dairy products, protein foods, fresh produce.
Campylobacter jejuni—Bacteria	Nausea, vomiting, fever, diarrhea, abdominal pain, headache, and muscle pain.	Meats and poultry, unpasteurized milk and dairy products.
Hepatitis A—Virus	Fatigue, discomfort, fever, headache, nausea, loss of appetite, vomiting, jaundice.	Water, ice, salads, coldcuts, sandwiches, shellfish, fruit, fruit juices, milk and milk products, vegetables.
Norwalk Virus	Cramps, nausea, headache, fever, vomiting.	Water, raw vegetables, fresh fruit, salads, shellfish.
Trichinosis—Parasite	Abdominal pain, nausea, diarrhea, fever, swelling around eyes, thirst, sweating, chills, fatigue, hemorrhaging.	Pork, nonpork sausages, wild game.
Shigellosis—Bacteria	Abdominal pain, diarrhea, vomiting, fever, dehydration.	Protein salads, lettuce, raw vegetables, poultry, shrimp, milk and milk products.
Listeriosis—Bacteria	Headache, fever, chills, nausea, vomiting, diarrhea, backache, meningitis, encephalitis.	Ice cream, frozen yogurt, unpasteurized milk and cheese, raw vegetables, poultry, meat, seafood.
Rotavirus	Abdominal pain, diarrhea, vomiting, mild fever.	Water, ice, salads, fruit, hors d'oeuvres.
Anisakiasis—Parasite	Tingling in throat, abdominal pain, coughing up worms, cramping, vomiting, nausea.	Fish, seafood.
Giardiasis—Parasite	Cramps, nausea, intestinal gas, fatigue, loss of weight.	Water, ice, salads.
Botulism—Bacteria	Constipation and diarrhea, vomiting, fatigue, vertigo, double vision, dry mouth, paralysis, death.	Underprocessed foods, canned low-acid foods, sautéed onions in butter sauce, baked potatoes, untreated garlic and oil products.
E. Coli—Bacteria	Severe abdominal cramps, diarrhea, vomiting, mild fever, kidney failure.	Raw ground beef, undercooked meat, unpasteurized milk and apple cider or juice, mayonnaise, lettuce, melons, fish from contaminated water.

The word **sanitation** means healthy or clean and whole. Sanitation also refers to healthy and sanitary conditions and effective sanitary practices. Foodservice professionals have an obligation to prepare food in a sanitary environment. Federal, state, and local health departments have established sanitation and food handling regulations. These regulations protect consumers from foodborne diseases.

In the foodservice industry, workers need to be aware of the types of food hazards that can occur. These hazards are biological, chemical, and physical. Any of these **hazards**, or sources of danger, can result in contaminated food.

BIOLOGICAL HAZARDS

Biological hazards come from microorganisms such as bacteria. Other types include viruses, parasites, and fungi. In addition to microorganisms, certain plants and fish can also carry harmful toxins. However, disease-causing microorganisms cause the majority of foodborne illnesses. For detailed information on specific foodborne illnesses, See Fig. 7-14 on page 167.

Foodborne Illness

As you have read, microorganisms, such as bacteria and viruses, are the root cause of foodborne illness. These microorganisms can grow in and on food when it isn't handled properly. Other conditions that can lead to foodborne illness are cross-contamination, poor personal hygiene, and food handler illness. For example, storing uncooked meats above cooked meats in the refrigerator can cause cross-contamination.

Each year the number of incidents of foodborne illness grows. Children, the elderly, and pregnant women are the most at-risk for getting foodborne illnesses. People who are chronically ill or who have weakened immune systems are also at risk. Fortunately, each of the conditions that breeds foodborne illness can be prevented. By following industry standards for safety, you can help eliminate the threat of foodborne illness.

RESPONDING TO AN OUTBREAK

If you have ever felt queasy after eating, you may have been a victim of a foodborne illness. An outbreak of foodborne illness happens when people become sick after eating the same food. If you suspect an outbreak, use these procedures:

- Inform the manager or supervisor of your suspicions immediately.
- Avoid panic. There are many reasons why people become ill, so it's best to let the health authorities investigate the situation.
- Save any food you suspect may be contaminated. Wrap samples in their original containers or in plastic bags. Clearly label them "Do Not Use."
- Report any information you may have about the situation to your supervisor. Your supervisor is responsible for contacting the appropriate authorities for an investigation.

Any outbreak of foodborne illness must be reported to the Department of Health. If you suspect an outbreak at your facility, a quick response is essential. An outbreak could cost the establishment thousands of dollars in legal fees, insurance costs, and loss of customers. It also could force the foodservice establishment out of business.

Fig. 7-15. Salmonella bacteria is one of the leading causes of foodborne illness. How could you help prevent the spread of salmonella in a foodservice operation?

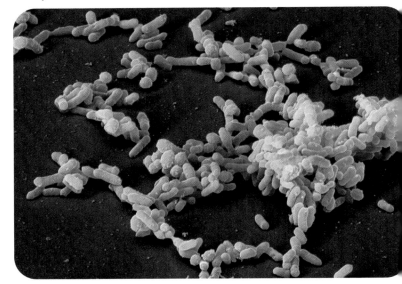

A laboratory analysis can tell which food made customers sick. In most areas, the public health department will investigate any outbreak of food-borne illness to protect public health. Their job is to learn how the illness was spread and how it can be prevented from spreading in the future. If you suspect an outbreak of foodborne illness, you should respond immediately.

■ **Bacteria.** Some forms of **bacteria** (back-TEAR-ee-ah), tiny single-celled microorganisms, can make people very sick if they find their way into food. See Fig. 7-15. People who have a bacterial illness may have symptoms that include nausea, abdominal pain, and vomiting. Other symptoms include dizziness, chills, and headache.

Bacteria are tiny and they multiply very rapidly. They can thrive in temperatures between 41°F and 135°F. Some bacteria do not need oxygen to grow. Instead, they rely on other food for energy. Bacteria prefer foods that are high in protein and moisture such as milk, meats, and seafood.

■ **Viruses.** Viruses are responsible for many food-related illnesses. In order to grow, viruses need a host, or another living cell. A host can be a person, animal, or plant on which another organism thrives. Once inside the host, the virus can multiply. Like bacteria, viruses can survive freezing and cooking. They can be transmitted easily from person to person, so they usually contaminate food when a foodservice worker uses poor hygiene. Poor hygiene may include sneezing or not washing your hands. Salads, sandwiches, milk, and other unheated food products are especially susceptible to viruses.

SAFETY & SANITATION

HEPATITIS A—Hepatitis A is a disease that causes inflammation of the liver. It can be transmitted to food by foodservice workers and by contact with contaminated water. Hepatitis A is one of the few foodborne illnesses that can be prevented. In addition to following effective hand-washing procedures, a vaccination for Hepatitis A can help protect you from infection.

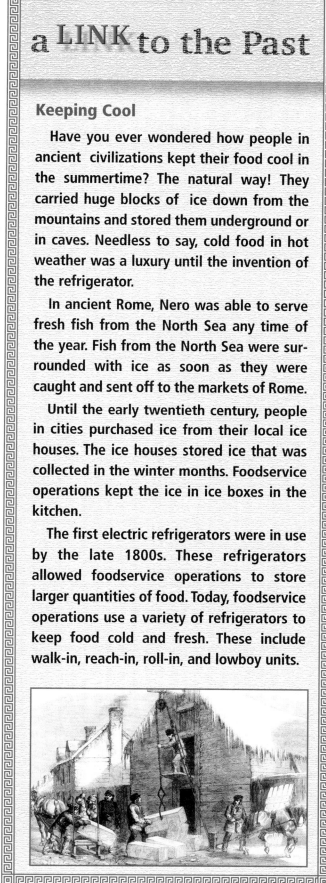

a LINK to the Past

Keeping Cool

Have you ever wondered how people in ancient civilizations kept their food cool in the summertime? The natural way! They carried huge blocks of ice down from the mountains and stored them underground or in caves. Needless to say, cold food in hot weather was a luxury until the invention of the refrigerator.

In ancient Rome, Nero was able to serve fresh fish from the North Sea any time of the year. Fish from the North Sea were surrounded with ice as soon as they were caught and sent off to the markets of Rome.

Until the early twentieth century, people in cities purchased ice from their local ice houses. The ice houses stored ice that was collected in the winter months. Foodservice operations kept the ice in ice boxes in the kitchen.

The first electric refrigerators were in use by the late 1800s. These refrigerators allowed foodservice operations to store larger quantities of food. Today, foodservice operations use a variety of refrigerators to keep food cold and fresh. These include walk-in, reach-in, roll-in, and lowboy units.

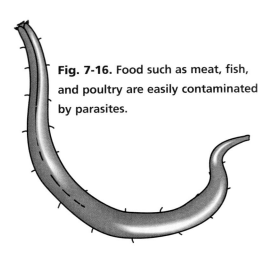

Fig. 7-16. Food such as meat, fish, and poultry are easily contaminated by parasites.

■ **Parasites. Parasites** (PAR-uh-sights) are larger than bacteria and viruses. They must live in or on a host to survive. Parasites are often found in poultry, fish, and meats. See Fig. 7-16. Some common parasites that invade food include:

• Protozoa.

• Roundworms.

• Flatworms.

Parasites can be eliminated from food by following proper cooking methods. Freezing the product for a number of days also can destroy parasites. Poultry, fish, and meat should be cooked until the minimum internal temperature is reached. You should check the food product in several different spots to be sure the safe temperature has been achieved. If the parasites are not eliminated, they can infect anyone who eats the contaminated food.

■ **Fungi. Fungi** (fun-GUY) are found in soil, plants, animals, water, and in the air. Fungi also are present in some foods. Some fungi can be large, such as mushrooms.

■ **Molds.** Molds are a form of fungus that you may have seen growing on bread or cheese. See Fig. 7-17. The fuzzy-looking spores produced by molds can be seen with the naked eye. Molds can grow at nearly any temperature, so they're often associated with food spoilage.

■ **Yeast.** Still another form of fungus is yeast. Yeast is most often associated with bread and the baking process. In this case, yeast is beneficial. However, if yeast is present in other foods, such as sauerkraut, honey, and jelly, it can cause spoilage.

Personal Hygiene

Microorganisms on tools, equipment, and cooking surfaces can get on the hands of foodservice workers. Then, when food is touched during preparation, the microorganisms can be transported from the hands to the food. The result is contamination. The key to avoiding bacterial and other biological hazards is good personal hygiene. Personal hygiene includes:

• Using proper hand-washing techniques.

• Practicing good grooming and cleanliness techniques.

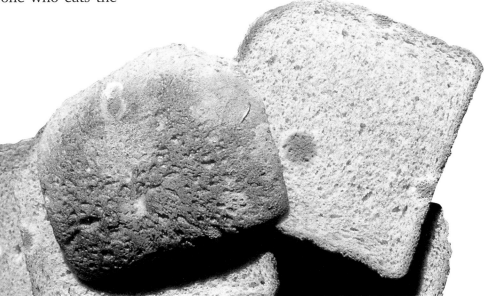

Fig. 7-17. Mold is a type of fungus. Why are some types of fungi safe to eat while others aren't?

- Wearing gloves and other protective clothing when required.
- Maintaining good health.
- Immediately reporting any illnesses or injuries to the supervisor.

⊠ CHEMICAL HAZARDS

Chemical hazards are caused by chemical substances such as cleaning supplies, pesticides, food additives, and toxic metals. If directions for a product's use aren't followed properly, the product could contaminate food. Customers could become very ill. Symptoms of food poisoning from chemical contamination can be felt immediately after the food is eaten. Material Safety Data Sheets (MSDS) must be kept on file.

Cleaning Products

Think about all the cleaning fluids and sanitizers that are commonly used in the foodservice industry. See Fig. 7-18. Some of these products are:

- **Detergents.** Used to clean walls, floors, prep surfaces, equipment, and utensils. Heavy-duty detergents are used to cut through grease.
- **Hygiene detergents.** Used to clean, deodorize, and disinfect floors, walls, and table tops.
- **Degreasers.** Degreasers are solvent cleaners. They are used on range hoods, oven doors, and backsplashes to remove grease.

- **Abrasive cleaners.** Used to scrub off soil that can be difficult to remove. Abrasive cleaners are used on floors and pots and pans to remove burned-on food. Use abrasive cleaners with caution.
- **Acid cleaners.** Used to remove mineral deposits in dishwashers and steam tables, for example. However, acid cleaners should not be used on aluminum. They will eat through the metal. Follow product directions and use with care.

To avoid possible contamination, each cleaning product should be used and stored properly. Cleaning products should not be stored near food. Cleaning products should always be kept in their original containers. They must be labeled so that employees know what's in each container. This will help prevent any possible mix-ups in the kitchen. Confusing a cleaning product for a cooking ingredient can be fatal. Disposal of cleaning products must be done according to local regulations. Local health departments will have suggestions for environmentally friendly disposal—call them for assistance.

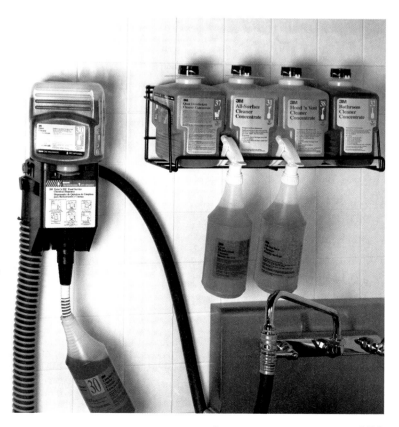

Fig. 7-18. Here are some examples of industrial cleaning products. How do industrial cleaning products differ from those used at home?

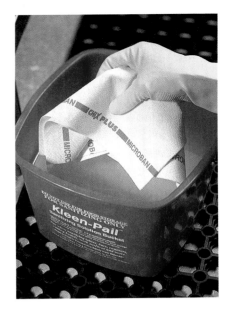

Fig. 7-19. It is important to use a sanitizing solution on all work surfaces as well as in the dishwashing process.

■ **Kitchen cleanliness.** Keeping the facilities clean and sanitary will help decrease the risk of contamination. Cleaning involves removing food and other soil from a surface. You should always clean as you work. Don't wait until all the work is done before cleaning or sanitizing. **Sanitizing** (SA-nuh-ty-zing) involves reducing the number of microorganisms on the surface. You must do both to eliminate contamination. Just because dishes, pots, pans, and work surfaces are clean, doesn't mean they're sanitary. See Fig. 7-19.

■ **Cleaning and sanitizing.** To maintain a safe environment, everything in a foodservice operation should be clean and sanitary. This means cleaning all pots, pans, and dishes, and all food contact surfaces. For example, a work surface should be thoroughly washed, rinsed, and sanitized after every use. You should clean and sanitize a surface:

• Before you use it to prepare another food product.

• If the tools you are using become contaminated by another food product.

Fig. 7-20. Salad bars are in continual use and must be kept clean to avoid contamination. What safety and sanitation practices can you identify in this photo?

• At four-hour intervals, or sooner, if the surface is continually in use. See Fig. 7-20.

Following these guidelines will help prevent cross-contamination. In addition, you can designate color-coded cutting boards and containers for use only with one type of food product. For example, a green cutting board would be used for cutting vegetables, but never for cutting chicken.

Pesticides

Many pesticides (PEHS-tuh-sides) are used in food storage and preparation areas to control pests. If used carelessly or in excessive amounts, chemical contamination can occur. As with cleaning products, it is important that pesticides be used according to directions. They should be stored properly, away from food, and in a locked or secure area. Be sure all pesticides are labeled correctly. Empty pesticide containers are considered toxic waste. Check local regulations before disposing of pesticides.

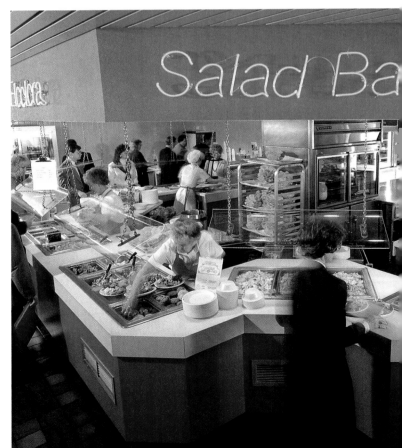

⊠ PHYSICAL HAZARDS

Physical hazards are caused by particles, such as glass chips, metal shavings, hair, bits of wood, or other foreign matter, that could get into food. Some physical hazards are found in food itself, such as bone shards or chips. However, most contamination occurs when foodhandlers do not follow proper safety and sanitation practices. Always use care when preparing, cooking, and serving food.

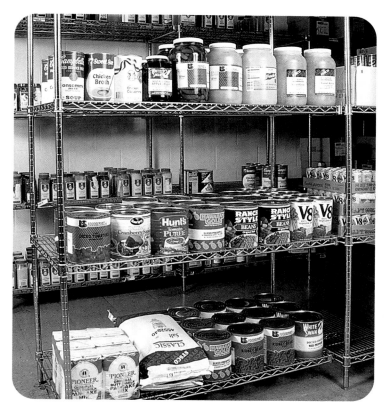

Pest Management

Wherever there is food, there is the possibility of insects and rodents. These pests can pose a serious threat to the safety of food products. Flies, roaches, and mice, for example, can carry harmful bacteria and spread disease. Once a facility is infested, it can be difficult to eliminate all pests. Therefore, establishing a sound pest management program is very important.

Most pests need water, food, and shelter. Denying mice and other pests these comforts can be an effective way to keep pests away. A clean and sanitary environment is not attractive to most pests. See Fig. 7-21. Pests seek out damp, dark, and dirty places. Make sure garbage is disposed of quickly and in the appropriate containers.

Even if you rigorously follow a good pest management program, the workplace may become infested. If so, using pesticides and other products near food can pose a risk of chemical contamination. If you suspect or see insects or rodents, report the situation to your supervisor.

Fig. 7-21. The storeroom can be a favorite feeding area for pests. What precautions should be taken to keep pests away from the storeroom and other kitchen areas?

SECTION 7-2 Knowledge Check

1. What is cross-contamination?
2. Explain the difference between biological and chemical hazards.
3. Identify the causes of foodborne illnesses.

MINI LAB

Working in teams, "swab" one area of the kitchen. Follow county health department rules and regulations. Share your team's findings with the class. Discuss how you can respond to the results.

SECTION SUMMARIES

7-1 Safety guidelines and equipment, such as wearing protective clothing, maintaining a floor free of clutter, and fire extinguishers and sprinkler systems, are used in the foodservice industry to keep workers safe.

7-1 Using precaution around gas appliances, storing oily rags properly, and keeping the workplace free of built-up grease are just three of the fire safety measures followed in a foodservice operation.

7-1 Knowing proper first aid measures prepares employees to treat emergencies such as burns, wounds, and choking.

7-1 Cardiopulmonary resuscitation is a life-saving technique used when a person is unresponsive. It involves applying firm compressions to the victim's chest.

7-2 Direct contamination occurs when raw foods are exposed to harmful organisms. Cross-contamination occurs when microorganisms are transported from one place to another.

7-2 There are three categories of hazards possible in a kitchen: biological, such as bacteria and parasites; chemical, such as cleaning products and pesticides; and physical, such as hair and metal shavings.

7-2 Prompt response to an outbreak of foodborne illness includes saving contaminated food in a plastic bag and reporting the situation to your supervisor.

CHECK YOUR KNOWLEDGE

1. Name three pieces of protective clothing.
2. What kinds of injuries can occur in the kitchen?
3. What are the four types of fire extinguishers found in most foodservice operations? When is each used?
4. What first aid measures should be followed for burns?
5. What procedure should you use to save a conscious adult from choking?
6. What is the most common source of cross-contamination?
7. What kind of potential hazard to food is yeast?
8. When is an illness considered an outbreak of foodborne illness?

CRITICAL-THINKING ACTIVITIES

1. Why do you think it's important to follow workplace safety guidelines? What could happen if people didn't follow the rules?
2. Suppose an outbreak of foodborne illness has occurred at the food service operation where you work. Why is it important to save and label the suspected contaminated food? How can this help control the outbreak?

WORKPLACE KNOW-HOW

Communication. As the manager of a cafeteria, you are responsible for ensuring that workplace safety guidelines are understood and followed. What checkpoints can you put into place to make sure employees follow these guidelines?

LAB-BASED ACTIVITY: Developing a Safety Manual

STEP ① **Working in teams, create a safety manual for a foodservice operation.** To create your manual, start by developing an outline that shows what information your team's manual will include.

STEP ② **Assign topics to each team member to ensure that everything is researched.**

STEP ③ **Decide if your team's manual will include artwork or illustrations.**

STEP ④ **Your manual should include:**
- A table of contents.
- An introductory paragraph on the importance of workplace safety.
- The role of OSHA and the EPA in ensuring workplace safety.
- The responsibilities of employers and employees in creating a safe workplace.
- Safe disposal of cleaning supplies and chemicals.
- Protective clothing checklist.
- Safety guidelines and checklist.
- First aid guidelines and a list of local emergency numbers.
- Safe disposal of pesticides.
- Personal hygiene tips.
- Cross-contamination prevention guidelines.
- Safe disposal of grease.
- Checklist of reusable containers and appropriate disposal of non-food containers.

STEP ⑤ **Complete your outline and conduct your research.**

STEP ⑥ **Write the manual.** Review the material in this chapter for information that you can use, and conduct additional research at your school library or on the Internet. You may want to contact the American Red Cross and the American Heart Association for additional information. Select pictures to include in your manual to help illustrate what you are writing.

STEP ⑦ **Share your team's safety manual with the class and display it in the classroom.**

STEP ⑧ **If you have access to the equipment, create a PowerPoint® presentation that could be used to market your team's safety manual.**

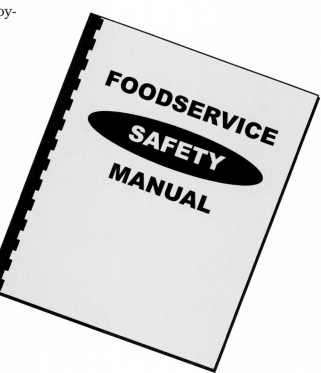

FOODSERVICE SAFETY MANUAL

HACCP Applications

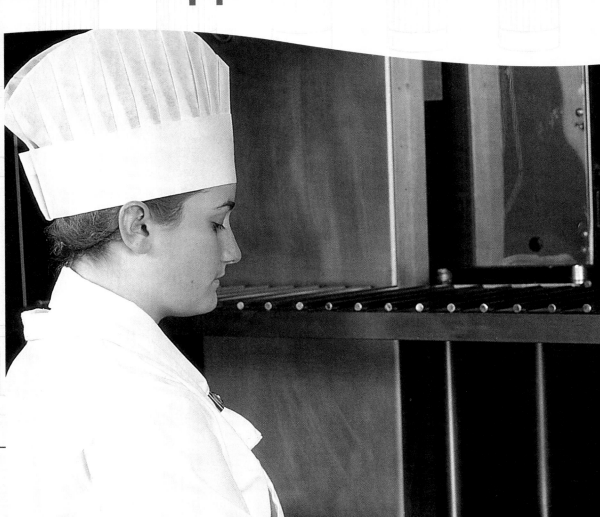

The Safe Foodhandler

KEY TERMS

• foodhandler

• hand sanitizers

OBJECTIVES

After reading this section, you will be able to:

• Demonstrate appropriate grooming for the workplace.

• Explain when and why gloves are used in the workplace.

• Demonstrate proper hand-washing procedures.

CROSS-CONTAMINATION causes foodborne illnesses. **Foodhandlers**, or workers who are in direct contact with food, usually are the cause of contamination and food-borne illnesses. Most customers expect foodservice establishments to employ workers who follow strict cleanliness guidelines. You can help prevent an outbreak of foodborne illness by practicing good grooming habits. You also must know proper hand-washing techniques. Other safety measures include wearing protective clothing and reporting illnesses.

GROOMING HABITS

Tiny microorganisms are a foodservice worker's enemy. They can be transmitted to food by food-handlers in a variety of ways. However, practicing good grooming habits is your best defense. Good grooming means bathing daily with soap and water. It also means washing your hair regularly. You should arrive at work clean. In addition you should always wear deodorant to work. Fingernails should be clean, trimmed neatly, and relatively short. It is never appropriate to wear fake fingernails or nail polish while working in the commercial kitchen. Fake fingernails can fall off into food, creating a physical hazard. Nail polish can chip off and contaminate food, posing a chemical hazard.

Clothes

Hands aren't the only way microorganisms are transferred. Clothes can also transfer bacteria to the food you handle. Dirt can be tracked into the workplace on your shoes and on your clothes.

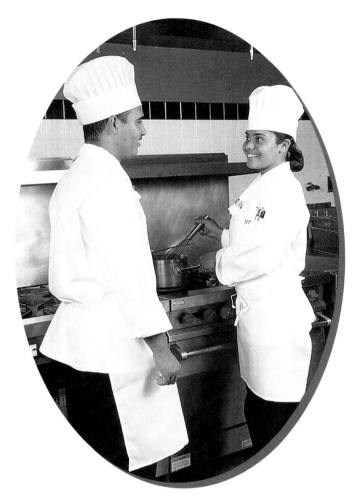

Fig. 8-1. Good grooming habits send a positive message to customers. What do you think might be considered poor grooming habits?

Always wear clean clothes to work. Most foodservice establishments will provide you with a uniform to wear. If you wear your uniform home, wash it before wearing it again. See Fig. 8-1.

Your shoes also should be appropriate for the workplace. Make sure they are comfortable. You will be on your feet for hours at a time. When selecting shoes, choose those with nonslip soles. They will help you avoid accidents. You should never wear open-toed shoes at work.

Jewelry

Believe it or not, the jewelry you wear can carry microorganisms that could make someone sick. Also, your jewelry could fall into the food, producing a physical hazard. Males and females should never wear jewelry while preparing or serving food. Remove it first. What should be removed? With the exception of a simple wedding band, all other rings, bracelets, necklaces, facial jewelry, earrings, and watches should be removed.

Hair

Many microorganisms live in human hair and can be easily transmitted to food. When you brush hair away from your face, microorganisms are transferred to your hands from your hair. When your hands touch food, the microorganisms are transferred to it. Foodborne illness can be the result.

Make it a habit to always have clean hair when you arrive at work. Dirty, oily hair is a breeding ground for microorganisms. Tie back longer hair in a hair restraint. See Fig. 8-2. Some foodservice establishments have regulations about the type of hair restraints to be used. In general, a good hair restraint, such as a hairnet, will keep your hair away from food. It also will keep you from having

Fig. 8-2. Hairnets help keep hair from falling into your face or onto food. Why is this important?

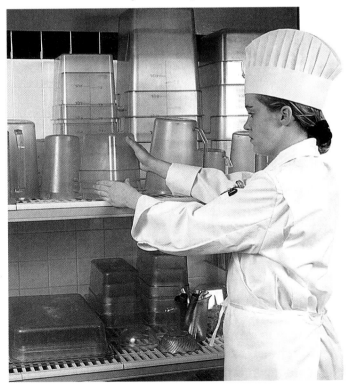

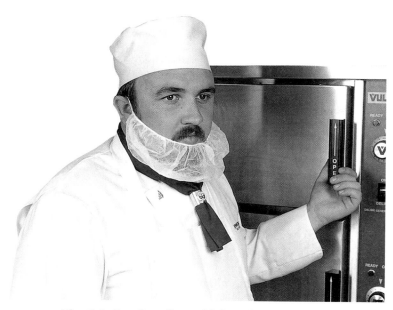

Fig. 8-3. Foodhandlers with beards are required to wear beard restraints such as the one shown here. What hazard might a beard pose to food?

to touch your hair while on the job. Foodhandlers with beards should wear beard restraints. See Fig. 8-3.

Protective Clothing

In addition to the clean clothes or uniform you wear to work, you will have protective clothing to wear. Protective clothing is worn to help minimize the possibility of food contamination. For example, if you work in preparation or clean-up areas, you'll need to wear an apron. Always make sure your apron is clean. Remove it whenever you leave the food preparation area.

Foodhandlers often wear gloves as a precautionary measure against cross-contamination. Gloves act as a wall between your hands and the food you handle. See Fig. 8-4. For

Fig. 8-4. Gloves act as a barrier between your hands and foods that will not be cooked.

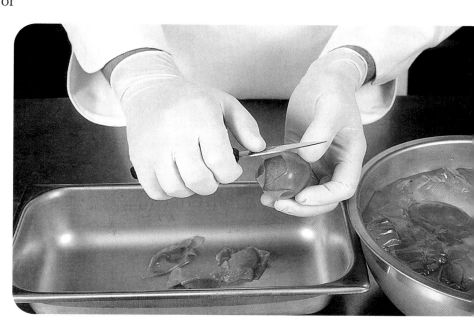

example, clear gloves are worn when serving food items in a cafeteria. This helps prevent cross-contamination. Never use soiled or torn gloves. You need to change gloves after each separate operation. You also need to change gloves approximately every four hours during continual use. Always change gloves immediately after handling any raw food.

HAND-WASHING PROCEDURE

You may think that wearing gloves can replace hand-washing. However, proper hand sanitation is extremely important in the foodservice industry. This is true even if you are wearing gloves for most tasks. Hand-washing is the most important thing you can do to prevent the transfer of food-borne bacteria.

At first, it may seem silly to think that you need to learn how to wash your hands. However, proper hand-washing techniques can mean the difference between a safe workplace and a potentially deadly one. This is because dangerous bacteria are so easily transmitted by hand.

To clean your hands and arms properly, thoroughly scrub any exposed surfaces with soap and warm water. Train yourself to always follow the steps in Fig. 8-5 on page 180.

Fig. 8-5. Proper hand-washing procedure.

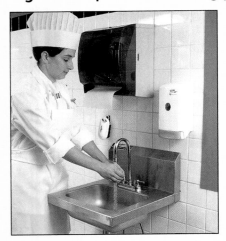

1. Wet hands and forearms with hot water.

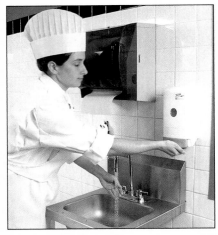

2. Apply enough soap to build up a good lather.

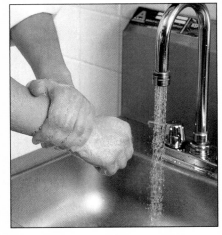

3. Rub hands and arms for at least 20 seconds.

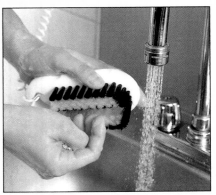

4. Clean fingernails with a brush.

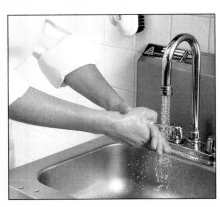

5. Rinse off soap thoroughly under running hot water.

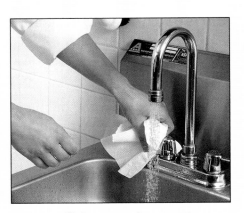

6. Turn off the water faucet using a paper towel.

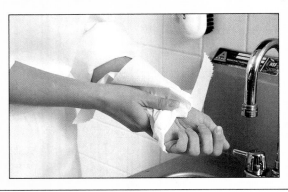

7. Dry hands and arms using a separate paper towel.

You should wash your hands every two hours to prevent cross-contamination. Always wash your hands:

- Before starting work.
- After any work breaks, including those to eat, smoke, drink, or chew gum.
- Before and after handling raw foods such as meat, fish, and poultry.
- After touching your hair, face, or body.
- After sneezing, coughing, or using a tissue.
- After using the restroom.
- After using any cleaning or sanitizing product.

- After taking out garbage.
- After cleaning dirty dishes and tables.
- After touching anything else that might contaminate food, such as a phone, money, door handles, or soiled tablecloths.

Several hand sanitizers are now widely available that can be used after washing. **Hand sanitizers** are special liquids that kill bacteria on your skin often without the use of water. While these products can reduce bacteria on hands, never use a hand sanitizer in place of hand-washing on the job.

PERSONAL HEALTH

Foodservice professionals need to be in good physical health when working with food. Otherwise, harmful bacteria can be spread from the foodhandler to the food that will be served. Foodborne illness could be the result.

■ **Illness.** If you have symptoms of a disease that can be transmitted, such as fever, sneezing, coughing, vomiting, or diarrhea, call your employer. You should not come to work sick.

If you feel ill while at work, it is your responsibility to immediately tell your supervisor. This is the only way to prevent contamination of the foods and work surfaces with which you come into contact.

■ **Wounds.** If you have a wound that may be infected, or a cut, burn, boil, or other sore, you might not feel sick. However, the bacteria in the wound could easily spread to the food you handle. Because of this, it's very important that you wash your hands thoroughly. Keep cuts completely covered. Make sure the bandage is kept clean and dry. See Fig. 8-6. If you have a wound on your hand, you may be reassigned to a work area where you won't come into direct contact with food.

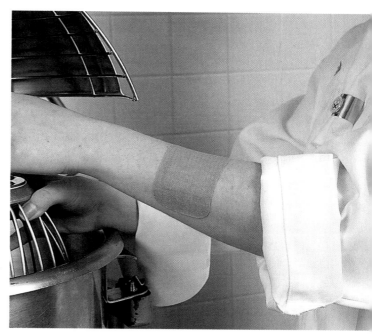

Fig. 8-6. If you must come to work with a wound, be sure it is clean and properly bandaged.

| SECTION 8-1 | Knowledge Check |

1. Summarize the grooming and personal hygiene habits all foodservice workers should follow.
2. List three instances when you should change gloves. How does this help improve workplace sanitation and safety?
3. When should you wash your hands at work?

MINI LAB

Choose a partner. Take turns demonstrating proper hand-washing procedure. Have your partner evaluate your hand-washing technique. Then, evaluate your partner's hand-washing technique. Practice until you both perform the technique correctly.

The HACCP System

KEY TERMS

- flow of food
- HACCP
- critical control point
- minimum internal temperature
- calibrated

OBJECTIVES

After reading this section, you will be able to:

- Explain the purpose of the HACCP System.
- State different hazards in the foodservice workplace.
- Describe the processes of monitoring, corrective action, record keeping, and verification.

A S food moves through a foodservice operation, it's important to be able to identify potential hazards. By using a time-tested system called HACCP, the flow of food can be monitored. The flow of food is the path food takes from receiving to disposal. Along this path, hazards can be controlled and dangers minimized.

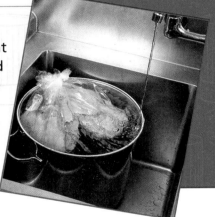

✕ WHAT IS HACCP?

Local health departments regularly inspect foodservice establishments. Your workplace also will use self-inspection steps to maintain sanitary conditions. **HACCP**, or Hazard Analysis Critical Control Point, is the system used by foodservice establishments. This system helps ensure food safety. HACCP combines:

- Food-handling procedures.
- Monitoring techniques.
- Record keeping.

The HACCP System was developed by the Pillsbury Company for the National Aeronautics and Space Administration (NASA) in the early 1960s. The system was designed to make food safe in outer space. HACCP was so beneficial, it was adopted by many segments of the food industry. Over the years, HACCP has been improved, and is now accepted worldwide. The HACCP System focuses attention on the flow of food through the foodservice facility at critical points. It helps foodservice employees:

- Identify foods and procedures that are likely to cause foodborne illness.
- Develop facility procedures that will reduce the risk of foodborne illness.
- Monitor procedures in order to keep food safe.
- Make sure that the food served is safe. See Fig. 8-7.

Fig. 8-7.

The HACCP System

Determine where food safety hazards might occur. For example, think about what food comes in contact with in the entire establishment.

▼

Find the critical control points in the flow of food that prevent a food safety hazard.

▼

Set boundaries or standards that are necessary for food to be considered safe. For example, set temperature limits for foods to be safe.

▼

Establish a procedure for monitoring the standards. For example, you might use a thermometer to check the temperatures of all foods and keep a record of these temperatures.

▼

Decide what to do if a standard is not met. For example, if a cooked food doesn't meet a standard you may decide to alter the cooking method.

▼

Evaluate your procedures regularly. You may need to modify your procedures in order to keep food safe.

▼

Develop a record-keeping system that identifies:
* Who documents the procedures.
* How documentation should be performed.
* When documentation should be performed.

HACCP Hazards

The first step of HACCP is to identify and evaluate hazards. These hazards could cause illness or injury if they're not controlled. The most frequently found hazards include:
* Poor personal hygiene.
* Contaminated raw foods.
* Cross-contamination.
* Improper cooking.
* Improper holding.
* Improper cooling.
* Improper reheating.
* Improper cleaning and sanitizing of equipment.

Any of these hazards can lead to an outbreak of foodborne illness. Because of this, it's critical that foodservice workers follow the HACCP System.

Critical Control Points

The next step in the HACCP System involves analyzing each control point. See Fig. 8-8. A **critical control point** is a step in the flow of food where contamination can be prevented or eliminated. For example, cooking food improperly allows bacteria and other harmful biological haz-

Fig. 8-8.
HACCP Analysis—The Flow of Food

POTENTIAL HAZARD	CONTROL POINT	CORRECTIVE ACTION
Selection of hazardous items; improper food preparation.	Menu Items & Recipes	Proper training.
Receipt and acceptance of contaminated food products.	Receiving	Inspect each delivery, reject contaminated goods.
Cross-contamination; improper storage resulting in spoilage; bacteria.	Storing	Follow FIFO procedures; maintain proper storage temperatures; discard old items.
Cross-contamination; bacteria.	Food Preparation	Good personal hygiene; gloves; hand washing; clean and sanitize utensils and work surfaces.
Bacteria not killed; physical and chemical contaminants.	Cooking	Achieve the minimum internal temperature.
Bacteria; physical contaminants.	Food Holding & Serving	Maintain proper temperatures, use clean serving equipment.
Bacteria.	Cooling	Apply rapid cooling methods; store food properly.
Bacteria.	Reheating	Heat food rapidly; don't mix old food with new food.

ards to grow. When a food such as poultry is cooked, the minimum internal temperature must be reached. If it isn't, microorganisms could survive and contaminate the food. This could make those who eat the food very sick. Cooking at high temperatures kills harmful microorganisms.

The same is true for cooling food. If food is cooled improperly, harmful bacteria can grow. Cooling food quickly prevents bacterial growth. According to the U.S. Centers for Disease Control, improperly cooled food is the most common cause of all reported foodborne illness. One technique used to cool food is as follows:

1. Place food in a shallow pan.

2. Place the pan of food into a large pan filled with ice. Do not stack more than one pan of food on top of the large pan of ice.

3. Use a thermometer to check the internal temperature of the food often. Foods that have an internal temperature of 140°F should drop to 70°F within 2 hours and to 41°F or below within 4 hours. Replenish ice as needed.

4. When the chilled temperature has been achieved, remove the pan of food from the pan of ice.

5. Dry the bottom of the pan of food and place the pan on the top shelf of the refrigerator.

6. Place a lid on the pan of food.

7. Label the pan of food with the date the food was prepared and its temperature at the time of storage.

Controlling Hazards

After you've identified the critical control points, it's important that you follow the procedures for minimizing hazards. For example, temperature and time control are two important measurements that impact food safety. The HACCP System has established standards for the internal cooking temperatures of foods. See Fig. 8-9.

The high temperatures you use when cooking food kill most of the food's harmful bacteria. The **minimum internal temperature** is the lowest temperature at which foods can be safely cooked. Below this temperature, microorganisms cannot be destroyed. This temperature varies from food to food, so it's important to learn the correct temperature for each food you prepare.

■ **Temperature danger zone.** The temperature danger zone is 41°F to 135°F. Foods must be thrown away after four hours if they are not held at 135°F or above. The four-hour time zone begins when food is received. Every time the food is within the temperature danger zone, the four-hour time zone decreases. It does not begin again. See Fig. 8-10.

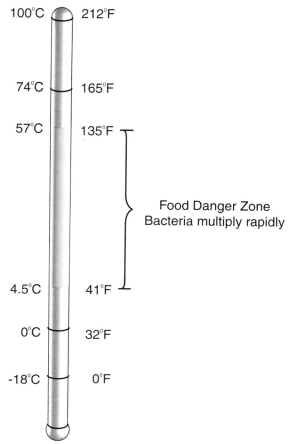

Fig. 8-10. The temperature danger zone is 41°F–135°F. What should you do with food that has been in the danger zone for more than four hours?

Fig. 8-9.
Safe Internal Cooking Temperatures

FOOD ITEM	TEMPERATURE	TIME
Pork, ham, bacon	145°F	15 seconds
Poultry, stuffed meats and pasta, casseroles, stuffings	165°F	15 seconds
Roasts (beef and pork)	145°F	4 minutes
Hamburger, ground pork, sausages, flaked fish	160°F	15 seconds
Steaks, veal, lamb	145°F	15 seconds
Fish	145°F	15 seconds
Eggs	145°F	15 seconds

Battle Against Bacteria

How can you tell if food has spoiled? Often, the odor of the food is the first sign. It was the odor of spoiled food that led French scientist Louis Pasteur to study the mysteries of bacteria. Born in France in 1822, Pasteur was a pioneer in the study of science and medicine. Pasteur was the first to show that living things come only from other living things.

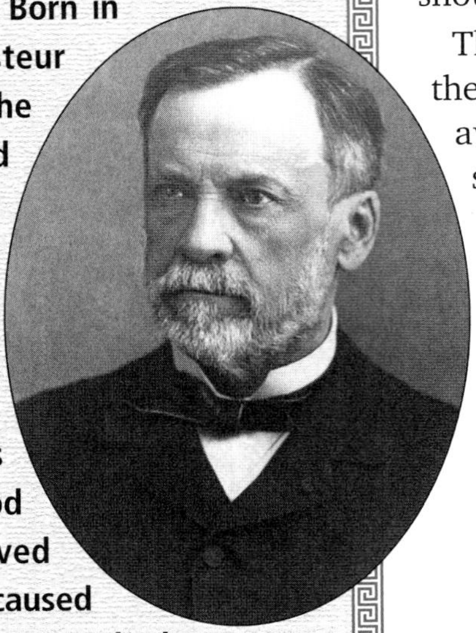

How does Pasteur's work affect the food industry? He believed something in the air caused food to spoil. Pasteur searched for living particles too small to be seen by the human eye. His search led to the discovery that bacteria in food multiply rapidly and cause the food to spoil. Pasteur suggested killing these germs by applying controlled heat. This process is known as *pasteurization*.

Today, pasteurization is commonly used for milk and other dairy products. Pasteurized foods that are placed in *aseptic* packages, such as drink boxes, do not need to be refrigerated. The aseptic packaging system works by filling a sterilized package with a sterile food product within the confines of a hygienic environment.

■ **Food thermometers.** There are a variety of food thermometers used to check the temperatures of foods. Both bi-metallic and digital thermometers are used in the foodservice industry. Fig. 8-11 shows several thermometers.

Thermometers are used to measure the internal temperature of cooked food. To do this, place the thermometer in the thickest part of the food. Take at least two readings in different places. Use thermometers to check the temperature of delivered foods, too. Fresh foods should be received at a temperature of 41°F or below. Thermometers should be accurate to within 2°F.

Thoroughly clean, sanitize, and air dry the thermometer after each use. This will help you avoid cross-contamination. Thermometers should be **calibrated** (ka-luh-brate-ed), or adjusted, before each shift or each delivery. A thermometer will also need to be recalibrated if it is dropped.

Fig. 8-11. Foodservice operations use a variety of food thermometers. What types of thermometers are shown here?

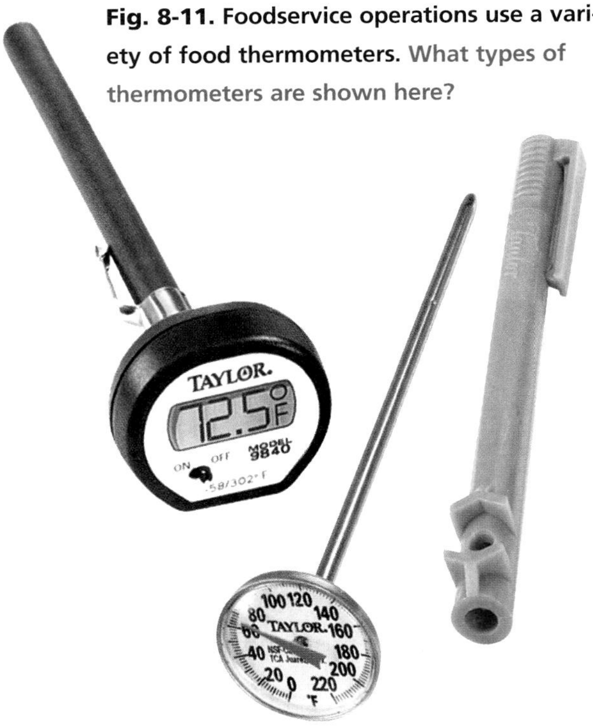

✖ MONITORING THE SYSTEM

Foodservice workers are responsible for monitoring, or checking, the systems in place. This allows them to ensure that proper procedures are followed in the flow of food. It can also help them spot potential problems.

For example, you should monitor the temperature of turkey breast when it is received. Make sure it is stored at the proper temperature of 41°F or below. You should also be concerned about contamination that could occur during storage. Raw turkey breast should be stored below cooked foods in the refrigerator and any ready-to-eat foods such as salads. This will prevent turkey juices from dripping on and contaminating any foods stored beneath them.

Corrective Action

When a potential hazard is found at a critical control point, you should take corrective action immediately. Refer to Fig. 8-8. It is the responsibility of each foodservice worker to make sure that the environment is a safe one.

For example, you see a foodhandler roasting whole chickens. You notice that he or she isn't checking the internal temperature of the food to determine that it has been reached. What should you do? Take immediate corrective action. Remind the foodhandler that the temperature needs to be taken before the food is served.

Chicken that is not cooked until the minimum internal temperature is met can carry harmful microorganisms. These microorganisms can be transferred to people when they eat the food. The result could be foodborne illness.

Verification

A very important step in the HACCP System is to verify that your system is working correctly. This ensures that the food you prepare and serve is safe. Foods should be traced through the operation at the end of each shift by the chef or manager. He or she should examine record-keeping logs of temperature and time, note any errors, and take any corrective action if necessary.

Record Keeping

Record keeping is an important part of maintaining an effective self-inspection system. Most record-keeping systems are simple to use and maintain. Record-keeping systems include:
- Flow charts.
- Policy and procedure manuals.
- Written logs.
- Spot-check temperature readings.

Logs are usually completed at the end of each shift or meal period. Be sure to find out which record-keeping systems are in use at your foodservice establishment. Follow directions for completing them thoroughly and carefully.

SECTION 8-2 | Knowledge Check

1. What is the purpose of the HACCP System?
2. Explain the food temperature danger zone.
3. Name three types of record keeping that might be used in a foodservice establishment.

MINI LAB

Divide into teams. Choose one HACCP critical control point. Role play how your team could avoid potential hazards related to your critical control point.

The Flow of Food

KEY TERMS

- **receiving**
- **storing**
- **FIFO**
- **pasteurized**
- **perishable**
- **holding**

OBJECTIVES

After reading this section, you will be able to:

- Explain why it is important to inspect all food products for damage and spoilage when they are received.
- Identify safety measures to take when preparing food.
- Identify safety measures to take when holding and serving food.
- Explain the steps involved in cleaning and sanitizing.

CRITICAL control points are steps in the flow of food. It's here that special attention is given to food products to prevent contamination. At each point in the flow of food, from **receiving**, or accepting deliveries, through serving, you'll need to be concerned with food safety and with sanitation.

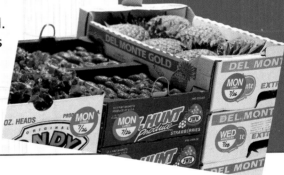

❎ RECEIVING & STORING FOOD SAFELY

Safety and sanitation procedures begin with receiving. No matter what food product you receive, it must be carefully inspected for damage. You also need to ensure that the food has been maintained at the proper temperatures during transit. As a foodservice professional, you will need to become familiar with these potential problem areas:

- Foods that have been thawed and refrozen.
- Foods that have insect infestation.
- Damaged foods or containers.
- Items that have been repacked or mishandled.
- Foods handled at incorrect temperatures.

Storing food, or placing food in a location for later use, is another control point where improper handling can result in contamination. All foods should be stored properly. This will prevent contamination, spoilage, and the growth of harmful bacteria. Always keep storage areas clean and dry. Make sure the temperature is monitored.

Different foods are stored in different places. There are three types of storage: dry, refrigerated, and frozen. The type of storage used depends on the type of food product being stored.

■ **Dry storage.** Foods that have a long shelf life are placed in dry storage. Flour, salt, dried beans, and canned foods are examples. The ideal temperature in a dry storage area is 50°–70°F. All stored food products should be kept at least six inches off the floor and six inches away from the wall.

- **Refrigerated storage.** Food products that need refrigeration should be kept at or below 41°F. Clearly label and date all containers. To prolong the shelf life of a product, use the "First In, First Out" inventory program, or **FIFO**. Store cooked foods and raw ingredients separately to prevent cross-contamination. If prepared or cooked and raw foods must be stored on the same side or shelving unit, always store cooked foods above raw foods. Frozen foods that are being thawed in the refrigerator should always be stored below prepared foods. Be sure to leave room for air to circulate.

- **Frozen storage.** Store frozen foods at 0°F or below. Clearly label and date all containers. Never put a hot food product into a freezer, because this will affect the temperature of the storage area. It could cause foods in the freezer to thaw and remain in the temperature danger zone for extended periods of time.

Seafood

Fish and shellfish are very sensitive to changes in temperature. If the correct temperature for seafood is not maintained, microorganisms will multiply rapidly.

Fresh, whole fish should be packed in ice at a temperature of 41°F or lower. See Fig. 8-12. The fish should have bright and shiny skin. The texture should be firm and the flesh should spring back when touched.

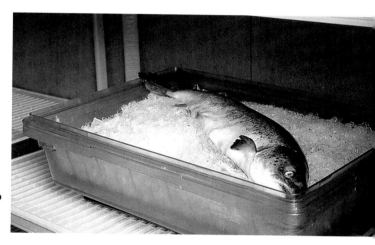

Fig. 8-12. When receiving fish and shellfish, check to ensure that the internal temperature is below 41°F.

THE KITCHEN "GLOW"

Due to the increase of foodborne illness, much research has gone into monitoring the cleanliness of foodservice operations. Although work surfaces, equipment, walls, floors, etc. may appear to "look clean," from a microscopic level, they may be contaminated. One way to determine the presence of bacteria is called adenosine triphosphate bioluminescence (ah-DEE-nah-seen try-FOSS-fate bi-o-lou-mah-NES-ents), or the "glow" test.

Adenosine triphosphate, known as ATP, is an energy molecule found in all living cells. So, a large concentration of bacteria will contain a large concentration of ATP molecules. In order to test the presence of ATP, an enzyme called luciferase (lou-SIF-eh-rase) is placed on the area to be tested. Luciferase is the enzyme found in the tails of fireflies. If luciferase comes in contact with ATP, light is emitted. A small portable machine, called a luminometer, is then used to test the amount of light output. The stronger the light that is produced, the more contaminated the area.

APPLY IT!

1. List four commonly known bacteria that contaminate a food environment.
2. Contact your local department of health to arrange a "glow" test demonstration.

The Food and Drug Administration (FDA) closely oversees the shipping of shellfish. Shellfish must be purchased from an approved FDA supplier. Shucked shellfish in packages of less than one-half gallon will have a sell-by date clearly shown on the label. Shucked shellfish have been removed from the shell. Packages with more than one-half gallon of shellfish will show the date the shellfish were shucked.

If you receive a container of live clams, oysters, or mussels, you must write the date they were delivered on the tag that is fastened to the container. These identification tags are kept for 90 days after the last shellfish has been used. This information is used to determine the source for possible contamination.

Fresh Meat & Poultry

Government agencies are responsible for inspecting fresh meat and poultry to make sure it is free from disease. They have strict quality standards and regulations that must be followed. However, microorganisms can still remain on a food product during processing. These microorganisms will multiply rapidly causing the food product to be contaminated.

To help ensure that this doesn't happen to your fresh meat and poultry, follow these guidelines:

- **Temperature.** The product should be delivered at 41°F or below.
- **Color.** Beef and lamb should be red; pork should be light pink. Poultry should not be a purple or green color. It shouldn't have dark wing tips.
- **Odor.** Meat and poultry should not have an offensive or sour odor.

- **Texture.** Meat should not feel slimy. Poultry should not be sticky under the wings or around joints.
- **Packaging.** Check for broken cartons, soiled wrappers, and leakage.

Meat and poultry also must be purchased from processing plants approved by the United States Department of Agriculture (USDA). Those products that have been inspected bear a seal of approval. See Fig. 8-13.

Eggs

Like meat and poultry, eggs must be purchased from USDA-approved processing plants. Make sure the eggs you receive and store bear the USDA inspection stamp. This stamp shows that the eggs have been purchased from a government-approved supplier. Eggs should be clean, dry, and uncracked.

When the eggs arrive at a delivery dock, they must be checked. Eggs should be received within a few days of the packing date. Store eggs immediately in a refrigerated storage area.

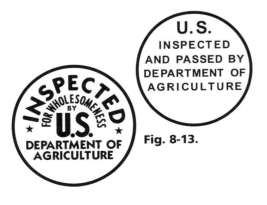

Fig. 8-13.

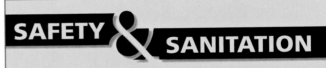

EGG SAFETY—Take the following extra precautions when preparing eggs:

- Always store eggs and foods that contain eggs separate from raw foods. Also avoid foods that may have an undesirable odor. Eggs absorb odors easily.
- Always wash your hands before and after working with eggs and foods that contain eggs.
- Wash, rinse, and sanitize utensils, equipment, and work surfaces after you prepare eggs or products that contain eggs.
- Make sure cooked eggs do not sit out for more than a very short period of time.

Fig. 8-14.

Unsafe Canned Goods

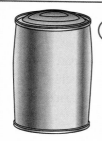

BULGES
Discard immediately. The can may have gas built up inside.

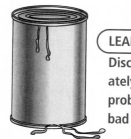

LEAKAGE
Discard immediately. The can probably has a bad seal.

RUSTY
Discard immediately. The can may be old.

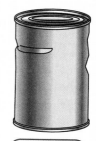

DENTS
Discard immediately. The can may have broken seams.

Dairy Products

Foodservice establishments should purchase and serve pasteurized dairy products. **Pasteurized** products have been heated at temperatures that kill bacteria. Unpasteurized products can contain dangerous levels of microorganisms that can cause foodborne illness. Milk and milk products labeled Grade A show that they meet FDA standards.

Dairy products, such as cheese, sour cream, yogurt, and butter, should be received at 41°F or below.

Refrigerated & Frozen Foods

Many foodservice establishments use some foods that have already been prepared before they are received at your facility. Refrigerated processed foods should be delivered at 41°F or below. Frozen foods should be received frozen. Always closely inspect packages, just as you would for meat and poultry, to check for damage.

All frozen foods should be frozen when they arrive at your facility. Check for signs that the food product has thawed and then been refrozen. You may be able to tell this by looking closely at the food. It may be discolored or dry. Another indication that the food may have thawed is liquid at the bottom of a product's container.

Dry & Canned Goods

Dry and canned goods have a longer shelf life than fresh meat, poultry, eggs, or produce. But that doesn't mean you shouldn't be concerned about food safety. Follow these guidelines for storing dried foods:

- Inspect packages for damage.
- Keep them in tightly sealed containers.
- Keep them dry.
- Watch for signs of insects and rodents.
- Check regularly for signs of spoilage.

Commercial canned goods also require your close attention. See Fig. 8-14 for signs of potential contamination.

Fresh Produce

The temperature for receiving and storing fresh produce varies depending on the product. Remember, however, fresh fruits and vegetables are perishable. **Perishable** (PAIR-ih-shuh-buhl) products are those that can spoil quickly, especially if not stored properly. Follow these general guidelines for receiving and storing fresh produce:

- Don't wash produce before storing.
- Wash produce just prior to preparing.
- Handle with care. Most produce bruises easily.
- Check produce for insects and insect eggs.
- Check produce for spoilage, such as mold, bruising, or wilting.

✖ PREPARATION & COOKING

You now know how to safely receive and store food according to the proper procedures. There are still several points in the flow of food at which food could become unsafe. One of those points is food preparation. Remember that you need to cook certain foods, such as poultry and meat, at specific temperatures in order to keep them safe.

Another way to keep food safe is to prevent cross-contamination and microorganism growth. Cold protein salads, such as chicken salad, can be the perfect vehicle for microorganism growth. Because raw and cooked foods are combined, not all of the microorganisms are killed by heat.

To avoid contamination during food handling, use recommended utensils, such as tongs or spatulas, rather than your hands. Hands can carry bacteria. Always make sure equipment, utensils, cutting boards, and other surfaces are cleaned and sanitized often. Keep foods covered when possible.

To avoid cross-contamination wash all fresh fruits and vegetables before preparation. Wash root vegetables and starches before and after peeling. Never prepare uncooked meats in the same area used to prepare fruits and vegetables.

Each type of food product you prepare is susceptible to a different kind of contamination. Knowing the risks of individual foods will help you prepare them safely for customers. See Fig. 8-15.

Fig. 8-15.

GENERAL PREPARATION AND COOKING GUIDELINES

- Use clean, sanitized cutting boards, knives, and utensils.
- Don't remove all the food product from the refrigerator at one time. Work with only as much product as you need for one hour.
- Always prepare produce on a separate area from raw meats, poultry, eggs, or fish.
- Clean and sanitize knives each time you prepare a different food product.
- Don't let food sit on the counter. Prepare or cook it immediately or return what is left to storage.
- Keep cold ingredients properly chilled in the refrigerator until you need them.
- Fully cook protein ingredients, such as chicken, before you mix them with other food products.
- Closely follow recipe directions when preparing foods.
- Cook food to the proper internal temperature.
- Don't mix leftover food with freshly prepared foods.
- Boil leftover sauces and gravies before serving.
- Thoroughly cook foods that have been battered or breaded.

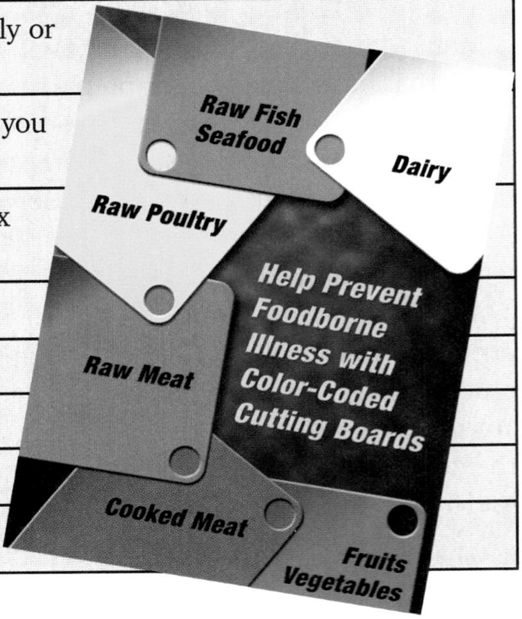

Raw Fish Seafood

Dairy

Raw Poultry

Raw Meat

Help Prevent Foodborne Illness with Color-Coded Cutting Boards

Cooked Meat

Fruits Vegetables

HOLDING FOOD SAFELY

In some foodservice establishments, foods may be cooked and served immediately. However, in other facilities, foods must be prepared ahead of time. Foods are then placed in an appropriate location. They are held, or kept warm, until someone orders it. This process is called **holding**. For example, you might prepare a bean soup for lunch, and the soup might be served over a three-hour lunch period. The soup would be held for service.

It's important that you learn how to hold foods properly. Foods are extremely susceptible to microorganism growth during holding. Here are general guidelines you can follow to ensure that food is held safely:

- Keep foods covered to reduce contamination.
- Take the internal food temperature regularly (a minimum of every two hours).
- Hold cooked foods at 135°F or above. If the temperature drops below 135°F, reheat the food to 165°F for 15 seconds. Hold it again at 135°F. If the temperature drops below 135°F for a second time, discard the food. Do not reheat it again.
- Hold cold food at 41°F or below.
- Stir hot foods regularly.
- Do not warm up cold food by placing it directly into a steam table.
- Never mix a fresh batch of food with food that's been in holding. Discard food after it has been held for four hours.
- Do not store cold food directly on ice. Put the food in a storage container and then put the container down in the ice until the food and the ice are at the same level.

SERVING FOOD SAFELY

You may recall that people are the main cause of cross-contamination. When food is served, the chances of contamination are high. It's important to learn the foodservice establishment's specific rules about how foods should be served.

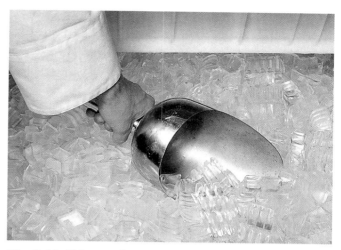

Fig. 8-16. Using tools properly helps prevent the spread of microorganisms.

However, there are several general guidelines that all foodservice workers should follow at this important step in the flow of food:

- Never touch ready-to-eat food with your bare hands.
- Never touch the food-contact surfaces of glasses, dinnerware, or flatware. Hold dishes by the bottom or an edge; hold cups by their handles; glassware by the lower third; and hold flatware by the handles.
- Never allow one plate of food to overlap onto another plate of food.
- Use tongs or scoops to pick up ice. Never use your hands. See Fig. 8-16.
- Cleaning cloths should only be used for cleaning.

COOLING FOOD SAFELY

The FDA recommends a two-stage method for cooling food safely. In the first stage, cooked foods are cooled down to 70°F within two hours. The second stage involves cooling the food down below 41°F in four hours. The two-stage method takes a total of six hours. However, some foodservice facilities use a one-stage, four-hour method, by which food is cooled to less than 41°F.

Refrigerators are not designed to cool hot foods. They are designed to hold cooled foods at cold

Fig. 8-17.

TYPE OF SANITIZER	AMOUNT TO USE	WHEN TO USE
Chlorine	1 t. per gallon	Soft or hard water at 75°F
Iodine	2 T. per 5 gallons	Hard water between 75°F–120°F
Quaternary Ammonia	About 1 t. per gallon	Soft water at 75°F

temperatures. Remember that the more dense, or thick, a food is, the slower it will cool. The container in which food is stored also determines how fast it will cool. Shallow stainless steel pans allow food to cool fast. Position labeled and dated pans so that air can circulate around them in the refrigerator.

⌧ REHEATING FOODS SAFELY

Reheating previously cooked foods must be done carefully. It must be reheated to an internal temperature of 165°F for 15 seconds within two hours of being removed from the refrigerator. If you are adding a previously cooked food to another food, such as tomato sauce to spaghetti, the whole mixture must be reheated to 165°F.

⌧ DISPOSAL POINT

The last stop in the flow of food is the disposal point. After foods have been prepared, cooked, and consumed, the remaining food must be disposed of properly. Cleaning and sanitizing are key actions taken at this point. Dishes, smallwares, utensils, and equipment must be cleaned and sanitized. The first step is to remove leftover food from dishes, equipment, tools, and smallwares. Food should be scraped into the garbage can. Then the dish or tool should be rinsed over the disposal before it is washed. Most foodservice operations use a combination of commercial sinks and dishwashers. Chemical sanitizers are used in both sinks and dishwashers to prevent bacteria growth. See Figure 8-17.

Manual Dishwashing

A three-compartment commercial sink is used for manual dishwashing. See Fig. 8-18. To wash items by hand, you must first scrape and pre-rinse them. Next, wash them in at least 110°F water and detergent. Then, rinse the dishes with clear water that is 110°F. Change the water as needed to keep it clear and hot. Sanitize items in at least 171°F water that contains a chemical solution for 30 seconds. Some health codes require 180°F water for sanitizing. Remove the items and allow them to air dry. Store items in a clean, dry area.

■ **Cleaning utensils.** To clean utensils, follow the manual dishwashing procedures. Never use steel wool or metal scouring pads on utensils. They can cause nicks and scratches. Bacteria can hide and multiply in these places. In addition, steel wool fragments may remain on pots or pans, creating a physical hazard if they make their way into food. Sponges should not be used because they are great hiding places for bacteria.

Fig. 8-18. A three-compartment sink is used to wash, rinse, and sanitize dishes. Be sure to use the proper proportion of sanitizer and water, and the correct water temperature.

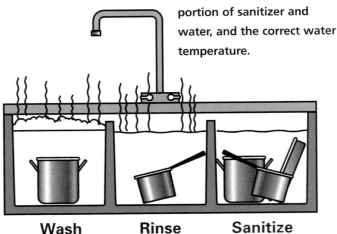

Wash   **Rinse**   **Sanitize**

Using a Commercial Dishwasher

Foodservice operations clean and sanitize a large volume of dishes. As you've read, dishes can be cleaned manually. However, it is more efficient to use commercial dishwashers for large amounts.

There are a wide variety of commercial dishwashers. See Fig. 8-19. They include: single-compartment, multi-compartment, carousel, recirculating, and conveyor.

These general guidelines can be followed when using a commercial dishwasher. They do not replace the need to read the instruction manual, however.

■ **Before running a dishwasher.** Before you can load dishes into a dishwasher, the following steps must be taken:

- Scrape and rinse soiled dishes and presoak flatware.
- Pre-rinse dishes to remove all visible food and soil.
- Rack dishes and flatware in a way that the water will spray all surfaces.

■ **Running a dishwasher.** To clean and sanitize the dishes effectively, run the dishwasher for a full cycle. Check the instruction manual for specific water temperatures required for each cycle.

Drying & Storing Items

After the dishes have been cleaned and sanitized, allow them to air dry. Do not touch dish surfaces that will come in contact with food. Be sure to wash your hands before storing items in a clean, dry area.

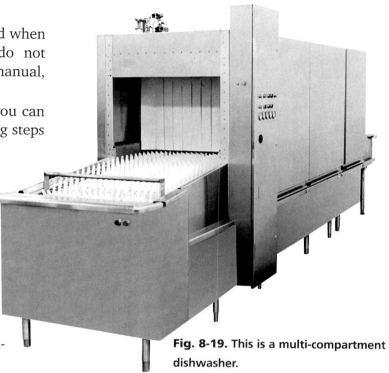

Fig. 8-19. This is a multi-compartment dishwasher.

SECTION 8-3 Knowledge Check

1. Explain how you can tell if fish is fresh.
2. How can you be sure the meat, poultry, and eggs you receive are from a government-approved supplier?
3. What are two things you can do when preparing fruits and vegetables to help reduce the growth of microorganisms?

MINI LAB

Working in teams, prepare four different cooked vegetables. Document the precautions your team takes to store the vegetable dish so that it is kept safe. Serve your dish the following day and share the precautions your team used.

CHAPTER (8) Review & Activities

SECTION SUMMARIES

8-1 Good grooming habits include bathing daily, wearing deodorant, and trimming fingernails.

8-1 In addition to hand-washing, gloves should be worn and changed often to prevent cross-contamination.

8-1 Hand-washing involves washing the hands, fingernails, and arms.

8-1 Foodhandlers need to be in good physical health to prevent the spread of foodborne illnesses.

8-2 HACCP was originally designed by NASA to ensure food safety for astronauts, and is now used in the foodservice industry as a self-inspection system.

8-2 Foodservice hazards can be biological, chemical, or physical.

8-2 Cooking and cooling foods are two critical control points in the flow of food.

8-2 For HACCP to be effective, foodservice professionals must monitor the systems they have in place and take corrective action where necessary.

8-3 All food products must be inspected carefully for signs of damage such as leaking packages, insect infestation, repackaging, and mishandling.

8-3 After food products are received, they must be stored quickly and properly to avoid contamination.

8-3 Cross-contamination is the greatest hazard to food during food preparation.

8-3 When food is being held or stored, bacteria growth is a possible source of contamination that must be monitored.

8-3 Cleaning and sanitizing are key actions taken at the disposal point in the flow of food.

CHECK YOUR KNOWLEDGE

1. What kind of hazard can human hair pose to food?
2. Name two articles of protective clothing worn at work.
3. Describe the hand-washing procedure.
4. What does HACCP stand for?
5. List the critical control points in the flow of food.
6. What is the temperature danger zone?
7. Name three types of food storage.
8. What does holding food mean?
9. Describe the process used to manually clean and sanitize dishes.

CRITICAL-THINKING ACTIVITIES

1. You are preparing soup in a stockpot on the range and notice a human hair floating in the soup. Why might this be a problem? How should you correct the problem?

2. As food moves through the various critical control points of the HACCP System, foodservice workers monitor the system to ensure standards are met. Why is this important? How do foodservice workers prove that the HACCP System is effective?

WORKPLACE KNOW-HOW

Problem Solving. A shipment of fresh tomatoes has just been delivered and you notice that one of the crates has a small hole in it. Upon closer inspection, you notice insects in and around the hole. What should you do?

196 UNIT 2 Quality Foodservice Practices

LAB-BASED ACTIVITY: Your HACCP System

STEP 1 Working in teams, create a HACCP system for the commercial kitchen pictured below. Use the HACCP critical control points on page 184 as your guide. Your system must address the following:

- Food-handling procedures.
- Monitoring techniques.
- Record keeping.

STEP 2 Develop a poster that explains how you will determine potential problems in each of the following areas:

- Receiving food.
- Storing food.
- Preparing and cooking food.
- Holding food.
- Serving food.

STEP 3 Have your instructor approve the team's poster.

STEP 4 Inspect your lab using your team's HACCP lab inspection system poster.

STEP 5 Report your team's findings to the class.

STEP 6 Discuss what each team's inspection system pointed out about the role of HACCP in keeping food safe.

STEP 7 Answer the following questions:

- Will you change the way you look for critical control points? Why?
- How can you be a better foodservice employee after this experience?

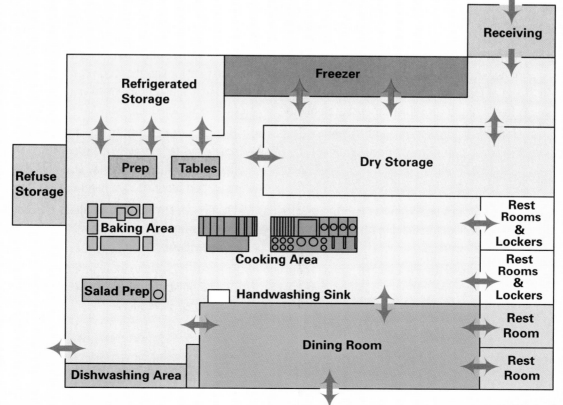

Research & Development

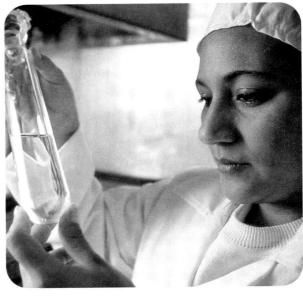

Have you ever wondered how the food products you eat everyday are created? A relatively new, yet rapidly growing, career path in foodservice is in research and development. Many food manufacturers are hiring experienced chefs and others with foodservice experience to assist in product development.

To succeed in research and development, you will need a culinary degree, a basic understanding of food science, excellent oral and written communication skills, and work experience. Research and development opportunities are varied and can be found in every part of the country.

Nutritionists often assist with the development of new food products. They also identify the kinds and amounts of nutrients in food products, and often develop consumer product statements.

Directors of recipe development create new recipes as part of menu development. Knowledge of food preparation techniques is necessary.

Food batchmakers set up equipment and modify recipes and formulas to produce specific flavors or textures. Solid math and organizational skills are essential.

Food scientists are involved in the production, processing, preparation, evaluation, and utilization of food. Strong skills in chemistry, biology, and psychology are necessary.

Packaging specialists develop packaging materials for specific food products. Strong skills in research and problem solving, and knowledge of packaging equipment are essential.

Product development technologists investigate ways to improve food products, such as flavor or shelf life. They may also help develop new food products that meet quality standards.

Quality assurance specialists check food products against quality, sanitation, and production standards.

Research chefs work with food scientists, manufacturing staff, and marketing departments to develop new products.

Working in the Real World...

RESEARCH CHEF

My name is David Horrocks, and I am a research chef for one of the largest flavor manufacturers in the world. I work in the flavor division with the savory group. My creative culinary ideas are used to sell flavors and seasonings to major foodservice and retail customers worldwide. Most of my days are spent cooking and tasting my own work.

My adventure with food started at a young age when I worked as a dishwasher, or "Dish Dog," in an Italian restaurant. Throughout my career, I was lucky enough to find myself employed by excellent chefs. They responded to my enthusiasm by teaching me more about food and advancing me to various positions in the kitchen. I worked in many different styles of food establishments, from fine dining, to high-volume food cafeterias. I have always had a passion for food, hard work, and life.

I graduated from Johnson & Wales University, with a bachelor's degree in Culinary Nutrition. The skills I obtained there were priceless. Not only did I learn about food, cooking, and nutrition, but I also learned about how the whole industry operates. Being a research chef involves experimenting, making presentations, traveling, attending meetings, and

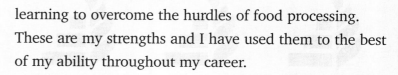

learning to overcome the hurdles of food processing. These are my strengths and I have used them to the best of my ability throughout my career.

In contrast to restaurant work, I now work a forty-hour week with holidays and weekends off. I love my job and I have more time to enjoy life, too.

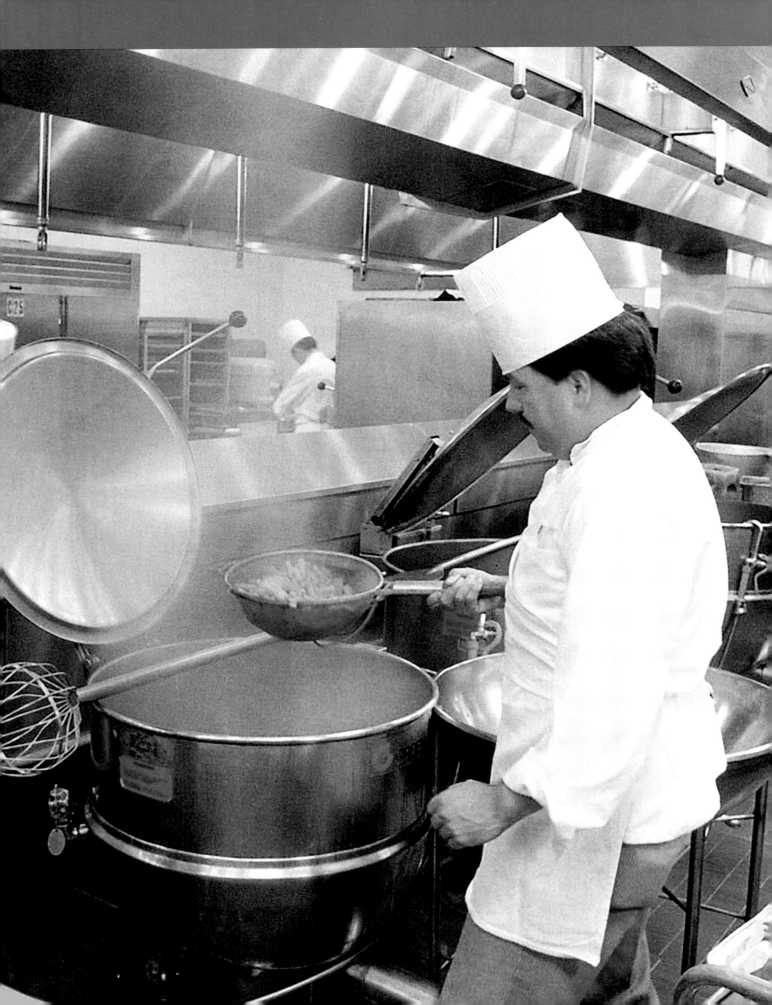

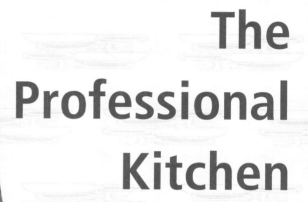

The Professional Kitchen

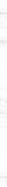

CHAPTER

9

Equipment & Technology

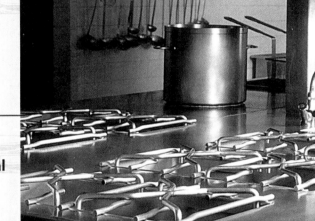

The Commercial Kitchen

OBJECTIVES

After reading this section, you will be able to:

• Identify work stations and work sections.

• Identify types of cooking lines.

• Explain the role of mise en place (meez ahn plahs).

• Demonstrate range of motion.

WORKING as a foodservice professional involves more than preparing and cooking food. It involves teamwork and cooperation among kitchen staff to create an efficient work environment. Before you step into a commercial kitchen and begin creating all types of interesting dishes, you need to become familiar with the kitchen. The layout of a commercial kitchen design is based on:

• The type of foodservice establishment.
• The amount of available space.
• The menu items to be prepared and the number of meals to be served.

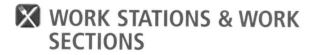

WORK STATIONS & WORK SECTIONS

The commercial kitchen is divided into work stations. A **work station** is a work area that contains the necessary tools and equipment to prepare certain types of foods. For example, onion rings are fried in a deep fryer. The work station where this takes place is called the fry station. Tongs and fry baskets would also be found in the fry station. See Fig. 9-1.

Each work station is arranged so that the kitchen staff does not have to leave their stations to perform their tasks. Work stations should have

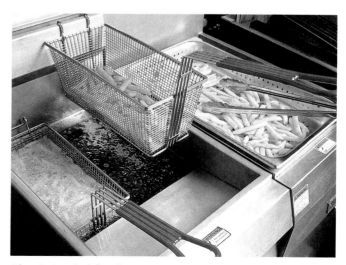

Fig. 9-1. Fried foods are prepared in the fry station.

Fig. 9-2.

SECTIONS	STATIONS
Beverage Section	• Hot Beverage Station • Cold Beverage Station
Garde-Manger Section	• Salad Station • Cold Platter Station • Sandwich Station
Short-Order Section	• Broiler Station • Griddle Station • Fry Station
Hot Foods Section	• Broiler Station • Fry Station • Griddle Station • Sauté Station • Dry Heat Station • Steam Station

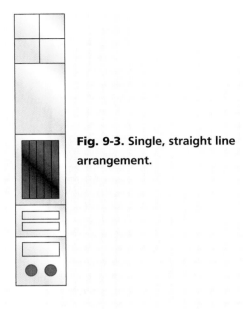
Fig. 9-3. Single, straight line arrangement.

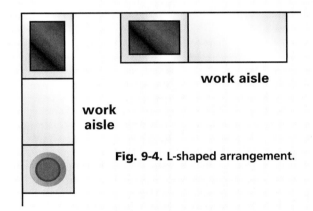
Fig. 9-4. L-shaped arrangement.

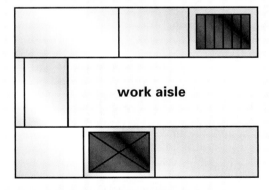
Fig. 9-5. U-shaped arrangement.

the necessary equipment, tools, work space, and power sources to operate efficiently. They also should have their own storage facilities.

Similar work stations are grouped into larger work areas called **work sections**. For example, a fry station and a griddle station would be part of the short-order section and the hot foods section. See Fig. 9-2.

⊠ THE COOKING LINE

Once the work stations and work sections have been identified, the **cooking line,** or arrangement of the kitchen equipment, is set up. Several arrangements may be used.

■ **Single, straight-line arrangement.** This type of arrangement allows equipment to be placed along a wall to form an island. This arrangement is used in larger kitchens. See Fig. 9-3.

■ **L-shaped arrangement.** The L-shape separates equipment into two major work areas. One side of the line may be used for food preparation, while the other side is used for cooking. See Fig. 9-4.

■ **U-shaped arrangement.** This type of arrangement is often used by establishments with limited space. It is also used in the dishwashing area of many commercial kitchens. See Fig. 9-5.

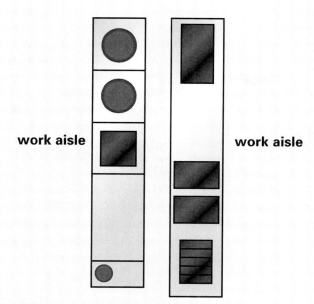

Fig. 9-6. Parallel, back-to-back arrangement.

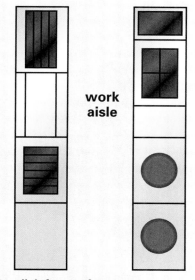

Fig. 9-7. Parallel, face-to-face arrangement.

■ **Parallel, back-to-back arrangement.** The parallel, back-to-back arrangement consists of two lines of equipment, sometimes divided by a wall. This arrangement is often used on ships and in hotels. See Fig. 9-6.

■ **Parallel, face-to-face arrangement.** This arrangement consists of two lines of equipment facing each other, separated by a work aisle. It is used in larger kitchens where constant communication between stations is necessary. See Fig. 9-7.

The cooking line arrangement determines what equipment and storage areas can be placed above, below, or across from the equipment. For example, some items may be stored on shelves above, below, or across from the cooking surface.

WORK FLOW

The layout of the kitchen has a direct effect on the work flow. See Fig. 9-8. **Work flow** is the orderly movement of food and staff through the kitchen. This movement helps reduce preparation and serving time. In addition to a well-designed kitchen, teamwork among staff and between work stations is essential for a good work flow. Having ingredients and equipment ready to use helps simplify tasks.

Mise en Place

Before you can prepare and cook the food, you have to get everything organized. **Mise en place** (meez-ahn-plahs) is a French term that means "to put in place." Mise en place includes assembling all the necessary ingredients, equipment, tools, and serving pieces needed to prepare food. This helps save time.

To effectively perform mise en place, work simplification techniques are used. **Work simplification** refers to performing a task in the most efficient way possible. Work simplification in the foodservice industry involves the efficient use of food, time, energy, and personnel.

- **Food.** Food can be prepared and cooked in a variety of ways, but not every method is efficient. For instance, you can chop an onion by hand, but a food processor will get the job done more quickly.
- **Time.** Time management in the kitchen results in prompt service. Different foods have different cooking times. By reviewing recipes prior to cooking, you can determine how much time is needed. Then you can plan your schedule by working back from the serving time. If making food for a large group, arrange food or plan set-up time to efficiently work in a production mode.
- **Energy.** Arrange your work station effectively. Hand tools and ingredients should be within reach. This allows for efficient range of motion. **Range of motion** means using the fewest body movements without unnecessary stress or strain. When your equipment, tools, and ingredients are easily accessible, you eliminate unnecessary stops and starts. An efficient range of motion eliminates wasted time and energy. See pages 440-441.
- **Personnel.** Hiring temporary or part-time employees helps management have the extra help they need during peak times. It also eliminates the expense of paying too many employees during non-peak times.

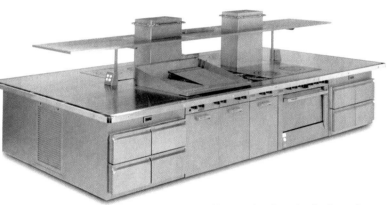

Fig. 9-8. An efficient kitchen is designed to maximize the allotted space.

SECTION 9-1 Knowledge Check

1. Name two decisions that need to be made before a kitchen can be designed.
2. Explain work simplification.
3. Explain how efficient range of motion impacts work simplification.

MINI LAB

Describe how you would perform mise en place prior to making a chef's salad for a party of six.

Receiving & Storage Equipment

OBJECTIVES

After reading this section, you will be able to:

• Identify receiving equipment.

• Explain first-in, first-out (FIFO).

• Identify storage equipment.

NOW that you know why a commercial kitchen is designed the way it is, you are ready to examine how food flows through a commercial kitchen. All products in the food flow begin with the receiving area. After they are received, they are stored.

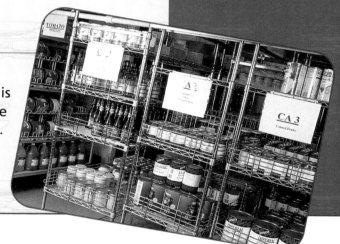

✖ THE RECEIVING AREA

Receiving involves more than just getting in an order. Receiving means checking that the ordered foods were received in the correct quantities at the right price. Foodservice professionals need to know what to check for when they receive orders. Many times, it's on the receiving end that problems occur. This is a big responsibility that should not be overlooked.

Receiving Equipment

The type of receiving equipment used is often determined by the size of the foodservice operation. Most operations have the following receiving equipment.

■ **Scales.** Receiving areas should have two types of scales: a platform scale and a counter scale. Both can be used to weigh boxes. Some foodservice operations also have portion scales. Portion scales are used to weigh cuts of meat.

■ **Thermometers.** Thermometers are used in the receiving area to check the temperature of frozen and fresh foods. These thermometers use infrared technology to check the temperature of food. They do not make direct contact with food products. Frozen foods should have a minimum internal temperature of 0°F or below. Fresh foods should be kept at 41°F or below. Food items that do not meet these safety standards should not be accepted.

- **Dollies.** Dollies are used to move items from the receiving area to the storage area. Dollies help foodservice professionals work more efficiently.

In addition, a good receiving area should also have a table large enough to hold boxes for inspection. A box cutter should be kept handy to open the packages and boxes. See Fig. 9-9.

When receiving shipments of food, you should follow these steps:

1. Check the purchase order against the actual shipment. Ensure that the order is correct and complete. Note any missing items.

2. Verify the invoice for accuracy. Check to ensure that the costs of the food items are correct, and that you were invoiced only for the items ordered. Note anything that is incorrect.

3. Inspect the food items for quality and reject any that do not meet quality standards.

4. Complete a receiving record. This should be a list that includes the quantity of items received, the item price, the date delivered, and the supplier's names.

5. Move the food items to the appropriate storage area. Each form of food—frozen, fresh, packaged, canned, and dry—must be handled and stored differently.

⊠ STORING FOOD

Food can be stored in refrigerators or freezers, on shelving units, or in storage bins and containers. The storage equipment used depends on the type and amount of food to be stored, the space available, and the type of foodservice operation.

Food must be stored properly to prevent it from spoiling and causing foodborne illness. When storing food items, foodservice professionals follow the First-In, First-Out (FIFO) rule. FIFO means that all food items should be used in the order they were received. Mark each item with the delivery date. Older items should be moved to the front of the storage facility. Newer items are placed in the back.

Refrigerators & Freezers

Fresh and frozen foods are stored in refrigerators and freezers. See Fig. 9-10. Commercial refrigerators and freezers are used to keep fresh and frozen foods, such as vegetables, dairy products, and meats, at the right temperature until used. There are three main types of commercial refrigerators: walk-in, roll-in, or reach-in units.

Walk-in refrigerators are basically refrigerated rooms. Reach-in refrigerators are not as large. Reach-in refrigerators are typically two- or three-door units with sliding shelves. Roll-in refrigerators have a rolling rack of sheet pans that can be rolled up a ramp and into the unit.

Food products that will be used often are stored in a **lowboy**. These half-size refrigerators fit under the counter in a work station.

Fig. 9-9. Receiving equipment.

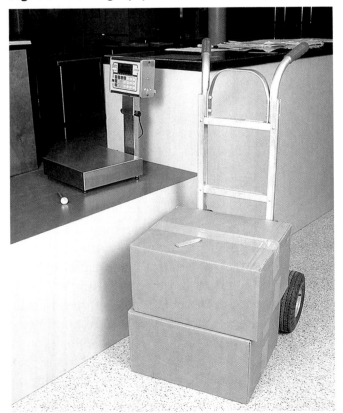

Fig. 9-10.

Refrigerators & Freezers

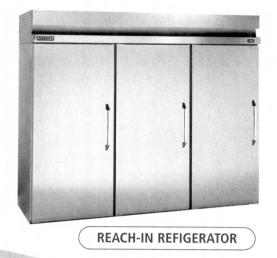

REACH-IN REFIGERATOR

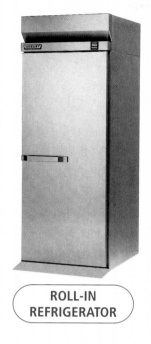

ROLL-IN
REFRIGERATOR

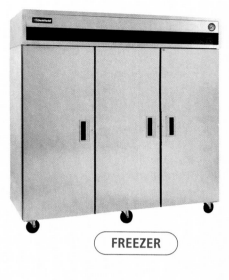

FREEZER

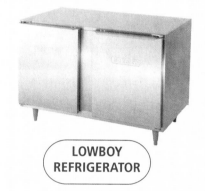

LOWBOY
REFRIGERATOR

Freezers are walk-in units that can store foods for long periods of time. At temperatures of 0°F or below, foods can be kept from one to six months, depending on the type of food and kind of packaging used. Foods that will be stored in the freezer must be covered well in airtight wrapping to avoid freezer burn. **Freezer burn**, light-colored spots on frozen food where surface drying has occurred, can ruin foods. As with all food products, frozen foods should also be labeled and dated.

Shelving Units

Shelving units are used to store various dry goods prior to use. There are several types of shelving units used in a commercial kitchen. For example, 6-ft. tall, stainless steel, wire shelving units are often used to hold food items, such as bread and boxed dry goods. All food should be stored at least six inches above the floor.

Some shelves fit into corners to maximize space. Overhead shelves are located in each individual work station. Overhead shelves can also be used to hold spices, kitchen tools, and cookware.

There are also shelves designed to hold canned goods. This type of shelving unit typically has a top-load design that allows the cans to roll forward to the bottom rack when a can is removed. This makes FIFO easy to follow. New cans are loaded at the top of the rack and roll in behind the older ones. See Fig. 9-11.

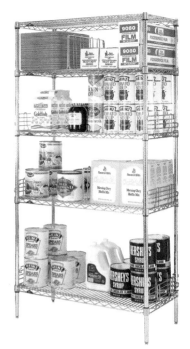

Fig. 9-11. Shelving units.

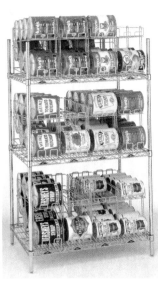

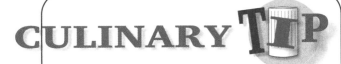

GLASS CONTAINERS—Glass is not recommended for storage containers because it can shatter. Aluminum is also not recommended because it reacts to acidic items, such as tomatoes.

Storage Containers

Smaller quantities of food are often placed in storage containers made of a sturdy, durable plastic. Labels identifying the contents and date of storage should always be clearly visible.

Storage containers should always have well-fitting, air-tight lids. Because these containers come in a variety of sizes, you can store different amounts of food with minimum exposure to air. This saves foodservice operations money by reducing the amount of food that spoils and must be thrown away. See Fig. 9-13.

Storage Bins

Storage bins are available in a variety of styles. Some storage bins are large, heavy plastic or polyurethane (pah-lee-yur-uh-thayn) bins with lids. They are used to hold dry ingredients like flour, beans, and rice. These storage bins are on wheels so they can be moved from one work area to another.

Storage bins can also be open wire bins that hold packaged items or canned goods. These types of bins can be positioned side-by-side or back-to-back, depending on the amount of available space. See Fig. 9-12.

Fig. 9-12.

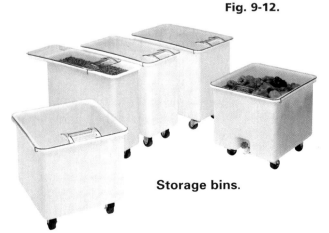

Storage bins.

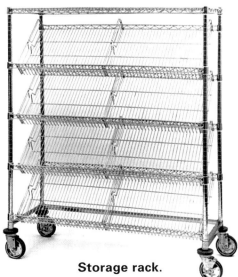

Storage rack.

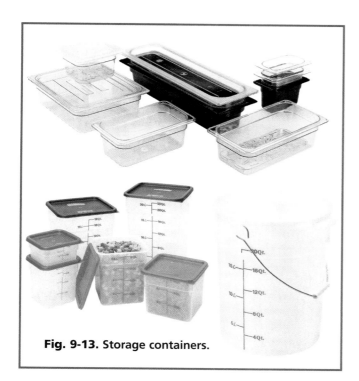

Fig. 9-13. Storage containers.

⊠ CLEANING & MAINTAINING EQUIPMENT

It is important to keep storage equipment clean. Clean equipment protects against contamination. When cleaning storage equipment, use the general guidelines that follow.

Refrigerators & Freezers

When cleaning and maintaining refrigerators and freezers:

- Maintain a regular cleaning schedule.
- Turn off the appliance and move all food to a cold storage area.
- For the reach-in and roll-in refrigerators and the freezer, wash the inside with a solution of baking soda and water.
- Clean the walk-in refrigerator as instructed by your supervisor.
- Wipe the outside with a damp cloth daily.
- Turn the appliance back on and refill with food.

Shelving Units & Storage Bins

When cleaning storage equipment, such as shelving units or storage bins, follow these general guidelines:

- Remove all food items from the storage unit. Using hot, soapy water, thoroughly clean shelves and storage bins.
- Rinse with clean water and then sanitize.
- Dry the storage unit thoroughly and replace the food items. Be sure to follow FIFO guidelines when placing food back in the storage units.

SECTION 9-2 | *Knowledge Check*

1. Explain FIFO.
2. Name three pieces of storage equipment.
3. Describe how you clean storage equipment.

MINI LAB

Imagine that a shipment of fresh, frozen, and dry food products has been delivered to the restaurant where you work. Create a list of 10 different food products that were delivered. Then determine where each product should be stored.

Preparation & Cooking Equipment

OBJECTIVES

After reading this section, you will be able to:

- Identify food preparation equipment.
- Contrast the heat sources used in cooking.
- Identify cooking equipment.
- Identify clean-up equipment.

HAVE you ever thought about how much equipment it takes to prepare and cook food for a simple meal at home? Now, imagine what is needed to prepare and cook food in a school cafeteria where hundreds of students eat every day. The preparation is time consuming, and special equipment is necessary to do the job well.

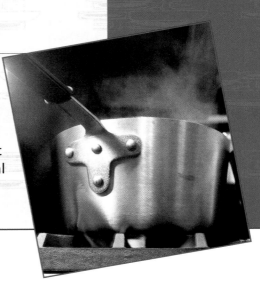

✖ PREPARATION EQUIPMENT

The equipment used to process, or prepare, food can streamline preparation time. Preparation equipment can be used to mix, chop, grind, grate, and slice large volumes of food. This equipment processes food, preparing it for cooking. Mixers, food processors, and slicers are common pieces of preparation equipment used in a commercial kitchen. See Fig. 9-14 on pages 213-214 (**Preparation Equipment**).

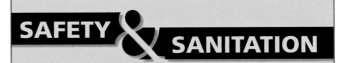

SAFETY & SANITATION

INSTRUCTION MANUAL—Equipment can be extremely dangerous if used improperly. Always refer to the instruction manual before operating any piece of equipment, and check with your supervisor before you start any equipment.

PREPARATION
Equipment

1. Slicer

A slicer has a 10 in. or 12 in. circular blade that rotates at high speed. It can be either automatic or manual. Slicers are used to slice foods into uniform sizes.

2. Bench Mixer

A mixer has a removable stainless steel bowl and a dough hook, paddle, and whip attachments. Counter models are available in 5-, 12-, and 20-qt. sizes. Floor models come in 30, 40, 60, 80, and 140 qts. The bench mixer is used to mix or whip doughs and batters. It can be used to slice, chop, shred, or grate foods by using different attachments.

3. Food Processor

A food processor has a removable bowl and an S-shaped blade. Food processors are used to grind, purée, emulsify, crush, and knead foods. Special disks can be added to slice, julienne, and shred foods.

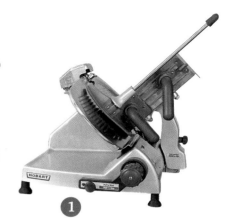

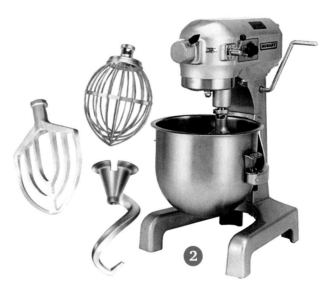

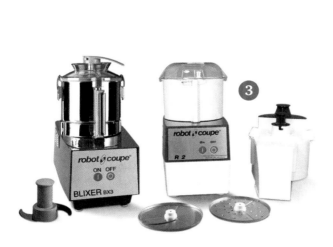

PREPARATION
Equipment (Cont'd.)

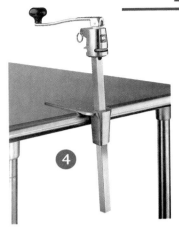

4. Table-Mounted Can Opener

Professional kitchens use heavy-duty can openers that are mounted on the edge of a table. Clean and sanitize can openers daily to prevent contamination. Replace worn blades immediately, as they can shed metal shavings into food.

5. Blenders

Blenders have stainless steel blades that can be used to blend and mix a variety of ingredients. They can also crush ice. Commercial blenders have removable thermoplastic or stainless steel containers.

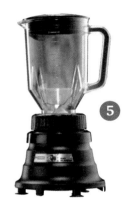

6. Commercial Juicers

Commercial juicers separate the pulp from the juice automatically. They have stainless steel blades and removable bowls.

7. Work Tables

Stainless steel and butcher block work tables are used in food production areas. Stainless steel tables are commonly used for food preparation. Butcher block tables are used more often at the bake station.

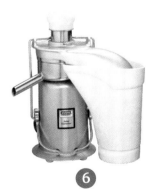

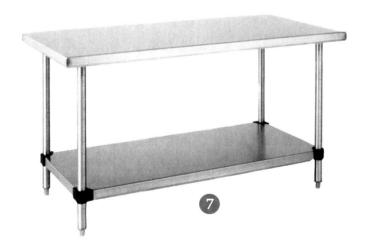

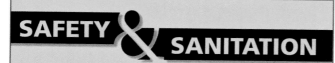
Cleaning Preparation Equipment

Safety precautions must be followed when cleaning professional equipment. Never place your hand or another object in a machine when it's running. Always turn it off first and unplug it. Refer to the instruction manual before cleaning any equipment.

The following provides general guidelines for cleaning preparation equipment. However, these guidelines do not replace instruction manuals or the guidance of your supervisor.

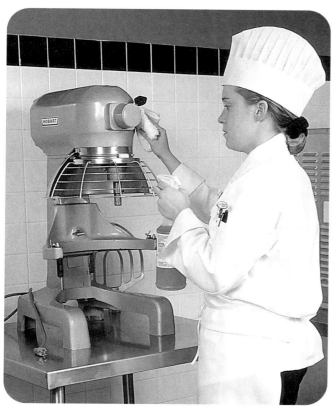

■ **The mixer and food processor.** To clean a mixer or food processor, refer to the instruction manual and follow these general steps:

1. Ensure that the equipment has been turned off and unplugged.

2. Remove the attachment and the bowl and wash them in hot, soapy water. Rinse and sanitize each piece. Dry them thoroughly.

3. Store attachments in an appropriate location.

4. Wipe the machine clean with a damp cloth. See Fig. 9-15.

■ **The slicer.** When cleaning a slicer, always follow safety precautions. The slicer is a dangerous piece of equipment. Refer to the instruction manual and follow these general steps:

1. Be sure the machine is turned off and unplugged.

2. Set the blade control indicator to zero.

3. Follow the instruction manual to take the slicer apart.

4. Wash the food carriage and blade in hot, soapy water. Use extra caution when cleaning the sharp blade. Rinse all pieces and let them air dry.

5. Wipe off the rest of the machine with a damp, soapy cloth. See Fig. 9-16.

6. Rinse with a damp cloth, sanitize, and dry. Reassemble the slicer. Immediately put the blade guard back in place.

7. Oil the slicer with nonedible oil as directed in the instruction manual.

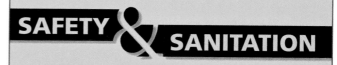
Fig. 9-15. This is the proper way to clean a bench mixer.

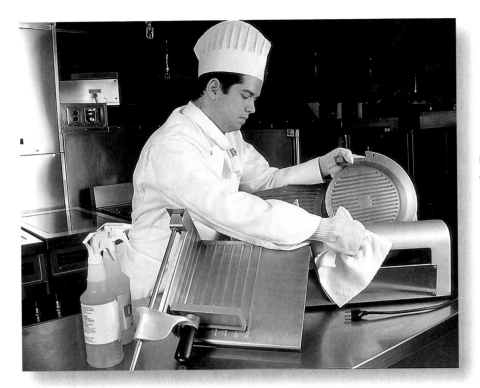

Fig. 9-16. This is the proper way to clean a slicer.

HEATING SOURCES

Food is cooked by heat that is generated through a number of sources: gas, electricity, radiation, microwaves, and light. Cooking equipment can use a number of these sources to generate heat.

■ **Gas.** Gas is a natural heat source that produces intense heat with a flame. It cooks food evenly. Ranges, ovens, and broilers can be gas operated.

■ **Electricity.** Like gas heat, electricity cooks food with intense heat, but depending on the type of metal the pot is made from, food may not cook evenly.

■ **Radiation.** **Radiation** cooks food by transferring energy from the cooking equipment to the food. The energy waves do not contain heat. Instead, these waves change to heat when they make contact with the food. Infrared and microwaves are examples of radiation energy.

■ **Microwave.** Another heat source used is a type of radiation called microwaves. **Microwaves** are invisible waves of energy that cause water mole-

cules to rub against each other and produce the heat that cooks food. Microwave ovens are an example of equipment that uses this heat source.

■ **Light.** Infrared lamps and FlashBake ovens use light waves as a heat source. The light waves do not contain heat, but heat is generated when the energy contacts the food. Infrared lamps are used to keep food hot until it is ordered by customers. FlashBake ovens are used to prepare small or individual servings quickly.

COOKING EQUIPMENT

Today's commercial kitchen uses a wide variety of equipment to cook food quickly and efficiently. Ranges, broilers, and ovens are just a few pieces of cooking equipment you will find in a commercial kitchen. Before you operate this equipment, you need to learn what the equipment looks like and how the equipment operates. See Fig. 9-17 on pages 217-219 (Cooking Equipment).

COOKING
Equipment

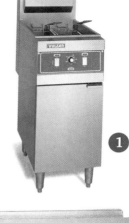

1. Deep-Fat Fryer

A deep-fat fryer cooks food at a constant temperature, which is controlled by a thermostat. Automatic or computerized fryers lower and raise food baskets in and out of fat at a preset time. Filtering allows the oil to be reused. Fryers are vital pieces of equipment in quick-service operations.

2. Open-Burner Range

An open-burner range has four to six burner units, each with individual controls. Each burner has its own heat source. This allows for more efficient use of heat than with a flat-top range.

3. Flat-Top Range

Also known as a French-top range, the burners of a flat-top range are arranged under a solid top that produces even heat over a large surface area. Flat-top ranges cannot be used as a griddle.

4. Griddle

Griddles can be flat or ridged. They can be a part of the range top, or a separate unit. Food is cooked directly on the surface of the griddle.

5. Microwave Oven

A microwave oven uses invisible waves of energy called microwaves to heat, reheat, defrost, and cook foods.

6. Broiler

Broilers cook food quickly from start to finish using intense, direct heat located above the food. They can be combined with a conventional oven as shown here, or stand alone as a separate unit.

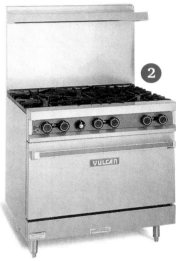

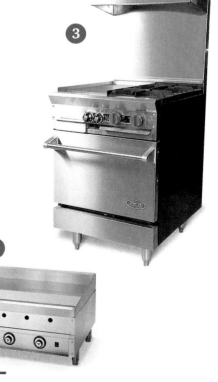

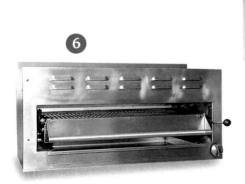

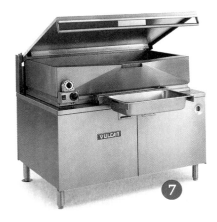

7. Tilting Skillet

The tilting skillet is the most flexible piece of equipment in a commercial kitchen. It is a large, flat cooking surface with sides to hold liquids. The skillet can be tilted to pour out liquid. It can be used as a griddle, fry pan, brazing pan, stockpot, bain marie, or steamer.

8. Steamer

A steamer cooks food quickly because it places the food in direct contact with hot water vapor.

9. Pressure Steamer

A steam pressure cooker works like a regular steamer except that the steam is under pressure. A pressurized door and a steam valve control the desired amount of pressurized steam.

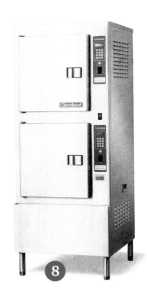

10. Steam-Jacketed Kettle

A steam-jacketed kettle also uses steam to cook foods quickly, but the steam does not come into direct contact with food. The steam is pumped between two stainless steel containers. The steam heats the inner kettle and cooks food quickly and evenly.

11. Trunnion Kettle

A trunnion (TRUHN-yuhn) kettle is a type of steam-jacketed kettle that can be tilted to empty contents by turning a wheel or pulling a lever.

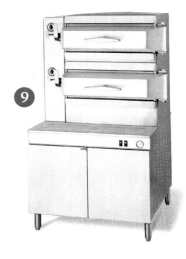

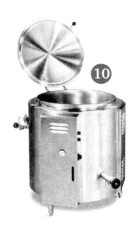

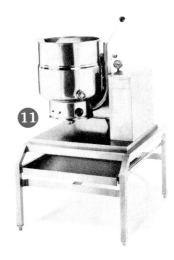

12. Combination Steamer/Oven

This steamer/oven uses a combination of cooking methods. It can use a fan to circulate air around the food like a convection oven. It can also use steam to cook food. Finally, it can combine convection and steam cooking. Combination steamer/ovens are used to bake, poach, grill, roast, braise, and steam foods.

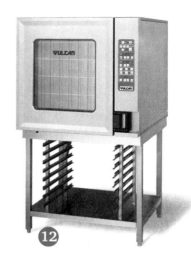

13. Deck Oven

A deck oven is also known as a stack oven. Electric deck ovens have separate baking controls for the lower deck and for the upper deck. Deck ovens are used for baking, roasting, and braising.

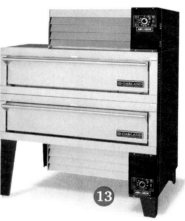

14. Convection Oven

A convection oven has a fan that circulates the oven's heated air. This fan allows you to cook foods in about 30% less time and at temperatures approximately 50°F lower than a conventional oven. Convection ovens are used for baking, roasting, and braising.

15. Salamander

A salamander is a small gas or electric broiler that is often attached to an open-burner range. Its heat source is also located above the food. Unlike a standard broiler, a salamander is used for browning, glazing, and melting foods.

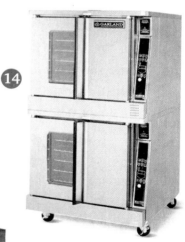

16. FlashBake Oven

A FlashBake, or infrared, oven uses both infrared and visible light waves above and below the food. Because the heat is so intense, foods cook very quickly without losing flavor and moisture. The FlashBake is used to bake smaller portions of food. It needs no pre-heating or venting.

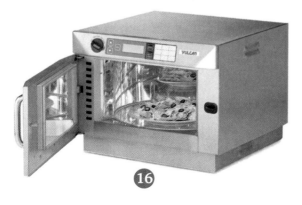

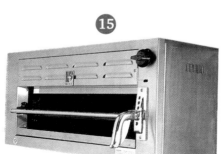

The Salamander

Commercial kitchens use salamanders (sa-luh-man-duhrs) for browning, glazing, and melting foods. Salamanders change the color of food by browning the outside layer, such as the crust of a casserole or pie. But how did the salamander get its unusual name?

Hundreds of years ago, salamanders, small amphibians (am-FIH-bee-uhns), were unknowingly carried into homes with the firewood. When the fire was lit, the animal would awaken and emerge from the flames, angry but unharmed. Thus began a popular myth that the salamander was able to endure great heat and could even live in fire. Therefore, the name *salamander* fits the small broiler used in commercial kitchens.

Today, the term *salamander* has been broadened to include other articles, such as an iron poker, a browning plate, and a small grill.

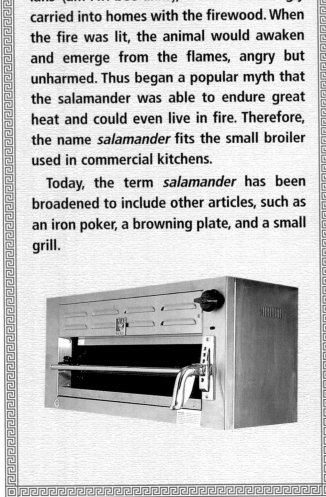

✕ CLEANING COOKING EQUIPMENT

When cleaning cooking equipment, always follow the instruction manual. Maintenance and repair needs can be handled through the manufacturer. Following are some general guidelines for cleaning equipment.

■ **Flat-top range.** To clean a flat-top range, loosen any burned food with a scraper. Then clean the rangetop with a damp, soapy cloth. Rinse it and wipe it dry.

■ **Open-burner range.** To clean an open burner, remove the grids and the drip pan. Soak them in hot, soapy water. While they're soaking, wash, rinse, and dry the rest of the range. Then wash, rinse, dry, and replace the grids and drip pan. See Fig. 9-18. Gas ranges have pilot lights, or continuously burning flames that light the burner when you turn on the range. Check to see that all the pilot lights are burning after you've cleaned the range. The flame should be blue, not yellow.

■ **Griddle.** To clean a griddle, polish the top with a special griddle cloth or stone. Polish in the same direction as the grain of the metal. Using a circular motion will scratch the surface of the griddle.

Fig. 9-18. Drip pans can be lined with foil to make cleaning easier.

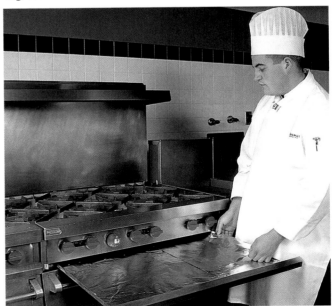

Wash the remaining area with warm, soapy water. Rinse and dry. Then recondition the top by coating it with a thin layer of nonedible oil. Heat the griddle to 400°F and wipe it clean. Repeat until the griddle is smooth and shiny.

■ **Broiler.** To clean a broiler, take out the grids and soak them in hot, soapy water. Remove caked-on food with a wire brush. Rinse, dry, and lightly oil with a nonedible oil. Scrape grease and burned food from the inside of the broiler. Wash the drip pans and put them back in place. Empty the grease trap, wash it, and replace it.

■ **Conventional and convection ovens.** When cleaning an oven, make sure the oven has cooled completely before cleaning it. Take out the shelves and wash them in hot, soapy water. Then rinse them and let them air dry. Wash the inside of the oven with warm, soapy water and dry it with a soft cloth. Wipe the outside of the oven with warm, soapy water. Rinse it with a soft, wet cloth and polish it with another soft cloth.

■ **Microwave oven.** To clean a microwave oven, let the oven cool completely before cleaning it. Wipe the inside and outside of the oven with a damp cloth and warm, soapy water. Then rinse and wipe dry. Make sure the microwave oven door seals tightly. If the door is loose or damaged, don't use the oven.

SAFETY & SANITATION

MAINTENANCE & CARE—Maintaining and caring for tools, utensils, and equipment is very important to the quality and safety of the food produced. Repair and replacement of equipment should be reported to your supervisor. Warranties should be kept in a safe place along with the instructions.

✕ CLEAN-UP EQUIPMENT

Foodservice operations see a constant flow of customers everyday. Customers expect cleanliness and efficiency in addition to good food.

■ **Commercial sinks.** Foodservice operations use several different types of commercial sinks. The most common type is the three-compartment sink. It is used to rinse, wash, and sanitize dishes. See Fig. 9-19A.

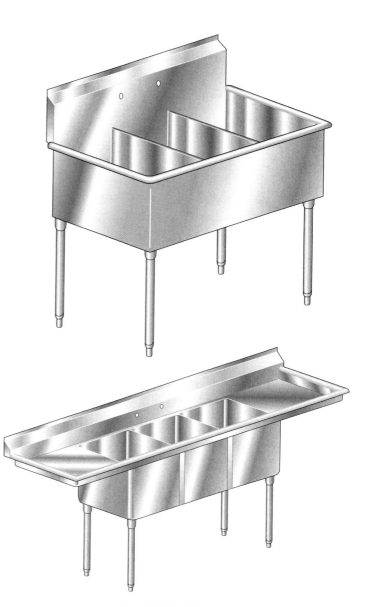

Fig. 9-19A. Three-compartment sinks.

■ **Garbage disposal.** Garbage disposals are mounted on sink drains. They are used to eliminate scraps of food leftover from preparation or scraped from plates. However, a garbage disposal does not replace the need for a garbage can. See Fig. 9-19B.

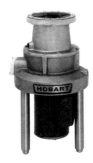

Fig. 9-19B. Garbage disposal.

■ **Commercial dishwashers.** A multi-tank, or carousel, dishwasher is common in large operations. Dishes are placed directly into racks on the conveyor belt. Hand-scraped, dirty dishes are rinsed and then manually loaded at one end of the machine, where they travel in a circle through areas that prewash, wash, rinse, sanitize, and dry them.

A single-tank dishwasher has only one compartment. Dishes that have been scraped by hand and rinsed can be loaded into its raised doors. As the doors are lowered, the washing cycle begins. Single-tank dishwashers are used to wash small loads of dishes. See Fig. 9-19C.

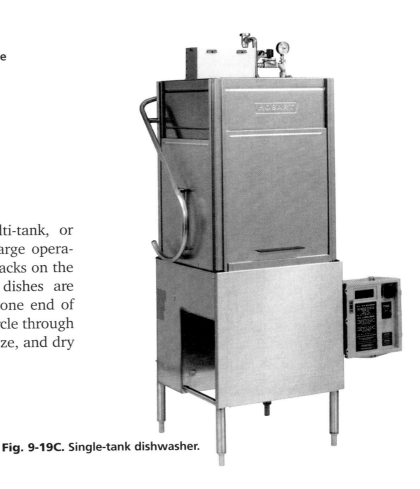

Fig. 9-19C. Single-tank dishwasher.

SECTION 9-3 Knowledge Check

1. Identify three common pieces of food preparation equipment.
2. Name five heat sources for cooking food.
3. Name four different commercial ovens.

MINI LAB

Divide into teams. Each team will clean and polish a large piece of equipment. Be sure to follow safety and sanitation guidelines.

Holding & Service Equipment

KEY TERMS

• steam table

• bain marie

• proofing/holding cabinet

OBJECTIVES

After reading this section, you will be able to:

• Identify the uses of hot food holding equipment.

• Describe the function of a steam table and a bain marie (bane mah-ree).

• Identify the uses of service equipment.

MANY times, foodservice operations cater meals or serve them buffet style. The challenge in these situations is keeping food hot over a period of time. Holding food that is prepared ahead of time requires special equipment. This equipment is designed to keep foods hot and safe. Serving customers also requires special equipment. Serving equipment helps staff provide quality service quickly.

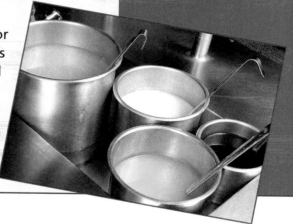

☒ HOLDING EQUIPMENT

Steam tables, a bain marie, overhead warmers, and proofing/holding cabinets are used to hold hot foods. See Fig. 9-20. Their purpose is to keep foods at a temperature of at least 135°F until the food is served. The high temperature prevents bacteria from growing. However, since the food is being kept warm at such a high temperature, the texture and color are likely to change. To prevent this, foods should be replenished frequently.

■ **Steam table.** A **steam table**, or food warmer, keeps prepared foods warm in serving lines. Foods are placed in hotel pans and placed into steam tables filled with steaming hot water. The pans are covered with either flat or domed lids. The temperature of the water is hot enough to keep foods warm while they are being served.

■ **Bain marie.** A **bain marie** (bane mah-ree), or water bath, is used to keep foods such as sauces and soups warm. Foods are placed in bain-marie inserts, which are then placed into a bain marie that is filled with hot water. You can also use either a single or double saucepan as a bain marie, depending on the food that will be placed in it. A bain marie also can be used to melt ingredients that will be used in other dishes. For these reasons, a bain marie is typically used in the production area rather than the service area.

■ **Overhead warmers.** Overhead warmers are used in the service area to keep foods hot until they are picked up by the serving staff and delivered to the customer. Some restaurants use overhead warmers to keep large cuts of meat hot before they are carved and served. Quick-service operations use them to keep pre-prepared foods warm so they can be served quickly. Food should only be kept under an overhead warmer for a short time. The heat can cause foods to dry out quickly.

■ **Proofing/holding cabinets.** A **proofing/holding cabinet** is an enclosed, air-tight metal container with wheels that can hold sheet pans of food. Temperature and humidity levels are controlled inside the cabinet. The internal climate of proofing/holding cabinets is ideal for proofing yeast-dough products. They are also used to keep food at 135°F or above during service.

✕ SERVICE EQUIPMENT

In addition to the equipment used to keep foods warm prior to serving, foodservice operations need to have a variety of service equipment. Service equipment can be used in the dining room, at a buffet, or at a catered function. Service equipment includes anything used to serve the customer. See Fig. 9-21 on pages 225-226 (Service Equipment).

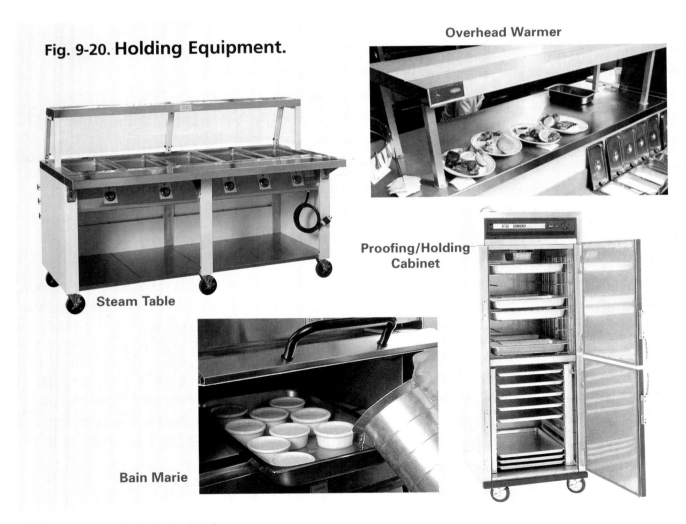

Fig. 9-20. Holding Equipment.

Overhead Warmer

Proofing/Holding Cabinet

Steam Table

Bain Marie

SERVICE
Equipment

1. Insulated Carriers

Insulated carriers are large boxes that can hold hotel pans and sheet pans filled with cooked food. Insulated carriers keep hot foods hot and cold foods cold. Some insulated carriers have wheels. If the carrier has a spigot, warm or cold beverages can be stored inside.

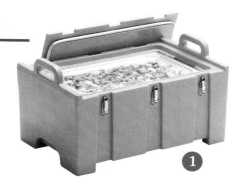

2. Chafing Dishes

Chafing dishes are typically stainless steel pans used to keep food hot during service. Hotel pans of food can be inserted into the chafing dish. Chafing dishes are available in a variety of sizes.

3. Canned Fuel

Canned fuel is used to keep food warm in chafing dishes. These small containers of solid fuel are ignited and placed beneath the chafing dish.

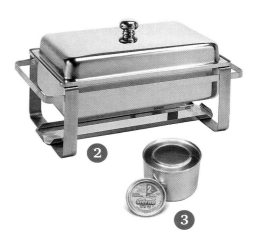

4. Coffee Systems

Coffee systems can brew coffee and keep it warm during serving time. A variety of models are available. Coffee systems consist of a water tank, thermostat, warming plate, and coffee server. Systems with a hot water spigot can also be used to make hot chocolate.

5. Scoops

Scoops are used to measure equal amounts of food. They have a lever to mechanically release the food and are numbered according to size. The number indicates how many level scoops it takes to fill a quart. The higher the number, the smaller the amount of food the scoop holds.

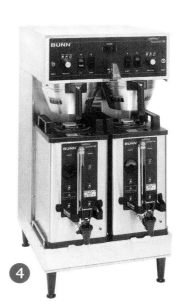

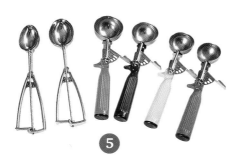

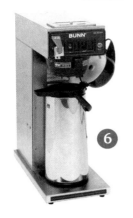

6. Airpot Brewing Systems

Airpot brewers are used to make hot beverages such as coffee. Airpots are tall, stainless steel containers with plastic lids and pump dispensers. They keep liquids hot for up to 10 hours.

7. Utility Carts

Utility carts are made of heavy-duty plastic or stainless steel. They are on wheels that allow them to be moved easily. Utility carts also have handles that allow them to be pulled or pushed. They are used to display or hold food, to bus tables, or to move heavy items from one location to another.

8. Hotel Pans

Hotel pans are stainless steel containers that are used to cook, serve, and store food. They come in many different sizes. Hotel pans fit in steam tables and other holding equipment. See Fig. 9-22.

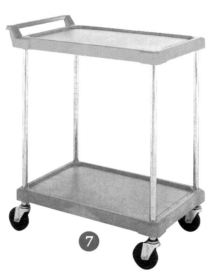

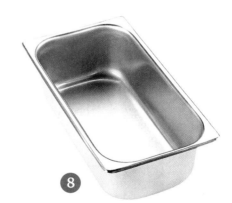

Fig. 9-22.

HOTEL PAN SIZE	APPROXIMATE CAPACITY	HOTEL PAN SIZE	APPROXIMATE CAPACITY
Full Size 20 ¾" × 12 ¾"	• 2 ½" deep = 8.3 quarts • 4" deep = 13 quarts • 6" deep = 20 quarts	**One-Third Size** 6 ⅞" × 12 ¾"	• 2 ½" deep = 2.6 quarts • 4" deep = 4.1 quarts • 6" deep = 6.1 quarts
Half-Size Long 20 ¾" × 6 ⁷⁄₁₆"	• 2 ½" deep = 3.7 quarts • 4" deep = 5.7 quarts	**One-Fourth Size** 6 ⅜" × 10 ⅜"	• 2 ½" deep = 1.8 quarts • 4" deep = 3 quarts • 6" deep = 4.5 quarts
Two-Third Size 13 ¾" × 12 ¾"	• 2 ½" deep = 5.6 quarts • 4" deep = 9.3 quarts • 6" deep = 14 quarts	**One-Sixth Size** 6 ⅞" × 6 ¼"	• 2 ½" deep = 1.2 quarts • 4" deep = 1.8 quarts • 6" deep = 2.7 quarts
Half Size 10 ⅜" × 12 ¾"	• 2 ½" deep = 4 quarts • 4" deep = 6.7 quarts • 6" deep = 10 quarts	**One-Ninth Size** 6 ⅞" × 4 ¼"	• 2 ½" deep = .6 quarts • 4" deep = 1.1 quarts

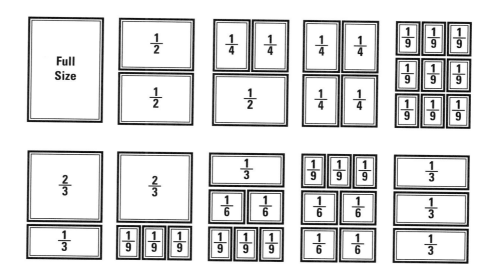

SECTION 9-4

Knowledge Check

1. Identify at least three pieces of holding equipment.

2. Explain when a steam table would be used instead of a bain marie.

3. Name at least five pieces of service equipment.

MINI LAB

Working in teams, practice using pieces of holding and service equipment.

SECTION SUMMARIES

9-1 Work stations and work sections are a way of organizing an efficient kitchen.

9-1 Kitchen equipment can be arranged into a number of cooking lines.

9-1 Effective work flow allows the orderly movement of food through the kitchen.

9-1 Range of motion is facilitated by a well-organized work station.

9-2 Receiving equipment, such as scales, are used to check food orders.

9-2 Applying the FIFO rule helps ensure food safety in the workplace.

9-2 Storage equipment is used to keep foods fresh and organized until they are ready for use.

9-3 Preparation equipment is used to perform a variety of tasks including shredding, grating, grinding, and slicing.

9-3 Cooking equipment can use any of the following sources to generate heat: gas, electricity, radiation, microwaves, and light.

9-3 Commercial kitchens use a wide variety of cooking equipment including ranges, ovens, and steamers.

9-3 Equipment used for cleaning includes commercial sinks and dishwashers.

9-4 Holding equipment keeps foods hot until they are used.

9-4 Service equipment is used to serve customers in the dining room, at the buffet, or at a catered function.

CHECK YOUR KNOWLEDGE

1. Identify three types of work stations.
2. Define mise en place.
3. Which piece of receiving equipment would be used to ensure that food products meet safety standards?
4. Define FIFO.
5. Name three types of refrigerators.
6. Identify pieces of preparation equipment that use attachments.
7. Explain how microwaves generate heat to cook food.
8. Identify five pieces of cooking equipment.
9. Explain how you would use a bain marie.
10. List five pieces of service equipment.

CRITICAL-THINKING ACTIVITIES

1. Explain how the layout of a commercial kitchen affects work flow.
2. You are employed at a small foodservice operation. The manager doesn't follow FIFO because of the small amount of business his establishment handles. Why is it important to always follow FIFO?

WORKPLACE KNOW-HOW

Problem Solving. You are a chef in a local restaurant. The convection oven you have been using is not working. You need to prepare roasted chicken for 20 customers. What other piece(s) of equipment could you use instead? Why?

LAB-BASED ACTIVITY: Commercial Kitchen Design

STEP 1 Use the menu below to determine:

- The tasks that will need to be performed.
- The type of foodservice equipment needed.
- The work stations needed.

STEP 2 Select the appropriate commercial equipment needed. Review the menus items, tasks to be performed, and the work stations needed.

STEP 3 Create a sketch of the kitchen, showing work stations and the cooking line. Label each piece of equipment on your sketch.

STEP 4 Answer the following questions:

- Did you select too much or too little equipment?
- Did you allow enough work space?
- How did your cooking line affect work flow?

Sample Menu

Breakfast

Juices & Fruits

Apple, Orange, or Grapefruit Juice $1.25

Breakfast Entrées

Two Eggs with Bacon or Sausage..............$4.95
French Toast with Maple Syrup.................$4.50
Hot Oatmeal $2.95

Sides

One Egg ....$.75
Toast ....$.75
Bacon or Sausage Links $2.50
Hashbrown Potatoes or Grits $1.25

Lunch

Soups & Salads

Chicken Noodle Soup ....Cup $1.25 Bowl $2.25
Soup of the Day.............Cup $1.25 Bowl $2.25
Tossed Green Salad $1.50
Chef Salad...$4.95

Sandwiches

Turkey Club with Fries $4.50
Cheeseburger with Fries...........................$3.50
Tuna or Chicken Salad Sandwich.............$3.25

Sides

French Fries $1.50
Creamy Coleslaw.......................................$1.25

Lunch Entrées

Fish & Chips..$5.95
Chicken Pot Pie $5.95

Desserts

Ice Cream..$1.50
Cheesecake..$2.50

Beverages

Coffee or Hot Tea (free refills) $1.25
Iced Tea & Assorted Soft Drinks $1.35
Milk...$1.25

CHAPTER

Knives & Smallwares

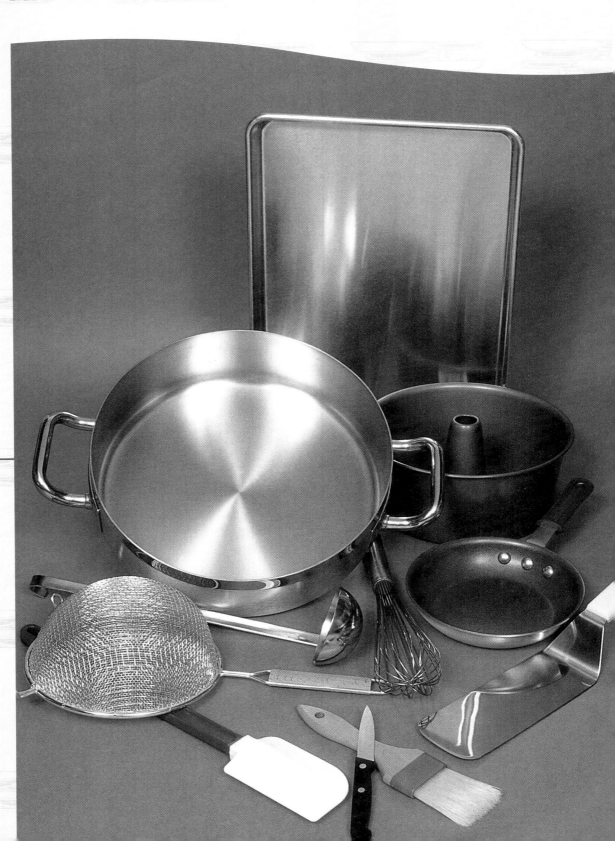

Knives

OBJECTIVES

After reading this section, you will be able to:

- Identify parts of a knife.
- Select appropriate knives for specific tasks.
- Perform basic cutting techniques.
- List important knife safety and sanitation guidelines.
- Explain proper knife storage guidelines.

KNIVES are the most commonly used kitchen tools, which is why they are such an important part of any chef's tool kit. A kitchen tool is an implement used in the kitchen. Accomplished chefs can perform countless valuable tasks with a sharp knife. To perform these tasks, however, chefs must be familiar with knife construction and type. They must also utilize proper cutting techniques and knife safety. Finally, chefs must know how to care for knives properly so they'll last.

✖ KNIFE CONSTRUCTION

In order to know which knife to use for a specific task, you must have a working knowledge of the different parts of a knife. See Figure 10-1.

Blade

The blade of a high-quality, professional knife is made of a single piece of metal that has been cut, stamped, or forged into its desired shape. The metals most often used for the knife blade are stainless steel and high-carbon stainless steel.

Stainless steel is a hard, durable metal made of chromium and carbon steel. It doesn't rust or discolor. Stainless steel also won't transfer a metallic taste to foods. The main drawback is that it's hard to sharpen.

High-carbon stainless steel is a mix of iron, carbon, chromium, and other metals that combines the best features of stainless steel and carbon steel. This expensive, high-carbon stainless steel doesn't rust or discolor and can be sharpened easily. This is the most common metal used for knives in the professional kitchen.

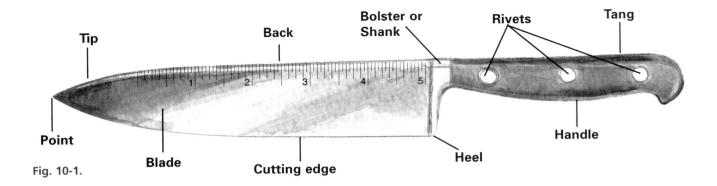

Tip

Back

Bolster or
Shank

Rivets

Tang

Point

Blade

Cutting edge

Heel

Handle

Fig. 10-1.

Tang

The **tang** is the part of the blade that continues into the knife's handle. Some knives have full tangs while others have partial tangs. A full tang is as long as the whole knife handle. Knives that are used for heavy work, such as chef's knives and cleavers, should have a full tang. Knives used for lighter work, such as paring knives and utility knives, may have a partial tang that does not run the entire length of the blade.

Handle

Knife handles can be made of several types of material, including hard woods such as rosewood and walnut. Other materials include plastic and vinyl. Because you'll be holding the knife for long periods of time, be sure that the handle feels comfortable in your hand. Your hand may cramp from using a handle that is either too small or too large. Manufacturers make various sizes of handles, so try different sizes to find one that fits your hand.

Rivet

The tang is attached to the knife handle with **rivets**. Rivets are metal pieces that fasten the handle to the tang. For comfort and sanitation, the rivets should be smooth and lie flush with the handle's surface.

Bolster

Some knives have a shank or **bolster** in the spot where the blade and handle come together. Knives with a bolster are very strong and durable. The bolster helps prevent food particles from entering the space between the tang and the handle.

❌ TYPES OF KNIVES

Chefs use a variety of knives to perform specific tasks. The chef chooses knives according to the type of food that she or he is preparing. For example, chopping onions requires a different knife than slicing bread. The following list describes the basic types of knives and their uses. See Fig. 10-2.

■ **Chef's knife.** The chef's knife, also called a French knife, is the most important knife in the chef's tool kit. This all-purpose knife with an 8–14 in. triangular blade can be used for peeling, trimming, chopping, slicing, and dicing. The 10-in. chef's knife is used for general work in a commercial kitchen. A skilled chef can also use this knife to cut large foods, such as meat, poultry, and fish, into smaller pieces. A smaller knife, but similar in shape to a chef's knife, is the *utility knife*—an all-purpose knife with a 5–7 in. blade. It's mainly used for peeling and slicing fruits and vegetables.

Fig. 10-2.

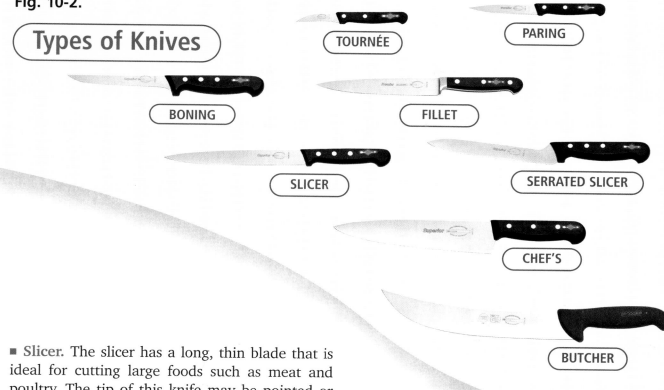

Types of Knives

TOURNÉE

PARING

BONING

FILLET

SLICER

SERRATED SLICER

CHEF'S

BUTCHER

■ **Slicer.** The slicer has a long, thin blade that is ideal for cutting large foods such as meat and poultry. The tip of this knife may be pointed or rounded. The blade may be rigid or flexible. The slicer's blade may also be **serrated** (suhr-ray-tuhd), or toothed like a saw. You can use a serrated slicer to slice coarse foods, such as bread and cake, without tearing them apart.

■ **Boning knife.** A small knife with a thin, angled 5–7 in. blade, the boning knife is used to remove bones from meat, fish, and poultry. You can also use this knife to trim the fat from meat. The boning knife's blade may be rigid or flexible. Rigid blades are used for heavier work. Flexible blades are used for lighter work.

■ **Paring knife.** The paring knife has a rigid blade that is only 2 to 4 inches long. You can use this knife to pare, or trim off a thin outer layer or peel from, fruits and vegetables.

■ **Tournée knife.** Similar in size to the paring knife, the tournée (toor-nay) knife has a curved blade that looks like a bird's beak. It is used to trim potatoes and vegetables into shapes that resemble footballs.

■ **Fillet knife.** The fillet knife has an 8–9 in. blade with a pointed tip. The blade may be rigid or flexible. It is mainly used to fillet fish.

■ **Butcher knife.** The butcher knife has a 6–14 in. rigid blade whose tip curves up at a 25° angle. It is sometimes called a scimitar (sim-ih-TAR) because its curved blade resembles a saber by that name. You can use the butcher knife to cut meat, poultry, and fish.

✖ KNIFE SKILLS

One of the most important skills you'll learn is how to use a knife properly. You'll use a knife to perform many different tasks, from boning fish to paring fruits, slicing bread, and dicing or mincing vegetables. The more you practice, the more efficient you'll become.

■ **Grip.** You can grip the knife in several different ways. Comfort and the task at hand will help you determine which grip to use. As a general rule, grip the knife firmly but not so tightly that your hand gets tired. Fig. 10-3 shows some basic gripping styles. Avoid placing your index finger on the top of the blade.

Fig. 10-3. Gripping styles.

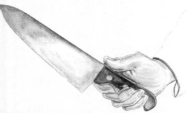

A: Grip the knife by placing four fingers on the bottom of the handle and the thumb firmly against back of the blade.

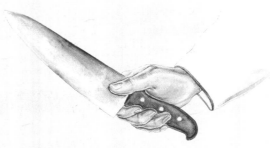

B: Grip the knife by placing four fingers on the bottom of the handle and the thumb against the side of the blade.

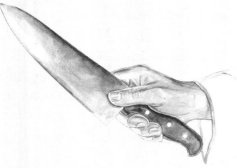

C: Grip the knife by placing three fingers on the bottom of the handle, the index finger flat against the blade on one side, and the thumb on the other side. This grip offers extra control and stability.

■ **Control.** To make safe, even cuts, you need to guide the knife with one hand while you hold the food firmly in place with the other hand. Use the sharp edge of the blade to do the cutting. A sharp knife is the safest knife to use. Use smooth, even strokes, and never force the blade through the food. Fig. 10-4 shows two safe ways to cut.

KEY Math SKILLS

MEASURING ANGLES

Common angle measures are often referenced to help you visualize how to hold a knife. You may recall that two non-collinear rays, with a common endpoint, form an angle. The measure of an angle is stated using the degree (°) symbol.

Common reference angles are 0°, 45°, 90°, and 180°. Angles measuring 0° and 180° are otherwise known as straight lines. A 90° angle is commonly referred to as a right angle, and a 45° angle is an angle halfway between a straight line and a right angle.

— 180° or 0°   ∠ 45°   ∟ 90°

Another method for remembering common reference angles is to think of the hands on a clock. At 12:00 and 6:00, the hands on a clock form a 180° angle, and at 3:00 and 9:00, the hands form a 90° angle.

Remembering these common reference angles will help you quickly estimate the correct handling position for a knife. For example, cut an item holding the knife at a 20° angle. For a visual picture of this angle, think of 20° being about halfway between a 0° angle and a 45° angle. If the angle happens to be at 100°, think of an angle slightly larger than a 90° angle. If in doubt, use a protractor to give you a concrete image of the angle.

TRY IT!

1. Sketch a 10° angle and a 60° angle.
2. Practice cutting each of these angles on a raw potato.

Fig. 10-4.

Cutting Method A:

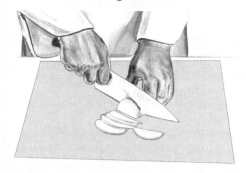

1. With your fingertips curled back, grip the food to be cut with your thumb and three fingertips. Holding the knife in your other hand, keep the tip of the knife on the cutting board, and lift the knife's heel.

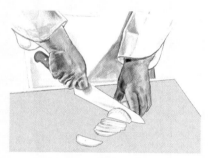

2. Use the second joint of your index finger as a guide as you slice with a smooth, even, downward motion. To make slices of equal size, adjust your index finger as you work. As you slice, move your thumb and fingertips down the length of the food, using the tip of the knife as the support.

Cutting Method B:

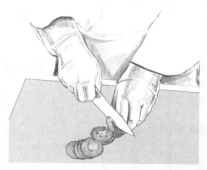

1. Use the same grip as described in Step 1 to the left. Slice the food into the desired thickness by using the second joint of your index finger to guide you. Lift the tip of the knife and cut by moving the knife slightly toward you and down through the food.

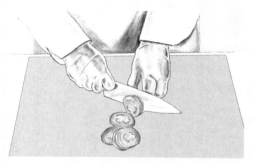

2. Use your wrist, not your elbow, to move the knife. Don't apply too much downward pressure. Your wrist serves as the support for this slicing method. The weight of the knife should be doing most of the work.

✖ KNIFE CUTS

The purpose of using a knife is to make a food smaller and to shape a food. It's important to cut foods in uniform pieces so that they cook evenly. Uniform sizes also make the finished product more visually appealing. The basic cutting techniques include slicing, mincing, and dicing.

Slicing

When slicing food, you will use a chef's knife to cut it into large, thin pieces. To slice safely, make sure the flat side of the food is down so it won't slip. If necessary, cut a piece of the food to create a flat surface. You can make various specialty slices including chiffonade, rondelle, and diagonal cuts.

- To **chiffonade** (shif-o-NOD) means to finely slice or shred leafy vegetables or herbs. This cut is often used to make certain garnishes. See Fig. 10-5.
- A **rondelle** (ron-dell), or round, is another type of slice. These disk-shaped slices are made from cylindrical fruits or vegetables, such as cucumbers or carrots. See Fig. 10-6.
- A diagonal cut results in an oval or elongated slice of a cylindrical fruit or vegetable. The technique used to slice a diagonal is similar to the one used for a rondelle except that you must hold the knife at an angle of approximately 60°. See Fig. 10-7.

Mincing

Food that is cut into very small pieces is minced (mihnsd). This technique is used most often on items such as shallots and garlic. See Fig. 10-8.

Dicing

When you dice a food, you'll use a chef's knife to cut it into ⅛- to ⅝-in. cubes. To make the cubes, you will need to cut the food into sticks, called julienne and batonnet, first. See Fig. 10-9.

Fig. 10-5. Chiffonade cut.

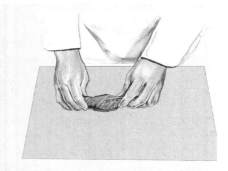

1. Wash and de-stem the vegetable's leaves as needed. Stack several leaves on top of one another and roll them tightly.

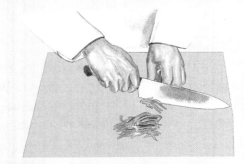

2. Holding the rolled leaves tightly, finely slice them.

Fig. 10-6. Rondelle cut.

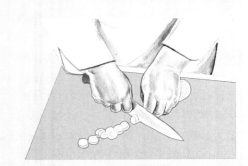

Peel the food if desired. On a cutting board, hold the knife perpendicular to the food and make even slices.

Fig. 10-7. Diagonal cut.

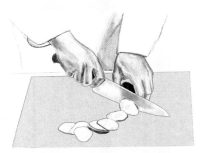

Peel the food if desired. On a cutting board, hold the knife at the desired angle to the food being cut and make even slices.

Fig. 10-8. Mincing.

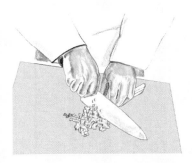

1. Dice celery using the same technique you would use to peel and dice an onion.

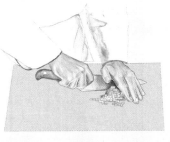

2. Hold the tip of the knife on the cutting board with a flat hand. Use a rocking motion to mince the celery with the knife's heel.

- **Julienne** (ju-lee-en) cuts are ⅛-in.-thick matchstick-shaped cuts. Carrots are often cut julienne.
- **Batonnet** (bah-toh-nah) cuts are thicker than julienne cuts. Batonnet cuts are ¼-in.-thick matchstick-shaped cuts. Some restaurants serve batonnet-cut fried potatoes.
- **Brunoise** (broon-WAZ) cuts are ⅛-in.-thick cubes. These are often cut after a vegetable has been cut julienne.

Fig. 10-9. Dicing.

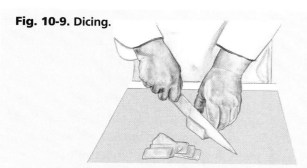

1. Peel the food if desired and square off the sides. Trim the food to the proper length for the slices you're making. Cut slices of the desired thickness.

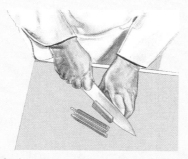

2. Stack the slices and cut them into uniform sticks. These sticks should be of the same thickness as the slices.

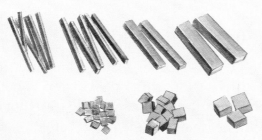

3. To make a small dice, make a ¼-in. cut perpendicular to the length of a batonnet. A ⅜-in. cut from a ⅜-in. stick makes a medium dice. A ⅝-in. cut from a ⅝-in. stick creates a large dice. Making a ⅛-in. cut from a julienne makes a cube called a brunoise.

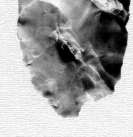

KNIFE-USE GUIDELINES—Here are some important safety guidelines that you must keep in mind when using knives:

- Always use the correct knife for the task.
- Always use a sharp knife. You're more likely to cut yourself with a dull knife because you'll need to use more force.
- Always cut with the blade facing away from your body.
- Always use a cutting board.
- Never let the knife's blade or handle hang over the edge of a cutting board or a table.
- When carrying a knife, hold it by the handle with the point of the blade straight down at your side. Make sure that the sharp edge is facing behind you. See Fig. 10-10.
- Don't try to catch a falling knife. Step away and let it fall.
- When you're passing a knife to someone, lay the knife down on the work surface or pass it by carefully holding the dull side of the blade with the handle facing out toward the other person.

Fig. 10-10.

- Never use a knife to perform inappropriate tasks, such as opening a can or a bottle or prying something apart. These tasks could damage or even break the blade.
- Never leave a knife in a sink filled with water. Someone could reach into the sink and be cut by the knife.
- Carefully wipe the blade from its dull side.
- Always wash, sanitize, and wipe knives before putting them away.

✖ KNIFE SAFETY & CARE

Now that you know which knives to use for which tasks and how to use them safely, you need to know how to care for them properly. To keep your knives in good condition, keep them sharp and clean. Sanitize knives after each use and always store them properly.

Sharpening Knives

You'll use a sharpening stone, or **whetstone**, to keep your knives sharp. A whetstone is made of either silicon carbide or stone, and may have up to three sides with grains ranging from coarse to fine.

1. Using four fingers to guide the knife, hold the knife at a 20° angle against the whetstone. If you're using a three-sided whetstone, start with the coarsest surface and end with the finest. See Fig. 10-11.

2. Press down on the blade, keeping it at the 20° angle. Gently draw the knife across the stone.

3. Continue moving the knife across the stone.

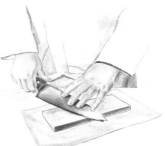

Fig. 10-11.

4. Gently bring the knife off the stone.

5. Turn the knife over and repeat Steps 1-4, using strokes of equal number and pressure.

Trueing Knives

After you've sharpened your knife, a steel is used to keep the blade straight and to smooth out irregularities. This process is called **trueing**.

1. Hold the steel with the hand that you don't write with. Place your arm in front of you at a 60° angle.

2. Hold the knife in the hand that you do write with. Rest the blade against the inner side of the steel at a 20° angle.

3. Keeping the knife at a 20° angle, slowly draw the blade along the entire length of the steel. See Fig. 10-12.

4. Repeat these steps several times on each side of the blade until the knife edge is straightened.

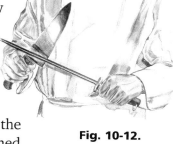

Fig. 10-12.

5. After using a steel, wipe the blade to remove any particles of metal.

Sanitizing Knives

Keeping knives clean is important. Wash knives in hot, soapy water after every cutting task and before storing them. Let knives air-dry thoroughly after washing and rinsing them.

To avoid cross-contamination and destroy microorganisms, sanitize knives after every use. Wipe down the blade and clean with sanitizing solution. There are also special sanitizing pads that can be used for wiping blades and handles.

Storing Knives

To prevent damage to blades or to people, knives must be stored safely. A convenient way to store knives is in a slotted knife holder. Because of the danger of exposed blades, a slotted knife holder should be hung on a wall, not on the side of a table. See Fig. 10-13.

A knife kit is a safe, handy storage unit for a large knife collection. Individual slots keep each knife safely in place. Most chefs prefer vinyl cases because they're easy to clean and sanitize.

Custom-built drawers are another storage option. As with knife kits, special slots hold each knife in place. Magnetized bars, which can be hung on the wall, are yet another way knives are stored in commercial kitchens.

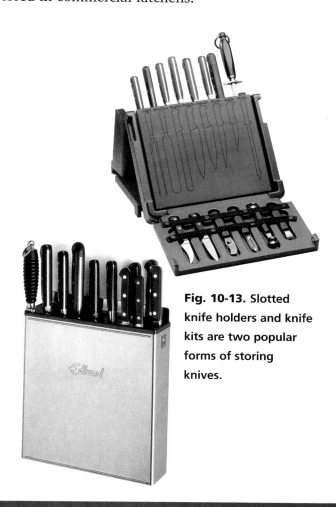

Fig. 10-13. Slotted knife holders and knife kits are two popular forms of storing knives.

SECTION 10-1 Knowledge Check

1. Contrast a chef's knife and a paring knife.
2. Contrast slicing, mincing, and dicing.
3. Explain why knife sanitation is important.

MINI LAB

Imagine that you've been asked to prepare a three-course meal that includes a garden salad, beef stew, and strawberry shortcake. Explain which knives and cutting techniques you'll use to prepare each course.

Smallwares

KEY TERMS

- **smallwares**
- **hand tools**
- **Parisienne scoop**
- **cookware**
- **heat transfer**

OBJECTIVES

After reading this section, you will be able to:

- Explain NSF certification standards and how they relate to smallwares.
- Select hand tools for specific tasks.
- Select cookware based on its heat transfer rating and specific use.
- Demonstrate proper cleaning and sanitizing of smallwares.

EVERY restaurant has a supply of hand tools, pots, and pans used for cooking called **smallwares**. Stainless steel and wooden hand tools, aluminum pots, and copper-bottomed pans are some of the smallwares that a cook uses. How will you know when to use which smallware? Becoming familiar with smallwares will help you prepare food in an efficient manner.

HAND TOOLS

Handheld items used in a foodservice operation to cook, serve, and prepare food are known as **hand tools**. The more you practice working with hand tools, the faster and more effectively you will use them.

The majority of hand tools are made of stainless steel, aluminum, or plastic. Several factors determine which material is used, including its durability, ease of use and cleaning, ability to transfer heat, and price. The following figure shows the hand tools used most frequently in professional kitchens. See Fig. 10-14 on pages 241-245 (**Hand Tools**).

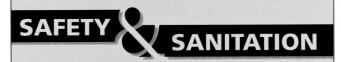

SAFETY & SANITATION

CUTTING BOARDS—Clean and sanitize all cutting boards after every use to prevent contamination. Different color-coded, plastic cutting boards have unique uses. Yellow is for poultry, red is for raw meat, blue is for fish, green is for produce, white is for dairy, and tan is for cooked meat. Using a different colored cutting board for each type of food helps prevent cross-contamination.

Hand Tools

1. Vegetable Peeler

A vegetable peeler is commonly used to shave the skin off fruits and vegetables. It can also be used to make delicate garnishes, such as carrot curls and chocolate curls.

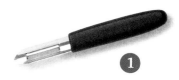

2. Apple/Fruit Corer

Push the corer through the center of the fruit so that the core comes out in one long, round piece. Small corers can be used on such fruits as apples and pears, while large models are used on such fruits as pineapples and grapefruits.

3. Tomato/Fruit Corer

A tomato corer is used to core and remove stems of tomatoes. It is also useful for removing vegetable markings, apple seeds, and potato eyes.

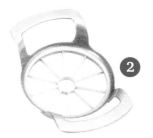

4. Kitchen Shears

Kitchen shears are used to tackle a variety of cutting chores, such as snipping string and butcher's twine, trimming artichoke leaves, and dividing taffy.

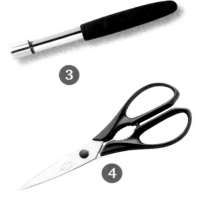

5. Cutting Boards

Cutting boards are made from wood or a composition of plastic or similar materials. They should have a smooth surface free of any deep scratches, nicks, gouges, or scars.

6. Cheese Slicer

A cheese slicer is used to cut slices from hard or semihard cheeses.

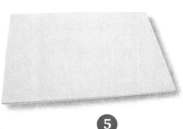

7. Butter Cutter

The surfaces of a butter cutter produce garnishes ranging from curls to grooves to marble-sized balls. For clean garnishes, make sure the butter is cold and the cutter has been warmed in hot water.

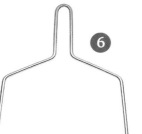

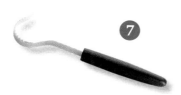

Hand Tools (Cont'd.)

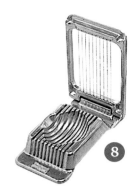

8. Egg Slicer

There are two kinds of egg slicers. One makes round shapes and the other makes wedge shapes. An egg slicer works by placing a peeled, hard-cooked egg in the hollow of the slicer. Push the tool down and the wires will slice the egg or cut it into wedges.

9. Pizza Cutter

For cutting baked pizza into serving pieces, no other tool slices more sharply and cleanly than a pizza cutter. It can also be used to cut pies and quiches.

10. Zester

A zester is used to remove tiny strips from the outer surface of citrus peels, which add visual interest and flavor to foods. It can also be used on vegetables, such as carrots and radishes, to add shavings to salads. Zesters work best on fresh, firm fruits and vegetables.

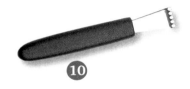

11. Melon Baller

A melon baller is used to scoop out smooth balls from many foods, such as cheese, butter, and melons. A melon baller with a scoop at each end, one larger than the other, is called a **Parisienne** (pah-ree-see-ehn) **scoop**. The scoops range in size and shape and sometimes have scalloped edges.

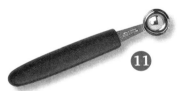

12. Whisks

Balloon whisks are light and bouncy with a rounded end. They are ideal for beating egg whites or light batters. Rigid whisks are longer and more rigid and made with heavier, thicker wires. Rigid whisks can tackle thick, dense sauces and batters.

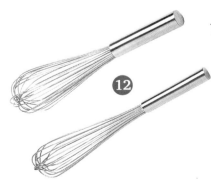

13. Solid, Perforated, and Slotted Spoons

Spoons are used to scoop, skim, mix, and serve. Perforated and slotted spoons are used to lift and drain foods from the liquid in which the food cooks.

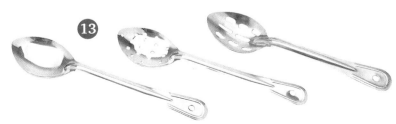

14. Rubber, Straight, and Offset Spatulas

A rubber spatula has a broad, flexible rubber or plastic tip on a long handle. It is used to scrape food from the inside of bowls and pans. It is also used to fold in whipped cream or egg whites. A straight spatula, or palette knife, has a long, flexible blade with a rounded end. It is useful for scraping bowls and spreading icing on cakes. An offset spatula, or turner, has a broad stainless steel blade that is bent to keep the user's hand off hot surfaces. It is used to lift and turn foods, such as pancakes, so they can cook on both sides.

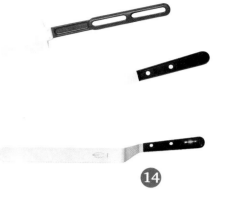

15. Chef's Fork

A chef's fork, also known as a braising fork, is used to lift and turn large cuts of meats and other items. It is also used to hold heavy pieces of food while they are being carved.

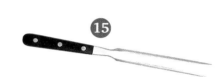

16. Skimmer

A skimmer has a flat, perforated surface for removing food from stocks and soups. It is also used to skim impurities from the tops of liquids.

17. Tongs

Tongs are spring-action or scissor-type tools used to pick up items such as meats, vegetables, or ice cubes.

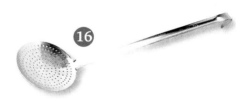

18. Meat Tenderizer

Each side of a meat tenderizer has different-sized toothlike points that are made of aluminum or steel. These points tenderize meat by breaking up and bruising the fibers.

19. Strainers

Strainers have a cup-shaped body made of perforated mesh. The holes range from extra fine to coarse. Strainers can be used to drain pasta, vegetables, and stocks after cooking.

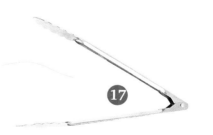

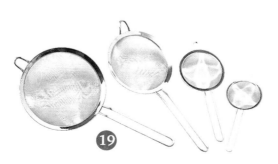

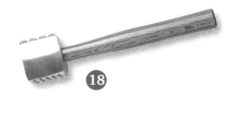

Hand Tools (Cont'd.)

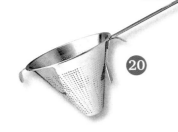

20. Chinois or China Cap

A chinois (sheen-WAH) or China cap is a cone-shaped metal strainer used for straining sauces and stocks. A pestle (PEHS-tuhl), or a round, batlike instrument, can be used to press very soft food through the China cap.

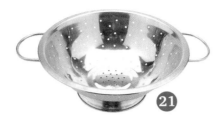

21. Colander

A colander is a large, perforated bowl used to rapidly drain water from cooked foods. It is also useful for rinsing food items before cooking.

22. Food Mill

A food mill is a bowl-like container used to purée and strain food. To use this tool, place food in the mill and turn the handle to force food through the disk. Disks are available with varying degrees of coarseness or fineness.

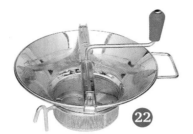

23. Box Grater

The most common type of grater is four-sided. Each side has different-sized holes that determine the size of the grated food pieces, from slices to shreds to crumbs.

24. Funnel

A funnel is used to pour liquid from a large container into a smaller container, such as from a pot into a bottle. Funnels are available in several different sizes and materials.

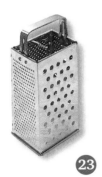

25. Pie Dividers

Pie dividers are circular tools that contain six openings, each the size of a piece of pie. Pressing the tool over the pie divides, or marks, the dish into the designated number of slices.

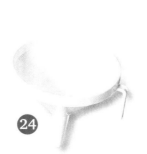

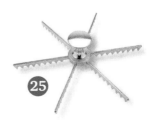

26. Pastry Tools

Pastry bags are filled with icing or other soft foods for hand-squeezed pastry decorating and assembly. They can be made of nylon, plastic-lined cotton, or disposable paper. Pastry tips fit onto the pastry bags and shape the flow of food as it is squeezed out of the bag. Pastry tips are available in different shapes and sizes, such as a star. A pastry brush is used to brush beaten egg, butter, or any other liquid onto dough before, during, or just after baking.

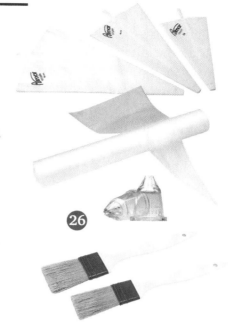

27. Rolling Pins

A rolling pin is used to stretch and roll dough, such as pie crusts, cookies, and biscuits. Most rolling pins are made of hardwood, but marble may be used because it is less likely to pick up the dough. Rolling pins with grooves that add patterns or fancy designs to dough are also available. French rolling pins do not have handles.

28. Bench Scraper

This hand-held rectangular tool has a stainless steel blade and a sturdy handle. The bench scraper can be used to scrape surfaces and cut dough into equal pieces.

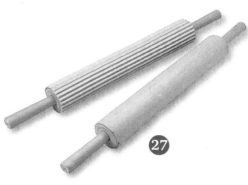

29. Food Molds

Food molds can turn foods such as gelatins, custards, and puddings into eye-catching shapes. Food in liquid form is poured into the mold and allowed to set. The food is removed by inverting a plate over the mold and turning the plate and mold over. The mold is then gently lifted away.

30. Vegetable Brush

With their short, tough bristles, vegetable brushes are useful for cleaning dirt off vegetables.

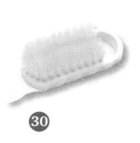

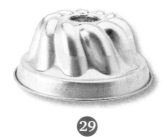

SELECTING APPROPRIATE TOOLS

The tools in a professional kitchen may look similar to the tools in a home kitchen. However, most home kitchen tools cannot withstand the heavy use of a foodservice operation.

Foodservice professionals select tools that are well constructed, comfortable to hold, and safe. NSF International, an organization previously known as the National Sanitation Foundation, tests these qualities. Many states require that foodservice operations use only smallwares and equipment that have been NSF-certified.

NSF Standards

NSF reviews tools and equipment based on certain design, construction, and installation standards. These standards reflect the following requirements:

- Tools, equipment, and their coatings must be nontoxic and should not affect the taste, odor, or color of food.
- Surfaces that come into contact with food must be smooth.
- Tools and equipment need to be easily cleaned.
- External corners and angles must be smooth and sealed.
- Internal corners and edges must be smooth and rounded.
- Waste must be easily removed from tools, equipment, and their coatings.
- Coatings and exposed surfaces must resist chipping and cracking.

MEASURING EQUIPMENT

Accurate volume measures are essential to the success of quantity recipes. Precisely measuring ingredients also helps control portion size and costs. You can take the guesswork out of measurements by using devices designed to accurately measure foods.

Measurements are usually needed for an item's weight or volume. Weight is the heaviness of a substance, while volume is the space occupied by a substance. Sometimes you will also need to measure temperature. See Fig. 10-15 on page 247 (**Measuring Equipment**) for the most common measuring devices used in food service.

SELECTING COOKWARE

Cookware plays an essential role in the professional kitchen. **Cookware** in any well-equipped kitchen includes pots, pans, and baking dishes. Pots and pans may be made of stainless steel, aluminum, copper, cast iron, or ceramics. The chef usually chooses his or her own cookware according to the restaurant's production needs. The following figure shows a range of cookware you'll find in most commercial kitchens. See Fig. 10-16 on pages 248-250 (**Cookware**).

CULINARY TIP

ALUMINUM WARNINGS—Be careful not to use stainless steel utensils with aluminum cookware. Stainless steel utensils can scrape off a thin layer of aluminum and cause certain foods to become discolored. Tomatoes and other foods that are high in acid should not be cooked in aluminum because of chemical reactions.

MEASURING
Equipment

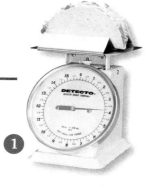

1. Portion Scale

A portion scale is a type of spring scale used to determine the weight of an ingredient or portion of food. It can be reset to zero so you can measure individual ingredients.

2. Electronic Scale

An electronic, or digital, scale weighs an item when it is placed on its tray. The weight is displayed in numbers on a digital readout rather than by a needle. This readout is more accurate than a portion scale.

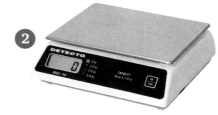

3. Balance Scale

A balance scale is used to measure most baking ingredients. The ingredients being weighed are placed on one side while weights are placed on the other side. When the two sides are balanced, the ingredients weigh the same as the weights.

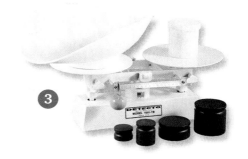

4. Volume Measures

Volume is measured in 8-, 16-, 32-, 64-, and 128-oz. quantities. Volume measures are made of metal, which can stand a lot of use.

5. Liquid Measures

Liquid measures also measure volume, and come in 1 c., 1 pt., and 1-, 2-, and 4-qt. sizes. The lip or spout of the measure helps prevent spills and makes pouring easier.

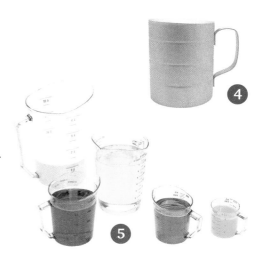

6. Measuring Spoons

Measuring spoons are available in sets and usually include measurements of ¼, ½, 1 tsp., and 1 tbsp. for volume. Stainless steel is recommended because it is less likely to warp or change shape.

7. Ladle

A ladle is used to portion liquids such as sauces and soups. Its long handle enables you to reach to the bottom of a deep pot or pan. The capacity, ranging from 1–16 oz., is marked on the handle.

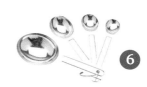

Cookware

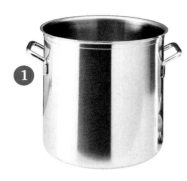

1. Stockpot
A stockpot has straight sides and is taller than it is wide. A stockpot is used to cook large quantities of liquid on the range, such as stocks or soups. Some stockpots have a spigot at the bottom so liquid can be drained off without lifting the pot.

2. Saucepot
The saucepot is similar in shape to a stockpot, only not as deep. The saucepot is used for rangetop cooking.

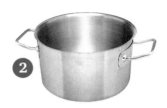

3. Saucepan
A saucepan has a long handle and straight sides. Primarily used for heating and cooking food in liquid, saucepans come in many sizes in order to accommodate a variety of needs.

4. Sauté Pans
There are two types of sauté pans: a pan with straight sides and a pan with sloped sides. Both are used to sauté and fry foods. The slope-sided pan allows the chef to flip items without using a spatula.

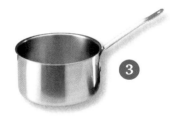

5. Wok
A wok is useful for fast rangetop cooking. The wok's height and sloped sides are well-suited for tossing ingredients, an essential step in stir-frying. Once food has been cooked, it can be pushed to the side of the pan, leaving the hot center free for new ingredients.

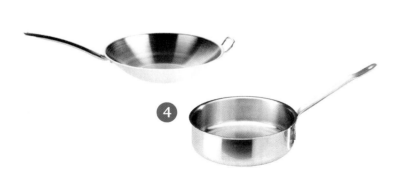

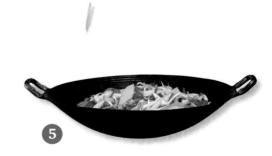

6. Cast-Iron Skillet

A cast-iron skillet is a heavy pan that can withstand high degrees of heat. It is useful for frying and sautéing a variety of items when steady, even heat is desired.

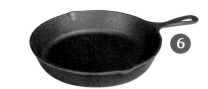

7. Hotel Pans

The cooked foods in a steam table are held in hotel pans. Hotel pans are often used to store refrigerated food and hold casseroles during baking. They come in many different sizes.

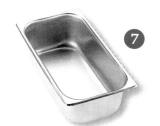

8. Roasting Pan

A roasting pan is used to roast various types of meat and poultry. A lift-out rack that fits in the bottom of the pan allows fat and juices to drain off the food.

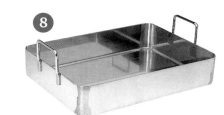

9. Sheet Pan

Sheet pans come in half and full sizes. They can be used to bake biscuits, cookies, sheet cakes, rolls, and meats such as bacon and sausage.

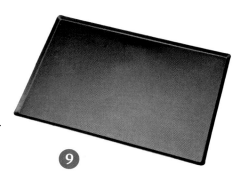

10. Stainless Steel Mixing Bowls

A well-equipped kitchen has a quantity of different-sized, stainless steel mixing bowls. These are used to combine, mix, and whip ingredients.

11. Springform Pan

A springform pan is used to bake soft, sticky mixes, such as cheesecake. It has an insert that rests in the bottom of the pan, and the sides are closed with clasps. Opening the clasps gently releases the cake.

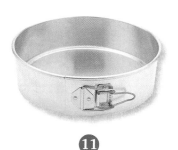

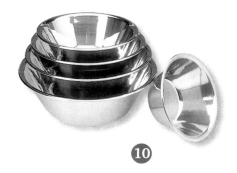

Cookware (Cont'd.)

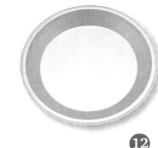

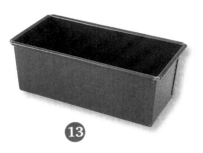

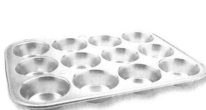

12. Pie Pan

Traditional pies are baked in pie pans. Deep pie pans are slightly wider to accommodate deep-dish fruit and meat pies.

13. Loaf Pan

A loaf pan, also known as a bread pan, is used to bake loaf-shaped foods, such as pound cake, meat loaf, and some breads.

14. Muffin Pan

Different kinds of muffins and cupcakes can be baked in muffin pans. Pans come in various sizes that yield from miniature to giant muffins.

15. Tart Pan

A tart pan is used to bake items with delicate crusts, such as tarts and quiches. The sizes range from 4.5 to 12.5 in. in diameter, and from 0.75 to 1.25 in. high. It has either fluted or smooth sides.

16. Tube Pan

An aluminum tube pan is used to bake tube-shaped desserts, such as angel food cake. It has a removable bottom.

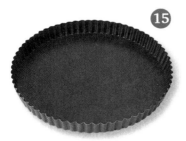

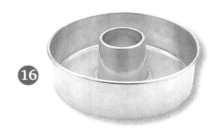

✖ HEAT TRANSFER

You need to consider more than size, shape, and quality when selecting cookware. **Heat transfer**, or how efficiently heat passes from one object to another, must also be kept in mind. The gauge, or type and thickness of the material, determines how well it conducts heat.

No single type of cookware will fit all your needs. For example, although silver is the best heat conductor, it is too costly to use for everyday purposes. Silver has a heat transfer rating of 100%. Copper also has a high heat transfer rating. It, too, is expensive and difficult to clean. That's why many kitchens use aluminum-clad or stainless steel-clad pots and pans. Some kitchens also use cookware with copper-lined bottoms. Cast-iron cookware is also popular.

■ **Aluminum.** Aluminum is a common metal used for commercial cookware because it is lightweight, inexpensive, and rust-free. It also is fairly heat efficient.

■ **Stainless steel.** Stainless steel is a popular choice for commercial cookware because it is virtually rust-free. However, it's a poor and uneven heat conductor. Stainless steel pots often have an added layer of aluminum or copper on the bottom for better heat efficiency. Sometimes iron is added so that the pot can be used on induction ranges.

✖ CLEANING & SANITIZING SMALLWARES

Thoroughly cleaning and sanitizing smallwares (tools and utensils) is an essential step in preventing the spread of bacteria. Even if smallwares look clean, they could still harbor harmful bacteria.

Smallwares need to be washed thoroughly in hot water, rinsed, and then sanitized using a sanitizer, such as chlorine or iodine. This can be done effectively by hand. Follow these steps to hand-wash and sanitize smallwares in a three-compartment sink:

1. Scrape and prerinse smallwares.
2. Fill the first sink with 110°F water and detergent. Wash the smallwares thoroughly with a brush. Drain and refill the water as needed.
3. Fill the second sink with water at about 110°F or use running water with an overflow. Rinse the smallwares to remove all traces of detergent.
4. The third sink is used to sanitize smallwares. Fill it with 171°F water. Some health codes require 180°F. Add the sanitizing agent in the amount listed on the container. Submerge the smallwares for about 30 seconds.
5. Remove and air-dry smallwares in a clean area. Towel drying can recontaminate smallwares.

SECTION 10-2 Knowledge Check

1. Name and describe two tools that measure volume.
2. Why are the bottoms of stainless steel pots and pans usually lined with another type of metal?
3. Explain how to clean and sanitize smallwares (tools and utensils) using a three-compartment sink.

(MINI LAB)

Suppose you work in a deli that wants to start offering chocolate chip cookies. Describe the specific smallwares you would need to measure, mix, bake, and serve the cookies.

SECTION SUMMARIES

10-1 The main parts of a knife are the blade, tang, handle, rivet, and bolster.

10-1 The types of knives that a chef uses to prepare food include: chef, slicer, boning, paring, tournée, fillet, and butcher.

10-1 Basic cutting techniques include: slicing, dicing, and mincing.

10-1 Some knife safety and sanitation rules are: use the knife that correctly suits the job, use a sharp knife, and sanitize the knife after every use.

10-1 Store knives in a knife kit, slotted knife holder, or custom-built drawers.

10-2 Some NSF standards for smallwares include: they must be made of nontoxic materials, be easily cleaned, and their coatings must resist chipping and cracking.

10-2 The efficiency of a pan's heat transfer is determined by the pan's thickness and the type(s) of metal it's made from.

10-2 Proper sanitizing procedures for smallwares need to be followed after every use, regardless if they appear clean.

CHECK YOUR KNOWLEDGE

1. Describe each part of the knife.
2. Explain why high-carbon stainless steel is the most common material used in professional knives.
3. List each type of knife and its main use.
4. Contrast chiffonade, rondelle, and diagonal cuts.
5. Describe the process of sharpening a knife on a whetstone.
6. Identify two types of whisks and explain when they are used.
7. Contrast a strainer and a colander.
8. Why is it important to use smallwares that are NSF-certified?
9. Define weight and volume.
10. Describe heat transfer in cookware, and identify which type of metal is the best all-around choice to cook with.

CRITICAL-THINKING ACTIVITIES

1. Assume you are joining two of your friends, who are also chefs, to cater a party. It is your responsibility to create the vegetable appetizers. Which knives will you need and why?
2. While measuring ingredients to make a cake, you decide to use a portion scale. Why?

WORKPLACE KNOW-HOW

Problem solving. When you consider purchasing quality knives, which two would you start with if you had a limited budget? Why?

LAB-BASED ACTIVITY: Choosing Knives & Smallwares

STEP ❶ Consider what you would need in order to open a sandwich shop that serves simple lunches and dinners. You don't have much kitchen space, so consider knives and smallwares that could be used for more than one job whenever possible. Also, decide whether you will prepare most of the food or if you will have some food prepared and delivered.

STEP ❷ Determine which of the following knives below will be needed for preparing sandwiches and accompaniments.

STEP ❸ Determine which of the smallwares below you will need for your sandwich shop.

STEP ❹ Write your answers to the following questions on a separate sheet of paper:

- Describe why you believe you need the knives, hand tools, and cookware that you chose to use in your sandwich shop.
- What equipment would you need to care for your knives and smallwares?
- Describe maintenance techniques for smallwares (tools and utensils).

Knives and Smallwares

Knives:
- Chef's Knives
- Utility Knives
- Slicer
- Boning Knives
- Paring Knives
- Tournée Knives
- Fillet Knives
- Butcher Knives

Hand Tools:
- Fruit Corer
- Vegetable Peeler
- Kitchen Shears
- Cutting Board
- Cheese Slicer
- Egg Slicer
- Zester
- Melon Baller
- Whisks
- Large Spoons
- Spatulas
- Chef's Fork
- Straight Tongs
- Strainers
- Funnel
- Vegetable Brush
- Can Opener
- Scales
- Liquid Measures
- Volume Measures
- Measuring Spoons

Cookware:
- Stockpots
- Saucepots
- Saucepans
- Wok
- Cast-Iron Skillet
- Hotel Pans
- Bain-Marie Inserts
- Roasting Pans
- Baking Pans
- Sheet Pans
- Stainless Steel Mixing Bowls

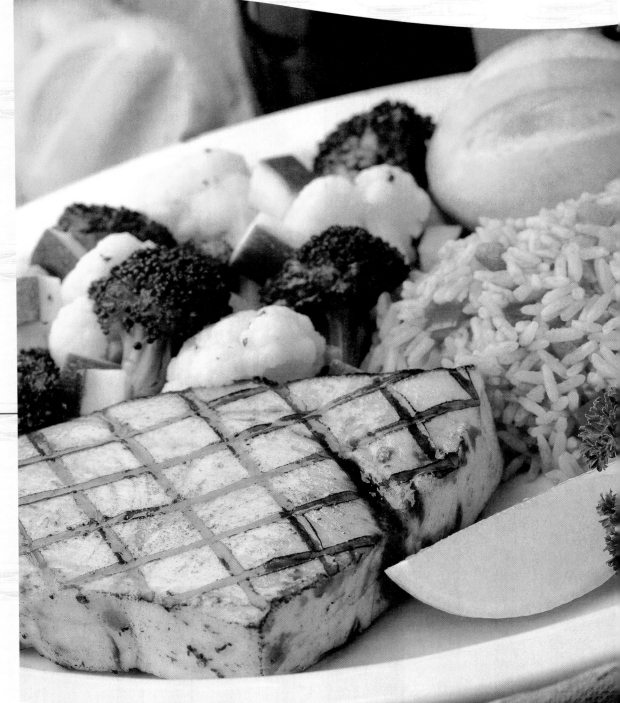

Culinary Nutrition

Nutrition Basics

KEY TERMS

• nutrients
• carbohydrates
• legumes
• amino acids
• cholesterol
• cardiovascular
• saturated fats
• monounsaturated
• polyunsaturated
• hydrogenation
• additives

OBJECTIVES

After reading this section, you will be able to:

• Define the six categories of nutrients.

• Describe the sources and functions of each nutrient category.

• Identify nutritious meals and the preparation methods used to prepare them.

• Describe the types and uses of food additives.

IMAGINE that some employees have complained that the cafeteria doesn't offer enough healthful choices on its menu. Before you make any suggestions to make menu items more nutritious, you need to understand the basics of nutrition. You can then use what you've learned to suggest more healthful menu items.

✖ THE NUTRIENTS

The human body requires food for growth and maintaining life. An important factor in meeting this need is a food's nutrient content. **Nutrients** are chemical compounds that help the body carry out its functions. There are more than 40 nutrients in food. They are grouped into six categories: carbohydrates, proteins, fats, vitamins, minerals, and water.

Carbohydrates

Carbohydrates are the body's main source of energy, or fuel. Simple carbohydrates, or sugars, include both natural and refined, or processed sugars. Natural sugars are part of foods like fruits,

vegetables, and milk. Foods with these sugars also carry other important nutrients. Refined sugars, such as those shown in Fig. 11-1, are sugars used primarily as sweeteners. These sugars provide little more than calories.

Complex carbohydrates are starches, such as pasta, grains, cereals, and **legumes**, or the seeds and pods from certain plants. Beans, lentils, and peas are examples of legumes. Foods high in complex carbohydrates contain many other nutrients your body needs, such as vitamins and minerals. The body breaks down simple and complex carbohydrates into a usable energy source known as glucose. Glucose gives your body the energy it needs to work properly.

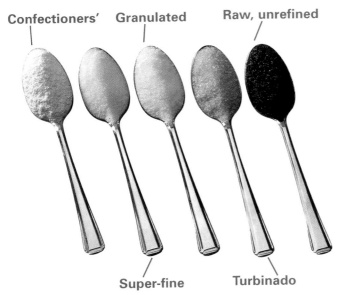

Confectioners'   Granulated   Raw, unrefined

Super-fine   Turbinado

Fig. 11-1. Refined sugars are simple carbohydrates.

■ **Fiber.** A unique form of a complex carbohydrate that does not provide energy is fiber. There are two types of fiber: soluble fiber, which dissolves in water, and insoluble fiber, which absorbs water. Fiber is key to the functioning of the digestive system and the elimination of wastes. Its main advantage is that it can't be digested. As it passes through the body, fiber helps remove harmful wastes. Insoluble fiber is found in the outer coating of whole grains. Soluble fiber is found in foods such as oat bran and grains. Soluble fiber has been associated with the prevention of heart disease and some cancers. See Fig. 11-2.

Fig. 11-2. Cabbage is a source of soluble fiber. Nuts provide insoluble fiber.

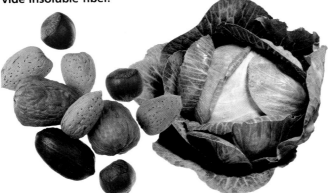

Proteins

Protein builds, maintains, and repairs body tissues. It is essential for healthy muscles, skin, bones, eyes, and hair, and it plays an important role in fighting disease. If a person doesn't eat enough carbohydrate and fat, the body will use protein for energy.

Through digestion, protein is broken down into small units called **amino acids**. There are 22 amino acids which can be combined in certain ways to produce complete proteins. Some amino acids can be created by the body, while others cannot and must be obtained from food. Animal foods, such as fish, meats, poultry, eggs, milk and milk products, provide all of the essential amino acids. They are called complete proteins. Most plant foods, such as vegetables, grains, nuts, and dry beans, lack some of the essential amino acids. Because of this, they are referred to as incomplete proteins. However, by combining nuts or dry beans and grains, a person can eat all of the essential amino acids. For example, peanut butter on whole wheat bread includes all essential amino acids. See Fig. 11-3.

Fig. 11-3.

COMPLETE PROTEIN FOOD COMBINATIONS
• Lentil salad, sunflower seeds, and beans.
• Garbanzo beans and sesame seeds.
• Rice and red beans.
• Refried beans and corn tortillas.
• Split pea soup and whole wheat bread.
• Peanut butter and whole wheat bread.
• Baked beans and brown bread.
• Pasta and beans.
• Wheat noodles with peanut sauce.
• Barley or couscous and garbanzo beans.

WHAT IS FAT?

Fat is a compound containing a chain of carbon and hydrogen atoms. All carbon atoms have four bonds, or links, to other atoms. Some of the bonds are single bonds and some are double bonds. Single bonds are formed when two atoms share one pair of electrons. Double bonds are formed when hydrogen bonds are missing. Without hydrogen, carbon cannot form single bonds. To make up for a missing hydrogen atom, a carbon atom will form a double bond with another carbon atom. Therefore, two carbon atoms that are each missing a hydrogen atom will bond to each other by forming a double bond.

Basically, fats are characterized by their chemical structure. All saturated fats have single bonds. Unsaturated fats are classified by the number of double bonds that form. For example, monounsaturated fat is missing two hydrogen atoms, which in turn create one double bond between the carbon atoms. Likewise, a polyunsaturated fat contains more than one double bond.

Two Fat Molecules

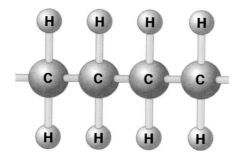

**Saturated Fat
(single bonding)**

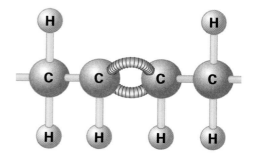

**Unsaturated Fat
(double bonding)**

APPLY IT!

Complete the following experiment to determine whether a food substance contains fat. You will need a brown paper lunch bag, cooking oil, an orange, peanut butter, mayonnaise, and water.

1. Cut the paper lunch bag into five sections. Label each section with the name of one of the ingredients listed and place it on a table or countertop.

2. Use your finger to rub a small amount of oil on one of the sections.

3. Repeat the process with each of the other ingredients listed.

4. When you are finished, lift each section of paper up to a light. Which foods caused the paper to become transparent?

5. Make a chart of each substance you test and record your observations.

6. Which substances appear to contain fat?

7. Select three more items and test them to determine if they contain fat.

Fats & Cholesterol

Fat and cholesterol play an essential role in keeping the body healthy. However, there is strong evidence that shows a diet higher than 30% in fat and cholesterol can put you at risk for such diseases as heart disease and cancer. Fat regulates bodily functions and helps carry fat-soluble vitamins. It is a source of stored energy and a cushion for body organs. Fat makes foods taste good. Fats are divided into three categories: saturated (SA-chuh-ray-tuhd), mono-unsaturated (mah-noh-uhn-SA-chuh-ray-tuhd), and polyunsaturated (pah-lee-uhn-SA-chuh-ray-tuhd).

■ **Cholesterol.** Found in all body cells and in all animal foods, such as meat, egg yolks, and dairy products, **cholesterol** (kuh-LES-tuhr-ol) is a fatlike substance. The body needs and does make its own cholesterol to produce cell membranes, hormones, Vitamin D, and bile acids, which help digest fats. Some cholesterol circulates through the blood stream in chemical packages called lipoproteins (LIH-poh-PROH-teenz). There are two types of lipoproteins. They are low-density lipoproteins (LDL) and high-density lipoproteins (HDL).

Too much LDL, or bad cholesterol, can contribute to **cardiovascular** (KAHR-dee-oh-VAS-kyuh-luhr), or heart-related, problems because it can build up on artery walls. This buildup slows or prevents the flow of blood to the heart and other vital organs. Higher HDL, or good cholesterol, helps lower the amount of cholesterol in the blood. Making wise food choices can help reduce the amount of harmful cholesterol in the blood.

■ **Saturated fats.** Fats that tend to increase the amount of cholesterol in the blood and are solid at room temperature are called **saturated fats**. Saturated fats include items such as lard, butter, whole-milk products, the visible fat on meat, and tropical (coconut, palm, and palm kernel) oils. Saturated fats have been linked to an increased risk for heart disease and other cardiovascular problems.

■ **Monounsaturated fats.** Usually liquid at room temperature, olive and peanut oils are **monounsaturated fats**. Unsaturated fats (poly and mono) are considered more healthful than saturated fats

because they generally do not raise cholesterol levels. Peanut oil is also a monounsaturated fat.

■ **Polyunsaturated fats.** Corn, sunflower, and soybean oils are **polyunsaturated fats** and are usually liquid at room temperature. Nuts, seeds, and fish also contain some polyunsaturated fats. Soybean oil is also a polyunsaturated fat.

Many fats, such as those found in margarine and shortening, have gone through a hydrogenation process. **Hydrogenation** (hy-DRAH-juh-NAY-shun) is a process in which hydrogen is added under pressure to polyunsaturated fats, such as soybean oil. Hydrogenation changes liquid oil into a solid fat.

Vitamins

Vitamins help regulate many bodily functions and assist other nutrients in doing their jobs. Fruits and vegetables are excellent sources of vitamins. Vitamins are divided into two types: water-soluble and fat-soluble. Both types of vitamins are vital for normal growth and bodily functions.

■ **Water-soluble vitamins.** Because they dissolve in water, water-soluble vitamins must be consumed every day since the body loses them in waste fluids. Water-soluble vitamins include Vitamin C and all the B vitamins. See Fig. 11-4A.

■ **Fat-soluble vitamins.** Unlike water-soluble vitamins, fat-soluble vitamins are stored in the liver. Vitamins A, D, E, and K are fat-soluble. If taken in large quantities for a long period of time, fat-soluble vitamins can accumulate and cause disease or even death. See Fig. 11-4B.

Minerals

Minerals are an essential part of your bones and teeth. They also regulate body processes, such as nerve function, and are needed in very small quantities. Minerals are divided into two categories: major and trace. The body needs more of the major minerals than it does of the trace minerals, but both types are equally important. Fig. 11-5A lists the major minerals, their functions, and sources. Fig. 11-5B lists the trace minerals.

Fig. 11-4A.
Water-Soluble Vitamins

VITAMIN	FUNCTION IN THE BODY	FOOD SOURCES
Thiamin (THIE-uh-muhn) (Vitamin B$_1$)	• Helps use carbohydrates for energy. • Promotes normal appetites.	Dry beans, pork and other meats, whole and fortified grains.
Riboflavin (ri-buh-FLAY-vuhn) (Vitamin B$_2$)	• Keep skin and eyes healthy. • Helps use carbohydrates, fats, and proteins for energy.	Dairy products, meat, poultry, fish, whole and fortified grains, eggs.
Niacin (NY-uh-suhn) (Vitamin B$_3$)	• Keeps skin and nervous system healthy. • Enables normal digestion. • Helps use nutrients for energy.	Meat, poultry, fish, liver, shellfish, dry beans, nuts, whole and fortified grains.
Vitamin B$_6$	• Assists in building red blood cells. • Helps use carbohydrates and proteins. • Keeps nervous system healthy.	Meat, poultry, fish, liver, shellfish, dry beans, potatoes, whole grains, some fruits and vegetables.
Vitamin B$_{12}$	• Assists in building red blood cells. • Keeps nervous system healthy. • Helps use carbohydrates, fats, and proteins.	Eggs, meat, poultry, fish, dairy products, shellfish, some fortified foods.
Folate (FOH-layt) (Folic Acid)	• Helps prevent birth defects. • Assists in building red blood cells. • Helps use proteins.	Dark green, leafy vegetables; dry beans; orange juice; seeds; whole and fortified grains; fruits.
Vitamin C [Ascorbic (uh-SKOR-bihk) Acid]	• Strengthens immune system. • Keeps teeth, gums, blood vessels, and bones healthy. • Helps heal wounds and absorb iron.	Citrus fruits such as oranges and grapefruits, kiwi, cabbage, strawberries, broccoli, tomatoes, cantaloupes, green peppers, and potatoes.
Biotin (BY-uh-tuhn)	• Helps use carbohydrates, fats, and proteins.	Dark green, leafy vegetables; liver; egg yolks; whole grains.
Pantothenic (PANT-uh-THEN-ik) Acid	• Helps use carbohydrates, fats, and proteins for energy. • Promotes growth and development. • Helps produce cholesterol.	Dry beans, meat, poultry, fish, eggs, milk, whole grains, fruits and vegetables.

Fig. 11-4B.

Fat-Soluble Vitamins

VITAMIN	FUNCTION IN THE BODY	FOOD SOURCES
Vitamin A	• Keeps skin and hair healthy and strengthens immune system. • Protects eyes and enables night vision.	Dark green, leafy vegetables such as spinach; yellow-orange fruits and vegetables such as carrots, pumpkin, and apricots; dairy products; liver; egg yolks.
Vitamin D	• Helps body absorb and regulate calcium and phosphorus for strong bones, teeth, and muscles.	Fortified milk; fatty fish such as salmon, liver, egg yolks; exposure to sunlight causes the body to produce vitamin D.
Vitamin E	• Protects other nutrients. • Helps create muscles and red blood cells.	Dark green, leafy vegetables such as spinach; vegetable oils; nuts; seeds; whole grains; wheat germ.
Vitamin K	• Assists in blood clotting.	Egg yolks; dark green, leafy vegetables such as spinach; liver; wheat germ and wheat bran.

Fig. 11-5A.

Major Minerals

MINERAL	FUNCTION IN THE BODY	FOOD SOURCES
Calcium	• Builds and renews bones and teeth. • Needed for muscle contraction. • Assists in blood clotting. • Regulates nervous system and other processes.	Dairy products; dry beans; fortified juices and cereals; dark green, leafy vegetables such as kale; turnips; canned sardines and salmon.
Magnesium (mag-NEE-zee-uhm)	• Builds and renews bones. • Helps nervous system and muscles work.	Whole grains; dry beans; dark green, leafy vegetables; nuts; seeds; fish; shellfish.
Phosphorus (FAHS-fuh-ruhs)	• Builds and renews bones and teeth. • Helps use nutrients for energy.	Dairy products, nuts, dry beans, whole grains, poultry, meat, fish, egg yolks.
Potassium (puh-TA-see-uhm)	• Helps maintain blood pressure and heartbeat. • Maintains fluid balance in body.	Fruits such as bananas, oranges, and cantaloupes; meats; dry beans; poultry; fish; vegetables; dairy products.
Sodium	• Helps regulate blood pressure. • Maintains fluid balance in body.	Salt, foods that contain salt, soy sauce, MSG.

Water

Water is essential for sustaining life. Water makes up about 60% of an adult's body weight. It cleans toxins from the body, cushions joints, and increases the body's ability to transport nutrients. Healthy adults need to drink 64–80 oz. of water a day. Those 8–10 glasses can come from any substance that is mostly water, such as juice, gelatin, soup, milk, and ice. However, water-based beverages that contain caffeine, such as coffee, tea, and soft drinks, cause the body to eliminate water.

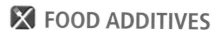 FOOD ADDITIVES

Additives are substances added to foods to improve them in some way. Different additives can extend a food's shelf life or improve its flavor, texture, or appearance. See Fig. 11-6 for additives commonly used in the foodservice industry.

The FDA is ultimately responsible for regulating additives that are put into foods. In some cases, the approval of additives can take many years. Food manufacturers must test an additive for its effectiveness, detection, measurability, and overall safety. The results are then submitted to the FDA for review and approval. Additives are periodically evaluated by the FDA. No additive has permanent approval.

Fig. 11-5B.

Trace Minerals

MINERAL	FUNCTION IN THE BODY	FOOD SOURCES
Chloride (KLOHR-yde)	• Works with sodium to balance fluids. • Helps nerve transmittal.	Salt, foods that contain salt, soy sauce, meats, milk.
Iron	• Helps cells use oxygen. • Helps the blood carry oxygen.	Meat; fish; shellfish; dry beans; egg yolks; dried fruit; whole and fortified grains; dark green, leafy vegetables.
Iodine	• Helps use energy.	Iodized salt, saltwater fish, shellfish, breads.
Zinc	• Assists in growth and maintenance of tissues. • Helps heal wounds and form blood. • Helps use carbohydrates, fats, and proteins. • Affects taste and smell.	Whole grains, poultry, fish, shellfish products, legumes, dairy products, eggs.
Copper	• Assists iron in building red blood cells. • Keeps nervous system, bones, and blood vessels healthy.	Meat, fish, shellfish, whole grains, nuts, seeds, dry beans.
Fluoride (FLAWR-yde)	• Strengthens teeth and prevents decay.	Fish, shellfish; fluoride is often added to drinking water.
Selenium (suh-LEE-nee-uhm)	• Helps heart function normally.	Fish, shellfish, eggs, liver, whole grains.

Fig. 11-6.

TYPE OF ADDITIVE	NAME OF ADDITIVE	FOOD IN WHICH ADDITIVE IS USED
Thickeners and Stabilizers	• Modified food starches • Cornstarch • Flour	• Fruit fillings, pie fillings, puddings. • Sauces, instant foods. • Sauces.
Gelling Agents	• Gelatin • Pectin	• Baked desserts, fillings. • Sherbets; fruit jellies, preserves, jams; glazes.
Nutrients	• Iron, vitamin C, thiamin, Riboflavin	• Enriched foods, such as breads, cereals, flour, juices, flavored beverages.
Coloring Agents	• Annato (uh-NAHT-oh) • Citrus Red No. 2, Red No. 3, Green No. 3, Yellow No. 6	• Cheese. • Soft drinks, baked items, cereals, candy.
Flavoring Agents	• Vanilla, almond, lemon • MSG	• Baked items, ice cream, candy. • Asian foods, soups.
Fat Substitutes	• Olestra™ (oh-LEHS-trah) • Simplesse™ (SIHM-plehs)	• Snack foods, such as potato chips. • Frozen desserts, such as ice cream; sour cream; margarine; salad dressings.
Sugar Substitutes	• Aspartame (AS-puhr-taym) • Saccharin (SAH-kuh-ruhn) • Acesulfame K (uh-SUHS-uhl-faym) • Sucralose (SOO-kruh-lohs)	• All-purpose sweetener used in all foods and beverages. • Used as a table-top sweetener and in a variety of foods and beverages. • Gelatin, pudding, candy, chewing gum, and as a table-top sweetener. • Dairy products, carbonated beverages, jams and jellies, chewing gum, syrup, and as a table-top sweetener.

SECTION 11-1   Knowledge Check

1. Define each of the six major categories of nutrients.

2. List the functions and food sources of two vitamins and two minerals.

3. What are three methods a foodservice operation can use to prepare and offer healthful meals?

MINI LAB

Suggest a more healthful alternative for each of the following foods: fried chicken, French fries, a cheeseburger, white rice, coconut oil, whole milk, and scrambled eggs. Explain how each change would improve the food's nutritional value.

Guidelines for Meal Planning

KEY TERMS

- daily values
- nutrient-dense
- glycogen
- dehydration
- vegetarians
- lacto vegetarians
- ovo vegetarians
- lacto-ovo vegetarians
- vegans
- phytochemicals

OBJECTIVES

After reading this section, you will be able to:

- Explain the purpose of the Dietary Guidelines for Americans, nutrition labels, and the Food Guide Pyramid.

- Describe how age, activity level, lifestyle, and health influence dietary needs.

- Apply knowledge of special dietary needs to menu planning.

WHEN planning menus, government guidelines and recommendations can help you create well-balanced meals. The Dietary Guidelines and Food Guide Pyramid are just a few. In addition, you need to be aware of the factors that influence a person's dietary needs. These factors include age, activity level, lifestyle, and health.

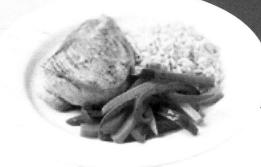

✖ GOVERNMENT GUIDELINES

For almost 100 years, the United States government has provided dietary guidelines and recommendations to help consumers make healthful food choices. Foodservice professionals must be familiar with these guidelines so they can meet the demands of health-conscious customers.

The Recommended Dietary Allowances

The Recommended Dietary Allowances (RDAs) for the essential nutrients are developed by the Food and Nutrition Board of the National Academy of Sciences. The RDA of each nutrient is designed to meet the nutritional needs of the majority of healthy Americans. RDAs are updated about every five years.

Nutrition Labels

Under the Nutrition Labeling and Education Act of 1990, most foods must include nutrition labels. Nutrition labels provide information on serving size, calories, and nutrients. Nutrients are measured in two ways: grams and daily value percentages. **Daily values** are the amount of nutrients a

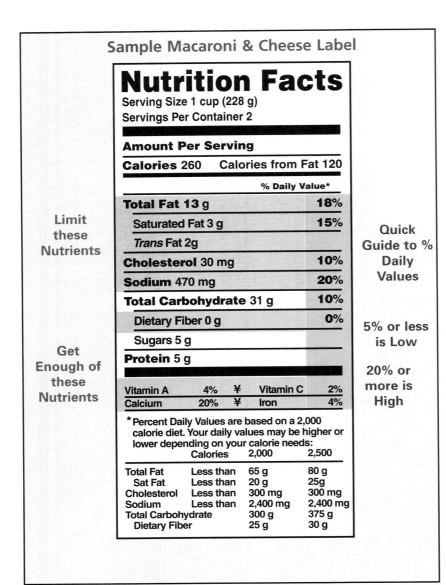

Sample Macaroni & Cheese Label

Nutrition Facts

Serving Size 1 cup (228 g)
Servings Per Container 2

Amount Per Serving

Calories 260   Calories from Fat 120

	% Daily Value*
Total Fat 13 g	**18%**
Saturated Fat 3 g	**15%**
Trans Fat 2g	
Cholesterol 30 mg	**10%**
Sodium 470 mg	**20%**
Total Carbohydrate 31 g	**10%**
Dietary Fiber 0 g	**0%**
Sugars 5 g	
Protein 5 g	

Vitamin A	4%	Vitamin C	2%
Calcium	20%	Iron	4%

*Percent Daily Values are based on a 2,000 calorie diet. Your daily values may be higher or lower depending on your calorie needs:

Calories		2,000	2,500
Total Fat	Less than	65 g	80 g
Sat Fat	Less than	20 g	25g
Cholesterol	Less than	300 mg	300 mg
Sodium	Less than	2,400 mg	2,400 mg
Total Carbohydrate		300 g	375 g
Dietary Fiber		25 g	30 g

Limit these Nutrients

Get Enough of these Nutrients

Quick Guide to % Daily Values

5% or less is Low

20% or more is High

Fig. 11-7. The Nutrition Facts panel has two parts. The top section contains product-specific information that varies with each food product. The bottom part provides general dietary information about nutrients.

person needs every day based on a 2,000-calorie diet. This number serves only as a guide, since each person's calorie needs are different. For example, if you ate one cup of macaroni and cheese, it would provide 18% of the total fats and 10% of the total carbohydrates you need each day. This percentage would be higher or lower if you eat more or less than 2,000 calories a day. See Fig. 11-7.

The nutrients listed first on a nutrition label are the ones most people eat in adequate amounts. The nutrients at the bottom of the label—Vitamin A, Vitamin C, calcium, and iron—are the nutrients many people lack in their diets.

Dietary Guidelines for Americans

The 2005 Dietary Guidelines for Americans are published by the USDA and the U.S. Department of Health and Human Services. These guidelines offer recommendations on how to make healthful daily food choices from the following USDA MyPyramid food groups: Fruit Group, Vegetable Group, Grain Group, Meat & Bean Group, Milk Group, and Oils. These guidelines can help you make healthful choices to meet your nutrient requirements while eating the number of calories that support a healthful body weight. See Fig. 11-8.

Fig. 11-8.

Summary of the Dietary Guidelines for Americans

MAIN TOPIC	KEY RECOMMENDATIONS
Adequate Nutrients Within Calorie Needs	• Eat a variety of nutritious foods and beverages. • Choose foods that limit saturated and *trans* fats, cholesterol, added sugars, and salt. Adopt a balanced eating pattern.
Weight Management	• Balance calories consumed with calories used for energy needs to maintain a healthy weight. Adjust calories and activity to prevent weight gain.
Physical Activity	• Engage in regular physical activity and reduce sedentary activities. • Include cardiovascular conditioning, flexibility, and resistance exercises for muscle strength and endurance.
Food Groups to Encourage	• Consume a variety of foods from the different food groups. Eat the recommended amounts each day balanced with energy needs.
Fats	• Consume less than 10 percent of calories from saturated fat and less than 300 mg/day of cholesterol. • Keep total fat intake between 20 and 35 percent of calories, with most fats coming from sources of polyunsaturated and monounsaturated fatty acids. • Choose lean, low-fat, or fat-free when selecting and preparing foods. Limit intake of fats and oils high in saturated and trans fat.
Carbohydrates	• Choose fiber-rich fruits, vegetables, and whole grains often. • Choose foods and beverages with little added sugars. • Practice good oral hygiene and consume sugar- and starch-containing foods and beverages less frequently.
Sodium and Potassium	• Consume less than 2,300 mg of sodium (about 1 teaspoon of salt) per day by choosing and preparing foods with little salt. • Consume potassium-rich foods, such as fruits and vegetables.
Alcoholic Beverages*	• Alcoholic beverages should not be consumed by some people, such as those who cannot restrict their intake, women who are pregnant or could become pregnant, children and adolescents, individuals taking medications that can interact with alcohol, and those with specific medical conditions. • Avoid alcoholic beverages when participating in activities that require attention, skill, or coordination.
Food Safety	• Avoid microbial foodborne illness by cleaning hands, food contact surfaces, and fruits and vegetables. • Keep raw, cooked, and ready-to-eat foods separated. • Cook foods to a safe temperature to kill microorganisms. • Refrigerate perishable foods promptly and defrost foods properly. • Avoid raw (unpasteurized) milk or milk products, raw or partially cooked eggs or foods containing raw eggs, raw or undercooked meat and poultry, unpasteurized juices, and raw sprouts.

Under-age consumption of alcoholic beverages is illegal and is not promoted by these guidelines.

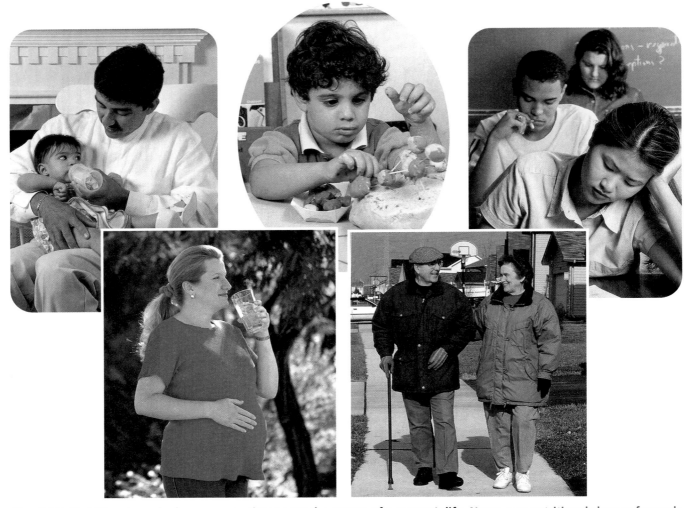

Fig. 11-9. Nutritional needs change many times over the course of a person's life. Name one nutritional change for each stage of life shown.

✖ MEETING DIETARY NEEDS

The Dietary Guidelines are useful tools for planning balanced menus for healthy adults. However, foodservice professionals need to be aware that these guidelines do not apply to everyone. Many factors can influence dietary needs, including age, activity level, lifestyle, and health.

Age

Nutritional needs change over a person's life span. Infancy, childhood, adolescence, and pregnancy are all periods of growth that require extra nutrients. Also, as people age, their dietary needs continue to change. See Fig. 11-9.

At each stage of life, it is important to eat nutrient-dense foods, such as fruits and vegetables. **Nutrient-dense** foods are low in calories, but rich in nutrients. Broccoli, carrots, sunflower seeds, and whole wheat bread are examples of nutrient-dense foods.

■ **Pregnant women.** A woman's nutritional habits before and during pregnancy influence her health and the health of her baby. Pregnant women should slightly increase their calories and eat more nutrient-dense foods. Mothers who decide to breastfeed need to follow these same guidelines and drink plenty of fluids.

■ **Infants.** Babies grow more during their first year than at any other time of their lives, so they need a plentiful supply of nutrients that contribute to growth. Generally, the only food babies need for the first four to six months is breast milk or formula. Infants then move to iron-fortified cereals, strained vegetables and fruits, and eventually cut-up table foods.

■ **Children.** Children need a wide variety of foods served in small portions. Because their stomachs can't hold much food at once, they need snacks between meals to supply all their nutrients. Snacks may include fresh fruit, half of a sandwich, or yogurt. It is normal for a child's appetite to vary. Children may eat more than usual during growth spurts and less than usual during periods of low growth.

■ **Teenagers.** The many psychological and physical changes that occur during adolescence lead to an increased need for almost all nutrients. Teenagers also begin to make their own food choices at this time.

■ **Elderly.** People lose muscle and bone mass as they age. The functioning of body organs also declines. Other factors that can influence the nutritional needs of the elderly include health problems, loss of teeth, a decreased appetite, and an inability to prepare nutritious meals.

Activity Level

Physical activity requires energy. The type of activity and its duration, frequency, and intensity determine how much energy is needed.

The nutritional needs of an athlete differ from those of a less active person because of the amount of energy each uses. Your body breaks down carbohydrates into glucose for energy. It converts extra carbohydrates into **glycogen** (GLY-kuh-juhn), a storage form of glucose. When exercising for long periods of time, the body uses glycogen for energy. Eating plenty of complex carbohydrates ensures that the body will have a steady supply of glycogen.

It is also important to drink plenty of water before, during, and after exercise. See Fig. 11-10. A large amount of water is lost through perspiration. Not replenishing this water can lead to **dehydration** (dee-hi-DRAY-shun), or fluid imbalance. Dehydration can cause health problems, such as heat stroke or heat exhaustion.

Lifestyle

Many Americans are adopting a vegetarian lifestyle. **Vegetarians** (veh-juh-TEHR-ee-uhns) do not eat meat or other animal foods. Instead, they eat plant-based foods, such as vegetables, grains, fruits, and beans. Vegetarian diets are generally lower in fat, saturated fat, and cholesterol than typical American diets. There are four types of vegetarians.

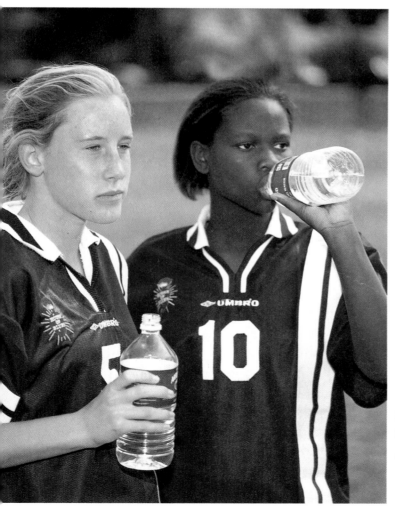

Fig. 11-10. Fluid is lost through perspiration, so it is important to drink plenty of water before, during, and after exercise.

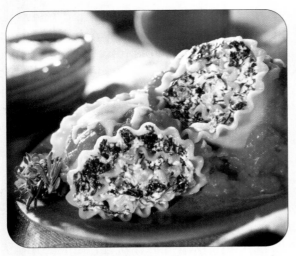

Fig. 11-A. Lacto Vegetarian.

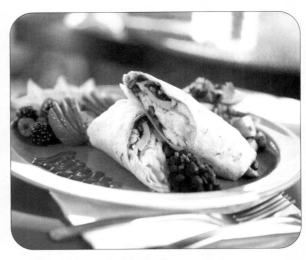

Fig. 11-B. Ovo Vegetarian.

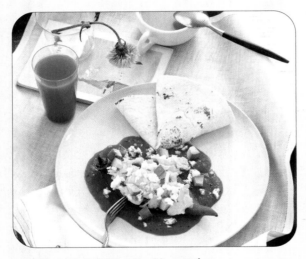

Fig. 11-C. Lacto-ovo Vegetarian.

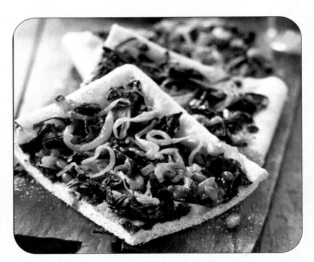

Fig. 11-D. Vegan.

- **Lacto vegetarians** eat or drink some dairy products, such as cheese and milk, but don't eat eggs.
- **Ovo vegetarians** eat eggs in addition to foods from plant sources.
- **Lacto-ovo vegetarians** include dairy products (lacto) and eggs (ovo) in their diets.
- **Vegans** (VEE-guns) do not eat any meat or animal products.

Most vegetarian diets are nutritionally complete if the vegetarians include a variety of foods. Vegetarians must be careful to combine foods in order to eat enough protein. The Vegetarian Food Pyramid is similar to the Food Guide Pyramid. However, the meat, fish, and poultry group has been replaced with dry beans, nuts, seeds, and meat alternatives such as soy products. See Fig. 11-11.

Health

Diet is key in preventing and treating many health conditions. Some of these conditions include cardiovascular disease and cancer.

■ **Cardiovascular disease.** Over time, cholesterol can block arteries and result in a stroke or heart attack. High blood pressure can also impact cardiovascular disease. Large intakes of salt or sodium can increase high blood pressure. The first step in treating high cholesterol or high blood

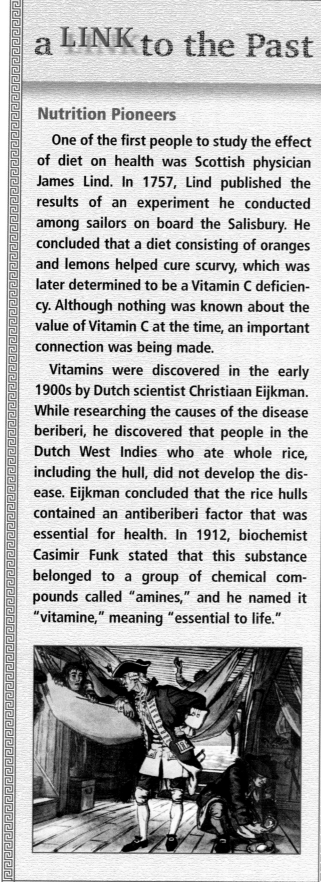
pressure is to modify the diet and increase exercise. People with high cholesterol are advised to reduce their fat, saturated fat, and cholesterol intake and increase their soluble fiber intake. People with high blood pressure need to limit their salt intake and the number of processed foods they eat, which tend to be high in salt.

There are many ways a foodservice operation can help people with high cholesterol and high blood pressure meet their dietary goals. For example, plan meals around dishes rich in complex carbohydrates and fiber, such as dry beans and whole grains. Feature lots of fruits and vegetables cooked with little or no fat or salt. Offer moderate portions of lean meats and fish. Limit the use of fats, especially saturated fats. Use alternatives such as olive oil instead of butter and skim milk instead of whole milk. Use seasonings, other than salt, that are rich in flavor.

■ **Food allergies.** Foodservice operations must provide information to customers about foods that may cause allergic reactions. Avoiding an allergy-causing food is the only way to prevent allergic reactions. Symptoms of an allergic reaction can include headaches, hives, difficulty breathing, nasal congestion, gastrointestinal distress, and even death.

It is important for menu descriptions to list a dish's ingredients. For example, if a chef uses peanuts in a sauce, it should be stated on the menu. This way customers who are allergic to peanuts can avoid ordering the dish. The illustration on page 288 in Chapter 12 shows some common foods that can cause allergic reactions.

■ **Cancer.** Cancer is the unrestrained division and growth of cells that interferes with normal body functions. It is the second leading cause of death in the United States. Research shows that a low-fat diet rich in fruits, vegetables, and fiber should be part of people's daily diets. Eating too much fat and saturated fat can increase the risk of cancer. A low-fat diet rich in fruits, vegetables, and fiber is thought to decrease the risk of cancer.

■ Phytochemicals. Natural chemicals such as those found in plants, fruits, vegetables, grains, and dry beans are called **phytochemicals** (FY-toh-KEHM-eh-kuhls). They seem to have anti-cancer properties. Each of these foods seems to have a different mix of phytochemicals. Thus, eating a variety of these foods provides the best nutritional benefit. For example, fruits and vegetables may help eliminate cancer-causing substances from the body. See Fig. 11-12.

Fig. 11-12.

PHYTOCHEMICAL	FUNCTION IN THE BODY	FOOD SOURCES
Flavonoids (FLAY-vuh-noyd)	• May function as an antioxidant. • Lowers the risk of cancer.	• Apples and grapefruit.
Resveratrol (ruhs-VEHR-a-trahl)	• Can prevent carcinogens. • May lower cholesterol.	• Grapes.
Limonene (LIH-muh-neen)	• Releases detoxification enzymes in the liver.	• Citrus fruits such as oranges, limes, and lemons.
Ellagic Acid (uh-LAH-jihk)	• Triggers the production of enzymes that fight carcinogens.	• Blackberries, cranberries, and strawberries.
Lycopene (LEYE-kuh-peen)	• Can function as an antioxidant. • May lower the risk of heart disease and cancer.	• Tomatoes and watermelon.
Capsaicin (kap-SAY-uh-suhn)	• May prevent carcinogens. • Diminishes blood clotting.	• Hot peppers.
Allyl Sulfide (A-luhl SUHL-fyd)	• Facilitates the production of enzymes that combat carcinogens.	• Onions, garlic, leeks, and shallots.
Isothiocyanates and Indoles (I-suh-thy-oh-sy-a-NAH-tuhs) (IHN-dohls)	• May increase the fabrication of enzymes that decrease carcinogens from harming DNA.	• Broccoli, cauliflower, brussels sprouts, and cabbage.

SECTION 11-2   Knowledge Check

1. Identify three ways that the Dietary Guidelines, nutrition labels, and the food pyramid can help you plan nutritious menus.

2. Explain how age, activity level, and lifestyle affect a person's dietary needs.

3. Explain how diet impacts health.

MINI LAB

Write down today's school lunch menu. How does the menu address the food pyramid and the Dietary Guidelines for Americans? What suggestions could you make to complete your food intake for the day?

Culinary Principles

OBJECTIVES

After reading this section, you will be able to:

- Explain how nutrients in food are affected by time and water.

- Prepare, cook, and store food to retain nutrients.

- List ways to reduce the amount of fat, cholesterol, and sodium in recipes.

SUPPOSE a pregnant woman dining at a restaurant orders red beans and rice. She knows that beans are an excellent source of iron, which is essential for a healthy pregnancy. What she may not know, however, is that the nutritional value of the beans may vary depending on how they are prepared. A food's nutrients can be lost through improper preparation, cooking, and storage. Knowing how these techniques impact nutrients will enable you to retain the maximum amount of nutrients in foods you cook.

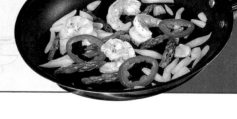

✖ PREVENTING NUTRIENT LOSS

How foods are prepared, cooked, and stored is critical to their nutritional content. The techniques that destroy nutrients can also destroy a food's color, texture, and flavor. By learning how to properly care for and prepare foods, you can ensure that the food you're serving is of the highest nutritional value possible.

From the time a food product is separated from the land or water, the possibility for nutrient loss begins. However, the way a food is prepared can speed up or slow down this process.

■ **Time.** Foods lose nutrients with age, so use them as soon as possible. Most foodservice operations use fresh produce and meats within three or four days and fresh ground meats within one to two days.

■ **Water.** Nutrients, especially water-soluble Vitamins B and C, will **leach**, or dissolve, into the water. For this reason, avoid letting vegetables rest in water before or after cooking. When cleaning produce, do not soak items in water for longer than necessary. See Fig. 11-13.

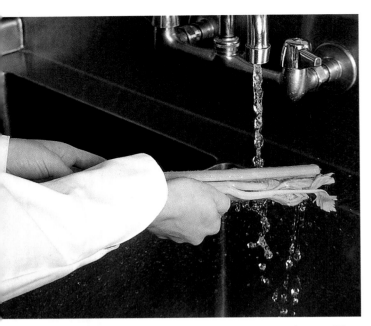

Fig. 11-13. If produce is soaked in water, nutrients will leach into the liquid. How can you prevent this from happening?

Cooking

The same elements that can harm food during preparation can harm it as it's being cooked. Follow these general guidelines while cooking:

- High temperatures can destroy vitamins in foods, such as deep-fried potatoes. Cook foods at the specified temperature.
- Prolonged cooking also contributes to nutrient loss. Do not overcook food items, such as boiled vegetables.

Healthful Cooking Techniques

It is the responsibility of foodservice operations to provide the public with tasty, healthful food choices. Menus should offer a variety of foods to fit people's different dietary needs. For example, cooking with less fat and sodium and using fresh, high quality foods help provide customers with flavorful, healthful foods.

Certain cooking techniques also are more effective than others at retaining a food's full nutritive value. These techniques include steaming, grilling, poaching, stir-frying, and microwaving.

- **Steaming.** This technique uses steam to cook food. Steaming can be done in a steam jacketed kettle or pots with special steamer inserts. In methods such as boiling, vitamins are quickly lost into the liquid. Sometimes part of the liquid can be mixed into a sauce or soup, but valuable nutrients are usually lost. Few nutrients are lost, however, when steaming.
- **Grilling.** Foods that are grilled are cooked on a gridlike surface above a heat source. Grilling requires little or no fat and, if done correctly, results in tender foods with a charbroiled flavor.
- **Poaching.** Poaching involves gently simmering food in just enough liquid to cover the item. No fat is added, and the small amount of liquid minimizes the effects of leaching. The liquid can also be incorporated into a sauce or soup.
- **Stir-frying.** Stir-frying is a technique that quickly cooks food in a minimum amount of oil. It results in crisp, colorful vegetables with minimal nutrient loss.
- **Microwaving.** Microwaving is often used in foodservice operations to reheat foods quickly. Foods can be prepared, stored, and then reheated in a microwave when they are needed. This retains a food's nutrients by eliminating the need to keep the food hot for a long period of time. It is also healthful because no added fat is needed.

Storage

Nutrients can still be lost after food is cooked. Storage exposes food to the harmful effects of water, light, air, and time. Using cool temperatures, lessening holding time, and cooking in smaller batches will minimize these effects.

- **Temperature.** Cool temperatures can slow down the processes that destroy a food's nutrients. One way to achieve this is to plunge cooked vegetables into cold water to stop the cooking process. Do not leave items in the water because the nutrients will leach out. Storing covered foods in the refrigerator is another way to slow down nutrient loss. See Fig. 11-14.

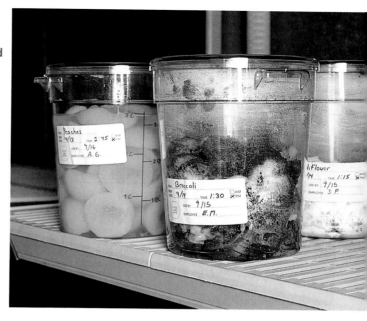

Fig. 11-14. Cool temperatures, such as those in a refrigerator, can slow the processes that destroy nutrients. **How else can cool temperatures be used in cooking?**

- **Holding.** Food should not be held in a steam table for a long period of time. Exposure to heat and water will eventually remove some of the food's nutrients.

- **Batching.** One way to lessen food storage problems is to use batch cooking. **Batch cooking** is the process of preparing small amounts of food several times throughout a foodservice period. This decreases the amount of food that will have to be kept warm and allows the kitchen to turn out freshly prepared meals for customers to enjoy.

USING FATS & OILS

Fat plays an important role as both a nutrient and a food. As a nutrient, it helps the body perform many important functions. Fat adds an enjoyable taste and texture to meals. Keep in mind that all vegetable oils except olive oil have an average smoking point of 400°F. The smoking point of olive oil is slightly lower. Fig. 11-15 lists the most common cooking oils and their uses.

Reducing Fat

One way to improve a recipe's nutritional content is to reduce the amount of fat and cholesterol with the following suggestions:

- **Reduce total fat.** The total amount of fat and oil in many recipes can be reduced with little effect to taste. Taste, however, is still the first concern of most diners.

- **Reduce fat.** Choose lean cuts of meat, trim the fat from them, and remove skin from poultry. Use non-stick or cast-iron pans so food can be cooked in less fat. See Fig. 11-16.

- **Reduce saturated fat.** Oils rich in flavor, such as olive oil, can be substituted in smaller amounts for saturated animal fats. Replace part of the but-

ter in a recipe with oil or sour cream with low-fat sour cream or yogurt.

- **Replace fat.** Where possible, replace part or all of the whole eggs in a recipe with egg whites or egg substitutes. Use high-quality, reduced-fat dairy products, such as reduced-fat cream cheese. Replace part of the fat in baking with puréed fruits. **Purées** are foods in which one or more of the ingredients have been ground in a food processor.

- **Offer plant-based foods.** In addition to lean meats, offer menu items based on pasta, rice, grains, and legumes. Also, increase the amounts of fruits and vegetables served with or included as part of an entrée. Plant-based foods appeal to vegetarians and people who want low-fat, high-fiber meals.

- **Change cooking techniques.** Techniques such as roasting, steaming, and baking require little or no added fat. They are more healthful than methods like deep-frying and pan-frying.

- **Use seasonings and flavorings.** Choose to season foods with fresh herbs and spices instead of butter or margarine. Use low-fat marinades to tenderize and add flavor to meats and seafood. Replace high-fat sauces with salsas or relishes.

Fig. 11-15.

COOKING OILS	DESCRIPTION	USES
Canola (kan-OH-luh)	• High in monounsaturated fat. • Neutral, light-colored oil with little flavor. • Also known as rapeseed oil because it comes from the rape plant.	All types of cooking, especially frying and baking.
Coconut	• High in saturated fat. • Little color.	Used in blended oils and shortenings.
Corn	• High in polyunsaturated fat. • Light, amber-colored oil. • Slight cornmeal flavor. • Sometimes marketed as "salad oil."	Frying, salad dressing.
Cottonseed	• High in polyunsaturated fat. • Pale yellow oil with sweet flavor. • Extracted from cotton plant seeds. • Quality depends on the season, type of fertilizer used, and the way it was extracted.	Shortening, salad dressing.
Olive	• High in monounsaturated fat. • Quality depends on soil, growing conditions, olive type, and the way it was extracted. • Extra-virgin olive oil, meaning it was made from the first pressing of olives, is the highest quality. • Ranges in color from deep green to pale yellow.	All types of cooking, salad dressing.
Peanut	• High in monounsaturated fat. • Amber-colored oil with nutty flavor.	Frying, deep-frying, salad dressing.
Safflower	• Very high in polyunsaturated fat. • Golden-colored oil.	Margarine, mayonnaise, salad dressing.
Sesame Seed	• High in polyunsaturated fat. • Two types: Middle Eastern, which is light with a mild flavor, and Asian, which is dark with a distinct, nutty flavor.	All types of cooking.
Soybean	• High in polyunsaturated fat. • Yellow oil. • Quality affected by season, climate, soil, and way it was extracted.	Margarine, salad dressing, shortening.

(Continued on next page)

Fig. 11-15 (Cont'd.).

COOKING OILS	DESCRIPTION	USES
Sunflower	• Very high in polyunsaturated fat. • Pale yellow oil with little flavor or odor.	All types of cooking, salad dressing, margarine, shortening.
Vegetable	• Polyunsaturated fat. • Products labeled "vegetable oil" are blended from many sources. • Other types of vegetable oil are corn, soybean, and cottonseed.	All types of cooking, salad dressing.

■ **Use special equipment.** Specially made equipment can make low-fat cooking easier. For example, nonstick pans and cast-iron pans allow food to be browned in a minimal amount of fat.

■ **Reduce portion size.** Limit portion sizes of meat, poultry, and seafood to 3–4 oz. (precooked weight). Increase amounts of vegetables, grains, beans, and pasta. Use a variety of colors and textures to add interest to the meal.

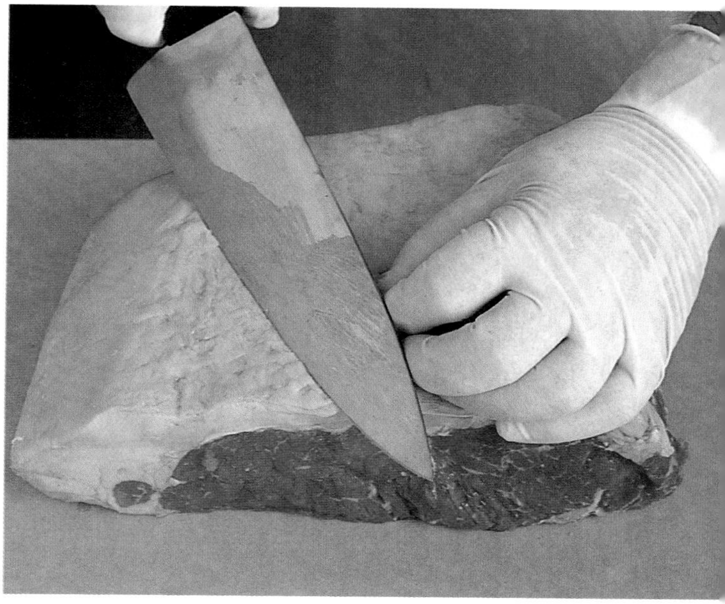

Fig. 11-16. Trimming the fat from cuts of meat is one way to reduce the amount of fat in a recipe.

SECTION 11-3 Knowledge Check

1. Name two ways to retain nutrients during preparation, cooking, and storage.
2. How do time and water impact foods?
3. Describe three methods for reducing the amount of fat in a recipe.

MINI LAB

Imagine you want to retain the maximum amount of nutrients in a spinach and mushroom salad. Describe how you would prepare and store the vegetables to keep the harmful effects of time and water to a minimum.

SECTION SUMMARIES

11-1 The six categories of nutrients—carbohydrates, proteins, fats, vitamins, minerals, and water—are each essential to the body in different ways.

11-1 Vitamins and minerals, which the body needs to function normally, can be found in many different foods. For example, the calcium found in dairy products keeps bones and teeth healthy, while iodine, found in iodized salt and shellfish, helps the body use energy.

11-1 Foodservice operations have many options for offering healthful meals, such as cooking with less saturated fat.

11-1 Some of the most common food additives used in food service are thickeners, sugar substitutes, and fat substitutes.

11-2 The Dietary Guidelines for Americans, nutrition labels, and the food pyramid are tools that help consumers make healthful, informed food choices.

11-2 Age, activity level, lifestyle, and health are factors that influence a person's dietary needs.

11-2 Foodservice operations need to accommodate different dietary needs by offering a variety of healthful foods on their menus.

11-3 How foods are prepared, cooked, and stored affects their nutritional content.

11-3 Time and water can cause foods to lose nutrients.

11-3 Reducing the amount of fat and cholesterol in recipes improves nutritional value.

CHECK YOUR KNOWLEDGE

1. Describe the functions of each of the six categories of nutrients.
2. How can the dining room staff help implement a nutritious menu?
3. List two benefits of using food additives.
4. Summarize the Dietary Guidelines.
5. Describe the dietary needs of the following people: pregnant woman, infant, child, teenager, elderly person.
6. What are the effects of a high activity level on dietary needs?
7. During food preparation, how can you avoid the harmful effects of time and water on nutrients?
8. What are two guidelines a foodservice employee could follow to retain a food's nutrients during cooking?
9. How can fat be reduced in recipes?

CRITICAL-THINKING ACTIVITIES

1. Why should the dietary needs of people with health problems be considered when planning a restaurant menu?
2. How do you think requiring nutritious labeling on foods has affected consumers?

WORKPLACE KNOW-HOW

Communication. Suppose that you are teaching restaurant servers about the nutritional content of menu items. List four questions a customer might have about nutrition. How would you instruct servers to handle these four questions?

LAB-BASED ACTIVITY: Planning Nutritiou

STEP ❶ Working in teams, plan a nutritious breakfast, lunch, dinner, and two snacks for an average healthy adult. The total calories a person needs to consume daily ranges from 1,000 to 3,000 depending upon the amount of physical activity. Food amounts range from:

Grain group	3 oz. to 10 oz.
Fruit group	1 c. to 2.5 c.
Vegetable group	1 c. to 4 c.
Milk group	2 c. to 3 c.
Meat & Bean group	2 oz. to 7 oz.

STEP ❷ Include a description of the following:

- Serving sizes of each item, using the Serving Sizes chart below as a guide.
- The overall appeal of each meal, including the variety of colors, textures, and flavors.
- Ways to prepare, cook, and store each item so that nutrients are retained.

STEP ❸ When finished, trade menus with another team.

STEP ❹ Evaluate the menu for nutritional value, variety, and appeal.

STEP ❺ Suggest foods that can be substituted or modified to reduce the amount of fat and cholesterol.

Portions

Bread Group
- 1 oz. slice of whole-grain bread
- ½ c. cooked cereal, pasta, rice
- 1 oz. ready-to-eat whole-grain cereal
- 1 small roll, biscuit, muffin
- ½ hamburger bun, English muffin

Fruit Group
- 1 medium apple, banana, orange
- ½ c. berries
- 6 oz. fruit juice
- ½ c. cooked, chopped, canned fruit

Vegetable Group
- ½ c. chopped raw vegetables
- ½ c. cooked dark green or orange vegetables
- 6 oz. vegetable juice
- 1 c. dark green, leafy raw vegetables

Milk Group
- 1 c. milk
- 1 c. yogurt
- 1½ oz. cheese

Meat & Bean Group
- 2–3 oz. cooked lean meat, poultry, fish
- ½ c. cooked dry beans
- 1 egg
- 2 tbsp. peanut butter
- ⅓ c. nuts (or 1½ oz.)

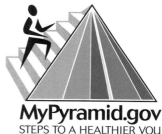

MyPyramid.gov
STEPS TO A HEALTHIER YOU

Creating Menus

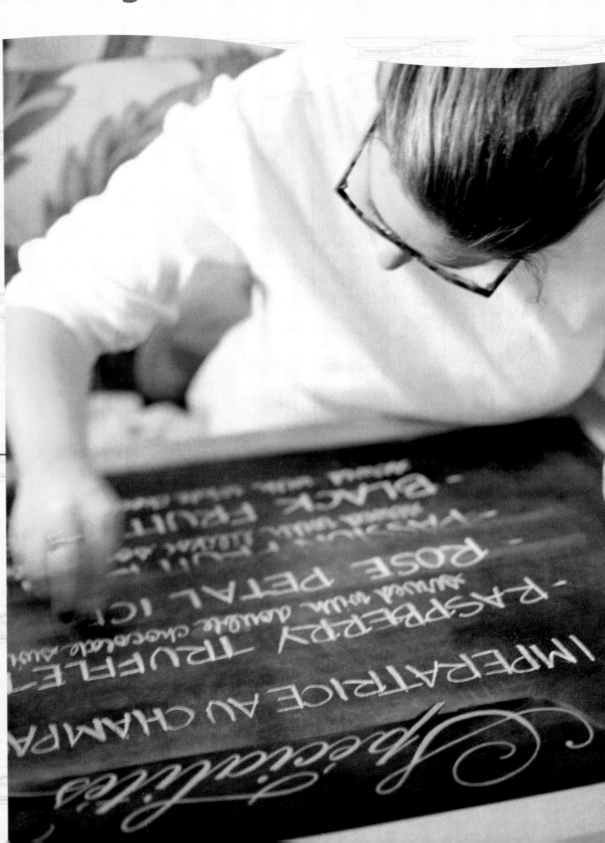

The Menu

KEY TERMS

- menu
- entrée
- fixed menu
- cycle menu
- à la carte menu
- semi-à la carte menu
- table d'hôte menu
- prix fixe menus
- continental menus
- accompaniments

OBJECTIVES

After reading this section, you will be able to:

- Explain the role of a menu.
- Summarize the factors that influence a menu.
- Describe the types of menus used by various foodservice establishments.

WHETHER you're craving stir fry or cheeseburgers, you go to a restaurant because you like the food it serves. You can find these food items on the **menu**, a listing of the food choices the restaurant offers for each meal. The menu, however, is more than just a list you look over before placing an order. It has a much larger role. In fact, it impacts every step of a foodservice operation. It determines the:

- Type of customer the establishment will attract.
- Layout and type of equipment needed.
- Workers needed and the skills they must possess.
- Type and number of supplies to be ordered.

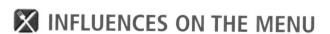 INFLUENCES ON THE MENU

If you were planning the menu for a restaurant, what would you choose? Menu planning isn't as simple as listing items that you like to eat. There are many other factors to consider when developing a menu.

■ **Target customers.** Think of the needs and lifestyles of the people you'll be serving. The menu is a restaurant's main marketing tool. For example, a lunch deli serves food that can be prepared quickly. See Fig. 12-1. A school cafeteria needs inviting and nutritious meals that will appeal to students. In both cases, foods need to be served in the most efficient way possible.

■ **Price.** People expect different types of establishments to offer food within a certain price range. Food items that are above or below this range will be out of place on the menu. For example, a $25.00 **entrée** (AHN-tray), or main dish, would be out of place at a family-style diner where most entrées cost around $8.95.

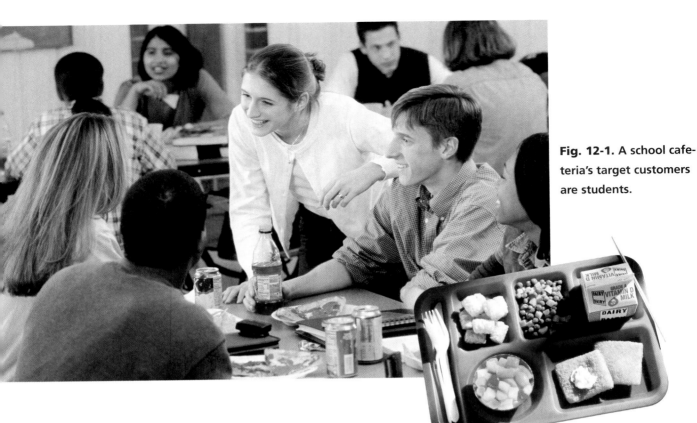

■ **Type of food served.** A menu is planned to reflect the type of food served in a particular restaurant. For example, people expect French food to be served at a French restaurant.

■ **Equipment.** The type of equipment available dictates what can be on the menu. For example, a specialty restaurant with a broiler can serve steak.

■ **Skill of workers.** Consider the skill level of the kitchen staff when selecting items for the menu. Employees at a quick-service restaurant will not be able to make the complex dishes that a four-star restaurant staff has been trained to prepare.

■ **Geography and culture.** The location of a foodservice operation can indicate its menu. For example, most coastal restaurants serve seafood, while beef and pork are common in Midwest eateries. The culture of various regions and ethnic neighborhoods can also impact the food choices available in restaurants. However, as people move around the country and the media promotes foods of different cultures, menus are becoming more varied.

■ **Eating trends.** Today's trend toward eating healthful foods has many restaurants offering more fruits, vegetables, grains, and legumes on their menus.

MENU TYPES

You can find just as many different kinds of menus as there are different kinds of foodservice operations. A menu can be a printed card that the server or host hands to customers. It can be a large sign behind a counter or a chalkboard menu that changes daily. The most popular types of menus include:

- Fixed and cycle menus.
- À la carte, semi-à la carte, and table d'hôte menus.
- Prix fixe menus.

Fixed & Cycle Menus

A fixed menu offers the same dishes every day for a long period of time. You will find fixed menus in dining places that serve different people every day, such as hotels, ethnic restaurants, and fast-food operations. See Fig. 12-2.

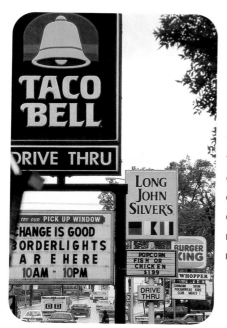

Fig. 12-2. Most fast-food restaurants use fixed menus because these restaurants serve different people every day. What other types of establishments might offer fixed menus?

A cycle menu is used for a set period of time, such as a week, a month, or even longer. At the end of this time period, the menu repeats daily dishes in the same order. For example, if a cycle menu is used weekly, it offers the same dishes on each Monday. You will find cycle menus in institutions that serve the same people day after day, such as schools, hospitals, factories, and military foodservice facilities.

À la carte, Semi-à la carte, & Table d'hôte Menus

In family-style and hotel restaurants, you will most often find foods listed three different ways on the menu. An **à la carte** (ah-lah-KART) **menu** offers each food and beverage item priced and served separately. In a **semi-à la carte menu**, you usually will find the appetizers and desserts priced separately. The entrée will likely include a salad or soup, potato or rice, vegetable, and possibly a beverage. A **table d'hôte** (tah-buhl DOHT) **menu** lists complete meals—everything from appetizers to desserts and sometimes beverages as well—for one set price. A set banquet menu is also an example of a table d'hôte menu, although in this case everyone is served the same meal for a set price.

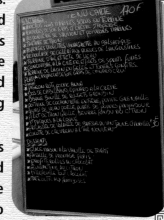

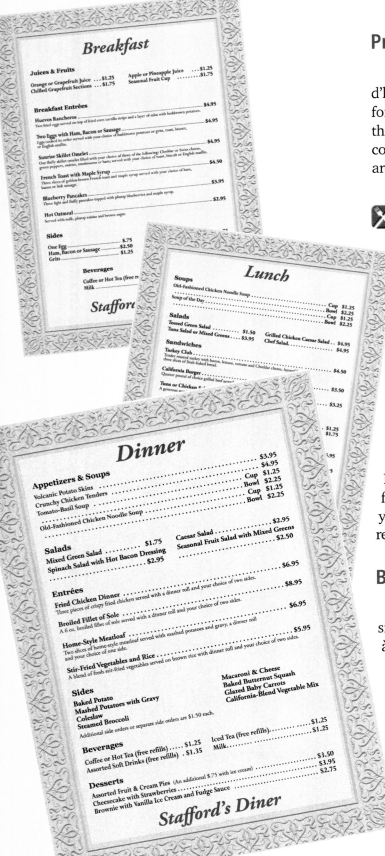

Fig. 12-3. This restaurant serves every meal of the day as shown by the menu. What type of menu is it?

Prix Fixe Menus

Prix fixe (pree feks) **menus** are similar to table d'hôte menus in that they offer a complete meal for a set price. With a prix fixe menu, however, the customer chooses one selection from each course offered by the restaurant. Prix fixe menus are sometimes used at elegant restaurants.

☒ MEAL-BASED MENUS

In addition to fixed and cycle menus, other types of menus include breakfast, lunch, dinner, and ethnic. Many foodservice operations have separate menus for breakfast, lunch, and dinner. If all three meals are available all day, some restaurants list them on the same menu. Breakfast, lunch, and dinner menus may be listed as à la carte, semi-à la carte, table d'hôte, or as prix fixe offerings. See Fig. 12-3.

■ **Ethnic.** Ethnic menus represent food from a specific country, such as China, Italy, Mexico, or France. Most people enjoy trying different ethnic foods for breakfast, lunch, or dinner, although you may find that preferences differ in various regions of the country. See Fig. 12-4.

Breakfast

Most breakfast menus are made up of inexpensive foods that are cooked to order. Menus may be à la carte or continental. À la carte menus price and serve each item separately. Some table d'hôte breakfast menus are also called continental menus. These menus provide mostly a selection of juices, beverages, and baked goods.

Breakfast menus usually include juices, fruits, cereals, eggs, French toast, pancakes, waffles, baked goods, beverages, and side items. Side items often include toast, potatoes, grits, or various breakfast meats.

Lunch

Lunch menus usually provide a diverse selection of à la carte items, but they also offer table d'hôte combinations, such as soup and salad or soup and sandwich. Lunch portions are usually smaller than dinner portions, so they are lower priced. Some food-service facilities offer daily lunch specials, while others operate a cycle menu of rotating lunch specials.

Lunch menus include appetizers, soups, salads, entrées, sandwiches, accompaniments, and desserts. **Accompaniments** are items that come with the meal, such as a choice of potato, rice, or pasta and a choice of vegetable.

Dinner

Dinner menus usually include the same food categories as lunch menus, yet require more complex preparations. However, dinner menus have more selections, offer larger portions, and have higher prices. Dinner is the most leisurely meal, since customers often have limited time for breakfast and lunch.

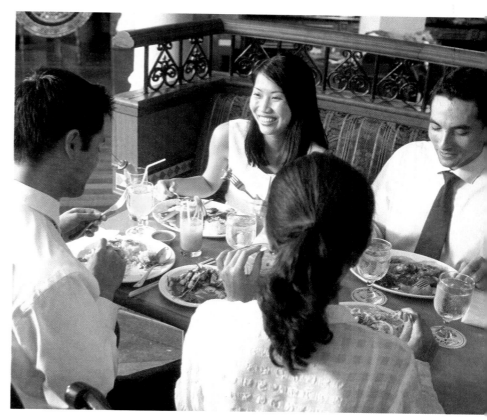

Fig. 12-4. Many people enjoy trying a variety of ethnic foods. Which ethnic foods are popular in your area?

SECTION 12-1 Knowledge Check

1. Explain four ways the menu impacts a foodservice operation.
2. List at least four factors that influence menu planning.
3. Describe the six types of menus.

MINI LAB

Evaluate a local restaurant menu. Does it respond to the factors that influence menu planning? Explain your responses.

Planning Menus

OBJECTIVES

After reading this section, you will be able to:

• List basic menu planning principles.

• Plan interesting menus that offer good nutrition and variety.

• Use truth-in-menu guidelines to write a menu description.

IMAGINE that you are responsible for planning and writing a menu for a foodservice operation. You'll want to create a clear and accurate menu that is easy to read. Foodservice professionals have created a set of principles that will guide you in planning a unique and appealing menu. Your menu will help your operation sell its food and meet customers' expectations.

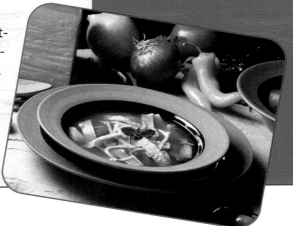

☒ WHO PLANS THE MENU?

A menu is the basic plan that a foodservice operation follows. The person responsible for deciding this plan depends on the type of facility.

In many foodservice facilities, the management staff plans the menu. In a large foodservice facility, such as a hotel, the executive chef works with management to create the menu. Registered dietitians (RDs), foodservice directors, and chefs write menus for hospitals, schools, nursing homes, and other institutions. For chain restaurants, the main office usually supplies the menu. However, the service staff as well as customers can also make good menu suggestions.

☒ MENU PLANNING PRINCIPLES

You have already learned about various factors that influence menu planning. Foodservice professionals have developed some additional principles for planning successful menus.

Variety

Some operations offer limited menus, such as a restaurant that specializes in gourmet pizzas or a school cafeteria that operates on a cycle menu. However, most customers expect to see variety in the menu listings.

Besides varying the types of food offered, you can also vary the way food is prepared. For example, appetizers might include deep-fried vegetables or a shrimp cocktail. Entrées may feature chicken, beef, and pork that are available roasted, baked, or broiled.

The visual appeal of your finished meal is also important. A meal without a variety of colors, shapes, sizes, temperatures, flavors, textures, number of items, and different arrangements lacks appeal. Imagine a plate containing broiled chicken, mashed potatoes, and steamed cauliflower. Now, imagine barbecued chicken, a baked potato sprinkled with chives, and crisp carrots. The second meal is more colorful and has a variety of textures and shapes. See Fig. 12-5.

Another way to add visual interest to meals is with garnishes. Garnishes are edible foods, such as a sprig of parsley or an orange slice placed on or around food to add color or flavor. A simple lettuce leaf and tomato slice brighten up an otherwise ordinary chicken sandwich. Garnishes can make customers feel that extra care has been used in preparing their meals.

Balance

Fruits, vegetables, starches, meats and other protein foods, and dairy products are all essential parts of a healthful diet. The menu should include foods from each of these groups.

When the menu offers meal options, think about how foods will look on the serving plate. Varying the flavors, shapes, colors, and sizes of foods adds to the visual appeal and sensitizes the taste buds. Think about the following items when planning which foods make a good combination on a plate.

- **Placement.** Visualize how the various foods will look on the plate and how the plate will be placed in front of the customer. Plating is key to eye appeal. Attractively plated food leads to enhanced customer satisfaction.

- **Serving size.** Do the portions of food look too small or too large on the plate? Will customers think they are getting their money's worth?

- **Proportion.** Is the **proportion**, or ratio of one food to another and to the plate, pleasing to the eye? For example, if a foodservice operation offers smaller portions of food for children and senior citizens, the portions should be balanced in size to each other and to the size of the plate.

- **Number of foods on a plate.** As a general rule, an odd number of foods on a plate is more visually pleasing than an even number of foods.

Truthfulness

Federal law requires that certain menu statements be accurate, especially those concerning nutrition, quantity, quality, grade, and freshness. These are called truth-in-menu guidelines.

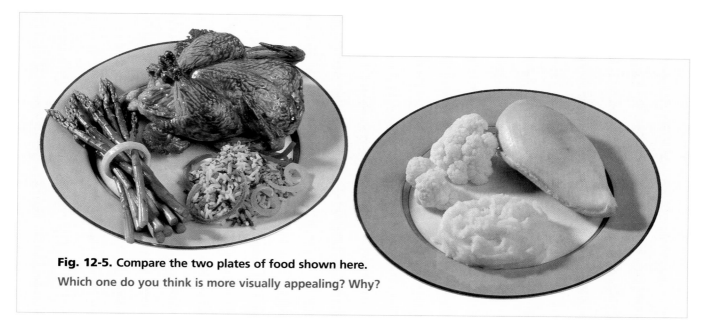

Fig. 12-5. Compare the two plates of food shown here. Which one do you think is more visually appealing? Why?

Fig. 12-6.
Truth-in-Menu Guidelines

GUIDELINE	EXAMPLES
1. **Brand names must be represented accurately.**	Examples of brand names of products on a menu are: Hunt's Ketchup®, Hellmann's Mayonnaise™, Green Giant Frozen Vegetables®, and Butterball Turkey®.
2. **Dietary and nutritional claims must be accurate.**	To protect customers from potential health hazards, the dietary structure of food must be correctly stated. For example, low-sodium or fat-free foods must be correctly prepared to ensure the protection of customers. All nutritional claims must be supported with statistical data.
3. **The preservation of food must be accurate.**	The preservation of food is as follows: frozen; chilling; dehydration; drying, such as sun or smoking; bottled; and canned. If a menu planner wishes to use the previous terms, the terms must be used correctly on the menu. For example, fresh fish is not frozen.
4. **Quantity must be accurate.**	If a sirloin is 16 oz., it must be stated on the menu that this is the weight prior to cooking.
5. **Location of ingredients must be accurate.**	If Dover Sole is on the menu, it must actually be from Dover, England. Pancakes with Vermont maple syrup must be served with Vermont syrup, not New Hampshire syrup.
6. **Quality or grade must be accurate.**	When listing quality or grade for meats, dairy products, poultry, and vegetables or fruits, accuracy is critical. For example, if you state "prime sirloin," it must be exactly that. You cannot use "choice" and say "prime" on the menu.
7. **Proper cooking techniques must be accurate.**	If broiled swordfish is on your menu, it must be cooked exactly that way. You cannot serve the swordfish baked.
8. **Pictures must be accurate.**	For example, apple pie à la mode must be apple pie with ice cream.
9. **Descriptions of food products must be accurate.**	If shrimp cocktail is described on the menu as four jumbo shrimp on a bed of crushed ice with a zesty cocktail sauce and lemon wedge, and the shrimp cocktail comes with medium-sized shrimp, the description is incorrect.

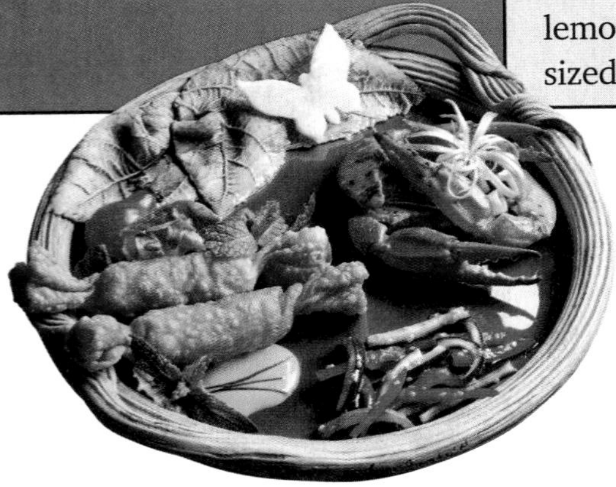

For example, "homestyle pies" must be baked in the establishment's kitchen, not purchased already prepared. "Fresh-squeezed orange juice" can't be made from frozen concentrate. "Louisiana frog legs" must have originated in Louisiana. However, some geographic names are accepted in the generic sense, such as French fries or New England clam chowder. Restaurants that don't follow these FDA guidelines can be required to pay a penalty.

Federal law also requires that nutritional statements like "low fat" or "light" be accurate. Many heart patients on restricted diets may order a meal based on its nutritional claim. What if a dish labeled "cholesterol free" on a restaurant menu is not really cholesterol free?

Foodservice operations must protect customers by ensuring that the food does meet its health claim. Restaurants must be able to prove nutritional claims made in advertising. See Fig. 12-6.

Nutrition

Regardless of the type of foodservice operation, menus should offer healthful food choices. If you are a menu planner at an institution, you have a responsibility to provide nutritious, appealing,

and well-prepared meals. People who eat at institutions usually can't go somewhere else if they don't like the food.

Nursing homes and hospitals must also offer a variety of foods for patients needing special diets, such as those following low-fat diets and people with diabetes or food allergies. See Fig. 12-7.

■ **Low-fat diets.** People follow low-fat diets for reasons such as heart disease, cancer, weight control, or just to maintain a healthful lifestyle. These people need foods that are high in fiber and low in fat and cholesterol. Examples of low-fat, high-fiber foods include fruits, vegetables, and whole-grain breads and cereals.

■ **Diabetes.** Almost 16 million Americans have **diabetes**, an illness that affects the body's ability to convert blood sugar into energy. People with diabetes must balance food, portion sizes, exercise, and medication to avoid complications and maintain a healthful lifestyle. Menu items appropriate for people with diabetes include fruits and vegetables; lean meats, poultry, and fish; low-fat and sugar-free food products; and whole grains. Making information available regarding the carbohydrate content of menu items is also helpful.

■ **Food allergies.** Employees in the foodservice industry must provide information to customers about foods that may cause allergic reactions. This includes providing detailed menu descriptions about the ingredients in menu items. Avoiding an allergy-causing food is the only way to prevent allergic reactions. See Fig. 12-8.

Flexibility

Menus need to change from time to time for a variety of reasons. The target market may change, as could the cost of various ingredients. Many menus have "specials" that offer customers additional choices. This flexibility also provides an opportunity to use seasonal foods such as squash, asparagus, watermelon, or cranberries.

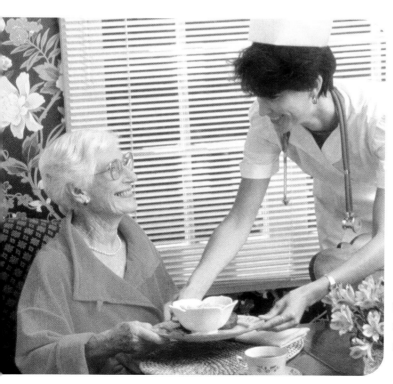

Fig. 12-7. Nursing home foodservice operations need to make sure that all foods meet the dietary needs of its residents.

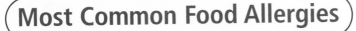

Most Common Food Allergies

Fig. 12-8.

Source: The Food Allergy Network

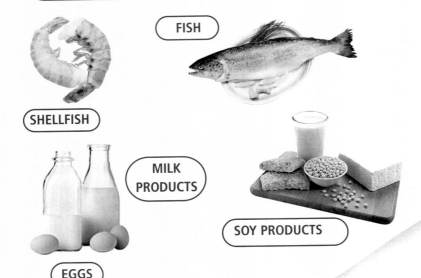

FISH

SHELLFISH

TREE NUTS
(such as walnuts
and pecans)

PEANUTS

MILK
PRODUCTS

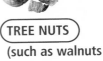

SOY PRODUCTS

EGGS

WHEAT

✖ WRITING MENU DESCRIPTIONS

Often, the basic menu list is given to someone who writes a description of each item. This lets the customer know exactly what each dish is, in the most appealing language possible. Because of limited space, each description should be as short as possible.

If customers don't understand what a dish is, they won't order it. Descriptions need to be clear and specific. For example, "fish" leaves too many unanswered questions. What kind of fish? How big is it? How is it cooked? How is it seasoned? "8 oz. Charbroiled salmon with dill sauce" is a much better menu listing. Effective descriptions can sell a menu item.

It's also important that the actual food match the printed menu description. The fish described above should indeed be salmon, weigh 8 oz. before cooking, be charbroiled, and come with dill sauce. Entice customers with honest descriptions of what they are going to get. If the meal they select from your menu doesn't meet their expectations, they will be disappointed.

SECTION 12-2   Knowledge Check

1. Who is responsible for planning the menu at a nursing home, a chain restaurant, and a hotel?

2. List the principles of menu planning.

3. Describe a situation that illustrates why a restaurant needs to follow truth-in-menu guidelines.

MINI LAB

You've just discovered that a support group for people with heart disease will be eating at your diner tonight. Today's special was supposed to be fried chicken, French fries, and sweet peas. Use those same ingredients to create a low-fat alternative.

Menu Design & Organization

OBJECTIVES

After reading this section, you will be able to:

• Identify the elements that influence menu style and design.

• Contrast basic menu formats.

• Describe the basic menu categories and how they are organized.

ONCE you know what types of food to include on a menu, you need to organize it in a way that is most appealing to the customer. Grouping dishes in categories makes it easier for customers to read through the menu and find items of interest. The look and feel of the menu will also influence how customers view the food.

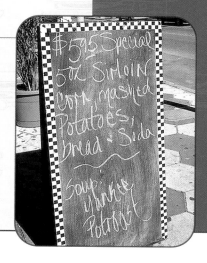

✖ MENU STYLE & DESIGN

You are given menus from two different restaurants. One is a thin piece of paper that doubles as a place mat. It features meals on the front and children's activities on the back. The other menu has a padded cover with the restaurant's name embossed in gold. The menu items are written in elegant letters on thick cream paper. Without even looking at the menu items, what are your impressions of these two restaurants? What kind of atmosphere would you expect to find if you dined at each of them?

The menu is the primary way in which a foodservice operation communicates with its customers. The factors that have the most impact on menu style and design are the influences on the menu discussed in Section 1: target customers, price, type of food served, equipment, skill of workers, geography and culture, and eating trends.

Influences on the menu help dictate how a foodservice operation chooses to convey a message to customers—through details such as the cover design, color, style of lettering, weight of the paper, and the way descriptions are worded. There are three common formats of menus. Each sets the tone for a meal. See Fig. 12-9.

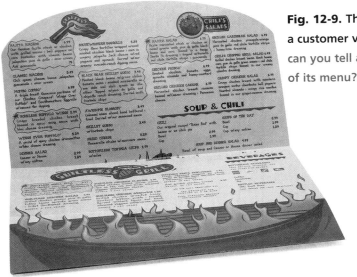

Some foodservice professionals believe that a spoken menu is friendly and increases conversation between customers and their servers. Others think that it doesn't allow the customer time to study the menu and make a decision. Many guests view spoken menus as a sign of well-trained servers.

Printed Menu Format

Printed menus are handed to customers as soon as they sit down. These menus often contain a list of specials, called **clip-ons**, fastened to the menu. Daily specials can also be written on folded cards that stand on the table, called **table tents**. A table tent can also be inserted in a stand that sits on the table. Besides listing specials, clip-ons and table tents allow restaurants to test new products and feature seasonal items. Printed menus can be changed daily using a computer and printer.

Menu Board Format

A **menu board** contains a hand-written or printed menu on a board on a wall or easel. It can easily reflect daily menu changes—for example, a chalkboard can be erased and a board with printed inserts can be changed. Its informality and flexibility make it perfect for use in cafeterias and fast-food restaurants. The chalkboard menu, though casual, can also be used in an upscale restaurant to emphasize freshness and creativity. See Fig. 12-10.

Spoken Menu Format

In some restaurants, after a customer is seated, a server states what foods are available and the prices of each. This **spoken menu** is often limited to a few items. Other restaurants present only the daily specials as a spoken menu.

✖ MENU CATEGORIES

Regardless of size and style, all printed menus are broken down into categories. The type of restaurant determines the categories and the order in which they are listed. Generally, categories are listed in the order in which they are consumed.

- **Appetizers.** Small portions of food meant to stimulate the appetite are called **appetizers**. They can be hot or cold and range from nachos to fruit salad to crab cakes. See Chapter 21 for more information on appetizers.
- **Soups.** On some menus, soups and appetizers appear in the same category. Cold and hot soup choices range from thin, savory broths to thick, creamy chowders. See Chapter 21 for more information on soups.

Fig. 12-10. A menu board can easily show daily menu changes.

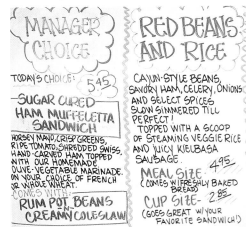

- **Salads.** This category refers to salads made with fresh, crisp vegetables and sometimes fruit or nuts. Some "house" salads come with a choice of dressings that are created by the restaurant. See Chapter 18 for more information on salads and dressings.

- **Cold entrées.** These entrées include salads topped with poultry, ham, or seafood, and cold meat, fruit, and cheese platters.

- **Hot entrées.** The ingredients and cooking methods for hot entrées vary greatly. Hot entrées usually include meat, poultry, fish, or seafood. They also can include casserole items, or **extenders**—items made from leftover low-cost ingredients. Vegetarian dishes like vegetable lasagna are also popular hot entrées.

- **Sandwiches.** Sandwiches, such as hamburgers and grilled cheese, are often shown only on lunch menus. They can be served either hot or cold and can be made from many different ingredients. Sandwiches often come with various breads, condiments, and spreads. See Chapter 19 for more information on sandwiches.

- **Accompaniments.** Vegetables and starches that serve as side dishes fall into this category. Vegetables provide a healthful, low-cost, colorful addition to meals. Starches include pasta, potatoes, rice, and other grains prepared in a variety of ways.

- **Desserts.** Desserts often are displayed on separate menus or dessert trays. Since many customers don't eat dessert at every meal, servers may need to spend extra time selling dessert.

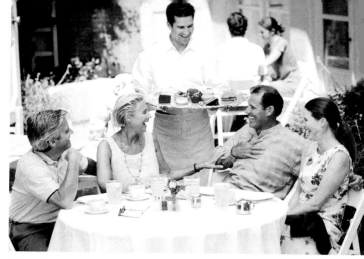

Fig. 12-11. Restaurants often display their desserts to entice customers to order them. Why would a server make an extra effort to sell desserts?

Desserts can include ice creams, puddings, and pastries. See Chapter 30 for more information on desserts. See Fig. 12-11.

- **Cheeses and fruits.** Cheeses such as Brie (bree) and Gouda (GOO-dah) are often listed with fresh fruits as an appetizer or dessert alternative.

- **Beverages.** This category lists beverage selections and prices. Beverages often include juices, milk, coffee, tea, and soft drinks.

Some restaurants use all of the menu categories but change the names to reflect a menu theme. For example, a restaurant with a sports theme might label their appetizers "First Inning." Other restaurants add and delete categories based on the type of meal they're serving. For example, a breakfast menu would not include appetizers, but it might include a section of "skillet" items.

SECTION 12-3 Knowledge Check

1. What elements influence menu design?
2. Describe three common menu formats.
3. List the traditional menu categories and give an example of a food item that could be found in each.

MINI LAB

You've been asked to design a menu for a new upscale restaurant. Think of a theme for the restaurant, and describe how you would incorporate that theme in the menu design. List menu items for each menu category.

Pricing Menu Items

KEY TERMS

• factor method

• markup-on-cost method

• competitors' pricing method

• psychological pricing method

OBJECTIVES

After reading this section, you will be able to:

• Identify the influences that impact menu prices.

• Use the factor method and markup-on-cost method of pricing correctly.

• Contrast the competitors' pricing method with the psychological method of pricing.

YOU'VE chosen your menu items, written enticing descriptions, and organized and designed your menu to impress even the most experienced diner. Now for the final step: setting prices. If prices are too high, you will lose sales or not attract customers. If prices are too low, you will lose money or not meet your operating costs. By choosing a pricing method best suited for your operation, you can help ensure a successful business.

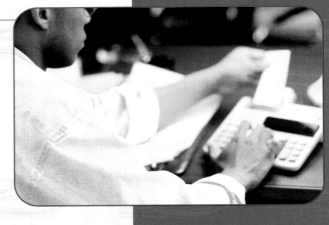

✕ WHAT INFLUENCES MENU PRICING?

Menu prices must cover the costs of operating your foodservice business while at the same time be fair to the customer. Many prices are influenced by labor, competition, customers, atmosphere, and location.

■ **Labor.** Menu items that require more time, care, and skill in preparation are often set at a higher price. In general, a menu prepared by an experienced kitchen staff is more labor intensive. These menu items tend to be more expensive.

■ **Competition.** Review competitors' menus to see what they are charging for similar items. Use your competition as a guide only, since details like portion size and ingredient quality may differ.

■ **Customers.** The types of customers your foodservice operation attracts will influence your menu prices. For example, you may charge less if your main customers are families rather than business professionals.

■ **Atmosphere.** The style of your foodservice operation helps determine prices. Customers expect fine-dining restaurants to be higher priced than casual, family-style establishments. This is due to a larger number of kitchen and service staff as well as a larger dining room area.

■ **Location.** It is important to consider the cost of living in the location of your foodservice operation. Restaurants in cities often serve people with a higher disposable income, so they can have higher menu prices than if they were located in small towns.

PRICING METHODS

There are many ways to price menu items. The most popular methods in the foodservice industry are the factor method, the markup-on-cost method, the competitors' method, and the psychological pricing method. See Fig. 12-12.

Factor Method

The **factor method** is a common pricing method for restaurants with successful past performance records. You must first determine what the food cost percent should be. To determine the food cost percentage, you divide the total cost of food by the total food sales. Then, take that food cost percent and divide it into 100%, which will result in your factor. Multiply the factor by the cost of the menu item. This will give you the menu selling price.

For example, if your food cost for the month is $5,000 and your total sales are $20,000, use the following formula to determine your food cost percentage:

```
                       .25 (food cost percent)
$20000.00. )$5000.00.
               400000.
               100000
               100000
                    0
```

Your food cost percent is 25%. If a hamburger and French fries cost $1.50 to make, you would compute the price as follows:

1.   4 (factor)
   .25.)1.00.

2. $1.50 (item cost)
    × 4 (factor)
    $6.00 (selling price)

You would sell the hamburger and French fries for $6.00.

Markup-on-Cost Method

Another common way to determine prices is the **markup-on-cost method**. To find the selling price, take the food cost of an item and divide it by the desired food cost percent.

For example, if you want the food cost percent to be 25%, and a grilled cheese sandwich and cup of tomato soup cost $1.25 to make, you would compute the price as follows:

```
        $5.00 (selling price)
.25. )$1.25. (item cost)
```

You would price the grilled cheese sandwich and tomato soup at $5.00.

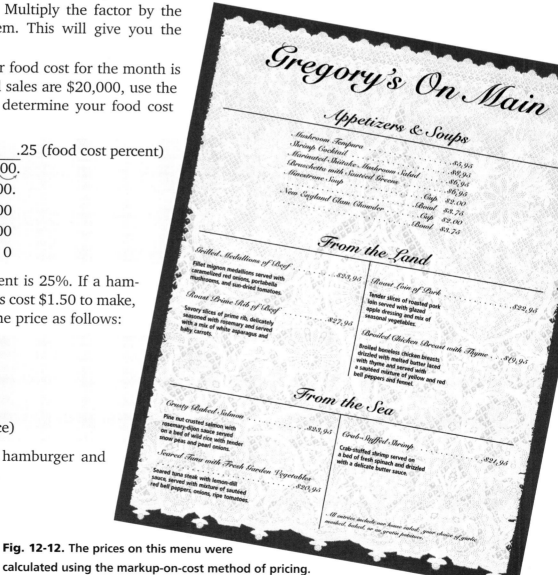

Fig. 12-12. The prices on this menu were calculated using the markup-on-cost method of pricing.

OPERATING WITH PERCENTAGES

A "percent" is a ratio that compares a number to 100. You can write a percent with the percent symbol or as a fraction or a decimal. A quick way to change a percent to a fraction is to divide the percent by 100 and simplify the fraction. A quick way to change a percent to a decimal is to divide by 100 by moving the decimal point two places to the left. For example, you can write 80% as:

$$\frac{80}{100} = \frac{4}{5} \text{ or } .80$$

People involved in food service use percentages in daily decision making. When beginning to determine menu selections and prices, you may first want to estimate the price of a meal. Then it will be quick to determine if the meal is worth placing on the menu.

You can estimate a percent of a number using compatible numbers and mental math. For instance, 28% of $19.85 is close to 30% of $20. Multiply 30% by $20 to get an estimate.

```
  .30
× 20
─────
  00
 60
─────
6.00
```

So, 28% of $19.85 is about $6.00.

You may find it helpful to estimate the percent of a number if you remember these equivalent percents, decimals, and fractions.

Percent	Decimal	Fraction
10%	0.10	1/10
20%	0.20	1/5
25%	0.25	1/4
33⅓%	0.33	1/3
40%	0.40	2/5
50%	0.50	1/2
66⅔%	0.66	2/3
75%	0.75	3/4
80%	0.80	4/5

TRY IT!

1. Estimate 42% of $8.99.
2. You need to price an entrée at $12.15 so you make a 31% profit. How much profit do you need to make on this entrée?

Competitors' Pricing Method

The **competitors' pricing method** charges approximately what the competition is charging. Some places charge slightly less in an attempt to attract more customers, or they charge slightly more in an attempt to appear more upscale. This method is risky because overhead costs such as rent, labor, food costs, and profit are different in every restaurant. See Fig. 12-13.

Psychological Pricing Method

Once the selling price is determined using other methods, the psychological pricing method can be used. The **psychological pricing method** is based on how a customer reacts to menu prices. For example, a customer may be more willing to order a $6.00 hamburger and French fries if you lower the price to $5.95.

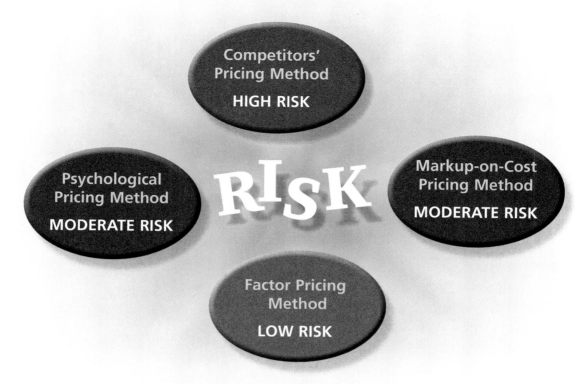

Fig. 12-13. There is a level of risk involved with every pricing method. Why shouldn't everyone always use the factor method of pricing?

Moving from one dollar category to another influences how customers view the value they are getting for their money. A price of $12.95 raised to $13.25 seems like a bigger increase than $13.25 raised to $13.75. In reality, however, the first increase is 30 cents, while the second increase is 50 cents.

Most restaurants start menu prices at the low end of a dollar category so they can adjust the prices several times without entering the next dollar category. For example, an item at $13.25 can be raised to $13.50, and then to $13.75 before moving into the $14 range.

Restaurants that emphasize quality food at low prices, such as diners and quick-service restaurants, often use psychological pricing methods. Few fine-dining establishments use this type of pricing because it doesn't fit their image of luxury and elegance. Customers who go to fine-dining restaurants usually are not as concerned with lower prices.

SECTION 12-4　Knowledge Check

1. List the influences that impact menu pricing.

2. Give an example that shows how to figure the markup-on-cost method of pricing.

3. What important factors are taken into account when using the psychological pricing method that are not used in the competitors' pricing method?

MINI LAB

Use the factor method to determine the selling price of a lunch consisting of a slice of pepperoni and cheese pizza and an iced tea. Your food cost percent is 30%. The item cost for the pizza is $3.00 and the item cost for the iced tea is 50¢.

SECTION SUMMARIES

12-1 The menu influences every step of a food-service operation.

12-1 Influences to consider when menu planning include your target customers, cost, the type of food served, the type of equipment, operational skills required, geography and culture, and eating trends.

12-1 Menu types include fixed, cycle, à la carte, semi-à la carte, table d'hôte, and prix fixe.

12-2 Menus are planned by management staff, executive chefs, registered dietitians, or foodservice directors.

12-2 Variety, balance, and truthfulness are some of the principles of menu planning.

12-2 Truth-in-menu guidelines require by law that descriptions of menu items be accurate.

12-3 The menu design, colors, lettering, paper, and wording all convey a message to the customer.

12-3 The three most common menu formats are menu boards, spoken menus, and printed menus.

12-3 Printed menu categories include appetizers, soups, salads, cold entrées, hot entrées, sandwiches, accompaniments, desserts, cheeses and fruits, and beverages.

12-3 Menu item categories are usually listed in the order they are consumed.

12-4 Menu prices must cover the costs of operating a foodservice establishment.

12-4 Pricing methods include the factor method, the markup-on-cost method, the competitors' method, and the psychological pricing method.

CHECK YOUR KNOWLEDGE

1. What role does the menu play in a foodservice operation?

2. Contrast fixed and cycle menus.

3. Define à la carte, semi-à la carte, table d'hôte, and prix fixe menus.

4. Describe two ways a restaurant can offer variety in their menu items.

5. What is meant by truth-in-menu advertising?

6. Describe the differences between a printed menu, menu board, and spoken menu.

7. How are food items listed on a menu?

8. List items that affect menu pricing.

9. Explain how to use the factor method and the markup-on-cost method of pricing.

CRITICAL-THINKING ACTIVITIES

1. Assume you will soon be opening your own restaurant. After careful analysis, which of the six types of menus would you choose for your establishment? Give five reasons for your choice.

2. Describe what might happen if a foodservice establishment failed to consider food allergies in menu planning. How might this impact the customer?

3. Why should customer response be considered when pricing menu items?

WORKPLACE KNOW-HOW

Communication. As the manager of a new restaurant, what instructions should you clearly communicate to the person who writes the menus? Why?

LAB-BASED ACTIVITY: Creating a Menu

STEP 1 Working in teams, create a menu for a new foodservice operation. Your team will need to determine:

- What type of facility the menu will represent.
- Who your target customers are.
- The type of food and menu that will be offered.
- The price range of menu items, which will reflect the type of facility.
- The equipment available to create the cuisine.
- The skill level of the workers.
- The local culture and geography.
- Current eating trends.

STEP 2 Determine the type of menu. Your team will also need to decide which meal of the day your menu will be for: breakfast, lunch, dinner, or a combination.

STEP 3 Be clear and concise in your menu descriptions. Make sure the menu you create offers a variety of nutritious options. Take into consideration that some of your customers may have special dietary needs.

STEP 4 Use the menu checklist at the bottom of this page to help organize the menu.

STEP 5 Determine selling price. Use the factor method, markup-on-cost method, psychological pricing method, or competitors' pricing method to determine each item's selling price.

STEP 6 Develop the menu layout. Using available resources, gather all of the menu information and put it in a menu format. You may want to look at several sample menus first. Display your team's finished menu.

Menu Checklist

Menu Influences:
- ✔ Target Customers
- ✔ Cost
- ✔ Type of Food Served
- ✔ Equipment
- ✔ Skill of Workers
- ✔ Culture and Geography
- ✔ Eating Trends

Menu Type:
- ✔ Fixed Menu
- ✔ Cycle Menu
- ✔ À la Carte Menu
- ✔ Semi-à la Carte Menu
- ✔ Table d'hôte Menu
- ✔ Prix Fixe Menu

Menu Style & Design:
- ✔ Cover Design
- ✔ Colors
- ✔ Style of Lettering
- ✔ Weight of Paper

Menu Format:
- ✔ Printed Menu
- ✔ Menu Board
- ✔ Spoken Menu

Kind of Meal:
- ✔ Breakfast
- ✔ Lunch
- ✔ Dinner
- ✔ Combination

Menu Categories:
- ✔ Appetizers
- ✔ Soups
- ✔ Salads
- ✔ Cold Entrées
- ✔ Hot Entrées
- ✔ Sandwiches
- ✔ Accompaniments
- ✔ Desserts
- ✔ Cheeses and Fruits
- ✔ Beverages

Using Standardized Recipes

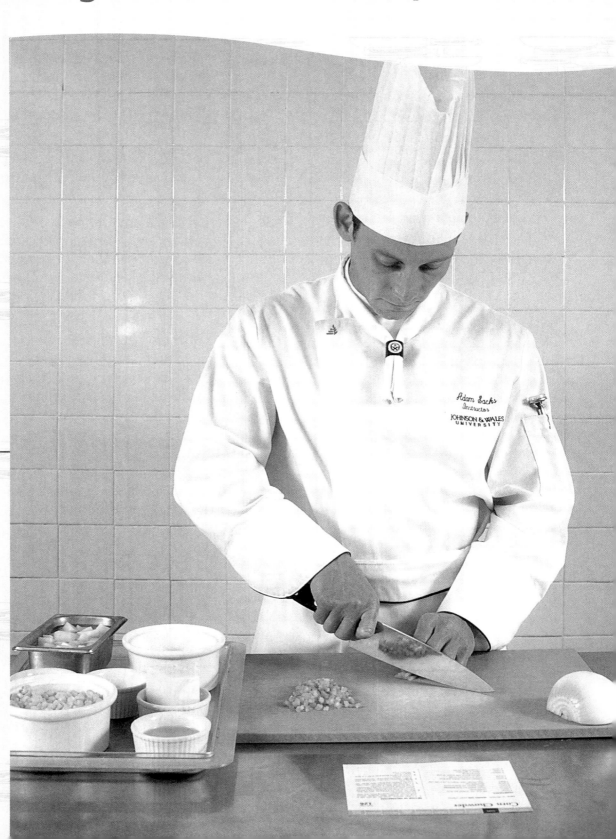

Why Use Standardized Recipes?

KEY TERMS

- recipe
- standardized recipe
- quality control
- yield
- portion size
- formula
- baker's percentage

OBJECTIVES

After reading this section, you will be able to:

- Explain the role that standardized recipes play in maintaining product consistency.
- Describe the parts of a standardized recipe.
- Contrast formulas and recipes.

RECIPES are important tools in the culinary profession. To get the desired result, you must carefully follow the specific directions contained in a recipe. The purpose of a recipe is to provide a set of written instructions for preparing a certain food. A recipe is not just a general set of instructions. Instead, a **recipe** is a precise set of directions for using ingredients, procedures, and cooking instructions for a certain dish. Following instructions and measuring ingredients accurately results in a consistent quality product of the same quantity every time it is prepared.

✖ STANDARDIZED RECIPES

A standardized (STAN-duhr-dyzed) recipe is customized to meet the needs of a particular food manufacturer or foodservice operation. In other words, a **standardized recipe** is a set of written instructions used to consistently prepare a known quantity and quality of a certain food for a food-service operation. Standardized recipes are based on the type of equipment used by a foodservice establishment.

The purpose of a standardized recipe is to direct and control the preparation of a particular food item. Each standardized recipe must go through quality control. **Quality control** is a system that ensures that everything meets the foodservice establishment's standards. This means that recipes are repeatedly tested for consistency in quality and quantity before they're used. To meet the consistency required for a standardized recipe, directions must be clear and easy to follow and ingredients must be listed accurately.

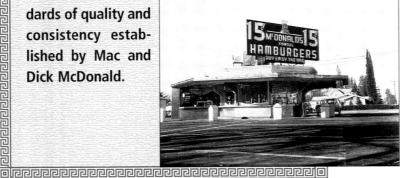
The benefits of standardized recipes include:
- Consistency in quality and quantity each time a recipe is made.
- Control of portion size and cost.
- Increased efficiency because of clear, concise instructions.
- Elimination of errors in food orders.
- Elimination of waste due to not overproducing food.
- Meeting customers' expectations each time the food item is prepared.

Although standardized recipes offer many benefits to foodservice operations, they can't solve problems caused by inconsistent purchasing and receiving of ingredients. Any substitutions in ingredients require retesting of the recipe. A recipe that is specific and uniform—producing the same model product each time—is the hallmark of a successful foodservice organization.

✖ PARTS OF A RECIPE

A successful standardized recipe is made up of the following parts. See Fig. 13-1.

■ **Product name.** Customers expect to receive what they order from a menu. The name of the recipe and the name on the menu should reflect the same product. Consistency with the product name helps eliminate confusion during preparation and serving.

■ **Yield.** The number of servings, or portions, that a recipe produces is the **yield**. The yield is an important factor in figuring cost per serving.

■ **Portion size.** The **portion size** is the amount or size of an individual serving. Standardized recipes indicate portion size.

Fig. 13-1.

Product Name {

Green Beans in Garlic Sauce

Yield { YIELD: 10 SERVINGS

Portion size { SERVING SIZE: 4 OZ.

INGREDIENTS

Ingredient Quantity {

3 oz.	Butter, melted
8 cloves	Garlic, peeled and minced
1 lb.	Canned crushed tomatoes
3 lbs.	Fresh green beans, washed, ends trimmed, and cut in half
1 pt.	White chicken stock, heated to a boil
	Salt and freshly ground black pepper, to taste

METHOD OF PREPARATION

Preparation Procedures {

1. In a saucepan, place the fresh green beans in boiling, salted water. Cook until done. Drain and shock in an ice bath. When cold, remove and drain.

2. In a sauté pan, heat the butter, and sauté the garlic. Add the crushed tomatoes, and sauté for 5 min.

3. Add the green beans and chicken stock to the tomatoes.

Cooking Time and Temperature {

4. Simmer at 180°F until done. Season to taste and serve, or hold at 135°F or above.

■ **Ingredient quantity.** Controlling quantity involves directions for measuring each ingredient. The quantity of each ingredient in the recipe should be followed closely during preparation. The recipe also lists exact yields and portion sizes.

■ **Preparation procedures.** The preparation procedures listed in standardized recipes are the result of careful testing by experienced culinary professionals. In order to consistently produce a high-quality product, you must follow these procedures carefully.

■ **Cooking temperatures.** You can literally ruin a recipe by using too high or too low a temperature. The temperature for rangetop cooking is indicated in recipes as low, medium, or high. It's indicated by specific temperatures for ovens and other appliances that have a thermostat to control cooking temperature. Most recipes require that the oven be preheated to a specific temperature. The time for preheating will vary with the type of oven.

■ **Cooking time.** Standardized recipes list the required cooking time. It's important to cook the food item for the recommended time, using the specified equipment.

FORMULA OR RECIPE

A **formula** is a special type of recipe used in the bakeshop. Although formulas and recipes are similar, there are three significant differences.

1. Recipes and formulas both contain a list of ingredients. In recipes, ingredients are listed in order of use followed by procedures to use for successful results. In formulas, however, ingredients are listed in order by decreasing weight and are often seen as percentages.

2. Precise weight measurements are used in preparing food products from formulas. This type of measurement, often called a **baker's percentage**, includes the percentage of each ingredient in relation to the weight of flour in the final baked product. Baker's percentages make it easy to increase or decrease the quantity of individual ingredients. Chapter 27 explains this in detail.

3. Formulas may not include the instructions required to prepare the product or dish.

RECIPE SUCCESS

The success of any recipe depends upon the experience level of the person following it. The desired effect cannot be achieved if the person using the recipe doesn't understand basic cooking techniques. An experienced cook learns to apply sound judgment as well as the appropriate techniques and principles to each recipe.

SECTION 13-1	Knowledge Check

1. Why are standardized recipes important to a foodservice operation?

2. List seven components of a standardized recipe.

3. Contrast a formula and a recipe.

MINI LAB

Select a standardized recipe and label the different parts. Read the recipe carefully. Would each team be able to get the same quantity and quality product? Why or why not?

Recipe Measurement & Conversion

KEY TERMS

- weight
- volume
- volume measures
- count
- recipe conversion
- conversion factor
- shrinkage

OBJECTIVES

After reading this section, you will be able to:

- Describe different recipe measurements and when each is used.

- Convert standard recipes.

- Explain the factors that affect recipe conversion.

RECIPES are designed and written to yield varying numbers of servings. Occasionally it is necessary to convert recipes, or adjust ingredient quantities, to meet the changing needs of the foodservice establishment. When the yield or portion size changes, it is necessary to convert a recipe before any preparation begins.

⊠ STANDARDIZED RECIPE MEASUREMENTS

No recipe can be successful if you are careless with measurement. Careful measuring helps achieve consistent quantity each time a recipe is prepared and served. For a successful end product, each ingredient must be measured precisely.

Standardized recipe measurements also make it quicker to increase or decrease a recipe when the need arises. Ingredients are measured by weight (lb., oz.), volume (c., tsp.), or count (2 eggs, 1 ear of corn).

Weight

In commercial food service, most ingredients are measured by weight. **Weight** is a measurement that tells how heavy something is. Measuring by weight is the quickest, easiest, and most accurate way of measuring foods such as flour, sugar, meats, and cheeses. Ounces and pounds are examples of common weight measurements.

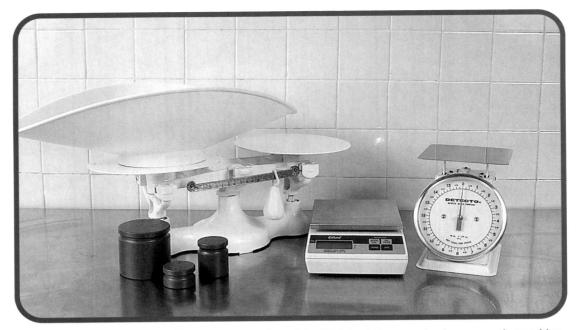

Fig. 13-2. Scales come in different types and models. Which of these scales is commonly used by bakers?

Fig. 13-3A.

MEASUREMENT	ABBREVIATION
Teaspoon	tsp. or t.
Tablespoon	tbsp. or T.
Ounce	oz.
Fluid ounce	fl. oz.
Pound	lb. or #
Cup	c.
Pint	pt.
Quart	qt.
Gallon	gal. or G.
Barrel	bbl.
Dozen	doz.
Bunch	bch. or bu.
Case	cs.

Scales for weighing come in various types, sizes, and price ranges. The types of scales generally used in food service are balance, portion or spring, and electronic or digital. See Fig. 13-2.

■ **Balance scale.** A balance scale, also called a baker's scale, has two platforms. One platform holds the item being weighed. The other platform holds weights. These weights are added or removed until the two platforms are balanced. Balance scales are used when precise measurement is important, such as in baking.

Fig. 13-3B.

MEASUREMENT	EQUIVALENT	
3 tsp.	= 1 T.	= ½ fluid oz.
16 T.	= 1 c.	= 8 oz.
2 c.	= 1 pt.	= 16 oz.
2 pt.	= 1 qt.	= 32 oz.
4 qts.	= 1 gal.	= 128 oz.
1 lb.	= 16 oz.	

- **Portion scale.** A portion, or spring, scale is similar to a bathroom scale. It weighs items by measuring how much the spring is depressed when an item is placed on its platform. A needle on a dial indicates the weight of the item. Spring scales are often used as portion scales. For example, you may use a spring scale to measure meats in a deli.

- **Electronic scale.** An electronic, or digital, scale is similar to a spring scale. It, too, has a spring that's depressed when an item is placed on its platform. However, the weight is displayed in numbers on a digital readout rather than by a needle. This readout is more accurate than a needle guide, but digital scales are more expensive than spring scales. An electronic scale is used as a portion scale.

Volume

The term **volume** refers to the amount of space that a substance occupies. **Volume measures** are used most often to measure liquids in food service. Volume measurements are expressed in cups, quarts, gallons, and fluid ounces. Fig. 13-3A and Fig 13-3B show common cooking abbreviations and equivalents.

Liquids are added to a recipe after being measured by volume. The volume measure should be placed on a level surface. Liquid should be filled to the specified line. Metal volume measures have measurement lines on both the outside and inside. See Fig. 13-4.

Count

The number of individual items used in a recipe to indicate the size of each item is referred to as the **count**. Measuring ingredients by count is done when a food ingredient comes in standard sizes.

For example, most recipes list eggs by count instead of by weight or volume. A cake recipe may ask for three large eggs or a cobb salad for one hard-cooked egg. The same recipe may also call for one small tomato, quartered, or three black olives, sliced. In contrast, shrimp is often sold by the pound, with the size of the shrimp determining the count. The smaller the count per pound, the larger the individual shrimp size. Each of these examples indicates count.

Fig. 13-4. It's important to measure liquids accurately when using volume measurements.
Why should volume measures always be placed on a level surface?

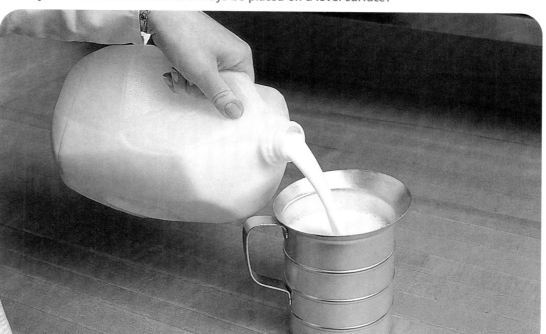

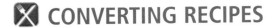 CONVERTING RECIPES

Sometimes you will need to alter a standardized recipe to produce more or less of a product. Changing a recipe to produce a new amount or yield is called a **recipe conversion**.

Total Yield Conversion Method

Before you increase or decrease the yield of a standardized recipe, a conversion factor has to be established. The **conversion factor** is the number that results from dividing the desired yield by the existing yield in a recipe. The conversion factor is obtained by using this simple math calculation:

$$\text{existing yield} \overline{)\text{desired yield}}^{\text{conversion factor}}$$

For example, if the existing recipe yield is 40 portions, but the yield needed is 80 portions, the formula will look like this:

$$\text{(existing yield) } 40 \overline{)80 \text{ (desired yield)}}^{2 \text{ (conversion factor)}}$$
$$\underline{80}$$
$$0$$

The recipe conversion factor is used to increase or decrease a standardized recipe. This is done by multiplying each ingredient quantity by the conversion factor to obtain the new quantity. If you decrease a recipe, the conversion factor will be less than one (a decimal). Whereas, if you increase a recipe, the conversion factor will be more than one.

For example, assume a recipe has a yield of 10 portions of Chicken Teriyaki requiring 3 lbs. of boneless chicken and 20 fl. oz. of teriyaki sauce. You need to convert the yield to 15 portions. Use the following steps:

Step 1: Determine the conversion factor.

15 (desired yield) ÷ 10 (existing yield) = 1.5
(conversion factor)

Step 2: Multiply the existing quantity by the conversion factor to obtain the new quantity.

existing quantity
× conversion factor
desired quantity

3.0 (lb. chicken)
× 1.5 (conversion factor)
4.5 (lb. chicken)

20.0 (fl. oz. teriyaki sauce)
× 1.5 (conversion factor)
30.0 (fl. oz. teriyaki sauce)

Recipe conversion is a skill you will use throughout your career in the foodservice industry. You will likely be called upon to convert recipes to different amounts and different portion sizes. Accuracy and consistency in making conversions is important in making a quality food product. The following passage takes you through the steps in converting portion size. See Fig. 13-5.

Converting Portion Size

A foodservice establishment may need to increase or decrease the portion size of a recipe. Perhaps customers are complaining that the portion is too small. Maybe the portion is so large that it's resulting in little or no profit for the establishment. In either case, it's important to know how to convert portion sizes as well as recipe yields. Here are the steps to follow in converting portion size.

Step 1: To determine the total existing yield, multiply the number of existing portions by the existing size of each portion.

existing portions
× existing portion size
total existing yield

Using the earlier Chicken Teriyaki recipe:

15 (portions)
× 5 oz. (portion size)
75 oz. (existing yield)

Step 2: To determine a new yield, multiply the desired portions by the desired portion size.

desired portions
× desired portion size
new yield

20 (desired portions)
× 8 oz. (desired portion size)
160 oz. (new yield)

Step 3: Divide new yield by existing yield to get the conversion factor.

$$\frac{2.13 \text{ (conversion factor)}}{\text{(existing yield) } 75 \overline{) 160.00 \text{ (new yield)}}}$$

Step 4: Multiply each ingredient in the existing recipe by the conversion factor to get the new ingredient yield.

existing yield
× conversion factor
new yield

4.50 lb. (existing yield, chicken)
× 2.13 (conversion factor)
9.58 lb. (new yield, chicken)
10.00 lb. (new yield, rounded up)

30.0 fl. oz (existing yield, teriyaki sauce)
× 2.13 (conversion factor)
63.9 fl. oz (new yield, teriyaki sauce)

64.0 fl. oz. (new yield, rounded up)

UNIT PRICES

Unit price is the cost per unit of measure. This may be per item, per pound, per quart, or any other unit measure. When buying food packaged in two different quantities, it is wise to know which is the better buy. To find the better buy, you will need to know the unit price.

Follow these steps to calculate the unit price of an item.

1. Divide the price by the number of chicken breast halves:

$$\frac{\$ \quad .83}{\text{(chicken halves) } 48 \overline{) \$ 39.99}}$$

2. Write it as a unit price. Each chicken breast half costs $ .83.

TRY IT!

Find the unit price of each:

1. 12 (#5) cans of beef broth for $6.50
2. 50 lbs. of cake flour for $18.75
3. 32 oz. of vanilla flavoring for $10.00

Determine the better buy:

4. ½ lb. of bread crumbs for $0.75
   OR
   3 lbs. of bread crumbs for $5.65
5. 3 qts. of pineapple juice for $7.45
   OR
   10 qts. of pineapple juice for $20.25

Fig. 13-5.

Southern Vegetable Soup

YIELD: 10 SERVINGS

SERVING SIZE: 8 OZ.

COOKING TECHNIQUES:
Sauté, Boil, Simmer

Sauté:
1. Heat the sauté pan to the appropriate temperature.
2. Evenly brown the food product.
3. For a sauce, pour off any excess oil, reheat, and deglaze.

Boil: (at sea level)
1. Bring the cooking liquid to a rapid boil.
2. Stir the contents, and cook the food product throughout.
3. Serve hot.

Simmer and Poach:
1. Heat the cooking liquid to the proper temperature.
2. Submerge the food product completely.
3. Keep the cooked product moist and warm.

GLOSSARY:
Brunoise: ⅛-in. dice
Chiffonade: ribbons of leafy greens
Marmite: stockpot
Render: to melt fat over low heat to separate it from the meat tissue

HACCP:
Hold at 135°F or above.
Reheat to 165°F for 15 seconds.

HAZARDOUS FOOD:
Beef

NUTRITION:
Calories: 180
Fat: 11.8 g
Protein: 8.7 g

INGREDIENTS

2 oz.	Salt pork, cut into small dice
10 oz.	Beef, bottom round, cut into small cubes
8 oz.	Canned peeled tomatoes, drained, seeded, and chopped
3½ qts.	Beef stock, heated to a boil
2 oz.	Frozen green beans
2 oz.	Red beans, cooked
4 oz.	Onions, peeled and diced **brunoise**
3 oz.	Celery stalks, washed, trimmed, and diced brunoise
6 oz.	Green cabbage, washed, cored, and **chiffonade**
3 oz.	Carrots, washed, peeled, and diced brunoise
2 oz.	Frozen corn kernels
2 oz.	Frozen okra, sliced
2 oz.	Zucchini, washed, trimmed, and cut in ½-in. dice
	Salt and freshly ground black pepper, to taste

METHOD OF PREPARATION

1. In a large **marmite**, place the salt pork, and **render** the fat, stirring frequently until browned. Add the beef, reduce the heat, and sauté until browned.
2. Add the tomatoes, and sauté for another 2 min.
3. Add the boiling stock, and simmer until the meat is slightly firm in texture.
4. Add all other ingredients, and continue to simmer until vegetables are tender.
5. Season to taste and serve immediately in preheated cups, or hold at 135°F or above.

Total Conversion Method

Southern Vegetable Soup

Existing Yield: 10 servings

Existing Portion Size: 8 oz.

New Yield: 35 servings

New Portion Size: 8 oz.

Determine the Conversion Factor:

$$\text{New Yield}\,)\overline{\text{Existing Yield}}^{\;\text{Conversion Factor}}$$

$$10\,)\overline{35.0}^{\;3.5}$$

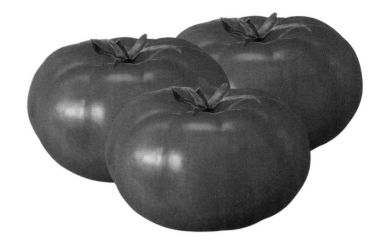

Ingredient	Amount	Multiplied By	Conversion Factor	Equals	New Yield
Salt Pork	2 oz.	×	3.5	=	7 oz.
Bottom Round	10 oz.	×	3.5	=	35 oz.
Peeled Tomatoes	8 oz.	×	3.5	=	28 oz.
Beef Stock	3½ qts.	×	3.5	=	12.25 qts.
Green Beans	2 oz.	×	3.5	=	7 oz.
Red Beans	2 oz.	×	3.5	=	7 oz.
Onions	4 oz.	×	3.5	=	14 oz.
Celery	3 oz.	×	3.5	=	10.5 oz.
Green Cabbage	6 oz.	×	3.5	=	21 oz.
Carrots	3 oz.	×	3.5	=	10.5 oz.
Corn	2 oz.	×	3.5	=	7 oz.
Okra	2 oz.	×	3.5	=	7 oz.
Zucchini	2 oz.	×	3.5	=	7 oz.

FACTORS THAT IMPACT CONVERSION

The conversion calculations do not take into account problems that may arise when you alter standardized recipes. These problems include adjustments to equipment, cooking times, cooking temperatures, and recipe errors. When you make adjustments to deal with these problems, be sure to write them down on your recipe.

Equipment

Recipes usually indicate the size of equipment needed to prepare the food item or product. If a recipe is increased or decreased, the size of the equipment may become a factor. The wrong equipment can affect the outcome of a recipe. It's important to use proper equipment to accommodate the recipe conversion.

Mixing & Cooking Time

Time is another important factor to consider when converting recipes. In general, the mixing time and cooking time are not increased when a recipe is converted. Certain changes, however, will affect mixing or cooking times. For example,

a formula that has been decreased could be affected by overmixing, and a formula that has been increased could be affected by undermixing.

Preparation times may also be affected by changes in equipment. For example, the Southern Vegetable Soup recipe on page 308 requires a large stockpot to prepare the existing yield of soup. When the recipe is decreased, a smaller pot will be needed to cook the new yield of soup. This smaller volume will likely change the cooking time. See Fig. 13-6.

Cooking Temperatures

Cooking temperatures can also be affected by a change in equipment. For example, imagine that the restaurant you work in has just bought a new convection oven. The recipe you're following was developed using a conventional oven. Because convection ovens bake much faster than standard ovens, the cooking time must be adjusted.

Shrinkage

Shrinkage is the percentage of food lost during its storage and preparation. Shrinkage is often caused by moisture loss. The amount of shrinkage affects not only cost but also portion sizes.

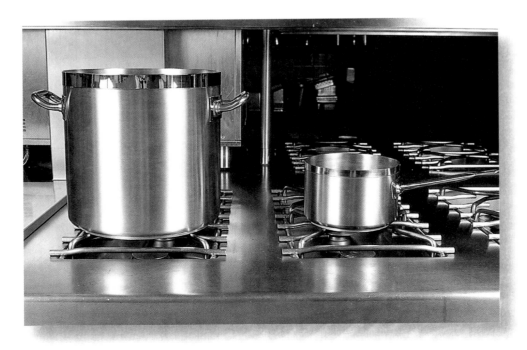

Fig. 13-6. The size of the equipment you use can affect cooking time.

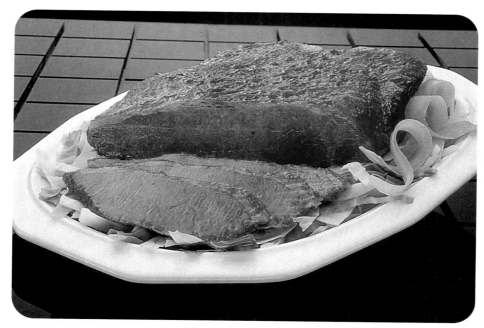

Fig. 13-7. Don't forget to consider shrinkage when you purchase food. What causes shrinkage?

Knowing ahead of time how much waste a product will have allows a foodservice professional to purchase the correct amount.

Corned beef, for example, shrinks when you cook it. You must consider this shrinkage when you purchase the beef. You will have to start with a larger amount in order to end up with an adequate portion. As a general rule, corned beef shrinks about 50%. If you need 10 lbs. of cooked corned beef, you'll need to purchase about 20 lbs. of uncooked corned beef. See Fig. 13-7.

Recipe Errors

Very often recipe errors are so minor that they don't affect the results. However, even minor errors can become major problems as the recipe is increased or decreased. To avoid this problem, recipes that have been adjusted need to be tested.

For example, a recipe may have mistakenly listed 2 oz. of cornstarch instead of 1 oz. The mistake may go unnoticed until the recipe is tripled and the amount of cornstarch affects both the appearance and the taste of the product. To eliminate problems such as this, recipes that have been converted must undergo testing.

SECTION 13-2 Knowledge Check

1. Explain the difference between weight, volume, and count measurement. Which is most accurate?

2. Describe a situation that might require an establishment to change portion sizes.

3. What problems might arise when converting recipes?

MINI LAB

Using the Southern Vegetable Soup recipe, make the following conversions:

- Increase the recipe to 50 servings.
- Increase the portion size to 10 oz.

SECTION SUMMARIES

13-1 A standardized recipe helps ensure consistency in quality, quantity, and portion size.

13-1 Every standardized recipe provides information for food services in planning, preparing, and using the food product.

13-1 Although a formula and a recipe both have a list of ingredients, they list these ingredients differently.

13-2 Recipes list ingredient portions by weight, volume, or count.

13-2 You must use the correct formula to adjust a standardized recipe's total yield or the portion size.

13-2 Many factors must be considered for the successful conversion of a recipe.

CHECK YOUR KNOWLEDGE

1. Describe a standardized recipe.
2. How does quality control ensure that standardized recipes meet a foodservice establishment's standards?
3. Explain the importance of the yield in a recipe.
4. How is the cooking temperature for range-top cooking indicated in recipes?
5. How are ingredients listed in formulas?
6. List the types of scales that might be used to weigh food ingredients.
7. What measurement is preferred for liquid ingredients?
8. List three food items that can be measured by count.

CRITICAL-THINKING ACTIVITIES

1. Give a specific example of a situation when a foodservice operation would need to retest a standardized recipe.
2. In what situations might a recipe need to be converted?
3. What conversion factor would you use to increase the portion size of a recipe that serves 10 people from 8 oz. to 10 oz.? Show how you arrived at your answer.

WORKPLACE KNOW-HOW

Cost analysis. Imagine that you're the manager of a restaurant specializing in locally grown produce. Because of severe winter weather, local fruits are very expensive. You may lose customers if you raise prices. What can you do?

LAB-BASED ACTIVITY: Weighing Dry Ingredients

STEP 1 Determine the amount of each ingredient needed to make a half sheet pan of corn bread for a fish fry. Using the chart below, list the ingredients on a separate sheet of paper and calculate the amount needed next to each ingredient. Use the following formulas:

$$\frac{\text{existing portions} \times \text{existing portion size}}{\text{existing yield}}$$

$$\frac{\text{desired portions} \times \text{desired portion size}}{\text{new yield}}$$

STEP 2 Calculate the total yield weight of the ingredients for a half sheet pan of corn bread.

STEP 3 Explain how to measure the dry ingredients for a half sheet pan of corn bread.

STEP 4 Determine the amount of each ingredient needed to make two sheet pans of corn bread. List the ingredients on a separate sheet of paper and write the amounts needed next to each ingredient. Use the following formula in your calculations.

$$\text{existing yield}\,\overline{)\text{new yield}}^{\text{conversion factor}}$$

STEP 5 Calculate the total yield weight of the ingredients for two sheet pans of corn bread.

STEP 6 Explain how you would measure the liquid ingredients to prepare two sheet pans of corn bread.

STEP 7 List the equipment needed to prepare two sheet pans of corn bread as compared to the equipment needed to prepare a half sheet pan of corn bread.

Corn Bread Ingredients	Yield: ___?___ ½ sheet pan	Yield: 9 lbs. 5¾ oz. 1 sheet pan	Yield: ___?___ 2 sheet pans
Flour, bread, sifted	?	1 lb., 12 oz.	?
Flour, pastry, sifted	?	12 oz.	?
Baking powder	?	2¾ oz.	?
Salt	?	1 oz.	?
Dry milk solids	?	6 oz.	?
Cornmeal	?	1 lb.	?
Sugar, granulated	?	1 lb., 10 oz.	?
Water	?	1 lb., 14 oz.	?
Eggs, whole	?	1 lb.	?
Oil, vegetable	?	12 oz.	?

14

Cost Control Techniques

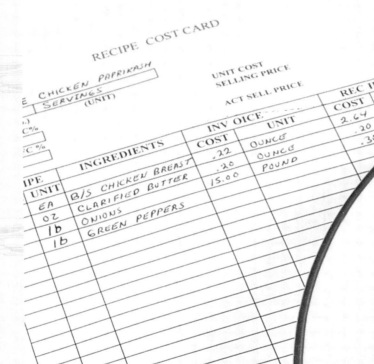

RECIPE COST CARD

						UNIT COST SELLING PRICE				RECIPE		TOTAL
CHICKEN PAPRIKASH								ACT SELL PRICE		COST	UNIT	13.20
	SERVINGS (UNIT)									2.64	EA	
					INVOICE					.20	OZ	
			INGREDIENTS			COST	UNIT			.30	lb	
						.22	OUNCE					
	UNIT		B/S CHICKEN BREAST			.20	OUNCE					
	EA		CLARIFIED BUTTER			15.00	POUND					
	OZ		ONIONS									
	lb		GREEN PEPPERS									
	lb											

Section 14-1
Calculating Food Costs

Section 14-2
Managing Food Cost Factors

Calculating Food Costs

OBJECTIVES

After reading this section, you will be able to:

• Describe methods of portion control and why it is important.

• Calculate unit cost, yield percentage, percent of shrinkage, and cost per portion.

• Complete a recipe costing form.

MONITORING food costs helps ensure that a foodservice facility covers its operating expenses. In this section, you will learn about factors that influence the cost of preparing menu items, such as portion size. You will also learn how to calculate and control food costs.

PORTION CONTROL

Customers expect their food to be uniform in size and quality. They're concerned with not only how the food looks and tastes but also the value they receive for their food dollars.

Serving consistent portions is essential to the success of a foodservice operation. The following guidelines help control portions:

• Purchase items according to standard specifications.

• Follow standardized recipes.

• Use standardized portioning tools and equipment.

Purchasing by Specifications

A foodservice operation must develop and implement standards to control food costs. These established standards must be followed to achieve consistency in daily operations.

One way of maintaining those standards is by purchasing food according to specifications. A **specification**, or spec, is a written description of the products a foodservice operation needs to purchase.

A foodservice facility can purchase products by count or number and expect to create a definite

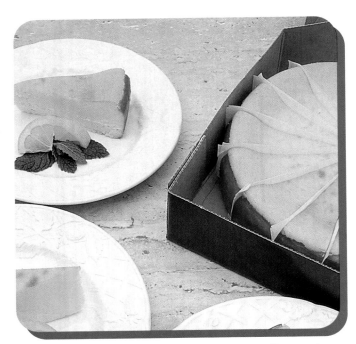

Fig. 14-1. This cheesecake was ordered according to the restaurant's specifications so that an exact number of portions could be created. Why is portion control so important to a foodservice operation?

number of food items from that amount. For example, whole cheesecakes can be purchased and then cut into a set number of individual servings. See Fig. 14-1.

A second way of purchasing by spec is to order products already divided into individual servings. For example, most facilities purchase single-serving pats of butter or packets of sugar or ketchup.

Following Standardized Recipes

Standardized recipes also help maintain consistent proportions. A standardized recipe includes the portion size and the total number of portions that will result when a recipe is prepared.

For example, if you prepare sauerkraut based on your facility's standardized recipe, you will end up with a specific number of servings. If you cook Polish sausage too long or at too high a temperature, the meat could shrink and result in smaller portions. It's important, therefore, to use the cooking time and temperature specified in the standardized recipe.

Portioning Tools & Equipment

If you use different-size ladles to fill soup bowls, you'll end up serving different amounts of soup. Using the same size ladle is one way to ensure that portions are consistent. Knowing the correct tools and equipment to use for each dish your facility prepares is an important aspect of portion control.

Scoops, or dishers, are commonly used to control portions during food preparation and serving. Use scoops to measure quantities of food such as cookie dough, mashed potatoes, or corn bread stuffing.

Scoops are available in a variety of sizes with color-coded handles. This helps foodservice employees match the appropriate scoop with a particular portion size. For example, a recipe for boneless stuffed chicken breasts may require use of one No. 12 scoop of stuffing for each chicken breast. However, this applies only to this particular foodservice operation. Another facility's version of this recipe may require use of one No. 8 scoop of stuffing for each chicken breast. See Fig. 14-2.

Other portion control tools and equipment include ladles, spoons, balance and portion scales, slicers, and volume measures.

Fig. 14-2. Scoops are color-coded in a variety of sizes to help employees serve the right portion.

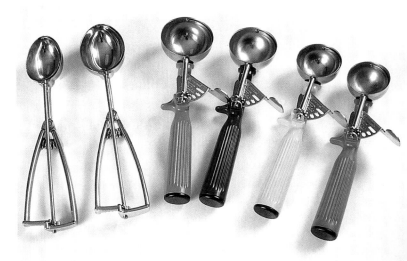

CALCULATING UNIT COST

Most foodservice facilities purchase food in **bulk**, or large quantities of a single food product. Buying in bulk is effective if storage space is available and food waste is avoided. Examples of bulk packages include a case of canned tomatoes, a flat of strawberries, or a 50-lb. bag of flour. Bulk items are divided into smaller quantities for use in individual recipes.

AS-PURCHASED PRICE

To find how much it costs to make one recipe, you must first determine how much the ingredients cost. Do this by converting the bulk price, called the **as-purchased (AP) price**, to the unit cost. The **unit cost** is the cost of each individual item.

For example, suppose a 50-lb. bag of granulated sugar costs $22.00. The Marinated Mushroom Salad recipe calls for several ounces of sugar. Therefore, the unit is ounces. To determine the unit cost of each ounce, first convert pounds to ounces by multiplying 50 by 16. There are 16 oz. in 1 lb. To find how much each ounce costs, divide $22.00 by 800 oz. The unit cost is $0.03 per ounce of sugar.

$$50 \text{ lb.} \times 16 \text{ oz.} = 800 \text{ oz.}$$

$$
\begin{array}{r}
.0275 \\
\text{(units) } 800.00. \overline{)22.00.} \text{ (AP price)} \\
\underline{1600} \\
6000 \\
\underline{5600} \\
4000 \\
\underline{4000}
\end{array}
$$

$0.0275 rounded up = $0.03 (unit cost)

The AP price is the cost of a food product when it is first purchased, usually in a large quantity. Some foods, such as deli meats, are used completely as they are purchased—there is no food waste. Other foods need some type of preparation, such as trimming or deboning, which results in waste.

PRODUCT YIELDS

Product yield is the amount of food product left after preparation. Many times, foods lose volume or weight as they are prepared.

A lot can happen to food to make the portion served to a customer smaller than the original product. For example, a roast can shrink up to one-third of its original size when it is cooked. The **as-served (AS)** portion is the actual weight of the food product that is served to customers.

EDIBLE PORTION

Many foods are reduced in size and weight during preparation and cooking. For example, carrots must be prepared before cooking. After preparation, the consumable food product that remains is called the **edible portion (EP)**. See Fig. 14-3.

You can see that what you buy isn't always what you serve. Foodservice buyers must consider the AP cost, EP cost, and AS portion when determining how much of a food product to purchase.

Fig. 14-3. The difference between AP and EP weight can be significant. What could be the consequences of underestimating the AP weight needed for a particular food?

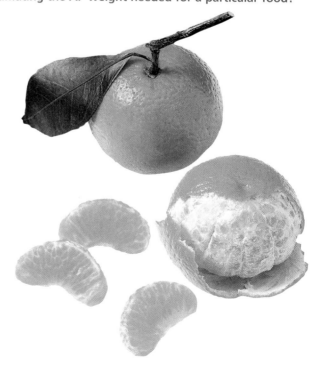

PERCENTS OF INCREASE & DECREASE

In some food cost calculations, you may be asked to find the percent of increase or decrease of a particular item. The percent of increase is important because it will show you how much an amount increased over the original amount. For example, if you are comparing an increase in cost of a food item from one month to another, you would use the percent of increase formula. The percent of decrease will show you how much an amount decreased from the original amount.

Use these formulas to determine the values:

$$\text{original amt.} \overline{)\text{final amt.} - \text{original amt.}}^{\text{percent of increase}}$$

$$\text{original amt.} \overline{)\text{original amt.} - \text{final amt.}}^{\text{percent of decrease}}$$

For example, find the percent of decrease for diced potatoes in a chowder. The original weight of the potatoes was 8.5 lbs. and the final weight is 6.9 lbs. Round the answer to the nearest whole percent.

$$\text{percent of decrease} = \frac{8.5 - 6.9}{8.5}$$

$$= \frac{1.6}{8.5} = 0.188$$

The percent of decrease is about 19%.

TRY IT!

1. What is the percent of increase of an item that was originally $5.95 and is now $8.10?

2. What is the percent of decrease of an item that was originally 10.2 lbs. and is now 7.3 lbs.?

⊠ YIELD PERCENTAGES

Product yield is the usable portion of a food product. A yield test is a process by which AP food is broken down into EP and waste. The **yield percentage** is the ratio of the edible portion of food to the amount of food purchased.

Yields vary depending on many factors. For example, how much a foodservice operation typically trims its meat products and whether or not these trimmings are used in other recipes will affect the yield.

Raw Yield Tests

Raw yield tests are used on food products that don't have any usable leftover parts, or by-products. For example, the outermost leaves of a head of lettuce are trimmed and discarded when cleaning the lettuce. The trimmings are never used. For foods like this that have no by-products, you must keep this loss in mind when determining yield.

To conduct a raw yield test for products without by-products, follow these steps:

1. Weigh the product before trimming. This number is called the AP weight.

2. Weigh the by-product material that was trimmed from the purchased product. This number is called the **trim loss**.

3. Subtract the trim loss from the AP weight. This number is the yield weight.

4. Divide the yield weight by the AP weight. This results in the yield percentage.

For example, you take two whole red bell peppers from the refrigerator in order to prepare Marinated Mushroom Salad. The two peppers weigh a total of 11 oz. After trimming the peppers, you have 3 oz. of trim loss, or unusable waste. To find the yield percentage, subtract the trim loss (3 oz.) from the AP weight (11 oz.). Then divide the yield weight by the AP weight. The yield percentage of 11 oz. of fresh red bell peppers is 73%.

```
       11 (AP weight)
      − 3 (trim loss)
       8 (yield weight)


                 .727
11 (AP weight) )8.00 (yield weight)
                 77
                 30
                 22
                 80
                 77
                  3
```

.727 rounded up = .73 or 73% (yield percentage)

Because each foodservice operation has its own standards for how workers should trim products, yield percentages will differ.

Cooking Loss Test

To determine how cooking affects yield percentage, follow these steps:

1. Identify the net cost and net weight of the raw food product.

2. Note how many portions are produced from the product after cooking.

3. Multiply the number of portions by the portion weight when served. This gives the total weight as served.

For example, the net cost of 20 lbs. of boneless turkey breast is $62.00. When cooked, the turkey breast results in 46 portions, each weighing 6 oz. To determine the total weight as served, multiply the number of portions (46) by the portion weight when served (6 oz.). The total weight of 20 lbs. of boneless turkey breast when served is 17.25 lbs.

```
        46 (number of portions)
       ×6 (portion weight)
       276 oz.
```

```
              17.25
16 (oz.) )276 (oz.)
              16
             116
             112
              40
              32
              80
              80
               0
```

17.25 lbs. = total weight as served

Shrinkage

Shrinkage may account for the weight loss that occurs when food is cooked. Shrinkage is the difference between the AP weight and the AS weight.

By finding the percent of shrinkage, you will know how much shrinkage affects the cost per lb. of a food product. To calculate this percent, divide the shrinkage by the AP weight.

```
                  percent of shrinkage
AP weight )shrinkage
```

Let's determine the percent of shrinkage of a hamburger patty. For example, the AP weight of a hamburger patty is 4 oz., while the AS weight of a cooked hamburger patty is 3.5 oz. The difference of 0.5 oz. is the shrinkage. Divide the shrinkage (0.5 oz.) by the AP weight (4 oz.). The percent of shrinkage for a 4 oz. hamburger patty is 12.5%. You would calculate the percentage as follows:

```
                  .125
4 (AP weight) )0.5 (shrinkage)
                  4
                 10
                  8
                 20
                 20
                  0
```

.125 = 12.5% (percent of shrinkage)

COSTING RECIPES

Determining the cost of a standardized recipe is an important part of cost control. Once the total recipe cost is calculated, a foodservice operation can figure how much each portion costs. The operation then uses this information to set menu selling prices.

Using a Recipe Costing Form

A Recipe Costing Form helps manage food purchasing and preparation. Fig. 14-4A shows a Recipe Costing Form. Here is an explanation of each part of the form:

A. **Recipe name.** The recipe name should be the same as the one listed on the menu.

B. **Portion size.** This is the standard amount of the food item that is served to each customer.

C. **Yield.** This is the number of servings that one preparation of the recipe yields.

D. **Menu category.** This refers to the menu category in which the food appears. See Chapter 12 for the traditional menu categories.

E. **Ingredients.** This is a list of each ingredient used in the recipe.

F. **Edible portion (EP).** This is the amount of an ingredient left after the waste product has been removed from the as-purchased amount.

G. **As-purchased (AP) amount.** This is the amount of the product that is purchased.

H. **Unit purchase price.** This is the price paid for each individual item in a bulk purchase. An item is measured in such units as pounds, gallons, or cans.

I. **Cost per unit.** To determine the cost per unit, divide the unit purchase cost by the number of purchase units, or quantity. For example, the mushrooms in the form on page 321 cost $12.20 for 10 lbs. Therefore, $12.20 ÷ 10 lbs. = $1.20.

unit purchase cost ÷ purchase unit = cost per unit

For some ingredients, you may need to convert the purchase unit to the type of unit used in the recipe. For example, although sugar is pur-

chased in 50-pound bags, the recipe amount is in ounces. To determine the cost of each ounce, first convert pounds to ounces as follows: 50 lbs. × 16 oz. = 800 oz. Then, use the formula above to determine the cost per unit.

J. **Ingredient cost.** To determine the cost for each ingredient used in the recipe, multiply the cost per unit by the AP amount.

cost per unit × AP amount = ingredient cost

For example, the mushroom cost per unit is $1.22. Therefore, $1.22 × 2 lbs. = $2.44, or the ingredient cost for the mushrooms.

K. **Ingredient cost total.** Add together the cost of each ingredient to get the ingredient cost total. For the Marinated Mushroom Salad on page 321, the ingredient cost total is $6.86.

L. **Q factor (1%–5%).** The Q factor, or the questionable ingredient factor, is the cost of an ingredient that is difficult to measure. Most foodservice operations have a preset Q factor percentage, such as 5%. That percentage is multiplied by the total cost of ingredients to find the Q factor dollar amount.

M. **Total recipe cost.** To calculate this cost, add the ingredient cost total (K) and the Q factor (L).

N. **Portion cost.** To calculate the portion cost, divide the total recipe cost (K) by the total number of portions that the recipe yields (C).

total recipe cost ÷ total number portions = portion cost

Fig. 14-4A.

| A. Recipe Name: Marinated Mushroom Salad | | | | | C. Yield: 10 servings | |
| B. Portion Size: 5 oz. | | | | | D. Menu Category: Salad | |

E. Ingredients		F. EP%	G. AP Amount	H. Unit Purchase Price		I. Cost Per Unit	J. Ingredient Cost
Quantity	Item	EP%	Quantity	Cost	Unit		
2 lb.	Button mushrooms, whole	100%	2.00 lb.	$12.20	10 lbs.	$1.22	$2.44
8 oz.	Diced red bell pepper	73%	10.96 oz.	$25.85	22 lbs.	$0.07	$0.77
1 oz.	Lemon juice	100%	1.00 oz.	$13.32	12 qt.	$0.03	$0.03
8 oz.	Olive oil	100%	8.00 oz.	$14.95	1 gal.	$0.12	$0.96
2 oz.	Granulated sugar	100%	2.00 oz.	$20.50	50 lbs.	$0.03	$0.06
1.5 oz.	Fresh basil, chopped	100%	1.50 oz.	$18.75	2.25 lbs.	$0.52	$0.78
1.5 oz.	Fresh oregano, chopped	100%	1.50 oz.	$4.70	12-oz. bag	$0.39	$0.59
1 head	Romaine lettuce, shredded	100%	1.00 head	$17.95	24 head	$0.75	$0.75
8 oz.	Green peas	100%	8.00 oz.	$0.89	1 lb.	$0.06	$0.48
	Salt & pepper to taste						

K. Ingredient Cost Total		$6.86
L. Q Factor (5%)		$0.34
M. Total Recipe Cost		$7.20
N. Portion Cost		$0.72

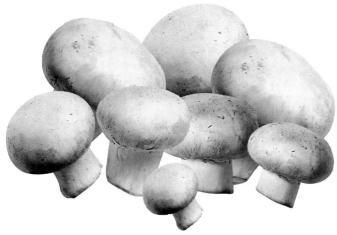

COST PER PORTION

Once you've completed a recipe costing form, you'll want to find the cost of individual portions of that recipe. The **cost per portion** represents the amount you would serve to an individual customer. To figure this, divide the recipe cost by the number of portions or servings.

The standardized recipe for Marinated Mushroom Salad results in 10 portions. You've added up the ingredient costs and found that the recipe cost is $7.20. To find the cost per portion, divide $7.20 by 10. The cost per portion of the Marinated Mushroom Salad is $0.72.

$$10 \text{ (portions)} \overline{\smash{)}7.20 \text{ (recipe cost)}} = .72$$

$$
\begin{array}{r}
.72 \\
10 \text{ (portions)} \overline{\smash{)}7.20 \text{ (recipe cost)}} \\
70 \\
\hline
20 \\
20 \\
\hline
0
\end{array}
$$

.72 = $0.72 (cost per portion)

RECIPE SOFTWARE

In order to streamline the recipe development and costing process, many restaurants and foodservice institutions often use computerized software. The benefits of this type of software include the prevention of costly pricing mistakes and increased speed in making changes to recipes that impact yield and cost.

Although a number of software programs exist, in general recipe software allows the foodservice personnel to:

• Create recipes.
• Alter the yield of recipes.
• Determine the cost per serving for recipes.
• Calculate menu costs.
• Average the costs for food, labor, and other overhead expenses into the total cost of producing recipes.
• Analyze the nutritional value of recipes.

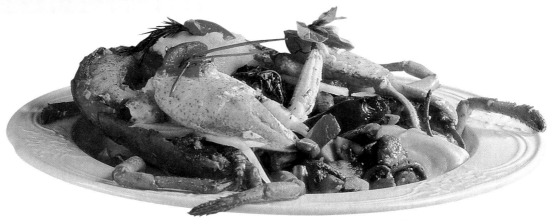

Fig. 14-4B. Marinated Mushroom Salad is often served as an accompaniment, as shown above.

SECTION 14-1 — Knowledge Check

1. List two ways a foodservice operation can control portion sizes.

2. How is shrinkage involved in food cost calculations?

3. What are two situations that would require you to use the Q factor?

MINI LAB

Calculate the following: (1) A facility pays $25.50 for a 30-dozen case of eggs. Find the unit cost of each egg. (2) The total recipe cost for Pecan Pie, which yields 8 servings, is $4.67. Find the cost per portion.

Managing Food Cost Factors

OBJECTIVES

After reading this section, you will be able to:

• Explain the steps, methods, and types of products involved in purchasing.

• Describe what tools and equipment to use and procedures to follow when receiving goods.

• Demonstrate techniques for storing and issuing goods.

• Summarize how kitchen waste and customer service affect cost control.

HOW can you best keep costs under control in a foodservice operation? You might be surprised by how many factors affect cost control. Menu pricing is important, but just as critical are purchasing, receiving, and storing methods. Another consideration is **issuing**, the process of delivering foods from storage to the kitchen as needed for use. Kitchen waste and customer service also impact an operation's bottom line. Knowing how to properly manage and control each of these factors is essential to the success of a foodservice operation.

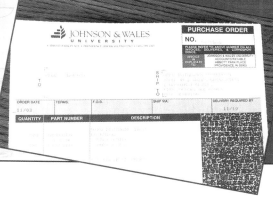

❌ MENUS

The menu is the foundation for the success or failure of a foodservice operation. A profitable menu must satisfy customers and stand up well against the competition. Careless changes to the menu can result in wasted ingredients and leftovers. Many factors influence the planning of a menu, including:

• **Space and equipment.** Is the available space and equipment adequate for making the menu items?

• **Ingredient availability.** Are ingredients readily available for each item?

• **Food costs.** Are the costs of food products and ingredients appropriate?

• **Employee skills.** Do employees have the skills needed to prepare the menu items?

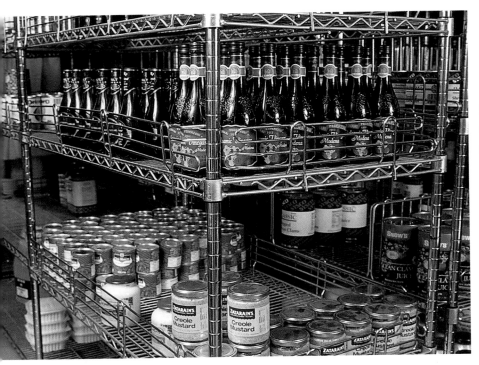

Fig. 14-5. Make sure to take available storage space into account when purchasing food products.

Consistent purchasing procedures help a foodservice operation in several ways. For example, they allow a facility to maintain an adequate supply of products at the lowest possible cost. They also ensure that quality products are purchased at the best price.

⊠ PURCHASING GOODS

Purchasing is more than buying products for a foodservice operation. It involves elements that directly affect a business's cost control. See Fig. 14-5. These elements include:

- Developing written specs for all items purchased.
- Determining the quantity of products needed.
- Assessing inventory stock levels.
- Establishing how much of each item to buy based on inventory and projected needs.

Once these functions have been performed, the purchasing agent can begin the purchasing process. Purchasing involves six steps:

1. Developing the order.
2. Obtaining price quotes from vendors.
3. Selecting the vendor and placing the order.
4. Receiving and storing the order.
5. Evaluating and following up on any errors with the order, if necessary.
6. Issuing products to the production team in the kitchen.

Types of Products Purchased

In the foodservice industry, four types of products are purchased: perishable (PEHR-ih-shuh-bul), semiperishable, nonperishable, and nonedibles. See Fig. 14-6.

- Perishable items have a relatively short shelf life. These include products such as fresh fruits, vegetables, meat, poultry, and seafood.

Fig. 14-6. Foodservice operations purchase many types of food products. How should each be stored?

Nonperishable

Semiperishable

Perishable

Nonedible

Perishable foods spoil easily. Therefore, they should be purchased in quantities that will be used quickly. Perishable items vary in price.

- **Semiperishable** products are perishable items that contain an inhibitor (in-HIH-buh-tuhr) that slows down the chemical breakdown of the food. These products include smoked fish, processed meats, and pickled vegetables.
- Nonperishable foods, such as canned goods and flour, have a long shelf life. The quality of these items is unchanged when they are stored for up to one year.
- **Nonedibles** are nonfood products. These include cleaning materials, paper goods, and smallwares.

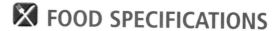 FOOD SPECIFICATIONS

A specification, or "spec," is a written, detailed description of products a foodservice operation needs to purchase. A spec acts as a quality control tool, helping a commercial kitchen correctly purchase exactly what's needed. Specs also communicate to vendors exactly what a foodservice operation expects to receive. For an example of a food spec, see Fig. 14-7.

Foodservice operations usually have a spec sheet for nonperishable products as well. The specs usually include the following information:

- Name of the supplier.
- Package size, quantity, or item count.
- Form of the item to purchase.
- Costs and quality limitations.

Food Purchasing Specification Order	
Exact Product Name:	Oranges
Packer Name:	N/A
Intended Use:	N/A
U.S. Grade:	Fancy
Product Size:	88 count
Type of Packaging:	Bulk
Package Size:	35-lbs. box
Form:	Fresh
Degree of Ripeness:	N/A
Additional Notes:	Firm and heavy in hand
Receiving Indicator:	No mold or chalk-white coating
Acceptable Substitute:	Navel for Valencia or Valencia for Navel
Point of Origin:	CA or FL
Price Per Unit:	
Comments:	

Fig. 14-7. A food spec tells vendors exactly what the foodservice operation expects to receive.

Using Yield Tests for Purchasing

In Section 1 of this chapter you learned how to calculate yield percentage, which is the ratio of the edible portion of food to the amount of food purchased. The results of yield testing greatly impact purchasing decisions. They tell how much food should be purchased in order to end up with the right serving of food on each customer's plate. Accurate yield tests help efficiently plan for a foodservice operation's purchasing needs.

Determining Purchase Quantities

There are several methods for determining exactly how much of a product to purchase. First, you must know how much of each product the chef expects to use to prepare menu items for a given sales cycle. The sales cycle is the period between deliveries.

The amount of available storage space and factors such as perishability, usage, and cost influence how much of a food product to purchase. Remember that perishable and semiperishable items are relatively expensive. Be careful when ordering larger quantities, as they may not be consumed before they spoil.

Vendor Relationships

The relationship between a foodservice operation and vendors must be based on mutual trust, honesty, and good business ethics. Establishing good vendor relationships is important to the success of a foodservice operation. An operation must be able to trust that vendors won't inflate prices or reduce the quality of the products they deliver. Vendors must provide a consistent supply of products according to a commercial kitchen's specifications. See Fig. 14-8.

Common Purchasing Practices

Foodservice operations use several methods of purchasing.

- **Open-market or competitive buying.** This is the most common method, in which a foodservice operation gets price quotes for identical items from several vendors. Open-market buying is often used for purchasing perishable foods.
- **Single-source buying.** In this method, a foodservice operation purchases most of its products from a single vendor. A discount is given when a large number of goods is purchased.

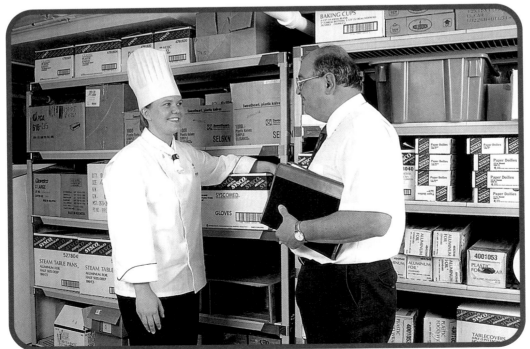

Fig. 14-8. Profitable foodservice operations have good relationships with their vendors. Describe two methods used to purchase goods from vendors.

Receiving Tools & Equipment

Make sure that the proper tools and equipment are available when goods are received. These include:

- Heavy-duty gloves with nonslip fingertips.
- Scales that are the proper size to weigh the food product received. Check that the scales are properly calibrated (KA-luh-brayt-uhd), or standardized, prior to use.
- A calculator to check total costs or add up total weights.
- Cutting devices for opening containers, packages, and boxes.
- Thermometer.

Checking the Purchase Order & Invoice

One of the most important steps in receiving food products is to make sure that the items received are the ones that appear on the purchase order. The purchase order lists the products the purchasing agent ordered. It should include the type of product ordered, the amount of product ordered and/or weight, and sometimes the unit price and total costs. In addition, confirm that the items listed on the invoice are the same ones that have been delivered. See Fig. 14-9.

Physical Inspection of Goods

Just because the products ordered are what show up on the receiving dock doesn't mean they should be automatically accepted. A critical step in the receiving process is inspection of goods.

First, visually inspect products, checking for quality, freshness, and damage. Depending on the product, you might also need to check for:

- Product tampering or mishandling.
- Improper storage practices. For example, look for evidence of thawing and refreezing, such as ice crystals or stains.
- Pest or rodent infestation.
- Dented, leaking, or misshapen cans.

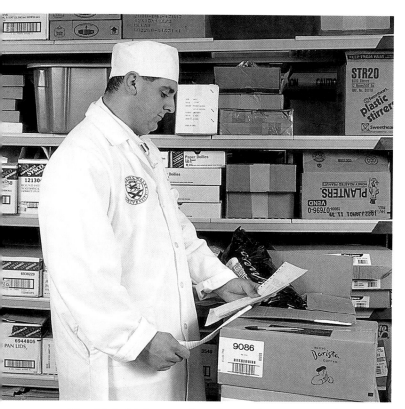

Fig. 14-9. Make sure that the products you receive always match the type, quantity, cost, and weight or volume listed on the purchase order.

❌ RECEIVING GOODS

After products are purchased, the next important function that occurs in a foodservice operation is receiving. Following certain procedures will keep foods safe during the receiving process.

Many foodservice establishments develop formal guidelines for receiving goods. Following these guidelines helps ensure that the products received are sanitary and correct as ordered.

- Package is intact and clean and has no evidence of stains or water damage.
- Package does not have a strange odor.
- Foods such as raw meat have been checked for cross-contamination.
- No large ice crystals are attached to the frozen food.
- Temperatures have been checked by placing a thermometer between or under packages. Perishables must be received at 41°F or below. Frozen foods must be received at 0°F or below.

Next, weigh the products and make sure their weights match what was ordered. Notify a manager immediately if errors are found.

INVENTORY CONTROL

Controlling inventory is an important cost control technique. Inventory should include everything that's needed to operate the business. For example, items such as food products, tableware, and equipment should all be monitored in inventory. A **physical inventory** is a list of everything that an operation has on hand at one time.

As soon as items are received, update the inventory control system. Many facilities use a perpetual inventory to track inventory. A **perpetual inventory** is a continuously updated record of what's on hand for each item. Many facilities have their perpetual inventory stored on a computer.

Computerized point-of-sale systems help monitor food inventories as food items are sold. At a glance you can see what products are in adequate supply and what products need to be replenished. See Fig. 14-10.

CULINARY TIP

TAKING INVENTORY—Inventory should be taken regularly and often. Most establishments determine their own standards, but some general guidelines to follow include:
- Perform an inventory of all food as necessary.
- Perform a costing inventory to check food cost.
- Have another person double-check to catch possible errors each time inventory is completed.

Fig. 14-10.

Perpetual Inventory Card

Name __Rice (White long-grain)__   Brand __China Rose__

Supplier __Lee Import co.__   Size __5 lb. sacks__

Date Rec'd	Quantity Rec'd	Date Issued	Quantity Issued	On-Hand	New Balance
9/26/01	10-5 lb. sacks			7-5 lb. sacks	17-5 lb. sacks
		9-28-01	1-5 lb. sack		16-5 lb. sacks

There is a delicate balance between having too much of a product in stock and too little. The amount of stock needed to cover a facility from one delivery to the next is called **parstock**. Such events as product shortages, delivery delays, and even the weather can affect the arrival of goods. With some products, such as coffee, sugar, and rice, it's important to keep a parstock on hand.

One way to decide how much goods to purchase is by using the **periodic-ordering** method. With periodic-ordering, a purchasing agent establishes how much product will be used in a given time period. The agent reviews the amount of product that is on hand, what will be needed, and how much parstock of the product is needed.

To use this method, add the parstock to the production needs, and subtract the amount on hand. This will give you the order amount.

parstock + production needs − stock on hand = order amount

Fig. 14-11. Use food products according to the First In, First Out (FIFO) system. How does FIFO help control costs?

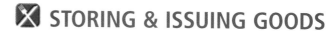

STORING & ISSUING GOODS

As soon as goods are received and the inventory control system is updated, the goods need to be properly stored. Label, date, and store perishable products appropriately. Some facilities use a bar code and computer system to keep track of inventory. With this method, all items are given a bar code sticker when they are received. This helps track the item through the inventory system.

Storeroom Controls

Goods should always be kept in their designated storage areas to help prevent spoilage, waste, and contamination. In general, the longer a food product is stored, the more its quality may deteriorate. To effectively manage food products, they must be rotated so that older items are used before newer ones.

■ **FIFO.** The system of rotating stock is called **First In, First Out**, or **FIFO**. In other words, items that are stored first should be used first. Foodservice facilities have established procedures for how to rotate food on storage shelves to ensure that the FIFO system is followed. See Fig. 14-11.

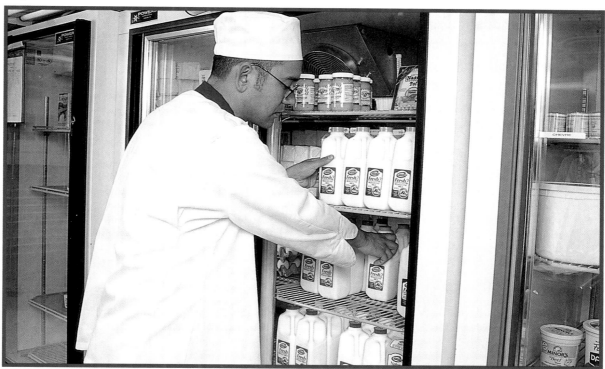

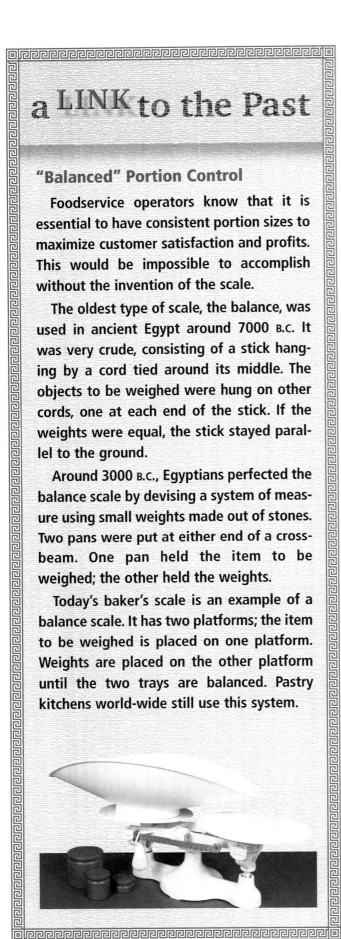
■ **Pest management.** Unfortunately, a food storage area can become a nice, cozy home for many insects and rodents. Remember that wherever there is food, there is the possibility of insects and rodents. Pests are a serious threat to food. To help make storage areas less attractive to pests:

- Keep storage areas clean, sanitary, and dry.
- Dispose of any garbage quickly.
- Keep food stored at least six inches off the floor and six inches away from walls.
- Remove as many items as possible from cardboard boxes before storing.
- Maintain appropriate temperature in storage areas.

Issuing Controls

Some facilities follow an issuing system that requires the use of a requisition. A **requisition** is an internal invoice that allows management to track the physical movement of inventory. It also helps calculate the cost of the food used each day. Complete requisition forms carefully, according to the facility's procedures. Record each item removed from storage. Accurate records are critical to a profitable foodservice operation.

For the most effective control, limit storage area access to as few people as possible. Theft is a problem for many foodservice operations. Keep the storage doors locked and only issue keys to authorized staff members.

⊠ MINIMIZING WASTE

The more food that's thrown out unused, the more profit is lost. A well-designed menu will allow chefs to use leftovers for a variety of food products. This reduces food waste.

Another way to reduce waste is to track the history of food products as they're prepared each day. Many commercial kitchens use a Daily Production Report form. The form shows how much food product was used, how much was sold, and how much was unused, or left over.

✕ CUSTOMER SERVICE

Suppose a restaurant serves the best spaghetti in town. The prices can't be beat, and the facility is always sparkling clean. So why are there empty tables? Even if a foodservice operation follows strict cost control and food management procedures, poor ser-vice can put it out of business.

Foodservice employees who interact with customers are responsible for serving orders courteously, accurately, and in a timely manner. The final bill should reflect only what the customer ordered and received. Properly trained staff who follow operational standards will make customer service and satisfaction a priority.

Foodservice facilities have found different ways to keep customers returning again and again. For example, some restaurants now offer free beverage refills, discounted or free birthday dinners, and huge desserts. The benefits of satisfied, repeat customers often outweigh the costs of offering "free" items. Creating interesting and cost-effective daily specials is another way to make dining experiences pleasurable. Most importantly, efficient, friendly service and quality food get customers to become frequent diners.

What are some other ways to analyze practices that improve customer satisfaction? Use the Internet to investigate customer service practices of various companies.

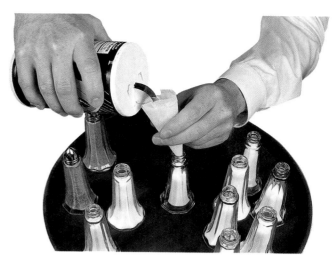

Fig. 14-12. Refill table condiments regularly.

Table Condiments & Paper Goods

Have you ever been served a plate of hot, crispy French fries and then had to wait forever for the server to return with the ketchup? If so, you probably didn't think too highly of the restaurant or its servers. Negative impressions like this don't have to happen. Keep frequently used table condiments such as ketchup and steak sauce on tables or within easy reach. Always make sure that salt and pepper shakers are full. No one wants to find a salt shaker empty. See Fig. 14-12.

Just as condiments need to be kept constantly refilled, so do paper products. For example, if straws and paper napkin dispensers are used, replenish the supply frequently.

SECTION 14-2   Knowledge Check

1. Name and define the four types of products a foodservice operation purchases. Give an example of each.

2. Describe two guidelines to follow when receiving goods.

3. What are two ways to prevent waste while foods are being stored?

MINI LAB

Identify the following as perishable, semi-perishable, nonperishable, or nonedible: canned green beans, salami, paper napkins, and fresh strawberries. Explain how to inspect each item for quality and safety. Which items should be stored first?

SECTION SUMMARIES

14-1 Portion control can help a foodservice operation cover its operating costs and improve customer satisfaction.

14-1 Portion control can be achieved through purchasing by specifications, following standardized recipes, and using portioning tools and equipment.

14-1 Unit cost, yield percentage, percentage of shrinkage, and cost per portion are methods used to calculate food costs.

14-1 Recipe costing forms are used to manage food purchase and preparation.

14-2 Purchasing involves elements that directly affect a business's cost control, such as determining the quality and quantity of products needed.

14-2 Following proper receiving procedures ensures that products received in good condition, correct as ordered, and properly handled.

14-2 Storeroom controls keep products safe to eat. Issuing controls help track products through the inventory system.

14-2 Controlled kitchen waste and excellent customer service help a foodservice operation control costs.

CHECK YOUR KNOWLEDGE

1. How does portion control affect customers?
2. List four types of tools or equipment that can be used to implement portion control.
3. Define and give two examples of food purchased in bulk.
4. Compare AP and EP.
5. How do you determine the cost per portion of a recipe?
6. What are the six steps involved in the purchasing process?
7. List information that could be included on a spec for a nonperishable good.
8. Name two ways you can check that products received have been properly handled.
9. What is a perpetual inventory?

CRITICAL-THINKING ACTIVITIES

1. Suppose a cook decided to ignore portion control guidelines. How would this impact the facility?
2. Draw conclusions about how a vendor might gain the trust of a foodservice operation.
3. What might happen to a foodservice operation if it didn't enforce issuing controls?

WORKPLACE KNOW-HOW

Decision Making. As a foodservice manager, you've decided to standardize portion control. What information, utensils, and tools will you use to aid in this process? What kind of staff training is needed?

LAB-BASED ACTIVITY:

Conducting a Yield Test

STEP ❶ In teams, conduct a yield test on one of the following foods:

- 10 carrots
- 4 apples
- 1 bunch celery
- 4 oranges
- 1 head cabbage
- 4 bananas
- 4 onions
- 1 coconut

STEP ❷ Weigh the food product on a food scale. This is called the AP weight. Record the number on a sheet of paper.

STEP ❸ Clean and trim the food product of any unusable parts.

STEP ❹ Weigh the parts, called the trim loss, and record the number.

STEP ❺ Subtract the trim loss from the AP weight. This number is the yield weight. Record it.

STEP ❻ Divide the yield weight by the AP weight. This will give you the yield percentage. Write it down.

STEP ❼ Compare your results with the results of other teams. Discuss possible reasons for results that differ from team to team.

STEP ❽ Form two teams—a vegetable team and a fruit team.

STEP ❾ As a team, combine your food products to create a menu item.

STEP ❿ Prepare the menu item and serve it to the other team.

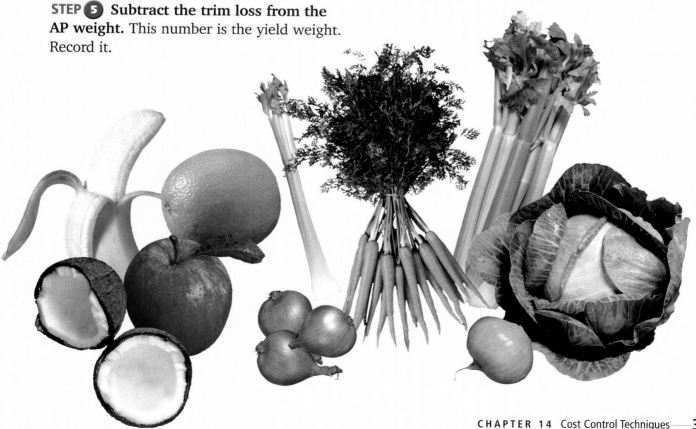

FOODSERVICE

Banquets & Catering

Careers in banquets and catering require strict attention to detail and the ability to transform a customer's wishes into an event to remember. A culinary background is helpful in understanding customer needs and communicating those needs to the kitchen staff. Being multilingual is often helpful.

Strong interpersonal and listening skills are key to successful catering operations. The ability to work diplomatically with different personalities and competing interests is crucial. Maintaining excellent customer service is a top priority in this business.

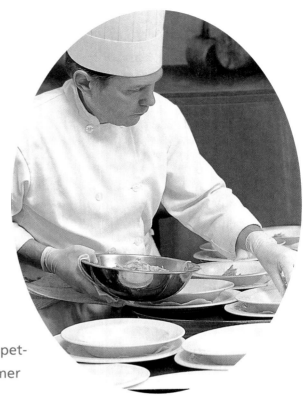

Banquet captains often host catered events and greet guests. They maintain contact with clients to make sure they are pleased before, during, and after the event. Other duties include overseeing table set-up and service.

Banquet managers are responsible for arranging and carrying out the foodservice plan. They help prepare menus, order equipment, coordinate room set-up, and schedule staff.

Chefs oversee food preparation activities and the kitchen staff for banquets and large catered events.

Catering directors ensure that all aspects of a catered event are carried out in a timely and orderly manner, making sure that all departments perform on schedule.

Catering sales managers work with customers in planning all aspects of an event, such as planning menus, table arrangements, and decorations.

Head servers coordinate all of the dining room activities for an event. They also supervise the wait staff and assist with executing banquet plans.

Menu planners work closely with the executive chef to select the menu items offered. A working knowledge of cost control, food preparation, and customer needs is essential.

Working in the Real World...

KEY SKILLS: Knowledge of foodservice industry; creativity; team player; excellent interpersonal and leadership skills; planning, organizational, and computer skills; background in business math, accounting, and inventory control.

AVERAGE SALARY: $32,000–$54,000

EDUCATION/TRAINING: Culinary degree; business, accounting, and management courses; restaurant experience a plus.

RECOMMENDED SUBJECTS: Food service, accounting, and marketing.

EMPLOYMENT OPPORTUNITIES:

- Openings will be plentiful through 2012 as the foodservice industry continues to expand.

- Advancing on this career path depends on skill, training, and work experience.

CAREER RESEARCH ACTIVITY

1. A catering director is in charge of the following events: a wedding for 600, a family reunion for 50, and a corporate awards ceremony for 250. Use print and Internet resources to research what would be involved in catering each of these events. Create a brochure advertising this caterer's skills.

2. Interview a professional caterer or banquet captain. Ask this person to describe his or her career path. Report your findings to the class.

CATERING DIRECTOR

My name is Rebecca Knopp and I am the catering director at NBC Studios in New York City. My employer is the Compass Group®—a world leader in foodservice management. I am responsible for all catering services at 30 Rockefeller Center.

I manage a catering department that delivers food to over fifty floors and handles the catering for the televison shows within the building. I also handle many high-profile events for the entertainment industry. From menu development, costing the rentals, and hiring temporary staffing, it is my responsibility to be involved in every aspect of planning to ensure successful events and satisfied clients.

Most days are very challenging. We receive many last-minute catering requests. This requires me to be extremely organized and able to make quick, effective decisions.

I attribute my success in the catering industry to the education that I received at Johnson & Wales. Persistence and dedication, along with my education, have enabled me to move up the ranks within the hotel, restaurant, and foodservice industry. I have held many positions in this field—offering me countless opportunities to grow as a professional.

Prior to my current position, I was under the impression that foodservice management was limited to hotels and restaurants. However, working here has shown me that you should always reach for the stars, or in my case feed them.

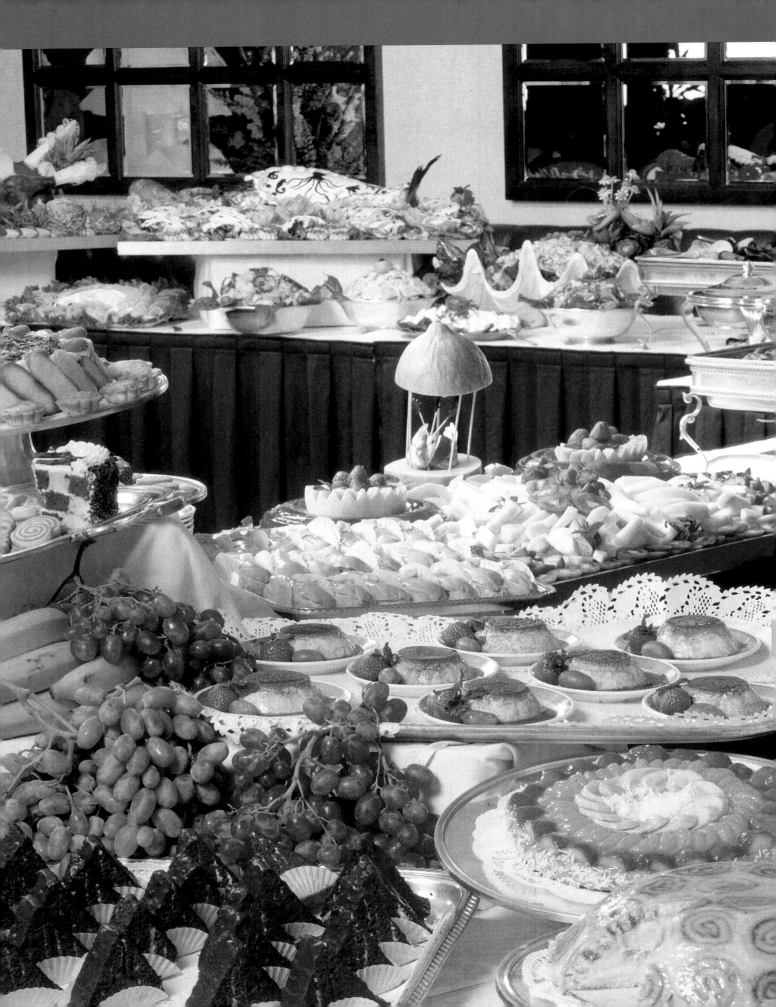

Culinary Applications

Cooking Techniques

How Cooking Alters Food

KEY TERMS

- dry cooking techniques
- evaporates
- moist cooking techniques
- combination cooking
- coagulate
- pigments
- caramelization

OBJECTIVES

After reading this section, you will be able to:

- Contrast different cooking methods.

- Explain how cooking affects a food's nutritive value, texture, color, aroma, and flavor.

SUPPOSE the restaurant where you work features chicken for dinner. There can be many different results, depending on how you choose to cook the chicken. The cooking technique used affects a food's nutritive value, texture, color, aroma, flavor, and appearance. To cook an egg, grill a steak, or stew tomatoes, you use very different cooking techniques. Although each technique involves heating the food, they all use a different process to make the heat transfer possible.

✖ COOKING TECHNIQUES

The degree of change that occurs during the cooking process depends on the length of cooking time, the temperature, and the cooking technique you use. The three cooking techniques are dry, moist, and a combination of both.

Dry Cooking

Dry cooking techniques use a metal and the radiation of hot air, oil, or fat to transfer heat. No moisture is used in this cooking process. Any moisture that comes from the food **evaporates**, or escapes, into the air. Baking is a dry cooking technique. See Fig. 15-1. You will learn more about dry cooking in Section 2 of this chapter.

Moist Cooking

Moist cooking techniques use liquid instead of oil to create the heat energy needed to cook the food. Boiling is a good example of this technique. You will learn more about moist cooking in Section 3 of this chapter.

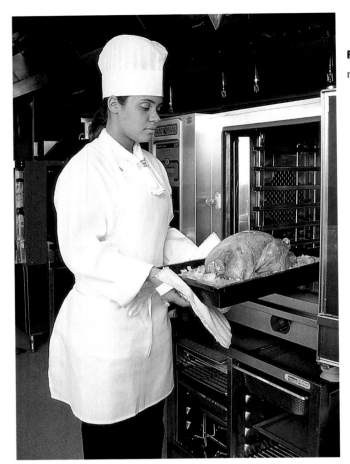

Fig. 15-1. Baking is a dry technique. What other cooking methods can you name that are dry techniques?

✖ NUTRITIVE VALUE

The length of time food is cooked and the cooking technique you use determine the nutritive value the food retains. Raw foods lose more nutritive value the longer they cook. In fact, certain cooking techniques actually speed up nutrient loss. For example, cooking green beans by boiling them extracts nutrients in two ways. Nutrients are destroyed simply because the food product is exposed to heat. Nutrients also are lost during boiling because they are diluted in the liquid used for boiling.

Combination Cooking

Combination cooking uses both moist and dry cooking techniques. This kind of cooking is a two-step process. You start cooking using one technique and finish with the other. For example, to prepare a tuna noodle casserole, you start by cooking the pasta, using the moist technique. Then you use the dry technique to bake the cooked pasta, mixed with the other ingredients. The objective of combination cooking is to build upon the food flavors. By understanding each cooking technique, you can begin to combine them in ways that create great tasting food.

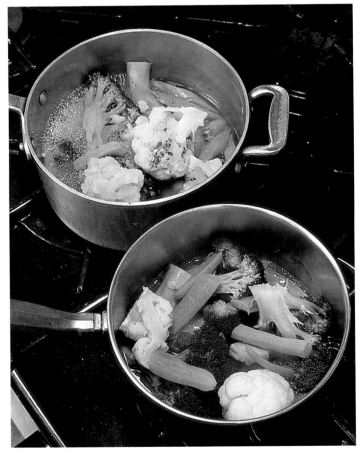

Fig. 15-2. Overcooking can make vegetables soft and mushy rather than fresh and crispy. Which pan of vegetables do you think has been overcooked? How can you tell?

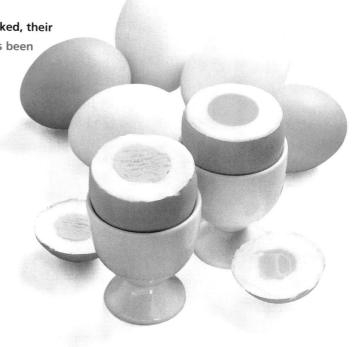

Fig. 15-3. When high-protein foods are cooked, their texture changes. Can you tell which egg has been cooked longer? How can you tell?

You might think that steaming the green beans would maintain all the nutrients. Although steaming vegetables is one of the best ways to minimize nutrient loss, exposure to heat still extracts some nutritive value from the food. However, because the vegetables are cooked by the steam, not water, all the nutrients aren't removed from the food.

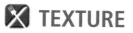 TEXTURE

If you've ever overcooked vegetables, you've seen how cooking can change the texture of food. See Fig. 15-2. During cooking, moisture is lost, food tissue breaks down, and proteins coagulate.

When heat is applied, the proteins in food **coagulate**, or change from a liquid or semiliquid state to a drier, solid state. The longer proteins are subjected to heat, the firmer and more solid they become. For example, compare the textural difference between a soft-cooked egg and a hard-cooked egg. Simmering an egg for 3–5 minutes produces a soft-cooked egg with a partly solid white and a semiliquid yolk. A hard-cooked egg with both a solid white and yolk, however, must be simmered for 8–10 minutes. See Fig. 15-3.

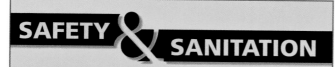

INTERNAL TEMPERATURES—Although you should be careful not to overcook food, it must be cooked to a minimum internal temperature to be considered safe. The thermometer shows the minimum safe internal cooking temperatures for various foods.

Coagulation also occurs in meat proteins as heat is applied to the meat. Meat proteins lose some moisture as the protein becomes more solid during cooking. Long, slow cooking and moderate heat combine to make meats tender, flavorful, and juicy. However, as with other protein foods, excessive heat can toughen the protein in meats because too much moisture is lost.

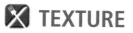 COLOR

The cooking process also affects the color of food. For example, certain ingredients commonly used when cooking vegetables, such as lemon juice and vinegar and baking soda, also can change the color of vegetables. You will learn about a cooking technique in Section 15-3 that helps maintain the color of many foods. Fruits and vegetables get their unique colors from naturally occurring pigments. **Pigments** are the matter in cells and tissue that gives them their color.

COLOR FADE

Do you know what gives green vegetables their color? Green vegetables, such as broccoli and spinach, contain two types of chlorophyll. One type of chlorophyll is a bright bluish-green color. The other type is a yellowish-green color. Green vegetables have about four times more of the blue-green type than the yellow-green type.

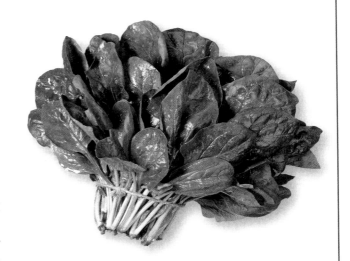

To maintain the color of a green vegetable, DON'T overcook it. When you cook green vegetables, the heat damages the vegetable's cells. This allows the acids within the once-living cells of the vegetable to be released. Magnesium in the chlorophyll is quickly replaced by hydrogen. Once exposed to this acid, the chlorophyll changes to a brownish-yellow color.

APPLY IT!

Complete the following experiment to determine which style of cooking provides a greener vegetable. You will need 4 broccoli stalks, a pot with a lid, and a second pot without a lid.

Bring 3 cups of water to a boil in each uncovered pot. Separate the florets, or flowers, of the broccoli. Place half of the broccoli in one pot and cover it with the lid. Place the rest of the broccoli in the other pot without a lid. Cook both pots of broccoli for 7 minutes. After 7 minutes, drain each pot and place the broccoli in two separate bowls.

Examine each bowl. Describe the color and the texture of the broccoli in each bowl.

1. Which dish has the greener broccoli?

2. Explain why you think one method of cooking had a greater impact on the color change than the other.

Pigmentation differs from one food product to another and varies depending on the cooking process used. Remember that the longer fruits and vegetables are cooked, the more their color will change.

Likewise, as meat cooks for extended periods of time, moisture is extracted and the meat loses its deep red color. These color changes happen at various temperatures. As the internal temperature of meat reaches between 140°F and 160°F, the redness decreases significantly. The same thing happens when the meat reaches an internal temperature between 168°F and 176°F. That's why the inside of a rare steak is red, a medium-rare steak is pink, and a well-done steak is brownish gray. Remember, using a thermometer is the only safe way to determine if meat is done.

✖ AROMA

The aroma created from cooking various foods can be as appealing as the flavor and presentation of the final product. Cooking techniques that use fat as an ingredient or as a way to transfer heat create an appealing aroma. **Caramelization** (KAR-ah-muh-leh-ZAY-shuhn), or the process of cooking sugar to high temperatures, is what creates these pleasing smells. As the sugar in the food turns brown a rich, flavorful aroma is produced. Caramelization can also affect the color and flavor of food. When pots and pans are washed, the caramelization is removed.

✖ FLAVOR

The cooking process also affects the flavor of food. If you've ever eaten overcooked meat or vegetables, you know that overcooking can ruin the flavor. However, applying the correct cooking technique can actually enhance the flavor.

For example, grilling meats over charcoal or woods such as hickory and mesquite gives them an appealing smoky flavor. Foods cooked with dry-heat methods taste rich because of the caramelization process. Moist cooking techniques help bring out a food's natural flavor.

Another way to enhance the flavor of food is to add seasonings and flavorings before, during, or after the cooking process. These seasonings and flavorings—which will be discussed in more detail in Chapter 16—include herbs, spices, and condiments. Knowing which seasoning to add, and when to add it, is an important part of your culinary training.

SECTION 15-1   Knowledge Check

1. Describe the key differences between the dry, moist, and combination cooking techniques.

2. How can you minimize nutrient loss when cooking foods?

3. Explain why the texture of foods can toughen after prolonged exposure to heat.

MINI LAB

Imagine that you are asked to prepare a colorful meal that will be photographed for a food magazine. Describe the meat, vegetable, and starch you'll choose and the cooking techniques that could be used to cook these foods.

Dry Cooking Techniques

KEY TERMS

- carryover cooking
- seared
- open-spit roast
- sautéing
- stir-frying
- dredging
- breading
- batter
- pan-fry
- deep-fried
- recovery time
- broiling

OBJECTIVES

After reading this section, you will be able to:

- Demonstrate dry cooking techniques.
- Demonstrate different methods of frying foods.

DRY cooking techniques include baking, roasting, sautéing, stir-frying, pan-frying, deep-frying, grilling, and broiling. Don't let the word "dry" fool you. It is called the dry cooking technique because no moisture is used in the cooking process. Any moisture that comes from the food evaporates into the air. Some dry cooking techniques use oil and fat to transfer heat. Others use metal and radiation of hot air to create the necessary heat. This section will introduce you to dry cooking techniques.

⊠ BAKING

Baking is a very popular dry cooking technique. Bread and chicken are foods that are commonly baked. Fish, vegetables, fruits, and pastry items can be prepared using this method.

To bake, you use dry heat in a closed environment, usually an oven. No fat or liquid is used. Any moisture that is created in the form of steam evaporates into the air because the food is cooked uncovered.

A large food product will continue to cook for 5–15 minutes after you remove it from the oven. This is called **carryover cooking**, or the cooking that takes place after you remove something from the heat source, which happens because the outside of the food is hotter than the inside of the food. This effect continues until the heat throughout the food becomes stable. It can add 5°F–15°F to the final temperature. There is no way to stop the carryover cooking that occurs in dry heat cooking. Just keep this in mind when you take something out of the oven. See Fig. 15-4.

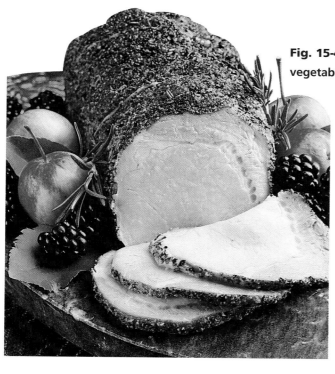

Fig. 15-4. Roasting adds a rich flavor to meats and vegetables. What other foods could be roasted?

and then turn the meat until all surfaces are browned. Place the pan in a hot oven to finish the cooking process.

When searing in the oven, place the food, such as a roast, in a pan in a 450°F–475°F oven. Cook for about 15–20 minutes, or until the outside begins to turn golden brown. Then reduce the heat to 325°F–350°F to finish the cooking process. Some meats should be basted during the cooking process to avoid dryness. Basting involves moistening foods with melted fats, pan drippings, or another liquid during the cooking time.

ROASTING

Like baking, roasting also uses dry heat in a closed environment. Foods commonly roasted include meat and poultry. These foods are placed on top of a rack that is inside a pan. This allows air to circulate all the way around the food. In general, roasting involves longer cooking times than baking. Carryover cooking also applies to roasting. Remove roasted foods from the oven just before they reach the desired doneness. Remember to use a thermometer to check the internal temperature. The remaining heat will complete the cooking process.

Roasting also differs from baking in that sometimes the outside of the food product is **seared**, or quickly browned, at the start of the cooking process. Searing locks in a food's juices, caramelizes flavors, adds color, and makes the food more tender. It also builds "body" in juice drippings that can be used to make sauces. Searing can be done two different ways, in a pan on the rangetop or in the oven.

When searing on the rangetop, place the food, such as a pork roast, in a pan that contains a small amount of heated oil. Brown the meat on one side

Open-Spit Roasting

Many cooks prefer to roast food over an open fire. This is called open-spit roasting. To **open-spit roast**, place the food, usually meat such as pork, on a metal rod or a long skewer, and slowly turn it over the heat source. Place a drip pan under the food to catch its juices. Check the internal temperature with a thermometer before removing food from the oven. Remember that the food will continue to cook 5–15 minutes after you remove it from the heat source.

SAUTÉING & STIR-FRYING

Sautéing (saw-TAY-ing) is a quick, dry cooking technique that uses a small amount of fat or oil in a shallow pan. Sautéing is generally used with delicate foods that cook relatively quickly. These foods include fish fillets, scallops, tender cuts of meat, vegetables, and fruit. Most sautéed foods are served with a sauce. See Fig. 15-5.

During sautéing, you'll want to seal the surface of the food. To do this, preheat a pan on high heat, then add fat or oil. When the fat or oil is heated and nearly smoking, add the food. Do not over-

a LINK to the Past

Cooking Through Time

Cave drawings dating back to the Stone Age show that prehistoric life centered around the gathering and preparation of food. When prehistoric people were hungry for cooked meat, they had no choice but to broil or roast their food on small open fires. As civilization evolved, people used clay pots to bake food on top of hot ashes.

During the Middle Ages, the cauldron was the main cooking pot in the kitchen. It was hung from a metal arm over hot coals. Stews or soups would cook in the pot while meat was broiled or roasted on a spit.

In the 17th- and 18th-century, people cooked their food over fire in kettles or on spits. Built-in ovens could be found on many fireplaces, allowing people to roast meat and bake bread.

The 19th and 20th centuries brought wood, coal, gas, and, finally, electric stoves. However, some of the practices that were used thousands of years ago—such as grilling meat on an open fire—are still in use today.

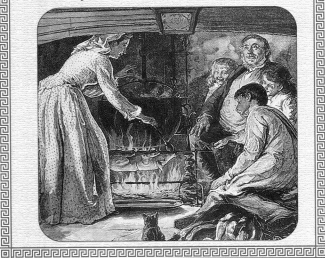

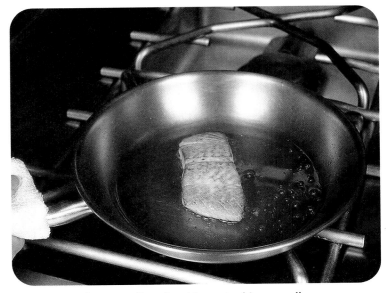

Fig. 15-5. When sautéing, food is cooked in a small amount of fat or oil. What types of food can be sautéed?

crowd the pan. Doing so will lower the temperature and cause the food to simmer. After the food is sealed, lower the temperature so the food cooks evenly. Foods may need to be turned occasionally.

A dry cooking technique similar to sautéing, called **stir-frying**, uses a wok, a large pan with sloping sides. Stir-fried foods require less cooking time than sautéed foods. Vegetables and tender, boneless meats are often stir-fried. To stir-fry, place a wok over high heat, add a small amount of fat, and then add small pieces of food. Because of the wok's size and shape, it's important to constantly stir the food as it cooks.

☒ FRYING

It's hard for most people to resist crispy foods, such as fried chicken and French fries. Foods like these are prepared using a dry-heat cooking technique called frying, in which foods are cooked in hot fat or oil.

During frying, the outside of the food becomes sealed when it comes in contact with the hot oil. The natural moisture in the food turns to steam, which bubbles up to the surface.

Foods can be dredged, breaded, or battered before frying.

- **Dredging.** One way to prepare foods for frying is to dredge them. **Dredging** means to coat foods with flour or finely ground crumbs.
- **Breading.** Another way to add texture and flavor to fried foods is to add a **breading**, or coating made of eggs and crumbs. Fig. 15-6 shows the breading process.
- **Batter.** Another tasty way to prepare fried foods is to batter them before frying to add texture and flavor. **Batter** is a semiliquid mixture that contains ingredients such as flour, milk, eggs, and seasonings. Dip the food into the batter right before frying.

Tips to Follow After Frying

After food has been fried, remove it from the oil and drain it well on an absorbent surface such as paper towels. You can also add seasoning at this time. Fried foods are best served and eaten immediately. If you can't serve the food right away, it can be stored under a heat lamp.

✕ PAN-FRYING

One way to fry food is pan-frying. To **pan-fry**, heat a moderate amount of fat in a pan before adding food. Use enough fat to cover about one-half to three-quarters of the food. The fat should not be so hot that it smokes. Instead, it should be hot enough to sizzle when food is added, usually 350°F–375°F. Because it's not completely covered, you'll need to turn the food after one side is done to allow for even cooking. Foods that are often pan-fried include chicken, potatoes, fish, and pork chops.

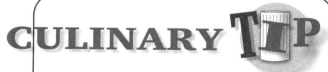

CULINARY TIP

PAN-FRYING—Chill cuts of meat before pan-frying so they will brown before the inside finishes cooking.

Fig. 15-6.

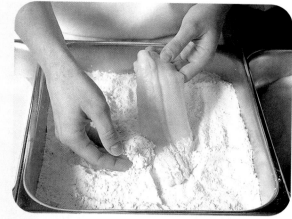

1. Dredge the food product in seasoned, dry flour by dipping it into the flour and coating it evenly on all surfaces. Shake off any excess flour.

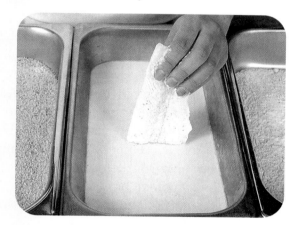

2. Immediately dip the food into an egg wash—a mixture of beaten eggs and a liquid such as milk or water—or other liquid. Coat the food completely. Shake off any excess.

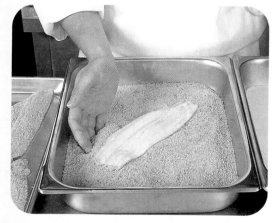

3. Quickly place the food into a container of dry crumbs and coat evenly. Crumbs can be made from bread, ground nuts, cereal, crackers, or shredded coconut.

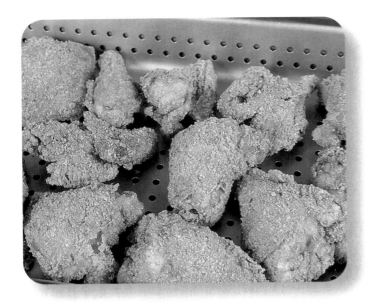

Fig. 15-7. Storing fried foods in a single layer helps keep them crispy.

GRILLING

Many commercial kitchens use gas, electric, charcoal, or wood-fired grills. Grilling is often used for tender foods that cook relatively quickly. To grill foods properly, you must first preheat the grill. Depending on the type of food you wish to grill, brush the food lightly with oil, and then place it on the grill. Don't move the food after you place it initially. This will help create the distinctive crosshatch markings of a grilled food product.

■ **Using a griddle.** Grilling can also be done on a griddle. A griddle is a flat, solid plate of metal with a gas or electric heat source. Griddles are commonly used to make sandwiches such as grilled cheese and breakfast items such as pancakes and eggs. Depending on the type of food being cooked, you may want to add a little fat to the griddle to keep the food from sticking. The temperature of a griddle is about 350°F. See Fig. 15-8.

DEEP-FRYING

Another way to fry foods is deep-frying. **Deep-fried** foods are cooked completely submerged in heated fat or oil at temperatures between 350°F and 375°F. Fried foods must be cooked until they are done on the inside. Temperature and timing on deep-fat fryers help you determine doneness. Fried foods will be a golden brown. Remove them and briefly hold them so the excess fat can drip off. See Fig. 15-7.

The most popular types of deep-fried foods are potatoes, onions, fish, and poultry. Many foodservice operations choose to purchase foods that are already breaded and ready to be deep-fried. In the foodservice industry, commercial fryers with fry baskets are commonly used. Commercial fryers have several advantages:

• There is less **recovery time**, or the time it takes for the fat or oil to return to the preset temperature after food has been submerged.

• The life of the fat or oil is maximized if correct temperatures are used.

Fig. 15-8. Cooking on a griddle is a very popular way to prepare breakfast foods. Name several other foods that can be cooked on a griddle.

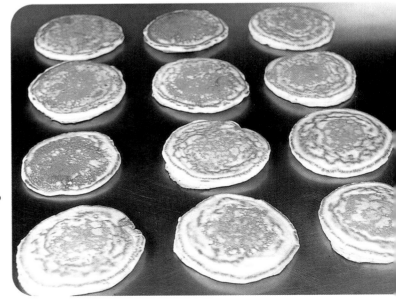

Food can also be grilled on a grooved griddle. This type of griddle has raised ridges. Although grooved griddles are similar in design to grills, they don't generate as much smoke as a grill. That's why food cooked on a griddle won't have the same smoky flavor as food cooked on a grill.

BROILING

Broiling means to cook food directly under a primary heat source. When you're broiling, the temperature is controlled by how close the food is to the heat source. Thicker foods should be placed farther from the heat source, and thinner foods should be placed closer to the heat source. This ensures that the inside and outside of the food will cook at the same rate.

Foods that are commonly broiled include meats and poultry. Unlike a grill, broilers are heated only by gas or electricity, so additional flavors cannot be added to the food by burning charcoal or wood. See Fig. 15-9.

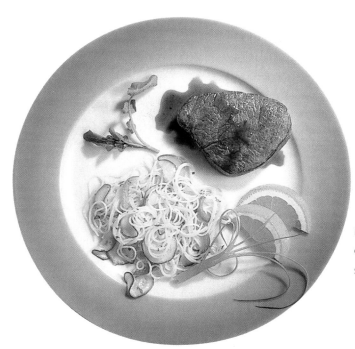

Fig. 15-9. Broiled foods are popular with many customers. Why do you think broiled foods are so appealing?

SECTION 15-2   Knowledge Check

1. Contrast roasting, baking, grilling, and broiling.
2. How do stir-frying and sautéing differ?
3. Describe different methods of frying.

MINI LAB

In teams, prepare a meal that includes three foods that are prepared with different dry cooking techniques. Have another team evaluate your meal. Explain how each item was prepared.

Moist Cooking Techniques

KEY TERMS

- boiling
- convection
- blanching
- parboiling
- simmering
- poaching
- steaming
- braising
- deglaze
- stewing

OBJECTIVES

After reading this section, you will be able to:

- Demonstrate moist cooking techniques.
- Demonstrate braising and stewing.

THERE'S more than one way to cook eggs. Some people like them hard-cooked, while others prefer their eggs lightly poached. Boiling and poaching are both moist cooking techniques. Cooking food using a moist technique involves heating food in a liquid other than oil. Moist cooking techniques include boiling, blanching, parboiling, simmering, poaching, and steaming. Sometimes, a moist cooking technique is applied to foods that have already been partially cooked using a dry cooking technique. This section will introduce you to moist and combination cooking techniques.

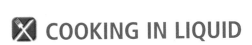

✖ COOKING IN LIQUID

When cooking foods in water or other liquids, foods are completely submerged. Boiling, simmering, and poaching involve cooking in liquid.

Boiling

Boiling is a moist cooking technique in which you bring a liquid, such as water or stock, to the boiling point and keep it at that temperature while the food cooks. The boiling point of water is 212°F at sea level. When liquid reaches the boiling point, food can be added and cooked. See Fig. 15-10.

When liquid boils, a process called convection occurs. During **convection**, the liquid closest to the bottom of the pan is heated and rises to the top, while the cooler liquid descends to the bottom of the pan. This sets off a circular motion in the pan that keeps the food in constant motion and keeps it from sticking to the pan.

Boiling cooks foods quickly. However, it can be harmful to some food. The rapid circular motion of the liquid doesn't harm pasta, but it can break apart a tender piece of fish. Because of this, very few food items are cooked completely by boiling.

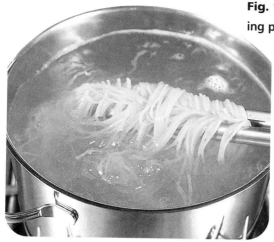

Fig. 15-10. Boiling is an effective method for cooking pasta since pasta holds its shape well as it cooks.

Blanching

Using the boiling method to partially cook food is also known as **blanching**. It is a quick way to change the flavor and keep the color in foods. Fig. 15-11 shows blanching as a two-step process:

1. Completely submerge the food in a boiling liquid and blanch, or briefly cook, it.

2. Then remove the blanched food from the liquid. If you want to make sure the food stops cooking as soon as you remove it from the liquid, plunge the food into ice water. This is called "shocking." It will completely stop the cooking process.

Remember that a blanched food item is only partially cooked, so a second stage of cooking is needed to complete the cooking process. For example, you might first blanch green beans and then sauté them in butter and herbs.

Blanching has many uses. In addition to simplifying the peeling process, blanching is sometimes used to:

- Precook foods before they are frozen.
- Soften herbs.
- Lock in the color of foods.
- Help preserve a food's nutrients.
- Remove excess salt from ham or pork.
- Remove blood from meats.
- Remove strong flavors from meats.

Fig. 15-11. Blanching is usually a two-step process. One way to cool the food immediately after boiling it is to plunge it into ice water. **What is the next step in the blanching process?**

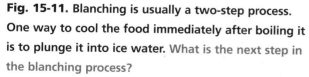

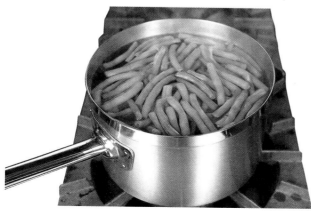

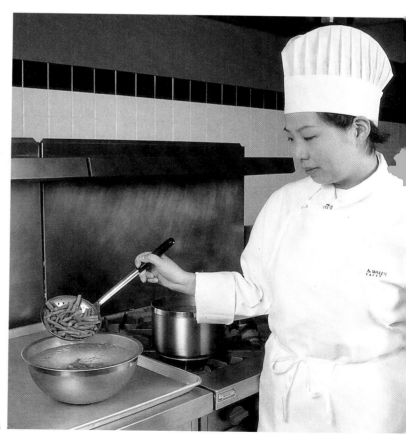

CULINARY TIP

PEELING TOMATOES—To make it easier to peel a fresh tomato, you can lightly blanch it. This process involves immediately plunging the tomato into ice water after blanching so that it doesn't continue to cook.

Parboiling

Parboiling is a moist cooking technique that is similar to blanching in that foods are put into boiling water and partially cooked. However, the cooking time for parboiling foods is longer than for blanching. Recipes that include parboiling will give you the exact timing for a particular food item. For example, ribs are often parboiled before they are grilled. This tenderizes the meat and reduces grilling time.

Simmering

Like boiling, **simmering** involves cooking food in liquid. However, when you simmer food, it cooks slowly and steadily in a slightly cooler liquid that's heated from 185°F–200°F. The bubbles in the liquid rise slowly to the surface of the liquid but do not break the surface.

Because of the lower temperature, not as much convection action occurs, so the cooking is a much gentler process. When simmering, foods such as yellow squash and zucchini should be fully submerged in the liquid. See Fig. 15-12.

The advantages of simmering include:

- Less shrinkage of the food.
- Less evaporation and better control over evaporation.
- Less breakup of fragile food, such as fish.

Simmering is also used to reduce, or decrease the volume of, a liquid. For example, you might want to simmer spaghetti sauce to make it thicker.

Poaching

Poaching is an even gentler method of moist cooking than simmering. To poach means to cook food in a flavorful liquid between 150°F and 185°F. Generally, tender or delicate foods such as fish and eggs are poached in just enough liquid to cover the food. You can poach food on the rangetop or in the oven. Sometimes the poaching liquid is used later to make a sauce that accompanies the food item when it's served.

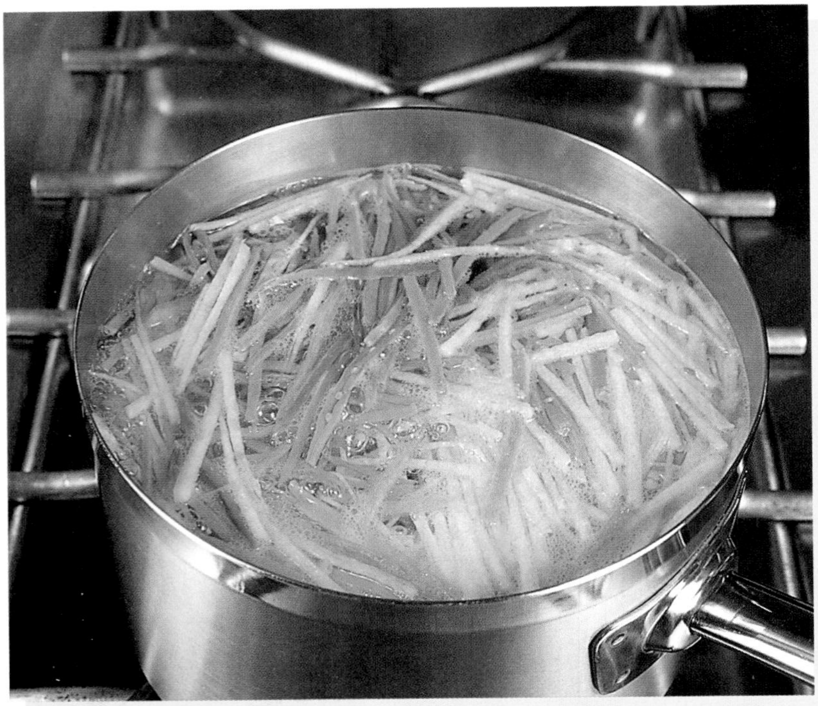

Fig. 15-12. Simmering cooks foods slowly. What are some of the advantages of simmering versus boiling?

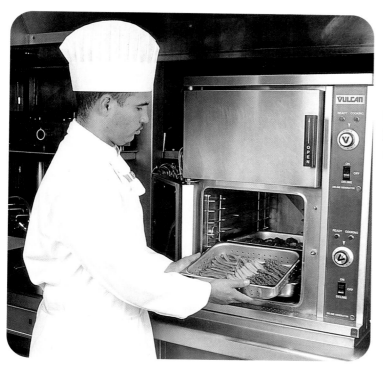

Fig. 15-13. These vegetables are being steamed just before serving. What are some advantages of steaming foods?

higher, cooking the food faster. A pressure steamer holds steam under pressure. As the pressure increases, so does the temperature. For example, if you're cooking asparagus at 10 pounds of pressure (10 psi) at 240°F, and you increase the pressure to 15 psi, the temperature will rise to 250°F. Steamers cook foods, such as vegetables, without dissolving the nutrients.

STEAMING

Steamed vegetables are both tasty and nutritious. **Steaming** involves cooking vegetables or other foods in a closed environment filled with steam, such as in a pot with a tight-fitting lid. Steam is created inside the pot when water reaches the boiling point and it turns into vapor and disperses as tiny drops in the air. Although the food never touches the liquid, the temperature inside the closed environment rises high enough to cook the food. Steaming is generally faster than other moist cooking techniques. See Fig. 15-13.

If pressure is added during the steaming process, the temperature inside the pot rises even

COMBINATION COOKING

Sometimes great things happen by combining the best of two techniques. Such is the case with combination cooking. As the term suggests, combination cooking combines two techniques you've already learned: moist and dry. Two major combination techniques are braising and stewing. Braising and stewing involve both a dry and a moist cooking process. The first step for both cooking methods is usually to brown the food using dry heat. Then the food is completely cooked by simmering the food in a liquid.

Cooking food using a combination technique is especially useful for tough, but flavorful, cuts of meat. The combination cooking process tenderizes the meat. It's also an excellent way to prepare large pieces of less tender meat.

Braising

Braising is a long, slow cooking process that can produce very flavorful results. It can make tough cuts of meat more tender. Follow the steps in Fig. 15-14 to properly braise a food product.

SAFETY & SANITATION

DON'T GET BURNED BY STEAM—Take special care when removing the lids from pots or containers that may have steam trapped inside. Always tip the lid open by lifting it away from your hand and body. Steam is at least 212°F and can cause severe burns.

Fig. 15-14. The Braising Process

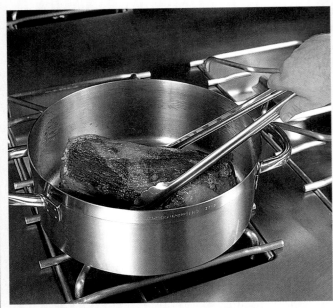

1. Begin by searing the food in a frying or roasting pan. When using meats, mirepoix is usually added to the pan when the meat is seared.

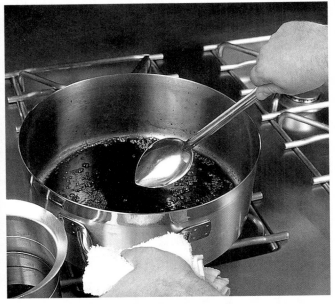

2. Remove the food from the pan and deglaze the pan. To **deglaze**, remove any leftover scraps of food from the pan; then add a small amount of hot stock or water and cook it on top of the range.

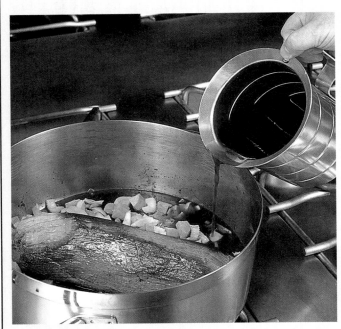

3. Return the seared food to the deglazed pan and add liquid, such as stock or sauce. Add enough liquid to cover no more than two-thirds of the food.

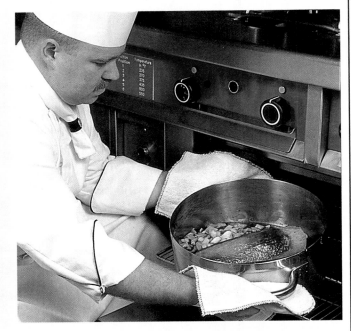

4. Place the pan in a 350°F oven, and cook the food slowly until it is fork tender. Turn the food every 20-30 minutes. Often, braised items are covered while cooking. Braising can also be done on the rangetop over low heat.

During the long cooking process, braising produces a very flavorful liquid. The flavors extracted from the food become highly concentrated. Imagine braising a piece of meat, such as a pork loin. The juices from the pork are slowly pulled away from the meat and mixed with the liquid in which the pork is being braised. The liquid, then, takes on the highly concentrated flavor of the meat's juices as it cooks.

Braised foods are always served with the cooking liquid. You'll want to strain, thicken, and add salt, pepper, or other spices to the liquid before serving. See Fig. 15-15.

Stewing

Stewing is another combination cooking technique. However, stewed foods are completely covered with liquid during cooking. Cooking time for stewing is generally shorter than for braising. That is because the main food item in stew is cut into smaller pieces before cooking. Follow these steps to stew foods:

1. First, sear the food product in a pan over high heat. Tender cuts of meat should not be stewed or they will become tough.

2. Completely cover the food with liquid.

3. Bring the stew to a simmer and cook until tender.

4. Add vegetables, if desired, partway through simmering the main food item. This will ensure that the vegetables will not be overcooked when the main food item in the stew is fully cooked.

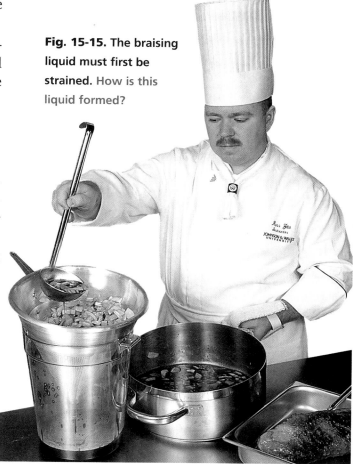

Fig. 15-15. The braising liquid must first be strained. How is this liquid formed?

SECTION 15-3 Knowledge Check

1. Give two reasons why you might want to simmer instead of boil a food product.

2. Explain why you would blanch foods.

3. Contrast braising and stewing.

MINI LAB

In teams, prepare a meal that includes three foods that are prepared with different moist cooking techniques. Have another team evaluate your meal. Explain how each item was prepared.

SECTION SUMMARIES

15-1 There are three different cooking techniques: dry, moist, and combination cooking techniques.

15-1 The cooking technique, the temperature, and the cooking time affect a food's nutritive value, texture, color, aroma, and flavor.

15-2 Baking, roasting, sautéing, stir-frying, pan-frying, deep-frying, grilling, and broiling are all dry cooking techniques.

15-2 Although no moisture is used in dry cooking techniques, these methods can improve the flavor and texture of foods.

15-2 There are two ways to fry foods: pan-frying and deep-frying.

15-3 Boiling, simmering, poaching, and steaming are moist cooking techniques.

15-3 To blanch a food, you partially cook it in boiling liquid.

15-3 Braising and stewing are combination cooking techniques.

15-3 Combination cooking techniques enhance the flavor of food by producing a flavorful liquid during the long cooking process.

CHECK YOUR KNOWLEDGE

1. How is heat transferred in dry cooking techniques?
2. How does cooking affect a food's nutrient loss?
3. What causes the pleasing aroma that occurs during cooking?
4. Why might you remove a roast from the oven a few minutes before it's done cooking?
5. Contrast pan-frying and deep-frying.
6. Explain the steaming process.
7. What are three uses of blanching?
8. What's the first step in braising and stewing?
9. Explain how the flavor of meat is extracted during braising.

CRITICAL-THINKING ACTIVITIES

1. Your server brings you a plate with a tough, grayish-brown piece of meat and limp, colorless vegetables. Explain what went wrong during cooking and why.
2. The pork loin roast you're planning to serve is extra lean. You're worried that it will be dry and tasteless. How will you prepare it? Why?

WORKPLACE KNOW-HOW

Communication. Imagine that you're the executive chef at a restaurant that's up for review by the local food critic. You want tonight's food to be perfect in flavor, nutritive value, texture, color, and aroma. What information should you clearly communicate to your staff about how cooking affects these important aspects?

LAB-BASED ACTIVITY:

Cooking a Meal

STEP 1 Working in teams, you will be preparing a three-course meal that involves dry, moist, and combination cooking techniques.

STEP 2 Your team will need to determine:
- What five menu items you will prepare.
- Which cooking technique you will use for each food item.
- The list of food ingredients needed to prepare all of the menu items.
- A work flow for team members to follow when preparing items.
- A preparation time schedule for your team.

STEP 3 Consider the following items when choosing the cooking techniques you will use:
- Nutritive value.
- Texture.
- Color.
- Aroma.
- Flavor.
- Appearance.
- Cooking time.

STEP 4 On your own paper, create a rating chart like the one below to evaluate your meal.

STEP 5 As a team, use the rating scale below to evaluate food items for texture, color, aroma, flavor, and appearance.
- How does each menu item rate?
- Which technique produced the best food product?

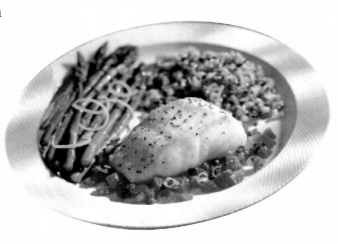

Cooking Techniques Rating Scale

QUALITY	Item A	Item B	Item C	Item D	Item E
Texture					
Color					
Aroma					
Flavor					
Appearance					
Total Score					

(1 = Poor; 2 = Fair; 3 = Good; 4 = Great)

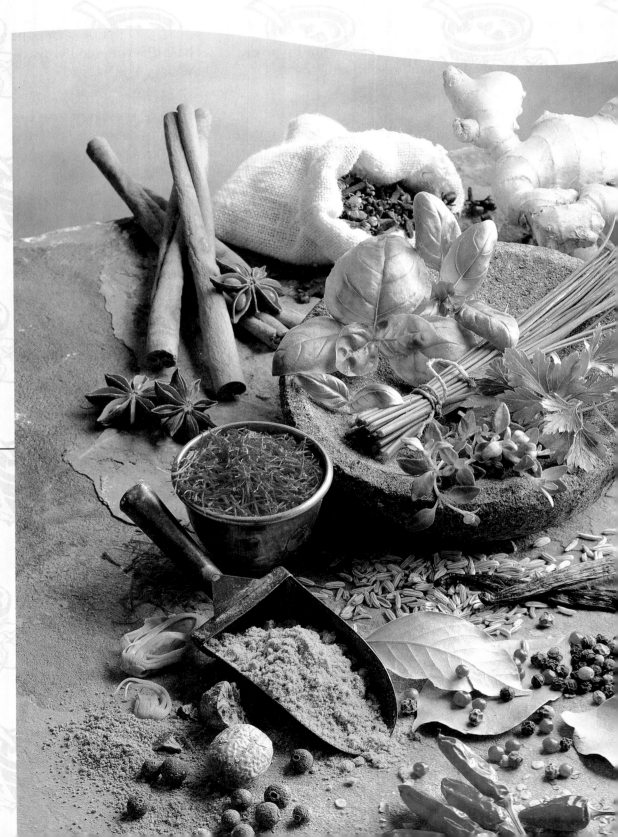

Seasonings & Flavorings

Enhancing Food

OBJECTIVES

After reading this section, you will be able to:

- Contrast seasonings and flavorings.
- Identify seven common ingredients used to enhance flavor.
- Explain when to add seasonings and flavorings to food.
- Contrast the characteristics of herbs versus spices.

IMAGINE eating food without any flavor, or several foods that all have the same flavor. This doesn't sound very appetizing, does it? Fortunately, foods have natural flavoring, but sometimes these flavors need to be strengthened. Seasonings and flavorings play a role in this. Enhancing the natural flavor of foods is part of the art of cooking. You need to understand how the flavor of food is enhanced in order to work in food production. Using seasonings and flavorings is a skill that develops over time. Tasting foods throughout the cooking process will help you develop this skill.

❌ SEASONINGS & FLAVORINGS

Both seasonings and flavorings improve or strengthen natural flavor. **Seasonings** are ingredients that enhance food without changing the natural flavor. If used correctly, the individual flavor of a seasoning cannot be detected.

Some seasonings are called flavor enhancers. **Flavor enhancers** increase the way you perceive the food's flavor without changing the actual flavor. They do not add flavor to a dish. Flavor enhancers achieve this by affecting your taste buds. Monosodium glutamate (mon-uh-SOH-dee-um GLOO-tuh-mayt), or MSG, is an example of a flavor enhancer.

Flavorings, on the other hand, are ingredients that actually change the natural flavor of the foods they are added to. Flavorings have their own distinct flavors. **Extracts**, or concentrated flavors, such as lemon and vanilla, are flavorings.

A wide variety of ingredients can be used as seasonings and flavorings. Salt and pepper are two of the most common. Others include onion, lemon, and MSG. A more detailed description of these ingredients follows.

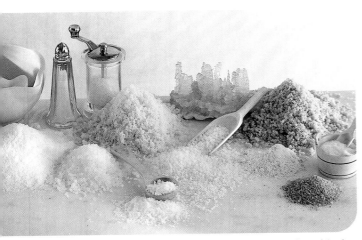

Fig. 16-1. Salt comes in many varieties. Name four kinds of salt most often used in food service.

Salt

Salt is the most commonly used seasoning today. It can be added to most foods to heighten flavor. Salt has a more distinctive taste on cooler foods than on hot foods.

Table salt is the most common type of salt used in food preparation. Rock salt usually is used as a bed during baking for foods such as clams, oysters, and potatoes. Sea salt is preferred by some chefs because it has a strong, distinctive flavor. Kosher salt is coarse and free of iodine or other additives. See Fig. 16-1.

The amount of salt added to food depends on the food being cooked. It also depends on the preference of the person who will be eating the food. Use care when adding salt. Taste food before adding more salt. You can always add more salt, but you can't remove it.

Pepper

Pepper is the most widely used spice in the world. **Spices** are flavorings that blend with the natural flavor of foods. Pepper is usually used in its ground form rather than whole pepper. Ground pepper brings out the flavor of foods and may be hard to see on some foods. Whole or cracked pepper, however, is in a large enough form to be detected in the flavor of the food when it is added. There is a wide variety of peppers that can be used. See Fig. 16-2.

■ **Black pepper.** Black pepper comes from the dried, unripe berries of the pepper plant. It is slightly hot, but not bitter. Black pepper stimulates juices in the lining of your stomach. It helps with digestion.

■ **White pepper.** White pepper comes from the kernel of ripe berries. It is an all-around seasoning that blends easily with most food, yet maintains a distinctive flavor. White pepper is a little hotter than black pepper.

■ **Green peppercorns.** Green peppercorns come from unripened berries. They are preserved in brine until they darken. Green peppercorns are expensive. They are used only in special recipes, such as grilled veal tenderloin with a delicate brown sauce.

■ **Red pepper.** Red pepper is not like black or white pepper. It is derived from the capsicum plant and is related more closely to the bell pepper family. It is used to add flavor to food, such as soups and sauces, without altering the food's natural flavor. Hot red pepper, such as cayenne, can be difficult to use because of its intense heat. It is easy to add too much to food. Paprika (pah-PREE-kuh) is a fine powder made from grinding sweet red pepper pods. Paprika can be sweet, mild, medium-hot, or hot.

Fig. 16-2. Shown here are various types of pepper. Why is pepper the most commonly used spice in the world?

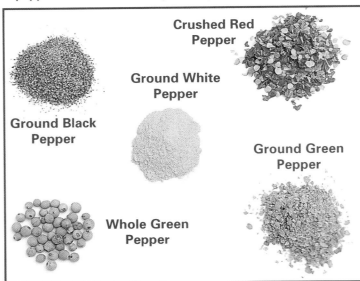

■ **Hot pepper.** Hot peppers are commonly referred to as chiles. They vary in their degree of hotness, color, and flavor. Hot pepper is often added to Indian and Asian foods.

Onion

Onions are a flavoring that can be added to just about any food dish. The onion family also includes scallions, leeks, shallots, chives, and garlic. See Fig. 16-3. All of these flavorings have a strong aroma.

When using foods from the onion family, keep in mind that, unlike herbs, fresh onions have a stronger flavor than dried ones. Depending on the form you are using, you may need to adjust the amount added to the food.

Lemon

The **zest**, or rind, of the lemon is another type of flavoring. It is added to dishes such as fish, meats, poultry sauces, vegetables, and desserts.

When cooking with lemon, use only the juice or the zest. Do not use the **pith** or white membrane, which is bitter. The juice and the zest contain the best flavor.

Fig. 16-3. The foods shown here belong to the onion family. How are they used to flavor different foods?

Monosodium Glutamate

Monosodium glutamate, or MSG as it is commonly known, is a flavor enhancer. MSG comes from seaweed. It intensifies the natural flavor of most of the foods it is added to. For example, MSG is often added to vegetables, poultry, and fish to bring out more flavor. However, MSG has no effect on the flavor of milk products or fruits.

CULINARY TIP

MSG ALLERGIES—Recent studies have shown that MSG is not dangerous to people unless they are sensitive to the substance. People who have food allergies, or are sensitive to certain ingredients, should avoid eating foods that contain those ingredients.

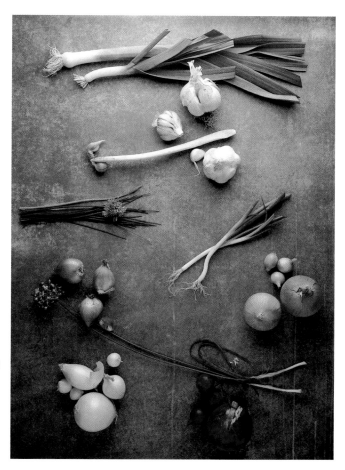

WHEN TO SEASON

As a general rule, you can season food at any time during the cooking process. However, certain forms of food lend themselves to seasoning at certain times. For example, when cooking a dish such as soup, you can add seasonings during the cooking process. However, you should wait until the end of the cooking process to add salt.

On the other hand, when cooking large pieces of food, such as a roast, you should add your seasonings at the beginning of the cooking process. Adding the seasonings early allows enough time for the seasonings to be absorbed effectively throughout the food.

If you choose to add your seasonings throughout the cooking process, be sure to taste the food and evaluate its flavor before adding more seasoning. Overseasoning can ruin the natural flavor of food. Dried seasonings should be added earlier in the cooking process than fresh seasonings.

Fig. 16-4. Spices such as nutmeg are added to liquids during cooking. Why are spices added early in the cooking process?

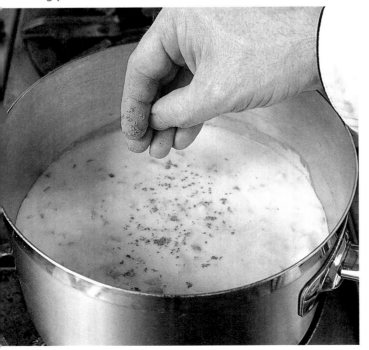

WHEN TO ADD FLAVOR

Flavorings also can be added to food at any time during the cooking process. However, the effects of flavorings are dependent on the length of the cooking time. You need to know how long the food must cook before you determine when to add the flavorings.

Flavorings require heat to release their flavors. They also need time to blend with the natural flavors of the food they are added to. For example, whole spices, such as ginger, take longer to be absorbed than ground spices. You will need to take this into consideration when adding flavorings. They should not be overcooked, however. Overcooked flavorings quickly lose their effect. See Fig. 16-4.

HERBS & SPICES

Herbs (urhbs) and spices are used to enhance the flavor of foods. Both blend with the flavors of other foods to create a new flavor. However, they differ in a number of ways. See Fig. 16-5.

Herbs are plants that grow in temperate, or mild, climates. The parts of the plant that are harvested and used as herbs are the leaves and the stems. Herbs can be fresh or dried. Fresh herbs aren't as strong in flavor as dried herbs. When using fresh herbs, you should use twice the amount of dried herbs called for in a recipe. Dried herbs should be stored in closed containers away from heat or excessive light. As they age, they lose their flavor.

Spices are obtained from the bark, buds, fruits, roots, seeds, or stems of plants and trees. Unlike herbs, spices are commonly used only in their dried form. Spices come in two forms: whole or ground into powder. Spices can be sweet, spicy, or hot. The flavor and aroma of spices are due to the oils found within the various parts of the plants. Some plants provide both an herb and a spice. For example, dill leaves are an herb, and dill seeds are a spice.

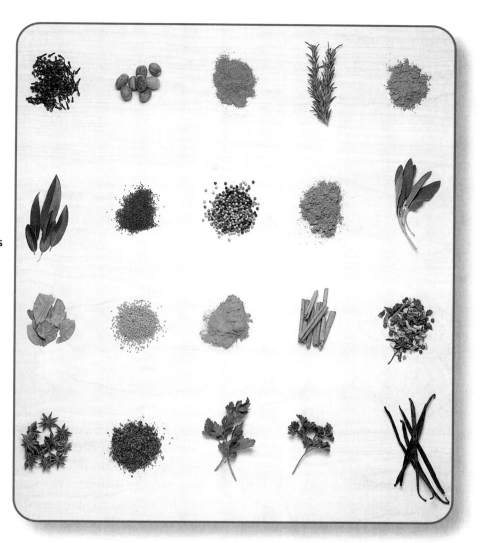

Fig. 16-5. Herbs and spices build the flavor of foods. Can you identify the herbs and spices shown here?

Some flavorings are considered **blends**, or combinations of herbs, spices, and seeds. Chili powder, curry powder, and garlic salt are examples of blends. These are ready-made dried products that can be purchased from a supplier or created in the commercial kitchen. When herbs are used with spices, they complement each other by enhancing flavor.

Knowledge Check

1. What is the difference between a seasoning and a flavoring?
2. Name three different flavorings.
3. How do herbs differ from spices?

MINI LAB

In teams, gather a total of six herbs and spices. Add one herb or spice to a clear broth or soup and taste it. Record the name and amount added. Continue to add items until your team likes the flavor.

Herbs & Spices

KEY TERMS

• sachet

• bouquet garni

• aroma

• paella

• risotto Milanese

OBJECTIVES

After reading this section, you will be able to:

• Identify different herbs and spices.

• Describe the various forms of herbs and spices.

• Explain how herbs and spices are used.

• Explain how to store herbs and spices.

PART of the job of a foodservice professional involves working with a great variety of herbs and spices. Can you tell the difference between parsley and chervil? Do you know how to recognize nutmeg and allspice? You need to know what they look like, the forms they are available in, their flavors and aromas, and how to use them with food. Herbs and spices enhance the flavor of food, but you must use them correctly. Incorrect use can ruin the flavor of foods. You need to know the effect of each herb and spice. Experience is your best teacher.

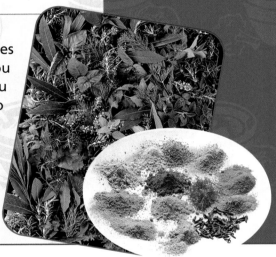

✖ HERB VARIETIES

Herbs are a flavoring that add color and aroma to foods. Herbs are grown in temperate climates. They can be fresh or dried. There are many different herbs that can be used in culinary preparation. Basil, chives, oregano, and sage are examples of herbs. Fresh herbs should be used whenever possible. Fresh herbs are most abundant in the summer. In the fall, fresh herbs can be dried and frozen for use during the winter. Knowing which to use, when to use it, and with what food is an important aspect of your job. See Fig. 16-6 on pages 365–367 (**Herbs**).

✖ USING HERBS

Herbs can be purchased in two forms: fresh and dried. Fresh herbs should be minced or crushed as close to cooking or serving time as possible. If used for cooking, they should be added at the end of the cooking process. If you are adding fresh herbs to uncooked foods, such as salads, you need to add them several hours before serving time. Herbs need plenty of time to release their flavor to cold foods. Dried herbs should be added at the beginning of the cooking process. Use a little and taste the food before adding more.

Herbs

1. Basil

Basil (BAY-zihl) is an herb from the mint family with tender, leafy stems. It is available in many varieties and has a mild, licorice-like flavor. Basil is available fresh or dried, as crushed leaves or ground. Basil is used in soups, tomato sauce, and salads. It is also used on pizza, vegetables, chicken, and pesto.

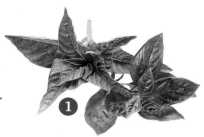

2. Bay leaf

Bay leaf is an herb that comes from the evergreen bay laurel tree. Bay leaves are commonly dried. They are used in soups, stews, vegetables, and meats. Bay leaves are generally removed from food before serving.

3. Chervil

Chervil (CHUHR-vuhl) is a slightly peppery herb that is shaped like parsley. It is available fresh or dried, as crushed leaves or ground. Chervil can be used in soups, sauces, salads, fish and shellfish dishes, and baked goods.

4. Chives

Chives (CHYVS) are the long, toothpick-like leaves of a perennial in the onion family. Chives have a delicate, onion flavor. Chives are available fresh, dried, or frozen. Chives can be used to flavor breads and soft rolls as well as soups, sauces, dips, and spreads. Chives can often be used in place of onions. They are often used to top off a baked potato with sour cream.

5. Cilantro

Cilantro (sih-LAHN-troh), from the coriander plant, has bright green leaves with longer stems. It has a distinct odor and a unique flavor. Cilantro is available fresh or chopped and frozen. Cilantro is used in sauces, salsa, and to add flavor to different dishes.

6. Dill

Dill (dihl) is a feathery-leaved herb. It has a strong, distinct flavor that is commonly associated with pickles. Dill comes in fresh or dried leaves. Dill is used in many soups, salads, and breads. It also is used to flavor various vegetable and fish dishes.

7. Garlic chives

Garlic chives are flat stems. They have a mild, garlic flavor and are available fresh. Garlic chives can be used to flavor breads, soft rolls, soups, sauces, dips, and spreads.

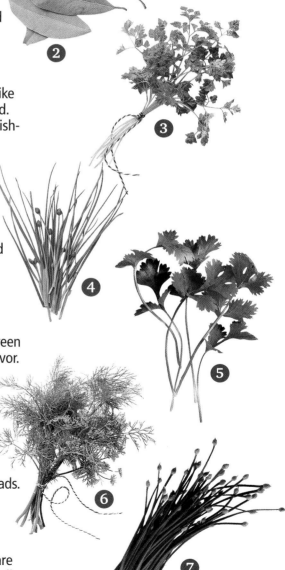

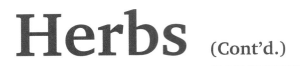

Herbs (Cont'd.)

8. Lemon grass

Lemon grass is a tough, fibrous grass. The base has a lemony flavor. It comes in fresh stalks. Lemon grass is used in curries and many spicy dishes.

9. Marjoram

Marjoram (MAHR-juhr-uhm) is a perennial plant of the mint family with a warm, mild flavor. It is available as fresh or dried, as crushed leaves or ground. Marjoram is used to flavor soups, stews, gravies, sauces, and many poultry, fish, and meat dishes.

10. Mint

Mint grows in many varieties, the most well known being peppermint and spearmint. Mint is available as fresh or dried leaves. Mint is used in sauces, sweet dishes, pastries, tea, and ice cream. It is often paired with chocolate. Mint is also used on lamb, peas, and in fruit beverages.

11. Oregano

Oregano (oh-REHG-uh-noh) is sometimes referred to as wild marjoram. It has a slightly bitter flavor. It is available as fresh or dried, as leaves or ground. Oregano is used in soups, sauces, tomato dishes, pizza, and meat and egg dishes.

12. Parsley

Parsley (PAHR-slee) is grown in many varieties. It has a soothing effect on your taste buds. It comes fresh or dried, as leaves or flakes. Parsley is widely used in soups, sauces, and dressings. It is often served as sprigs, or chopped and used to add color to foods.

Some herbs and foods are natural combinations. For example, lamb is often flavored with rosemary. Basil seems to go hand-in-hand with tomato sauce. Most pizzas are flavored with oregano. However, chefs often experiment with different combinations to create new and interesting dishes.

When cooking liquid dishes, such as soups, stocks, and sauces, fresh herbs can be added to the dish in a sachet or a bouquet garni. A **sachet** (sa-shay) is French for bag. To make a sachet, place your herbs in the center of a small square piece of cheesecloth. See Fig. 16-7. Pull the four corners together and tie the bag with twine. A sachet is usually tied to the handle of a stock pot with twine that is long enough to allow the sachet to be in the liquid. This also makes removing the sachet easy. See Fig. 16-8.

13. Rosemary

Rosemary, an evergreen shrub with needlelike leaves, is a member of the mint family. It has a strong flavor and aroma. It is available fresh or dried, whole or ground. Rosemary is used in soups, stews, sauces, and baked goods.

14. Sage

Sage is a member of the mint family. It has soft downy leaves that are fragrant and warm. It is available fresh or dried, whole or ground. Sage is often used in soups, stews, stuffings, and sausages. It is also used as a seasoning for poultry and pork.

15. Savory

Savory (SAY-vuh-ree) is another member of the mint family. It has a spicy taste and comes fresh or dried, as crushed leaves. Savory is used with meat and fish dishes, chicken, eggs, stuffings, and in many baked goods.

16. Tarragon

Tarragon (TEHR-uh-guhn) is an herb from the daisy family. Its flavor is a cross between mint and anise (AN-ihss) and is what gives béarnaise sauce its flavor. It comes fresh or as dried, crushed leaves. Tarragon is used to flavor salad dressings, mustards, marinades, vinegar, sauces, and soups. It can also be used with chicken, veal, and fish.

17. Thyme

Thyme (TIME) is a shrub of the mint family. It has a sharp and spicy flavor. It is available fresh or dried, as crushed leaves or ground. Thyme is used in meat, poultry, and fish dishes, as well as in soups and baked goods.

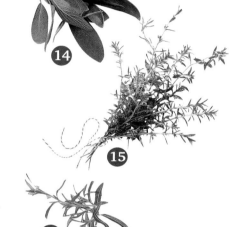

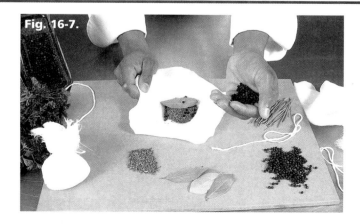

Fig. 16-7.

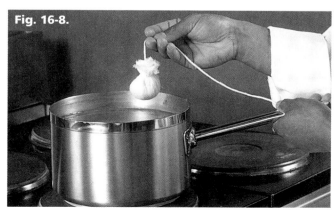

Fig. 16-8.

A **bouquet garni** (boo-KAY-gahr-NEE) is a combination of fresh herbs and vegetables tied in a bundle with butcher's twine. The bundle is dropped into the stock pot and allowed to simmer. Before the dish is served, the bouquet garni is removed. The most common ingredients in a bouquet garni are leeks, parsley, celery, and thyme.

STORING HERBS

Proper storage is essential to maintaining the flavor of herbs. Fresh herbs should be wrapped loosely in a damp cloth and refrigerated. Store at temperatures between 34°F and 40°F. Dried herbs should be kept in opaque, airtight containers. Store dried herbs in a cool, dry place at temperatures between 50°F and 70°F. Avoid exposing stored herbs to heat, light, and excess moisture. Exposure to air can weaken the flavor of herbs.

SPICE VARIETIES

Like herbs, there are a number of spices that you can add to the foods you cook. You should know each spice, its **aroma**—or distinctive pleasing smell, and its effect on food. You can achieve this by tasting foods as you experiment with adding spices.

You can easily add spices to hot foods such as soups, sauces, and broths with the help of a sachet. A sachet allows you to add the flavor of spices to the food without leaving the actual spice in the dish to be served. Typical ingredients include cloves, garlic, and crushed peppercorns. When mixed with herbs, parsley and thyme are often used. See Fig. 16-9 on pages 369-371 (Spices).

a LINK to the Past

The Spice of Life

Spices have played an important role in history. The search for better routes to the spice-rich lands of the East led to an era of great exploration and expansion. The spice trade was the major cause of medieval wars. In addition, spice fortunes financed much of the Renaissance in art.

Of all the spices in the world, pepper is the most popular. It was once so highly valued that it was traded for gold, ounce for ounce. In the Middle Ages, pepper was so rare and expensive that it was sometimes used as currency to pay taxes and rent.

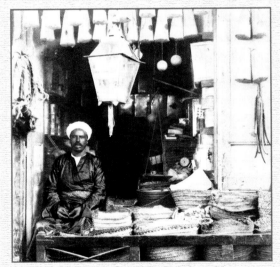

Spices were highly valued commodities not only in Europe, but also in America. Between 1780 and 1873, American ships made nearly 1,000 voyages to the Orient, returning to American ports with millions of pounds of spices. Through history, spices have played a vital role in food preparation, food preservation, and medicines.

Spices

1. Allspice

Allspice is the dried, unripe berry of the pimiento (pih-MYEHN-toh) tree, a tropical evergreen found in the West Indies and in Latin America. The berries are dried and either left whole or ground. The flavor of allspice combines the flavors of nutmeg, clove, and cinnamon. It is available dry, whole, or ground. Whole allspice is used with pickles, meats, fish, sausages, and sauces. Ground allspice is used in pies, cakes, puddings, relishes, and preserves.

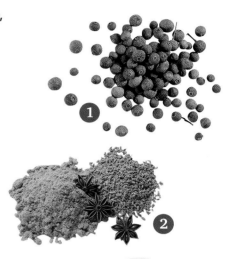

2. Anise seeds

Anise (AN-ihss) seeds are dried green-brown seeds with a strong, licorice-like aroma and flavor. They are dried and available whole or ground. Anise can be used to flavor a variety of dishes, including fish sauces, breads, cakes, cookies, and candies.

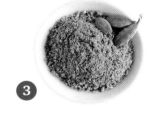

3. Cardamom

Cardamom (KAR-duh-muhm) is the seed from the fruit of an herb in the ginger family. It has a sweet, almost pepper-like flavor and aroma. It is the third most-expensive spice in the world behind saffron and vanilla. It is available whole or ground. Cardamom is used in curries, sweet dishes, yogurt, and baked goods.

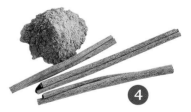

4. Cinnamon

Cinnamon is the thin, dried inner bark of two related evergreen trees of the laurel family. It is used in baking more than any other spice. Cinnamon has a warm, spicy aroma and flavor. It is available dried in sticks or ground. Cinnamon is used in cakes, cookies, pies, curries, sweet potatoes, meat stuffings, and preserves.

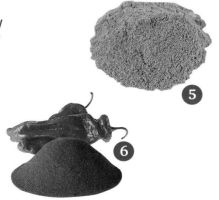

5. Celery seeds

Celery seed is a tiny, seed-like fruit with a strong celery flavor. It is available whole, ground, or mixed with salt. In its whole form, celery seed is used in sauces, salads, cole slaw, and pickling. Ground celery seed is used in soups, stews, and salad dressings.

6. Chili powder

Chili powder is a dried, ground blend of cumin, garlic, onion, and chile peppers. It is used in chili, egg dishes, and meat dishes.

Spices (Cont'd.)

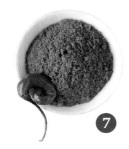

7. Cayenne

Cayenne (KY-yehn) comes from hot red peppers that are ground into powder. It has a strong flavor that gives food a "kick." It is dried and ground. Cayenne is used with meat, fish, eggs, and poultry. It is also used in soups, sauces, and salads.

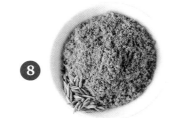

8. Cumin

Cumin (KUH-mihn) seeds are the dried, ripened fruit of an herb in the parsley family. It looks like caraway seed, but has a much different flavor and aroma. Cumin is available whole or ground. It is the spice that lends chili its distinctive flavor. Cumin is also used to flavor chicken, fish, curries, couscous, sausages, and hard cheeses.

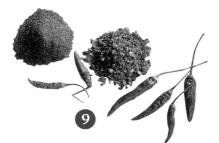

9. Chiles

Chiles are peppers that grow in a variety of shapes and sizes from round to oblong. They range in color from red, yellow, and green to purple. Chiles can be mild, sweet, or extremely hot. They are available fresh and dried. Chiles are used in a variety of dishes including salads, pickles, sauces, vegetable dishes, salsas, and meat dishes.

10. Dill seeds

Dill seeds are the small, dark seeds of the dill plant. They have a slightly sharp taste and distinct odor. Dill seeds are used in soups and salads. They are also used with sauerkraut and fish.

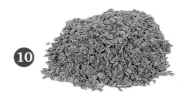

11. Fennel seeds

Fennel (FEHN-uhl) seeds are from a tall, hardy plant in the parsley family. In addition to fennel seeds, the fennel plant is used widely in cooking and pickling. Both have a mild, anise-like flavor. Whole fennel seeds are used in breads, crackers, and sausages. They are also used in tomato sauce, marinades, and with fish and shellfish.

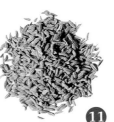

12. Saffron

Saffron (SAF-ruhn) is a yellow spice derived from the crocus plant. It has a sweet scent, but a bitter taste. Saffron is the most expensive spice in the world. It is available dried as whole threads or ground. Saffron is used to lend its color and flavor to dishes such as **paella** (pi-AY-yuh), a Spanish rice dish with meat or shellfish, and **rissotto Milanese** (rih-SAW-toh MIH-lah-neez), an Italian dish which includes rice sautéed in butter before adding stock.

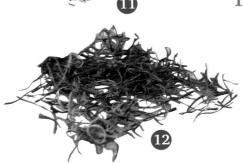

13. Pepper and Peppercorns

Pepper is a smooth, woody vine that climbs tree trunks to produce grapelike clusters of small berries. The berries start green and then turn red as they ripen. There are four varieties: green, black, white, and pink. Each has its own unique flavor. Pepper is available whole, as peppercorns, or ground. Pepper is used in all sorts of dishes.

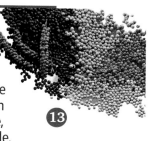

14. Nutmeg

Nutmeg (NUHT-meg) is the kernel of the fruit or seed of the evergreen nutmeg tree. Nutmeg is dried, removed from the shell, and either ground or kept whole for grating. Nutmeg has a sweet, warm, spicy flavor. Freshly grated nutmeg is superior in flavor to prepared ground nutmeg. Nutmeg lends itself to many baked items, soups, sauces, chicken, potatoes, and custards.

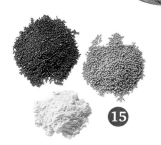

15. Mustard seeds

Mustard seeds are the small, round, smooth seeds of the watercress family. They have a tangy flavor. Mustard seeds are available whole, ground, or prepared as a condiment sauce. Mustard seeds are used in salads, salad dressings, and sauces. They are also used with meats, fish, cheese, and eggs.

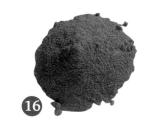

16. Paprika

Paprika (pa-PREE-kuh) is derived from dried, ripe, red sweet peppers. Its flavor is sweet. Hungarian paprika can be semi-hot or very hot. It is available fresh or dried, whole, canned, diced, or ground. Paprika is used in soups, stews, sauces, salad dressings, and tomato dishes. It is also used to accent fish and shellfish dishes.

17. Ginger

Ginger is the underground stem of a plant native to Asia. It can be used fresh or dried. Dried ginger is most often used in baking to flavor cookies and cakes. Fresh ginger has a stronger flavor than the dried form and should be peeled before it is used. Ginger has a strong, sweet, peppery flavor. It is available whole, in pieces, slices, or ground. Fresh ginger is used with fish, poultry, and curries. Dry, ground ginger is used in baked goods and with fruits.

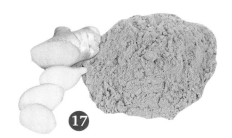

☒ USING SPICES

Spices can be used in a variety of forms, such as whole, ground, sliced, or in chunks. The form you use partially depends on the length of cooking time. For example, whole spices take longer to release their flavor. Therefore, whole spices should be added as early as possible to the cooking process. A 10-minute cooking time would not be long enough to use whole spices in the dish.

You can also use whole spices when poaching fruit or in a marinade (MEHR-uh-nayd). Regardless of the form used, spices should be added to cold food several hours before serving time. This will allow the flavor of the spices to be released into the food.

Ground spices release their flavor immediately. In this case, it is best to add ground spices near the end of the cooking process. This way the flavor won't be cooked away.

Whenever you cook with spices, you must measure them accurately. Strong spices, such as clove, cayenne, or cumin, can overpower the food if too much is used. As a rule of thumb, spices should not dominate the food but complement it, the exceptions being curries or chilis. Remember, spices are used to enhance the flavor of food.

☒ STORING SPICES

Spices should be stored in airtight containers away from direct sunlight. Light can rob spices of their flavor. Spices are best kept in a cool, dry place at temperatures of 50°–70°F. See Fig. 16-10.

Many factors in addition to sunlight and heat can affect the flavor of spices. The age, type, and source of the spice play a role in how long a particular spice can be stored. Check spices often to ensure their strength.

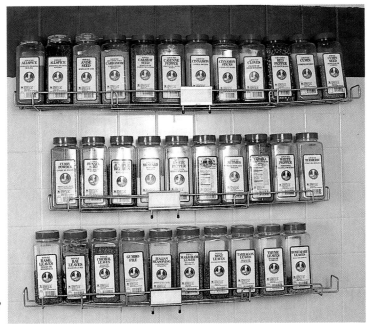

Fig. 16-10. Store spices in a cool, dry place.

Why is it important to store spices properly?

SECTION 16-2   Knowledge Check

1. Name five herbs and five spices and the forms in which they are available.

2. How should you properly store dry herbs?

3. When should spices be added to foods?

MINI LAB

Working in teams, compare the aroma and texture of three herbs and three spices. How do they differ? Find a recipe in which each herb and spice is used. Discuss what the recipes tell you about how the herbs and spices are used.

Condiments, Nuts & Seeds

OBJECTIVES

After reading this section, you will be able to:

• Describe various condiments and the foods they accompany.

• Explain how condiments are stored.

• Identify a variety of nuts and seeds.

• Describe how nuts are used.

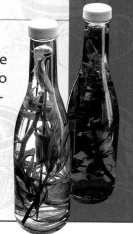

YOU'VE learned about herbs and spices, but what about the condiments, nuts, and salsas that can be served with food to enhance flavor? Salsa, ketchup, steak sauce, mustard, and vinegar are requested often by customers. Almonds and other nuts are often added to food during cooking. Poppy seeds and sesame seeds are used in many baked goods. As a foodservice professional, you will need to know which items are used in your establishment, and what foods they are served with.

❌ VARIETIES OF CONDIMENTS

Condiments are flavored sauces traditionally served as accompaniments to food. Their purpose is to complement food. There is a wide variety of condiments from which to choose. They vary from sweet and tart to hot and spicy, sour, or a combination of these sensations. Condiments can be purchased ready to use or created in the kitchen. Some condiments are used more often than others. See Fig. 16-11A and Fig. 16-11B.

■ **Salsa.** The Spanish word for sauce is **salsa** (SAHL-sah). A brand selection of salsas are available today. Salsas can be fresh or cooked mixtures of chiles, tomatoes, onions, and cilantro. Unopened, cooked salsas can be stored at room temperature for six months. Opened salsas should

always be tightly covered and refrigerated. Fresh salsas can only be refrigerated for five days.

■ **Ketchup.** Ketchup is a tomato-based sauce used throughout the world as a flavoring. Ketchup is typically bright red in color and has a tangy, sweet and sour taste. As ketchup ages, its color becomes dark and its flavor becomes stale.

■ **Steak sauce.** Steak sauce is a tomato-based sauce that is tangier than ketchup. It varies widely in color, from brown to dark red. Steak sauce is used with grilled and broiled meats.

■ **Prepared mustards.** Prepared mustards are a combination of ingredients, such as ground white, black, and brown seeds, vinegar, salt, and spices. Grinding the seeds releases an oil that gives mustard its unique flavor.

Fig. 16-11A.

CONDIMENT	DESCRIPTION	USES
Barbecue Sauce	A mixture of brown sugar, ketchup, chili sauce, green pepper, and vinegar.	Barbecue sauce is used on meats that are broiled, grilled, roasted, and baked.
Chili Sauce	Cooked, fresh, red chiles with spices, vinegar, salt, sugar, and garlic are combined in chili sauce.	It is used with seafood and meats.
Ketchup	A mixture of tomatoes, sugar, vinegar, and salt.	Ketchup is used on most fried foods, grilled meats, and hot dogs.
Steak Sauce	A mixture of tomatoes, vinegar, raisins, salt, spices, herbs, orange base, dehydrated garlic, and onions.	Steak sauce is commonly used on meats.
Salsa	Chile peppers, tomatoes, onion, cilantro, lime juice, salt, and spices are often combined in salsa.	It is used on chicken, grilled steak, potatoes, tortillas, tacos, and eggs.
Hot Sauce	A red pepper sauce.	Hot sauce is used in soups, stews, vegetables, and on eggs.
Chinese Soy Sauce	A salty mixture of soybeans, salt, and wheat make up soy sauce.	It is used on vegetables, rice, meat, fish, and in casseroles.
Sweet and Sour Sauce	A mixture of fruit, vinegar, and sugar.	Sweet and sour sauce is used on chicken, fish, pork, and as a glaze.
Mustards	A combination of ground white, black, and brown mustard seeds can be prepared into a sauce.	It is used on pork, beef, vegetables, cold cuts, sandwiches, and in salads and sauces.
Balsamic Vinegar	Made from red wine vinegar that has been aged in wooden barrels.	Balsamic vinegar is used in dressings, on salads, and in dips.
Cider Vinegar	Made from apple cider, cider vinegar is more acidic than white vinegar.	It is used in dressings and sauces.
Fruit-Flavored Vinegars	Produced by steeping fresh fruits, such as raspberries and strawberries, in vinegar.	Fruit-flavored vinegars are used on salads, in dressings, and in dips.

Prepared mustards have a variety of textures, from smooth to coarse to chunky. They also have a variety of flavors, from mild to hot. Prepared mustards are served with pork and beef. They are also used with vegetables, sandwiches, and salads. As mustards age, their flavor decreases.

■ **Pickles.** Pickles are made from vegetables that are **fermented** (fuhr-mehn-tuhd), or chemically changed, in brines or vinegars flavored and seasoned with dill, garlic, sugar, peppers, or salt. Cucumbers, tomatoes, and peppers are the most common pickled vegetables.

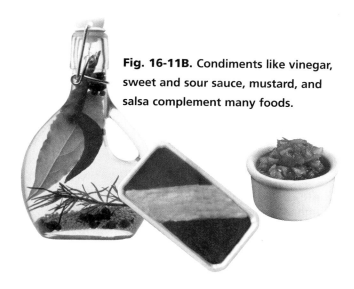

Fig. 16-11B. Condiments like vinegar, sweet and sour sauce, mustard, and salsa complement many foods.

■ **Relishes.** Coarsely chopped or ground pickled items are called **relishes**. The most common flavors are sweet relish and dill relish.

■ **Vinegars.** Vinegar is a sour, acidic liquid used in cooking, marinades, and salad dressings. Vinegar comes in a variety of flavors. Some common vinegars are white vinegar, red wine vinegar, balsamic (bahl-SAH-mihk) vinegar, and cider vinegar. Discard vinegars three months after they are opened.

■ **Flavored oils.** Flavored oils are those that have been enhanced with ingredients, such as herbs, spices, and garlic. The oils of these ingredients are extracted and then poured into olive or canola oil. This process creates a more flavorful oil than would result from adding the flavor enhancer itself to the oil. Flavored oils can also be used during cooking or added to food before serving. Flavored oils can be used as dressings or marinades, too.

Some flavored oils are created by the chef by simply adding the flavor enhancer, not the extracted oil, to olive or canola oil. In this situation, only prepare enough oil to use for one day to avoid foodborne illness.

Sometimes different vegetable oils are combined to create a different taste. For example, Szechwan-flavored oil is a combination of sunflower oil, canola oil, sesame seed oil, and natural flavorings, such as garlic, ginger, red pepper, and paprika. These flavored oils can be used during the cooking process with a variety of foods.

STORING CONDIMENTS

Unopened condiments should be stored in cool and dry areas. Temperatures should be between 50°F and 70°F. Opened condiments should always be stored in the refrigerator.

When using canned condiments, such as ketchup, barbecue sauce, and relishes, remove the condiments from the cans and transfer them into airtight plastic containers. Store condiments in the refrigerator once the original packaging has been opened.

NUTS & SEEDS

A variety of nuts and seeds can be used with many different foods to enhance natural flavor. Nuts and seeds also add color and texture to food.

Nuts are available shelled and unshelled. Nuts can be used in their natural form, blanched, toasted, or roasted. Seeds can be used in a variety of ways. Some seeds, such as cumin and coriander, are considered to be spices, and are used during cooking. Other seeds, such as sesame and poppy seeds, are used in baked goods.

Nuts and seeds can be used in a variety of foods to add flavor, color, and texture. Nuts are a good source of the B vitamins and of protein. When using nuts, be sure they come from the current year's crop. Nuts should be purchased in small quantities because they can spoil or become infested with insects easily. See Fig. 16-12 on pages 376-377 (**Nuts & Seeds**).

Storing Nuts & Seeds

To store fresh nuts and seeds, place them in an airtight container. The container should be placed in a cool, dry area with limited exposure to light. Nuts can also be refrigerated or frozen in airtight containers.

Nuts & Seeds

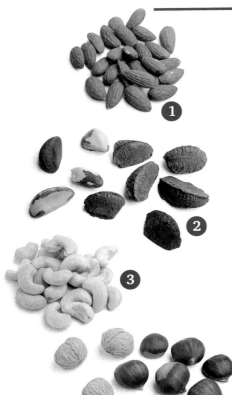

1. Almonds

A medium-brown nut that is white inside, almonds can be sweet or bitter. Sweet almonds are eaten; bitter almonds are used as a source for almond flavoring. Almonds are available whole in the shell, shelled, skinned, sliced, in pieces, or as a paste.

2. Brazils

Brazils are not actually nuts, but the seeds of a fruit. Brazil nuts are available whole in the shell or shelled.

3. Cashews

The cashew is the edible seed of a tropical evergreen tree. Most cashews are salted and roasted. They are available raw or toasted.

4. Chestnuts

Chestnuts are sweet nuts that contain more starch and less fat than other nuts. They can be roasted, boiled, or steamed. Chestnuts are available whole in the shell, dried, and canned in water or syrup.

5. Hazelnuts

Hazelnuts grow in clusters and are the nut of the hazelnut tree. They are sweet, rich, grape-size nuts and often are used in salads and main dishes.

6. Peanuts

Peanuts are small nuts that resemble peas. The two most common types are Virginia and Spanish peanuts. The Virginia peanut has larger kernels and more flavor than the Spanish variety. Many people are allergic to peanuts. Customers should be told which menu items include peanuts. Peanuts are available as dry roasted, granules, salted, unsalted, and in the shell.

7. Pecans

Pecans are the nut of the pecan tree. They have a very thin shell. Pecans are available whole in the shell, chopped, and in halves.

8. Pine nuts

Pine nuts are the kernels of pine cones. They taste like almonds and are available raw, toasted, and frozen.

9. Pistachios

Pistachios (pih-STASH-ee-ohs) are pale green to creamy white in color and have a mild flavor. Pistachios are available in the shell, shelled, roasted and salted, and dyed red.

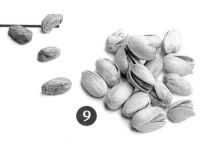

10. Walnuts

Walnuts are the fruit of the walnut tree. Sizes vary from small to large. Walnuts are available whole in the shell, shelled as halves, and chopped.

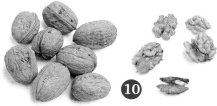

11. Poppy seeds

Poppy seeds are the dark black, dried seeds of the poppy plant. Poppy seeds are available whole.

12. Pumpkin seeds

Pumpkin seeds come from pumpkins. They are available in the shell, toasted, and raw.

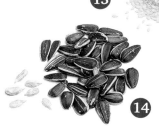

13. Sesame seeds

Sesame seeds are creamy-colored, flat, oval seeds that have a nutty flavor. They are available whole, roasted, and ground into paste.

14. Sunflower seeds

These seeds come from the sunflower. The whole seed can be eaten raw or cooked.

SECTION 16-3 — Knowledge Check

1. Name at least five condiments and the foods they are used with.
2. How should condiments be stored?
3. Describe five different types of nuts and five different types of seeds.

MINI LAB

Working in teams, select three nuts or seeds. Experiment with various ways to prepare them, such as blanching, roasting, or sugaring. Store them in airtight containers and refrigerate.

Sensory Perception

OBJECTIVES

After reading this section, you will be able to:

• Describe the sensory properties of food.

• Explain how the sensory property of flavor is a combination of three sensory experiences.

• Explain sensory evaluation.

• Identify the factors that affect sensory evaluation.

USING seasonings and flavorings successfully requires foodservice professionals to understand sensory perception. **Sensory perception** is how a person's eyes, nose, mouth, and skin detect and evaluate the environment. Sensory perception will help you improve your ability to taste. This, in turn, will allow you to increase your customers' enjoyment of food.

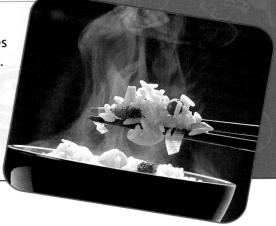

✖ THE SENSORY PROPERTIES OF FOOD

Sensory properties of food affect how people perceive food. These sensory properties are color and appearance, flavor, and texture. Each one is detected by four of five sense organs: the taste buds, nose, skin, and eyes. See Fig. 16-13.

When people eat, these sense organs evaluate the food. This is done with special **receptors**, or groups of cells, that detect **stimuli**, or things that cause an activity or response. When a stimulus is detected, nerve impulses carry the signal to the brain. The information is then processed. When the stimulus is food, the sense organs of taste and smell cause a reaction that increases the produc-

tion of saliva. Gastric secretions are also increased. These two fluids help aid digestion and the distribution of nutrients to the body.

Color & Appearance

The appearance of food is usually the first indication of how it will taste. The brighter and more colorful the food, the more visual appeal it has. The brain processes visual information about flavor and texture based on appearance alone. It then makes decisions about likes and dislikes. This occurs because of people's highly developed

Fig. 16-13.

SENSE	RECEPTOR	STIMULI	SENSATION
Taste Buds	Taste cells	Sugars, salts, acids, amino acids, and alkaloids	Taste
Nose	Olfactory cells	Odor chemicals	Smell
Skin	Free nerve endings; skin receptors	Chemicals; heat and pressure	Pain; touch
Eyes	Rods and cones	Light energy	Sight

sense of sight. In fact, our sense of sight is so highly developed that it may cause messages received from the other senses to be ignored. Therefore, foodservice professionals should ensure that the color and appearance of food will be visually appealing to customers.

■ **Lighting.** Different types of lighting affect the perception of color. Foodservice professionals should be aware that what they see in kitchen lighting may not be what the customer sees in dining room lighting. For example, when the color green is viewed under an incandescent light, it will appear more yellow than when it is viewed under fluorescent lighting. See Fig. 16-14.

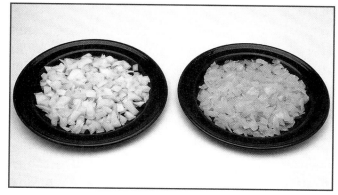

Fig. 16-15. Raw onions are opaque. Cooked onions are translucent. Why does this happen?

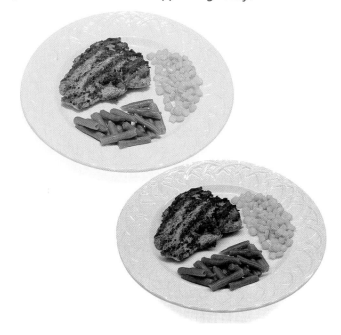

Fig. 16-14. Lighting affects the color of food. Which plate of food looks more appetizing? Why?

■ **Physical structure.** The physical structure of food affects color. For example, spinach is made of plant cells that contain a large amount of liquid. These plant cells are surrounded by air pockets. When raw spinach is cooked, air escapes from the pockets, and the plant cells burst. This causes the air pockets to fill with liquid. Likewise, because light reflects off liquids differently than it does air, cooked onions appear **translucent**, or clear, rather than **opaque**, or cloudy. See Fig. 16-15.

■ **Chemical structure.** The chemical structure of food also impacts appearance. For example, the pigments, or the chemicals that give vegetables their color, change during the cooking process. Pigments found in foods include red as in beets, white as in cauliflower, green as in broccoli, and yellow as in squash. When properly cooked, pigments remain bright. When overcooked, pigments become dull.

Flavor

The sensory property of flavor, or taste, is a combination of three sensory experiences: basic tastes, aromas, and feeling. People's perception of these three sensory experiences is chemical in nature. Salt, for instance, changes the chemistry of certain taste buds. This change in chemistry triggers a signal to the brain that travels through nerve fibers. The brain translates this signal into the perception of saltiness.

■ **Tastes.** The basic tastes are: sweet, salty, sour, and bitter. Sometimes savory (SAY-vuh-ree) is included. **Savory** means stimulating and full of flavor.

Tastes are detected by taste buds, cells scattered over the surface of the tongue. See Fig. 16-16. In addition to taste buds, saliva plays an important role in taste perception. Without saliva, the taste molecules—sweeteners, salts, acids, and bitter components—could not reach the taste cells.

■ **Aroma.** The perception of aroma is more complex than that of tastes. Humans can detect hundreds, even thousands, of distinctly different aromas. The perception of smell allows people to differentiate between similar flavors, such as an orange versus a tangerine. Therefore, people can "taste" the different flavors.

Fig. 16-16. The basic tastes are sweet, salty, sour, and bitter.

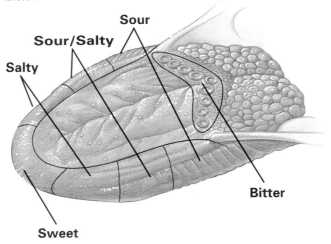

Sour
Sour/Salty
Salty
Sweet
Bitter

TASTE SENSATIONS

The tongue contains many tiny bumps called papillae (pah-PIH-lee). These bumps sense the basic tastes of bitterness, saltiness, sourness, and sweetness. Each bump contains over 200 taste buds. Typically, the taste buds responsive to sweet and salty foods are located at the tip of the tongue. The taste buds responsive to bitterness are often located at the back of the tongue, and the taste buds responsive to sour foods appear to be along the sides of the tongue.

APPLY IT!

Experiment with flavors to determine which part of your tongue is sensitive to bitter, sour, salty, and sweet foods. You will need four coffee stirrers, 1 tsp. salt, 1 tsp. sugar, 1 tsp. cocoa powder, one lemon, and a glass of water.

1. Draw a sketch of your tongue and divide it into four sections: the back, the right side, the left side, and the front.

2. Use the coffee stirrer to place a sample of salt on the tip of your tongue. Record whether it tastes sweet, sour, bitter, or salty.

3. Repeat the procedure on each section of your tongue, recording the taste. After you complete the experiment with the salt, rinse your mouth with water and repeat the experiment with the sugar, cocoa powder, and lemon. Be sure to rinse between each sample.

■ **Nerve endings.** Nerve endings that reside just below the skin throughout the mouth and nose are responsible for detecting flavors. They allow you to feel the menthol in peppermint and the carbon dioxide in carbonated beverages. In fact, people who have lost their sense of taste and smell often can still detect the presence of certain flavors with these nerve endings.

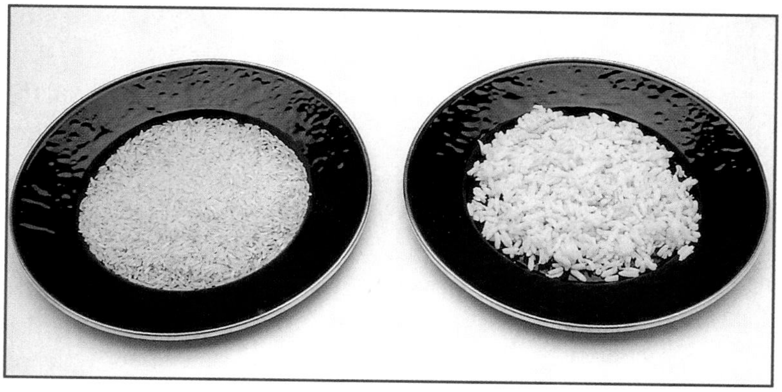

Fig. 16-17. Food can be categorized by texture. What textures do you see in this photo?

Texture

The last sensory property of food that must be evaluated is texture. The characteristics of texture can vary greatly. For example, cooked rice can be described as rough or smooth, sticky or slick, hard or soft, moist or dry, chewy or crumbly, depending on the way it was prepared and the type of rice. Sometimes one characteristic stands out, but foodservice professionals need to practice analyzing food as completely as possible. See Fig. 16-17.

When evaluating the texture of food, ask these questions:

1. How does the food feel against the soft tissue in the mouth?

2. How does the food react to being squeezed, pulled, bitten, or chewed? Is it hard? Does it bounce back like gelatin? Is it crumbly? When evaluating texture, you will need to see how food reacts to being eaten.

3. How does the food react to the warmth of the mouth? For example, the smooth textural characteristics of ice cream and chocolate depend in part on how quickly and completely they melt in your mouth.

4. Does the food leave a coating in the mouth and throat after swallowing? For example, shortenings, especially those with a high melting point, tend to leave a waxy coating in the mouth, while oils tend to leave a slick, greasy coating. Is the coating that you taste pleasant or unpleasant?

5. How does the food sound when chewed? Potato chips are not crispy and tortilla chips are not crunchy unless you can hear the crisp or crunch.

⊠ SENSORY EVALUATION

Sensory evaluation is the systematic tasting of food by consumers and foodservice professionals. Many foodservice operations conduct consumer taste tests to determine what their customers like and dislike. Therefore, food companies strive to design the taste to the customers' likings.

Customers test foods based on their likes and dislikes, but food taste testers need to evaluate food objectively. Their job is to describe only the sensory characteristics. To increase the objectivity of the evaluations, food products are tasted "blind." This means that the samples are not labeled so that the testers will not know which product they are tasting.

Much practice is needed to successfully recognize and identify the many interrelated sensory characteristics of food. While culinary skills involve putting flavors together, the process of sensory evaluation is one of taking things apart.

Product Factors

Different versions of the same type of food may taste or smell different from each other. For example, one vinaigrette (vihn-uh-GREHT) dressing may taste more sour than another even though they both contain the same amount of acid. This is because different food products have different characteristics. Several factors influence the characteristics of a food product.

■ **Flavor enhancers.** Flavor enhancers change the natural flavor of food without adding a flavor of their own. It is believed that flavor enhancers interact with certain taste chemicals and receptors, producing a different taste perception.

■ **Amount of oil and water.** The amount of oil or water in foods will affect the perception of taste and smell. A taste chemical that dissolves in oil will not fully dissolve in saliva and, as a result, little of it will reach the taste buds. When an odor chemical dissolves in water or oil, it will not evaporate to the olfactory cells where it can be smelled.

Plate Composition

Plate composition should be carefully planned even before the food is cooked to ensure success. This is done by presenting contrasts in color and appearance, height, shape, texture, flavor, and temperature of foods.

■ **Color.** The colors of food presented on a plate should be vibrant and contrasting. Don't choose only different shades of green, for example. Choose several colors to create an interesting plate. Good color can also be attained by carefully choosing the plate on which the food will be served. However, the plate should not detract from the food presentation.

■ **Height.** Often one of the most difficult elements to achieve in plate composition is varying the heights of food on a plate. Achieving this requires careful planning. For example, a poorly planned presentation of a steak, mashed potatoes, and corn on the cob might consist of simply placing each food product on the plate. A more effective presentation incorporates height. The mashed potatoes are neatly piped onto the plate in a circular pinnacle using a pastry bag fitted with a star tip. The grilled steak is then placed leaning slightly against the mashed potatoes. The cob of corn is then cut in half and stood on each side of the steak.

■ **Shape.** Vary the shape of foods in every presentation. Don't serve meatloaf in the form of a round patty with sautéed peas and boiled new potatoes.

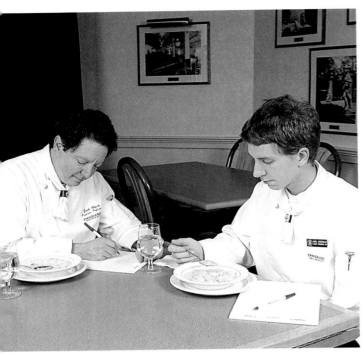

Fig. 16-18. Taste testing by foodservice professionals needs to be objective. What is the goal of testing food products?

■ **Type of ingredients.** Vinaigrette dressings are made of oil, vinegar, and herbs, and may contain the same amount of acid. However, if they contain different types of acid, they will not be perceived as the same. For example, if one contains vinegar and the other contains citric acid from lemons, the vinaigrette made from vinegar will seem more acidic.

■ **Product temperature.** Products that are warm typically have a stronger taste and aroma than those that are chilled.

■ **Product consistency.** Thicker products may have less flavor than thinner ones. This is because flavor molecules take longer to dissolve or evaporate in saliva when food products are of a thicker consistency. See Fig. 16-18.

■ **Presence of other factors.** You can suppress the ability to perceive flavor in foods by combining tastes or aromas. For example, if you add sugar to vinaigrette, it won't taste as acidic. This is true even if the amount of sugar added is so small that sweetness cannot be detected. Add acid to food to make it less sweet; salt to make it less sour; and sugar to make it less bitter.

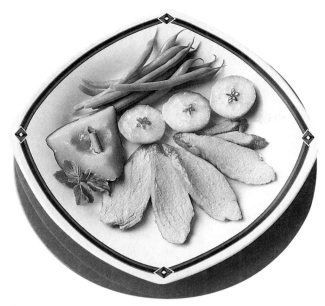

Fig. 16-19. Plate food with varying shapes.

These are all round forms. Instead, try serving the meatloaf with asparagus spears and diced, roasted potatoes to create a better variation of shapes. See Fig. 16-19.

■ **Texture.** Include a variety of textures in each plate composition by carefully choosing foods that may have soft, hard, chewy, crunchy, creamy, or meaty textures. The most common mistake made is serving too many soft foods on the same plate.

■ **Flavor.** Each element of food in a plate presentation should contribute to the overall flavor of the food. Flavor should be considered when choosing ingredients, the preparation and cooking methods, and the seasonings to be used.

■ **Temperature.** Foods should be served at the appropriate temperatures. Hot food should be served on hot plates, while cold food should be served on chilled plates.

■ **Garnishing.** Not all food presentations require a garnish. However, garnishes should compliment the food. For example, strawberry cheesecake is best garnished with a strawberry—not a twist of lemon. A garnish should be the crowning touch on a presentation of food. See Fig. 16-20.

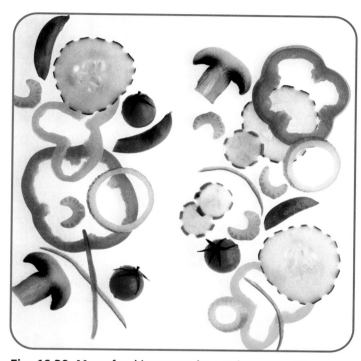

Fig. 16-20. Many food items can be used as a garnish.

SECTION 16-4   Knowledge Check

1. What are the sensory properties of food?
2. Name five factors that affect sensory evaluation.
3. What elements should be considered when plating food?

MINI LAB

Practice identifying seasonings by aroma. First, smell the seasonings and view their labels. Then identify the seasonings by aroma only. Repeat the lab using five different seasonings. Identify each one by taste alone.

CHAPTER 16 Review & Activities

SECTION SUMMARIES

16-1 There are several common ingredients used to enhance the natural flavor of food.

16-1 Spices and flavorings can be added to foods at any time during the cooking process, though certain forms of foods require the addition of seasoning at a specific time.

16-1 Herbs and spices, though different, are both used to enhance and flavor foods.

16-2 A large variety of herbs are available in frozen, fresh, or dried form.

16-2 To use herbs effectively, you need to know each herb's flavor and its effect on food.

16-2 Proper herb storage will ensure flavor retention.

16-2 Foodservice professionals need to know each spice's flavor, aroma, and effect on food in order to use each effectively.

16-2 The length of cooking time and the type of dish being prepared will determine the choice and form of spice to be used.

16-2 Spices must be carefully stored to retain their potency.

16-3 Condiments are flavored sauces that are served with food.

16-3 There are a number of nuts to choose from to add flavor, color, and texture to food.

16-4 Color, appearance, flavor, and texture of food should be evaluated to determine how each will affect the senses.

16-4 Foodservice professionals taste a variety of food products to evaluate, or analyze, their characteristics.

16-4 Food characteristics are affected by factors such as temperature and consistency.

CHECK YOUR KNOWLEDGE

1. What's the difference between seasonings and flavorings?
2. How are fresh seasonings different from dried seasonings?
3. How can you effectively add seasonings and flavorings to soups, sauces, or stocks?
4. What factors affect the potency of a spice?
5. Name six common condiments.
6. What types of nuts might be added to food?
7. What factors play a role in the color of food?
8. What factors impact the sensory characteristics of a food product?
9. How does plate composition affect the sensory appeal of food?

CRITICAL-THINKING ACTIVITIES

1. Assume you are asked to determine three seasonings to be used in the preparation of a new dish containing lamb. After careful thought, you make your selection. Which three would you choose? Why?
2. Why would foodservice operations use dried herbs and spices rather than fresh?

WORKPLACE KNOW-HOW

Problem solving. As a cook in a restaurant, you have been assigned by the chef to prepare a recipe using fresh herbs. As you begin, you realize that the restaurant is out of that fresh herb. However, there is a dried form of it available. What ratio would you use to measure the correct amount of the herb for this dish? Would you ask the chef if the dish should still be created? Why?

LAB-BASED ACTIVITY: Herbs & Spices in Action

STEP 1 Working in teams, use herbs and spices to create a new sauce. Your team will need to determine:

- What type of food will the sauce accompany?
- What enhancement will the sauce bring to the food?
- What will be the desired consistency of the sauce?
- What will be the base ingredient for the sauce?
- At what temperature will the sauce and the accompanying food be served?

STEP 2 Review the list of herbs and spices below and investigate how they are used in various foods.

STEP 3 Decide which spices or herbs will produce the flavor your team desires for your sauce.

STEP 4 Decide on the best time to add your seasonings to produce the maximum flavor.

STEP 5 Prepare your sauce and the food it accompanies. As your team works, write down the proportions of spices and herbs used, and the combinations experimented with to alter or enhance the taste. Remember to use all spices and herbs sparingly at first. You can always add more. Also, write down the amounts of other ingredients used to prepare your sauce and the food it accompanies.

STEP 6 When you are satisfied with your sauce, write out the recipe for others to use.

STEP 7 Share your team's sauce with the class. Evaluate each team's sauce for flavor, color, and texture. Use the following rating scale to score each team's sauce:

1=Poor; 2=Fair; 3=Good; 4=Great

Herbs & Spices

Herbs
- Basil
- Chervil
- Chives
- Cilantro
- Dill
- Garlic chives
- Lemon grass
- Marjoram
- Mint
- Oregano
- Parsley
- Rosemary
- Sage
- Savory
- Tarragon
- Thyme

Spices
- Allspice
- Anise seed
- Cardamom
- Cayenne
- Celery seed
- Chili powder
- Chiles
- Cinnamon
- Cumin
- Dill seed
- Fennel seed
- Ginger
- Mustard seed
- Nutmeg
- Paprika
- Pepper
- Saffron

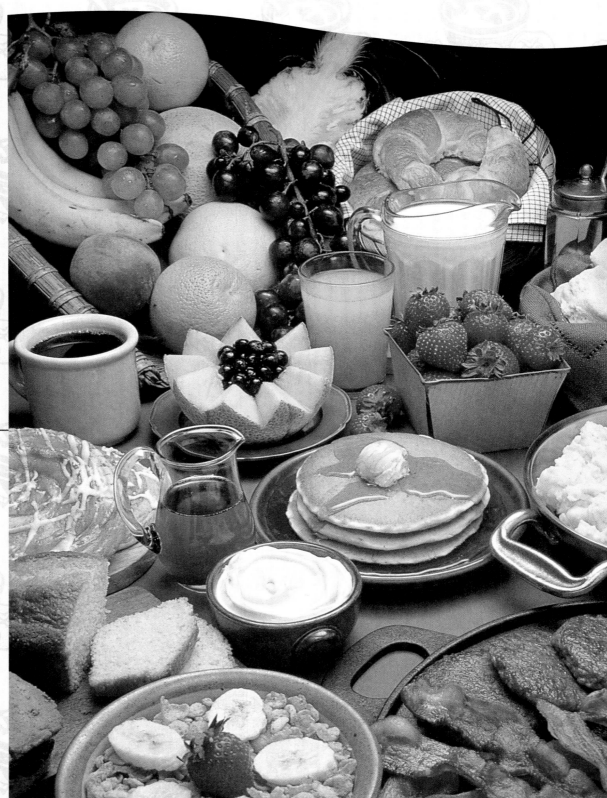

17 Breakfast Cookery

CHAPTER

Section 17-1
Breakfast Food Basics

Section 17-2
Meat & Egg Preparation

Section 17-3
Breakfast Breads & Cereals

386

Breakfast Food Basics

KEY TERMS

- albumin
- porous
- pasteurized
- soufflés
- dehydrated
- ready-made breads
- ramekins

OBJECTIVES

After reading this section, you will be able to:

- Identify basic breakfast foods.
- Explain the grading process of eggs.
- List types of breakfast meats, breads, and cereals.

BREAKFAST foods are not just for breakfast anymore! In the United States, many people eat breakfast foods at any meal. The standard menu includes eggs, meat, potatoes, breads, pancakes, waffles, cereals, fruit, and yogurt. Some restaurants offer customers more unusual choices, such as a special pizza or breakfast burritos. In short, anything goes!

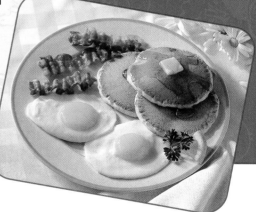

✖ BREAKFAST PROTEIN FOODS

Several breakfast protein foods are from the pork family—ham, bacon, and sausage. Eggs are another breakfast protein food. These protein foods are often served together, such as ham and eggs. Frequently, breakfast protein foods are served with a bread or potato choice to round out the meal.

Types of Meats

Typical breakfast meats on foodservice menus include ham, bacon, Canadian bacon, or sausage, although there are many other protein-based breakfast possibilities, such as smoked salmon, tofu, and turkey bacon. As in any aspect of food service, the best way to ensure a quality breakfast protein food is to start with high-quality meats.

■ **Ham.** Precooked ham is often used as a breakfast meat. Slices of ham are either baked or browned under a broiler.

■ **Bacon.** Most foodservice operations purchase pork bacon sliced, although it is available in whole slabs. In addition to pork bacon, turkey bacon is available in many restaurants for customers who desire a lower fat breakfast meat. Smoky flavored bacons, such as hickory smoked, are available in many operations. Bacon may be served thin- or thick-sliced. The thickness is specified by the number of slices per pound. The average number of slices is 18–22.

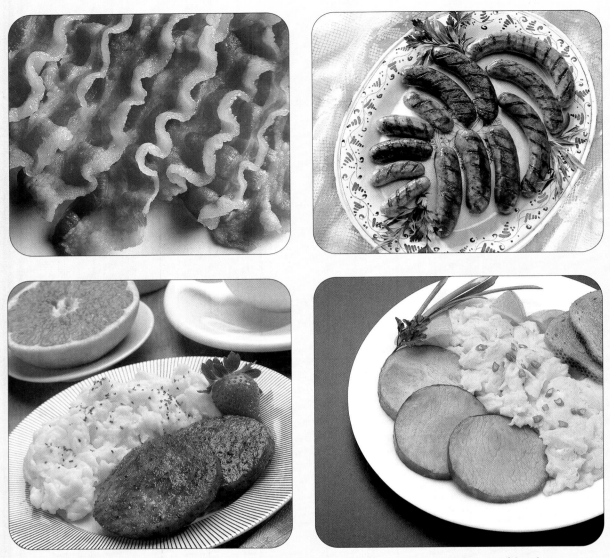

Fig. 17-1. Breakfast meats accompany many standard breakfast menu items. What combinations are most appealing to you?

■ **Canadian bacon.** Another breakfast meat, Canadian bacon, comes from boneless pork loin. It is smoked and brined, and has a thin layer of fat on its surface. Canadian bacon is cut smaller than ham slices, but it is cooked and served in a similar way. It is used in egg specialty dishes such as eggs benedict.

■ **Sausage.** Sausage is often made of ground pork that has been seasoned and stuffed into casings. Sausage is served in links or formed into patties. Links keep better than patties because the casings keep the links from drying out. Other types of sausage may be made from turkey. See Figure 17-1.

Egg Composition

Eggs seem to be the perfect breakfast food. They are an inexpensive source of protein and can be prepared in many different ways to suit various tastes and standards. An egg has three main parts: shell, yolk, and white.

■ **Shell.** Like any shell, an eggshell serves to protect the egg's content. Eggshells range in color from white to brown, and they vary in thickness and porousness. The color of the egg indicates the type of chicken. The color of the eggshell does not affect the interior color of the egg or the taste.

Fig. 17-2.

GRADE	CHARACTERISTICS	USES
AA	Yolk is firm, centered in the shell, holds its shape, and stands up high; white is clear and thick, so it doesn't spread out over a large area when broken in the pan; shell clean, normal shape.	Poaching, frying, hard- or soft-cooked.
A	Thinner than AA, so it spreads slightly when broken in the pan; fairly firm yolk; clear white.	Hard- or soft-cooked.
B	Less firm yolk and white, so the egg doesn't hold its shape in the pan and spreads over a wide area; yolk is large and flat; shell may be slightly stained or an abnormal shape.	Scrambled eggs; baking.

■ **Yolk.** The yolk, almost one-third of the egg's weight, contains fat and protein, along with vitamins and iron. Most of an egg's calories and all of its cholesterol and fat are found in the yolk. The color of the yolk depends on the diet of the chicken.

■ **White.** Two-thirds of an egg is made of the clear white, or **albumin** (al-BYOO-mehn). The thickest part of the white surrounds the yolk. Riboflavin (ry-buh-FLAY-vuhn) and over half the protein of the egg are found in the white. It is clear and soluble when the egg is uncooked, but becomes white and firm when cooked.

Eggs may look solid, but they are actually very **porous** (POHR-uhs). Porous means that flavors and odors can be absorbed through the shell and that the egg can lose moisture even when the shell is unbroken. For this reason, eggs need to be stored carefully. Eggs will keep for several weeks if stored at 36°F, but will quickly lose quality if left at room temperature. In fact, eggs will lose a full grade in quality in one day if they are left at room temperature. Remember these egg storage tips:

• Store eggs in their original containers or in covered containers.

• Store eggs away from foods with strong flavors or odors, such as onions.

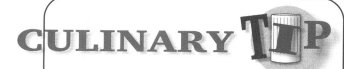

CULINARY TIP

USING LARGE EGGS—Most commercial kitchens use large eggs. Therefore, most standardized recipes assume that large eggs will be used. A large egg weighs at least 2 oz.

• Thaw frozen eggs in the refrigerator and use them in baked dishes that will be thoroughly cooked.

Egg Grades & Quality

The U.S. Department of Agriculture is responsible for grading eggs according to three designations. From highest to lowest, they are Grade AA, Grade A, and Grade B. These grades designate several qualities, such as an egg's appearance when it is cracked into a pan, and the characteristics of the yolk, the white, and the shell. See Fig. 17-2.

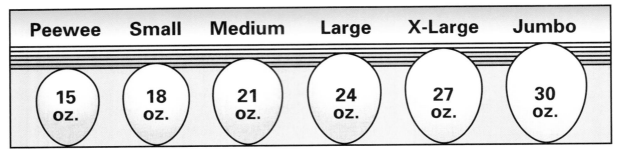

Fig. 17-3. The range of eggs is determined by the weight per dozen.

■ **Size.** Size is part of the grading process. There are six categories: jumbo, extra large, large, medium, small, and peewee. The size is not determined per egg, but by the weight per dozen. See Fig. 17-3.

Forms of Eggs

Eggs are sold in three forms: fresh, frozen, and dried. Each form has particular uses. Egg substitutes are available for people with dietary concerns such as high cholesterol. One egg substitute is made with albumin and a vegetable substitute for the yolk. Another substitute consists of soy products, making this a poor choice for recipes that require eggs as the thickening agent. Eggs are used in many recipes to thicken, bind, and add moisture, color, and flavor. Eggs are also a perfect breakfast food.

■ **Fresh eggs.** Fresh eggs are used in commercial kitchens and for home use. Because the yolk gets flatter as it ages, the appearance of a poached egg is better when the egg is fresh.

■ **Frozen eggs.** Frozen eggs are high-quality fresh eggs that are pasteurized (PAS-chuh-rized) and then frozen. **Pasteurized** egg products are heated at very high temperatures for a short time in order to destroy bacteria. They come in large containers

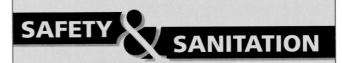

PREVENTING SALMONELLA—Salmonella bacteria are found in a chicken's intestinal tract. It is a serious health concern when using raw or undercooked eggs. To avoid salmonella poisoning:

• Refrigerate eggs immediately.
• Use only pasteurized egg products.
• Don't use eggs that are broken or cracked.
• Be careful not to drop any shell pieces in with the liquid egg.
• Wash work surfaces, tools, equipment, and your hands thoroughly.

and need to thaw for a couple of days in the refrigerator before they can be cooked. Frozen Grade A eggs are often used in commercial kitchens for scrambled eggs and other recipes that call for beaten eggs. For example, **soufflés** (soo-FLAYS), or puffed egg dishes, can be made with frozen eggs.

■ **Dried eggs.** Dried eggs are **dehydrated** (dee-HI-dray-tuhd), which means that the water is removed. They are used in commercial foodservice operations.

BREAKFAST BREADS & CEREALS

Bread may be an even more popular breakfast item than eggs. Toast, muffins, biscuits, scones, and bagels are some of the many choices. Nearly every customer who orders an egg item will want bread with it. Many customers choose a bread item as the mainstay of their favorite breakfast.

Cereals appear on all breakfast menus and are served either hot or cold. Cereals are made from grains such as wheat, corn, rice, and oats, and are a good source of carbohydrates. Breakfast cereals should be stored in airtight containers.

Quality Breakfast Breads & Cereals

Once breads are baked, they become stale quickly. It is necessary to consider how far in advance you will be able to prepare and bake breads before they are served.

■ **Ready-made breads.** Breads that are made in advance and delivered to foodservice establishments are called **ready-made breads**. The choice of quality pre-prepared breads on a breakfast menu is almost unlimited. Bagels, scones, doughnuts, muffins, croissants, and English muffins are just a few examples. The only breakfast bread items that are routinely prepared to order are toast, pancakes, French toast, and waffles. See Fig. 17-4.

■ **Hot cereals.** Hot cereals typically fall into two categories:

• Granular cereals, such as grits or farina.

• Whole, cracked, or flaked cereals, such as oatmeal and cracked wheat.

Hot cereals are served with milk or cream and white or brown sugar. Sometimes small ceramic bowls called **ramekins** (RAM-ih-kihns) filled with raisins, fresh fruit, or nuts are served with cereal. Hot cereals are a welcome menu choice for many older people as well as health-conscious people of all ages. See Fig. 17-5.

■ **Cold cereals.** Many cold cereals are purchased ready to eat. Some restaurants make their own special blend of granola (gruh-NOH-luh), a blend of grains, nuts, and dried fruits. Like hot cereals, cold cereals are served with milk or cream, sugar, and sometimes fresh fruit, such as sliced strawberries or bananas. Cold cereals are often a favorite breakfast choice for both children and adults. They are available in quantity portioning machines and as individual portions.

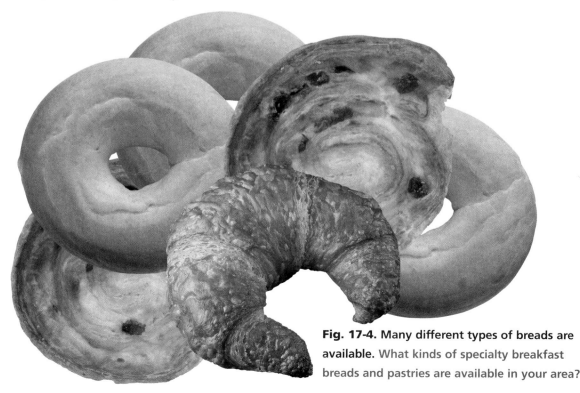

Fig. 17-4. Many different types of breads are available. What kinds of specialty breakfast breads and pastries are available in your area?

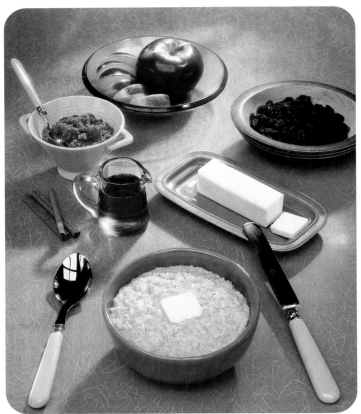

Fig. 17-5. There are many delicious accompaniments for hot cereal.

⊠ QUICK SERVICE BREAKFASTS

Most restaurants that serve breakfast offer a variety of similar options and combinations. Eggs are often served either scrambled, over easy, hard, basted, poached, or as omelets. Eggs usually come with a choice of toast, biscuits, or an English muffin. Egg dishes may also be accompanied by meat, such as bacon, ham, or sausage.

Breads such as pancakes, French toast, and waffles can be ordered in combination with eggs and a meat choice, or alone; for example, a stack of three to five pancakes with butter and syrup or fruit toppings.

Potatoes are often served as a side dish for breakfast such as home fries, hash browns, and cottage fries. Home fries are usually diced or sliced. Hash browns are shredded and may include onions and seasonings. Cottage fries are cut into ½-inch thick circles.

More often than not, breakfast items may be ordered á la carte so that the customers can create their own combination of foods. Learning to prepare breakfast items quickly and with skill is necessary for the successful foodservice professional.

SECTION 17-1   Knowledge Check

1. What are the four safety considerations to follow when storing and using fresh eggs?

2. Which grade of egg would you use in scrambled eggs, poached eggs, and hard-cooked eggs?

3. What are some reasons you might choose pre-prepared breads for a breakfast menu, and what exceptions would you make?

MINI LAB

Working in teams, create three different breakfast menus. Be sure to include eggs, meat, potatoes, and breads as menu selections. Challenge another team to regroup your menus into a fourth menu option.

Meat & Egg Preparation

OBJECTIVES

After reading this section, you will be able to:

- Prepare breakfast meats.
- Describe at least four ways to cook eggs.
- Prepare breakfast egg dishes.

BREAKFAST meats and eggs are easy to cook. Most breakfast meat and egg dishes can be prepared quickly and do not require much advance preparation. Nonetheless, timing breakfast meat and eggs with accompanying breakfast foods, such as pancakes or waffles, is a practiced skill.

✖ COOKING BREAKFAST MEATS

The most common breakfast meats—ham, bacon, and sausage—have relatively high levels of fat. Because bacon can be made of nearly 70% fat, it will shrink a great deal during cooking. Additional fat does not need to be added when cooking breakfast meats.

The best way to cook breakfast meats is on a low temperature. Do not overcook them. Meat becomes dry, tasteless, and tough if overcooked.

■ **Ham.** Precooked ham slices are typically served with breakfast dishes. The ham slices only need to be warmed and browned slightly under the broiler or on the griddle before serving.

■ **Bacon.** Most bacon served with breakfast is made from pork, although turkey bacon is sometimes offered as an alternative. To help reduce shrinkage, cook bacon on a low temperature, and use an oven when cooking bacon in quantity. Use the following steps to cook bacon:

Baked Ham Slices

YIELD: 50 SERVINGS   SERVING SIZE: 1½ OZ.

Bake:
1. Preheat the oven.
2. Place the food product on the appropriate rack.

HACCP:
Hold at 135°F or above.

HAZARDOUS FOOD:
Ham

NUTRITION:
Calories: 82.6
Fat: 5.71 g
Protein: 7.34 g

INGREDIENTS

5 lbs.	Ham, fully-cooked, boneless, trimmed of fat

METHOD OF PREPARATION

1. Preheat the broiler or oven to 350°F.

2. Slice the ham into 1½-oz. portions, and lay out on sheet pans.

3. Bake to an internal temperature of 145°F, or about 10 minutes. Remove, and transfer to hotel pans for service. Hold at 135°F or above.

---

1. Arrange the bacon in single strips on a sheet pan lined with parchment paper.

2. Cook at 300°F–350°F until the bacon is almost done.

3. Remove from the oven. Be very careful not to spill the hot grease.

4. Finish cooking the bacon on the griddle.

5. Blot to remove excess grease and serve.

■ **Sausage.** Sausage is generally made from fresh pork, although turkey and chicken sausage are also served at some restaurants. It comes in both patties and links. Sausage must be cooked until it is well done but not dry and hard.

In most restaurants, sausage is cooked in bulk. It is often first cooked in the oven and then finished to order on the griddle. Because sausage links are wrapped in casings that help hold in moisture, it is easier to prevent them from drying out when cooking than it is for sausage patties.

■ **Plating cooked meats.** Most breakfast meats are served in combination with eggs and potatoes on the same plate. Sometimes, especially with large omelets, the meat may be served as a side dish on a separate plate. Ham slices should be neatly sliced, and sausage and bacon should be attractively arranged on the plate.

✗ COOKING EGGS

Knowing how to cook eggs properly is important from taste and presentation standpoints, but it is a health issue as well. Overcooked eggs may be tough and rubbery, but undercooked eggs pose a serious health threat.

Cooking eggs at a moderate temperature is very important. Overcooking eggs at a high temperature results in a tough, rubbery, and discolored final product. In addition, the flavor may be affected. Likewise, eggs that are left in a steam table will turn green if they get too hot and begin to overcook.

■ **Protein coagulation.** It is important to understand that coagulation, or the temperature at which egg protein becomes solid, varies with different parts of the egg. In general, whole beaten eggs coagulate at about 156°F, with whites coagulating at a slightly lower temperature than yolks. Because of this, it is possible to make eggs sunny-side up, for example, that have soft yolks but cooked whites.

■ **Curdling.** When making scrambled eggs that are mixed with a liquid such as milk, the coagulation temperature increases to 180°F. Most burners set on "high" are much hotter than that, meaning

GREEN EGGS?

Have you ever wondered where the term *green eggs* comes from? When hard-cooked eggs are overcooked, a green ring may form around the egg yolks. The green color is simply the reaction between sulfur and iron compounds at the surface of the egg yolk. Green yolks in hard-cooked eggs can be avoided by using the proper cooking time and heat level, and by rapidly cooling the cooked eggs.

When preparing scrambled eggs, there is also the hazard of producing green eggs. Using stainless steel pans and low heat, cooking in small batches, and serving as soon as possible after cooking help keep scrambled eggs from turning green.

APPLY IT!

Divide into four teams. Each team will prepare a serving of eggs. Record your observations about cooking time, and the appearance and flavor of the eggs.

Team A. Prepare two hard-cooked eggs according to recipe directions for cooking and standing time.

Team B. Prepare two hard-cooked eggs following the recipe, but allow the eggs to stand 5 minutes longer than the recipe directions.

Team C. Prepare two scrambled eggs according to recipe directions using medium heat.

Team D. Prepare two scrambled eggs according to recipe directions, but use high heat.

Contrast the eggs prepared by each cooking method. What are the differences between the eggs cooked by teams A and B and the eggs cooked by teams C and D?

that eggs can easily become over-cooked at that setting. The eggs and solids may separate, or **curdle** (KUHR-duhl), resulting in a tough yet watery egg dish.

Fried Eggs

Fried eggs are the most popular breakfast egg dish. For best results, use Grade AA eggs in any fried egg dish. Fried eggs must be cooked to order and served immediately. In some quick-service operations, fried eggs are cooked in egg rings to produce a uniform shape. However, most fried eggs are cooked in a pan on the rangetop or on the griddle.

When turning an egg on the griddle, be sure to flip the egg by sliding the spatula underneath. Then lift one side up and over, leaving one edge of the egg touching the griddle. See Fig. 17-6.

Poached Eggs

Poached eggs are a popular breakfast choice. It's best to use very fresh eggs for poaching since they hold their shape better when the yolks and whites are firm. Break one egg at a time into a small dish. Then add each egg to simmering water that contains an acid such as vinegar. This will cause the egg to coagulate quickly. Avoid using boiling water to poach eggs because it causes the eggs to separate and become tough.

CHAPTER 17 Breakfast Cookery **395**

Fig. 17-6.

TYPE OF EGG	DESCRIPTION	METHOD
Sunny-side up	Egg is not flipped over during cooking, so the yellow yolk stands up. The yolk should be well-visible, highly mounded, and yellow.	Make sure you do not break the yolk when cracking the egg into the pan. Cook on medium heat for about 4 min. until the white is firm.
Basted	A type of sunny-side up egg. The yolk will have a thin cover of white on it.	Egg is cooked in butter over low heat. The butter is spooned over the egg as it continues to cook, "basting" it. **Variation:** Instead of basting with butter, add 1–2 tsp. of water and cover the pan so the steam cooks the top of the egg.
Over-easy	Egg is turned over during frying and cooked so that the yolk is still liquid when served and cut.	Cook about 3 min. on the first side over medium heat, then turn it and cook about 2 min. on the other side.
Over-medium	The yolk is partly cooked.	Cook a little longer than for over-easy.
Over-hard	The yolk is firm and fully cooked.	Cook until the yolk is completely firm but not overcooked and rubbery.

Scrambled Eggs

Scrambled eggs are usually made with whole eggs. However, egg whites can be substituted for customers who prefer fewer calories and less fat and cholesterol. See the step-by-step process for making scrambled eggs.

1. Break eggs into a bowl and whisk them until they are well blended. Stir in a little milk or cream if desired.

2. Heat butter in a sauté pan, or on a griddle if you are preparing many orders at once. When the butter sizzles, add the egg mixture.

3. Cook over low to medium heat, stirring slowly with a spatula by shifting portions of the egg mixture as it coagulates, allowing the uncooked egg to run underneath the cooked portion. See Fig. 17-7A to the right.

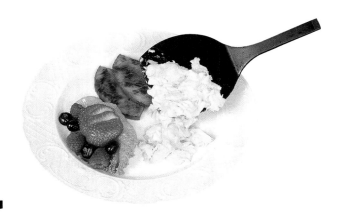

4. When eggs are set, but not overly hard, they are done. Scrambled eggs continue to cook a little after being removed from the pan.

5. Remove the eggs from the heat. The eggs will still be soft, shiny, and moist. They should not be green or brown. See Fig. 17-7B below.

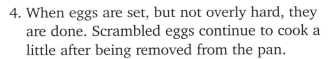

Omelets

The omelet (AHM-leht) is an egg specialty in many different countries. A seasoned omelet pan and high heat are required to make a beautiful omelet. When you **season**, or condition, a pan, you seal the surface with a layer of baked-on oil to prevent sticking.

■ **French and American omelets.** Both French and American omelets are folded omelets; however, the difference between these two types of omelets is that French omelets must be stirred and shaken simultaneously, which takes practice. Though French omelets require practice to prepare, they have two big advantages over American omelets:

- They are lighter and puffier in texture.
- They are faster to cook.

American omelets are made by following these steps:

1. Crack eggs into a bowl and whip with a wire whisk.

2. Place the pan on the burner and turn the burner on high heat. When the pan is hot, add clarified butter and swirl it around to coat the entire inside of the pan.

3. After pouring the beaten eggs into the hot pan, do not stir them or shake the pan. Simply lift up the edges of the egg mixture with a spatula to allow the uncooked portion to run underneath.

4. Once the eggs are set but still soft, add the filling and then fold the omelet neatly. Cook the omelet until lightly firm. See Fig. 17-8.

5. Slide the omelet out of the pan and onto a plate.

The ingredients used for omelet fillings are as broad and creative as your imagination. Vegetarian omelets are very popular.

■ **Soufflé omelets.** The three basic parts of a **soufflé** (soo-FLAY) omelet include the base, filling, and beaten egg whites. To make a

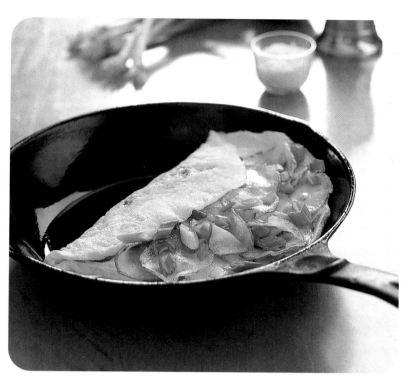

Fig. 17-8. Omelet fillings can vary. Try including sautéed vegetables, crumbled cooked bacon, smoked salmon, sliced mushrooms, grated cheese, or salsa.

CULINARY TIP

WHIPPING EGG WHITES—Sometimes egg whites are beaten to a light, frothy consistency to add lightness to scrambled eggs and omelets. To produce successfully beaten egg whites, remember these hints:

1. Egg whites will foam better if you allow the eggs to sit at room temperature for an hour before separating and whipping.

2. Use a clean metal or glass bowl when whipping egg whites. Residue on the bowl or the whisk will prevent egg foam from developing.

3. When breaking eggs, do not let any yolk break into the whites. If you do, they will not beat well.

4. Use beaten egg whites immediately.

Shallow-Fry:
1. Heat the cooking medium to the proper temperature.
2. Cook the food product throughout.
3. Season, and serve hot.

GLOSSARY:
Whisk: to aerate with a whip
Julienne: matchstick strips

HACCP:
Cook to 145°F.
Hold cooked eggs at 135°F or above.
Hold uncooked egg mixture below 41°F.

HAZARDOUS FOODS:
Eggs
Milk

NUTRITION:
Calories: 506
Fat: 41.9 g
Protein: 28.9 g

CHEF NOTES:
When the eggs have set in the sauté pan, place the pan under a broiler for 10–15 seconds to finish cooking the eggs; then roll the omelet out of the pan and onto a preheated serving plate. This creates a fluffier presentation and ensures that the eggs are well done.

Omelet with Cheese

YIELD: 10 SERVINGS   SERVING SIZE: 8 OZ.

INGREDIENTS

30	Eggs, cracked into a bowl
	Salt and ground white pepper, to taste
8 oz.	Milk
5 oz.	Clarified butter, melted
3 oz.	Fresh parsley, washed, excess moisture removed, and chopped
1 lb.	Cheese, **julienne**

METHOD OF PREPARATION

1. Season the eggs with salt and pepper. Add the milk, and **whisk** until the eggs are well combined.
2. Heat an omelet pan with ½ oz. of butter.
3. When hot, add a 6-oz. ladle of egg mixture.
4. Shake the pan, and mix the eggs until they begin to firm, lifting the edges to allow liquid egg to run underneath (see chef notes).
5. When the omelet is almost firm, or 145°F, turn it over.
6. Place the cheese in the center of the omelet, fold, and roll onto a preheated dinner plate. Serve immediately, or hold at 135°F or above.
7. Repeat the procedure until all of the eggs are cooked.
8. Garnish with chopped parsley.

soufflé omelet, a heavy sauce, such as a Béchamel (bay-shah-MEHL) sauce, is prepared and egg yolks are added to it. The filling is then added to the sauce and the egg whites are folded in. The mixture is baked in a soufflé dish and served immediately. If soufflé omelets are prepared in a restaurant, the base can be made ahead. Then the filling and egg whites can be combined with the base and the omelet finished.

■ **Frittatas.** Frittatas (frih-TAH-tuh) are flat, open-face omelets. They are not folded over like most omelets. Instead, the eggs are beaten and mixed with the precooked filling ingredients, and then cooked over low heat without stirring. A frittata can either be turned over and cooked on the other side, or placed under the broiler until the top is set and slightly browned. Frittatas are usually cut in wedges and served warm or cold. See Fig. 17-9.

■ **Quiche.** A quiche (KEESH) is a pie crust filled with a mixture of eggs, cream, cheese, and vegetables or meat. Quiche can be served for breakfast, lunch, or dinner.

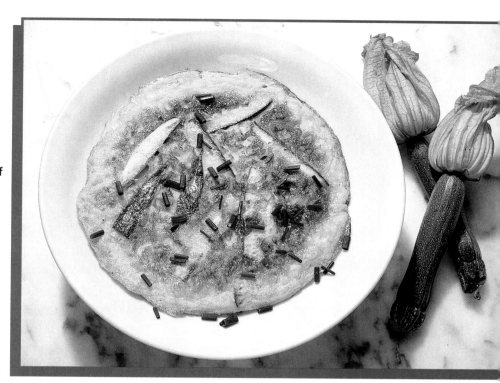

Fig. 17-9. Frittatas can be works of art. What ingredients do you think are a part of this frittata?

Shirred Eggs

Shirred (SHEHRD) eggs are covered with cream or milk and sometimes bread crumbs. They are usually prepared in ramekins lined with a variety of ingredients, such as spinach, bread, ham, bacon slices, or artichoke hearts. The egg is cracked into the center of the cup and topped with grated cheese, onion, and herbs. Sauces may also be added after baking. To make shirred eggs:

1. Butter the ramekins to keep ingredients from sticking.
2. Line the ramekins, if desired, with a slice of ham or other appropriate ingredient.
3. Carefully break an egg or two into the dish.
4. Sprinkle with salt and pepper, if desired.
5. Bake the eggs at 350°F until they begin to set.
6. Add grated cheese, onion, or fresh herbs, such as minced fresh thyme, parsley, or basil, to the top and finish baking.

■ **Serving shirred eggs.** Arrange garnishes on one side of the plate. Over the eggs, spoon sauces such as hot cream, mild green chili, mushroom, tomato, or brown sauces; or place asparagus tips, sautéed mushrooms, or crumbled bacon on top.

Simmering Eggs in the Shell

Soft-, medium-, and hard-cooked eggs are all cooked in the shell in hot water. These eggs are sometimes referred to as hard- or soft-cooked. Since boiling water can cause eggs to become tough and discolored, place the eggs in cold water. Then simmer the eggs until they reach the desired level of doneness.

Eggs prepared properly should have evenly cooked whites and yolks. The yolk should not be discolored, and the egg should not have an unpleasant taste. To make simmered eggs in the shell, follow this procedure:

1. Make sure the eggs have been at room temperature for an hour before cooking to prevent the shells from cracking as they cook.
2. Fill a saucepan with enough water to cover the eggs.
3. Simmer the eggs according to the level of doneness desired:

Soft-cooked	3 minutes
Medium-cooked	4–5 minutes
Hard-cooked	8–10 minutes

Plating Eggs

Fried eggs and scrambled eggs are often served with combinations of toast, meat, potatoes, and a garnish. Each item should be placed on the plate in an attractive and uncluttered manner. The garnish used most often is a twisted slice of orange or a slice of melon.

Shirred eggs are served in their individual baking dishes, which are then placed on a larger plate that holds the side dishes. The garnish will often be placed on top of the shirred eggs. Paprika, cinnamon, and parsley are common garnishes for shirred eggs.

Omelets must be attractively placed on a plate, with a simple garnish, such as a sprig of parsley. Because there may be many ingredients in an omelet, numerous side dishes are usually not required. Omelets can be served with meat or potatoes. Often, only toast is served.

Simmered eggs are usually served in egg cups in the shell, accompanied by side dishes and various garnishes. The customer uses a spoon to gently tap the top of the shell to break it and then scoops out the insides for eating. See Fig. 17-10.

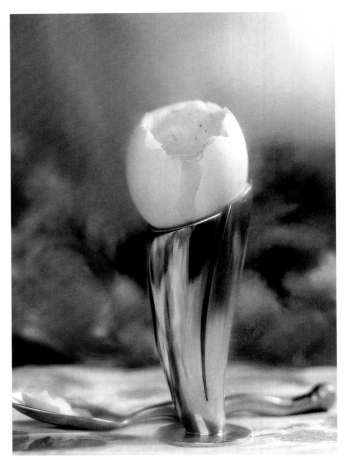

Fig. 17-10. For many people, eating soft-cooked eggs out of an egg cup is a special taste treat. Why do you think they are served in this fashion?

SECTION 17-2 Knowledge Check

1. Summarize how to cook the three most popular breakfast meats.
2. Name three things to remember when successfully whipping egg whites.
3. Describe four types of cooked eggs along with one important tip when preparing each of them.

MINI LAB

Working in teams, prepare and plate the following egg dishes: fried eggs, scrambled eggs, shirred eggs, omelets, and soft-, medium-, and hard-cooked eggs. Share what you learned about your team's experience in cooking eggs.

Breakfast Breads & Cereals

OBJECTIVES

After reading this section, you will be able to:

• List quick breads served with breakfast.

• Prepare pancakes, waffles, and French toast.

• Prepare hot cereals.

BREADS and cereals are an essential component of breakfast menus. Rarely is an order of eggs sold without a breakfast bread. Quick breads, such as pancakes and waffles, toast, and French toast are generally cooked to order. Many operations purchase ready-made pastries, muffins, and doughnuts. This section will introduce you to breakfast breads and cereals.

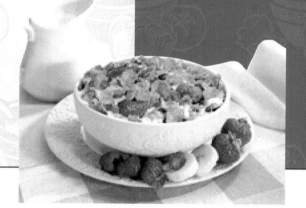

⊠ USING READY-MADE BREADS

Ready-made or convenience (kuhn-VEEN-yuhts) breads include pastries, doughnuts, and many kinds of quick breads, such as muffins.

Pastries

Pastries, also known as Danishes, are popular breakfast delicacies. They are made from yeasted, sweetened dough with butter, which gives pastries the rich flavor that makes them so appetizing. Egg is added to some kinds of pastries, which usually are filled with almond paste, fruit, cream cheese, or nuts. Bear claws and strudel are two of the more well-known types. Pastries can be made from scratch, frozen doughs, or purchased ready-made.

Doughnuts

Doughnuts are sweetened, deep-fried pastries that often are ring-shaped. There are two categories: cake and raised. Cake doughnuts are leavened with baking powder, while raised doughnuts get their leavening power from yeast. Cake doughnuts are heavier than raised doughnuts, and they tend to have spices or chocolate added to the mix as well.

Quick Breads

Many foodservice operations rely on **quick breads**, a type of bread made from quick-acting leavening agents such as baking powder. They are easy to make, even from scratch, because they do not need yeast. Chapter 29 covers quick breads in depth. In restaurants, they complement the main entrée or serve as the main part of a continental breakfast. Muffins are especially useful because they are so versatile. Varieties from corn muffins to seasonal berry muffins can add interest and nutrition to any breakfast menu choice.

While muffins are popular, loaf-style quick breads fulfill the same function and are very tasty. Cranberry nut bread, banana bread, and zucchini bread are just a few of the quick breads that can add interest and pizzazz to a breakfast menu. Biscuits are small, round quick breads. They are usually rich and savory, but can be sweet. Biscuits should have a light, tender, and flaky texture. **Scones** (SKOHNZ) are a type of quick bread similar to biscuits that are often cut into triangle shapes. See Fig. 17-11.

Quick breads are enhanced by servings of flavored cream cheese, jellies, and jams alongside them. These toppings and spreads are usually served in small ramekins on the side or in prepackaged, individual servings.

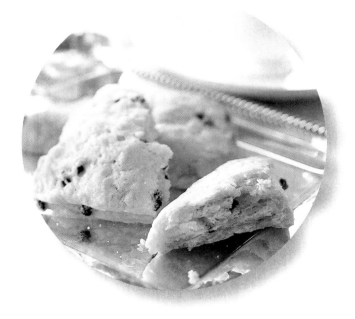

Fig. 17-11. Scones can add a special and creative twist to a breakfast menu. What condiments could be served with this quick bread, and how would you rate the overall presentation?

⊠ PREPARING PANCAKES & WAFFLES

Both pancakes and waffles are made from batters that can be mixed ahead of time and refrigerated. In general, wet and dry ingredients are mixed separately. The wet ingredients are then added to the dry ingredients and stirred until well moistened. Do not overmix.

■ **Pancake preparation.** Ladle ¼-cup portions onto a 375°F griddle that has been well greased. To ensure round pancakes, leave enough room for spreading. When bubbles appear on the top of the pancakes, it's time to turn them. You should only turn, or flip, a pancake once. If you turn it more often, the pancake will get hard. Cook pancakes until they are nicely browned on both sides.

■ **Waffle preparation.** Follow these steps in preparing waffles:

1. Mix the wet ingredients in one bowl and the dry ingredients in another. Add the liquid ingredients to the dry ingredients.
2. Beat the egg whites into soft peaks, add sugar, and beat until the peaks are stiff.
3. Fold the egg whites into the batter.
4. Pour the batter onto a preheated and lightly oiled waffle iron and then close the top.
5. Cook until the signal on the waffle iron indicates that the waffles are done.

■ **Plating pancakes and waffles.** Pancakes and waffles are cooked to order and should be served piping hot. Pancakes get tough and waffles lose their crispness when held too long. They may be served with a variety of condiments, including butter, hot syrup, cold flavored syrups, fruit toppings, whipped cream, or nuts. Pancakes and waffles are often served with a side order of breakfast meats, eggs, or both.

COOKING TECHNIQUE:
Bake

Bake:
1. Preheat the oven.
2. Place the food product on the appropriate rack.

HACCP:
Hold at 135°F or above.
Hold unused batter at 41°F or below.

HAZARDOUS FOODS:
Milk
Pasteurized eggs

NUTRITION:
Calories: 478
Fat: 11.6 g
Protein: 9.63 g

CHEF NOTE:
For best results, make pancakes to order.

Pancakes with Maple Syrup

YIELD: 50 SERVINGS

SERVING SIZE: 4 EACH

INGREDIENTS

1 qt.	Pasteurized eggs
3 qt.	Milk
2 tbsp.	Vanilla extract
6 lbs.	All-purpose flour
8 oz.	Sugar
6 oz.	Baking powder
1 lb.	Butter, melted
2 qt.	Maple syrup, heated and kept warm at 140°F

METHOD OF PREPARATION

1. Preheat the griddle.

2. In a mixing bowl, beat the eggs.

3. Add the milk and vanilla to the beaten eggs, and mix well. Set aside.

4. Mix all of the dry ingredients together. Add the egg mixture, and whisk to a smooth batter.

5. Stir the butter into the mixture.

6. Let the batter rest for 1 hour before using.

7. To cook, pour approximately 2 oz. of batter on a seasoned, lightly buttered griddle.

8. Cook until the bubbles appear on the top and the edges become dry.

9. Turn over, and bake the other side until done. Serve immediately, or hold at 135°F or above.

10. Hold the unused batter at 41°F or below if not used immediately.

11. Serve with warm syrup.

12. Repeat the procedure until all of the batter is used.

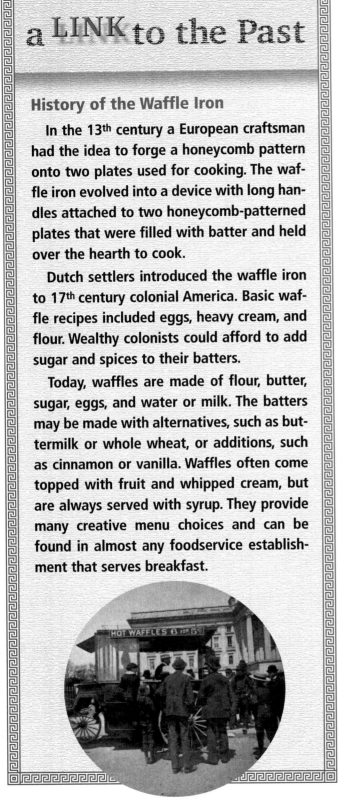
Fig. 17-12. Create an artful presentation by arranging the French toast and sprinkling confectioner's sugar over the top.

✖ PREPARING FRENCH TOAST

French toast is a favorite breakfast choice. It can be made with different types of bread, including white and sourdough. French toast is a good way for commercial kitchens to utilize day-old bread. Day-old bread is firmer and holds batter well when it's grilled.

Some establishments choose to serve crunchy French toast. After soaking the bread in the egg mixture, the bread is dipped in low-fat bran or corn cereal and then flash-fried. Crunchy French toast is often served with sliced bananas and low-fat syrup.

■ **French toast preparation.** Follow these steps for preparing and cooking French toast.

1. Slightly beat eggs.
2. Add milk, sugar, cinnamon, nutmeg, and vanilla to the eggs and stir well.
3. Dip each slice of bread into the batter, being sure to thoroughly coat each side. For crunchy French toast, dip in crushed cereal after battering.
4. Brown each side of the bread slices on the griddle to preferred doneness.

■ **Plating French toast.** French toast is cut in half diagonally, and the halves are arranged attractively on a plate. It may be served with hot or cold syrup, fruit toppings, jam or preserves, powdered sugar, or a combination of these items. French toast may also be served with a side of breakfast meat or with eggs. See Fig. 17-12.

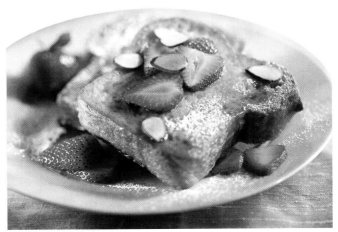

✖ PREPARING HOT CEREALS

Hot cereals are another popular breakfast choice for restaurant patrons. Whole, cracked, or flaked grains are the cereals most often served. To make hot cereal, follow the directions carefully. Here are some general guidelines:

1. Measure water in a cooking pot and bring it to a boil. Milk or cream can be used instead, but it is much more expensive.

2. Add a measured amount of cereal carefully, stirring it constantly.

3. As soon as it thickens, stop stirring. If you continue, the cereal will become gummy.

4. Cover, reduce the heat, and cook until done.

5. Keep the cereal covered until ready to serve.

■ **Plating hot cereals.** Hot cereals are served in a bowl that is usually placed on top of a plate. Milk, half-and-half, or cream may be served along with

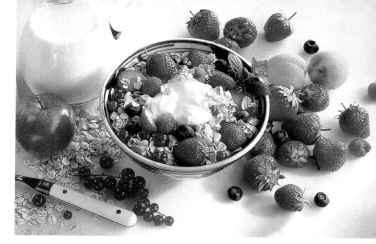

Fig. 17-13. An assortment of cereal toppings add both visual interest and flavor to cereal. **What do you think are customers' favorites?**

small ramekins of raisins, nuts, or fruit slices. Toast, English muffins, or a quick bread may also be served with hot cereals.

✖ SERVING COLD CEREALS

Cold cereals require no preparation. They are served with milk or cream, fruit, nuts, or sugar. Some restaurant owners offer their customers a wide variety of individual servings of boxed cold cereals, while other establishments may offer granola along with accompaniments, such as fruits, nuts, and yogurt. See Fig. 17-13.

■ **Plating cold cereals.** Cold cereals are served with milk, half-and-half, or cream and sliced fruit such as bananas or berries. Cold cereals are often accompanied by toast or quick breads.

> ## CULINARY TIP
>
> **PREVENTING LUMPY CEREAL**—To prevent lumps in hot cereals, add a small amount of cold water to the cereal before adding the cereal to boiling water. This keeps the grains separate. Be sure to factor in the amount of cold water to the total amount of water added in the cooking process.

SECTION 17-3 — Knowledge Check

1. List three kinds of quick breads served for breakfast.

2. Name four condiments to serve with waffles or pancakes.

3. Describe the steps for cooking hot cereal.

MINI LAB

In teams, prepare waffles, pancakes, French toast, or hot cereals. Serve your classmates and evaluate the results of each breakfast bread and cereal.

SECTION SUMMARIES

17-1 Breakfast foods include both hot and cold cereals, meats, breads, and eggs all prepared in a variety of combinations and styles.

17-1 Eggs are a basic ingredient to many breakfast foods.

17-1 Grading eggs allows the foodservice operations to choose the best grade of egg for their particular need.

17-2 Correctly preparing breakfast meats will help to retain their flavor.

17-2 Egg preparation varies from simply fried and seasoned eggs to whipped omelets that are blended with milk and folded over ingredients.

17-2 Types of cooked eggs include fried, poached, scrambled, omelet, shirred, and simmered.

17-3 Quick bread choices include muffins, biscuits, sweet loaf breads, and scones.

17-3 Because of the easy preparation of French toast, pancakes, and waffles, they are considered quick breads.

17-3 Hot cereals are often served with a variety of sides, which may include fresh fruit and milk.

CHECK YOUR KNOWLEDGE

1. What is the recommended limit of time eggs should be left at room temperature?

2. How is the size of the egg determined?

3. A restaurant placed its weekly order for eggs, ordering both Grade AA and B eggs. Why would two grades of eggs be needed?

4. List three ways to use frozen eggs.

5. What is the result of cooking breakfast meats at a lower temperature?

6. At what temperatures do the different parts of the egg coagulate?

7. Contrast an American omelet, a soufflé omelet, and a frittata.

8. Name four spreads or toppings to serve with quick breads.

9. How do cooks prevent hot cereals from becoming lumpy?

CRITICAL-THINKING ACTIVITIES

1. Currently there are not many low-calorie, low-cholesterol, or low-fat alternatives on your menu except margarine as a butter substitute. What recommendations would you make?

2. Why do you think that milk or cream is sometimes added in the preparation of scrambled eggs?

WORKPLACE KNOW-HOW

Problem solving. If you find eggs left out on the prep station over night, what would you do with them and why?

LAB-BASED ACTIVITY: Preparing an Omelet

STEP ❶ Working in teams, create an American omelet. You will need to determine:
- What type of fillings, if any, will be added to the omelet? See the choices below.
- What type of cheese, if any, will be added to the omelet?
- What type of bread choices will be served with the omelet?

STEP ❷ Determine what mise en place will be necessary for preparing the omelet.
- Will meats need to be cooked ahead of time?
- Will vegetables need to be diced and cheese grated?
- Prepare a list of tasks in logical order.

STEP ❸ Cook the omelet according to the method chosen, adding ingredients when appropriate.

STEP ❹ Plate your omelet and the bread choice.

STEP ❺ On a separate piece of paper, answer the following questions:
1. How did the mise en place contribute to the omelet's preparation?
2. When considering the end result of the omelet, is there anything you would do differently next time? Why or why not?
3. When considering the end result of the omelet, is there anything you would do to produce a different result?
4. What would you do differently and why?

Omelet Fillings

- Steamed or sautéed vegetables
- Chopped onion or scallions
- Grated cheese
- Crumbled cooked bacon
- Diced ham
- Smoked salmon
- Sour cream

- Minced chives
- Salsa
- Sliced avocados
- Sliced mushrooms
- Sliced green or black olives
- Creamed chicken
- Chopped tomatoes

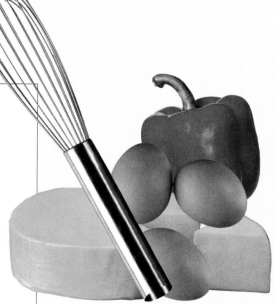

Garde Manger Basics

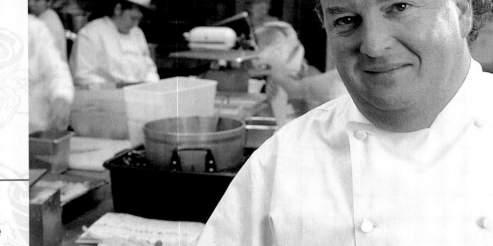

What Is Garde Manger?

KEY TERMS

- garde manger
- brigade
- garnish
- quenelle
- tournéed

OBJECTIVES

After reading this section, you will be able to:

- List the items a garde manger needs to consider in preparing food.
- Identify the types of food prepared in the garde-manger work station.
- Describe the tools and techniques used by a garde manger.
- Prepare decorative garnishes.

THE **garde manger** (gahrd mohn-ZHAY), also known as the pantry chef, is the person responsible for the planning, preparation, and artistic presentation of cold foods. These foods include salads and salad dressings, cold hors d'oeuvres (or DERVS), fancy sandwiches, canapés (KAN-uh-pays), and cold platters.

✖ GARDE MANGER FOODS

The garde manger plans dishes using many fresh ingredients, including vegetables, fruits, prepared meats, fish, seafood, breads, and cheeses. Simple ingredients are used to create and artistically present:

- Hors d'oeuvres.
- Salads.
- Canapés.
- Fancy sandwiches.
- Fruit, cheese, meat, relish, and combination trays.
- Garnishes for all types of dishes. See Fig. 18-1.

The garde manger manages the garde-manger department in restaurants, large hotels, and many catering operations. He or she manages a team of people called a **brigade**. Each member of the brigade specializes in a particular type of cold food preparation. In planning this kind of food, the garde manger brigade considers:

- The cost of ingredients and the time required to prepare dishes.
- The use of many different food items so the menu is interesting. See Fig. 18-2.
- The use of different colors and textures throughout the meal.
- The appeal of the food to the people eating the meal and the ability of the brigade to prepare the dishes.

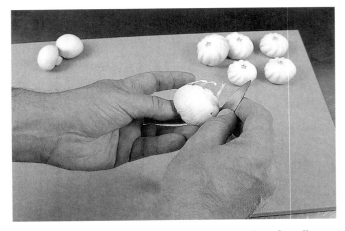

Fig. 18-1. The garde manger creates garnishes for all types of dishes.

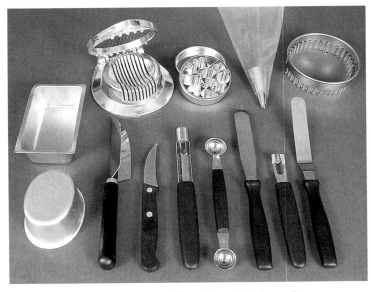

Fig. 18-3. In addition to a well-equipped kitchen, the garde manger needs specialized equipment.

✖ GARDE-MANGER EQUIPMENT

The garde manger needs a well-planned and well-equipped work area. Usually, the garde-manger work station will include:

- Walk-in and reach-in refrigerators and freezers.
- Several ranges to cook foods, such as roast beef and turkey, before they are served cold.
- Smoker.
- Ice-cube makers.
- Food slicer or mandoline.
- Food processor.
- Individual molds, pastry bags, a garnishing set that includes a variety of garnishing knives, offset spatulas, an egg wedger and slicer, and large cutters. See Fig. 18-3.

✖ PREPARING GARNISHES

Many garnishes are created in the garde-manger work station. The word **garnish** comes from the French word "garnir," which means "to decorate or furnish." In the culinary world, it means to use food as an attractive decoration. It is something that should add real value to the dish by increasing its nutritional value and visual appeal. See Fig. 18-4.

A simple garnish, such as a sprig of mint or a wedge of fruit, can be used to add eye appeal in the form of color and balance.

Fig. 18-2. The brigade's job is to create an interesting menu from varied ingredients.

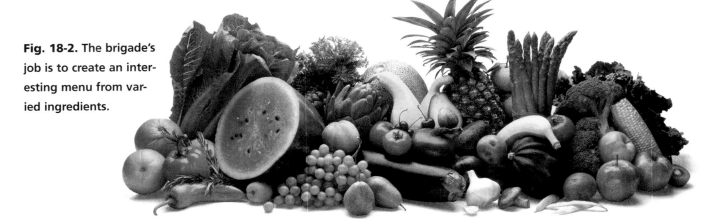

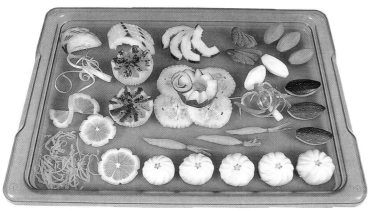

Fig. 18-4. Garnishes add that special touch. Can you name these garnishes?

A garnish should complement the flavors and textures of the meal. Mushrooms, cucumbers, scallions, pickles, radishes, and lemons are good examples of garnishes. A **quenelle** (kuh-NEHL), or a purée of chopped food formed into shapes, can also be used. See Fig. 18-5.

Having the appropriate tools will allow you to create all sorts of garnishes. You can make some garnishes with everyday tools, such as forks, spoons, and paring knives. For example, use a fork to score, or make ridges in a diamond-shaped pattern, on pies and meats. You can make quenelles by using two spoons to shape a purée. Fruits and vegetables can be cut into decorative shapes with a paring knife. For more elaborate garnishes, use the tools from a garnishing set as described in Fig. 18-6 on pages 412-413 (**Garnishing Tools**).

Fig. 18-5.

GARNISH NAME	INGREDIENTS
Clamart (clah-MAHR)	Peas
Crécy (kray-CEE)	Carrots
Doria (DO-ree-ah)	Cucumbers cooked in butter
Dubarry (doo-bah-REE)	Cauliflower
Fermière (fayr-MYAYR)	Carrots, turnips, onions, and celery
Florentine (FLOOR-en-teen)	Spinach
Judie (joo-DEE)	Braised lettuce
Lyonnaise (ly-uh-NAYZ)	Onions
Niçoise (nee-SWAHZ)	Tomatoes cooked with garlic and black olives
Parmentier (pahr-mahng-TEE)	Potatoes
Princesse (pran-SES)	Asparagus
Provençale (pro-vohn-SAHL)	Tomatoes, garlic, parsley, and mushrooms or olives
Vichy (VEE-shee)	Carrots cooked and glazed
Bouquetière (boo-kuh-TYEHR)	Bouquet of vegetables
Jardinière (jahr-duh-NIHR)	Garden vegetables
Primeurs (pree-MUH'R)	First spring vegetables
Printanière (prin-tan-YAIR)	Spring vegetables

Garnishing Tools

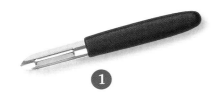

1. Vegetable Peeler

Although this tool is used mainly to shave the skin from fruits and vegetables, it's also an important garnishing tool. Use it to make decorative carrot curls and chocolate curls.

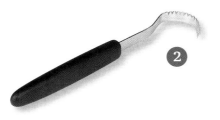

2. Butter Cutter

This tool has four surfaces that can be used to make a range of garnishes, from curls to grooves to marble-size balls. For best results, use ice-cold butter and a butter cutter that has been warmed in hot water.

3. Zester

To add eye appeal and flavor to your dish, use the zester to remove small strips of the colored part of citrus peels. You can also use this tool to shave pieces from colorful vegetables, such as carrots and radishes.

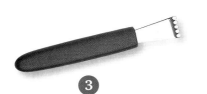

4. Melon Baller

A melon baller or a Parisienne (puh-ree-zee-EHN) scoop can be used to scoop out balls of cheese, potatoes, butter, and melons.

5. Tournée Knife

You can use this small knife with a curved blade to make **tournéed** (toor-NAYD), or turned, vegetables that have an oblong shape with seven equal sides and blunt ends.

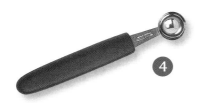

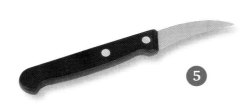

6. Channel Knife

This odd-shaped knife can be used to pare strips of peel from citrus fruits and thin grooves from carrots and cucumbers.

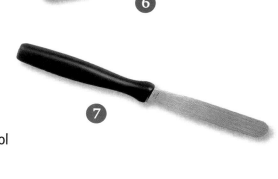

7. Decorating Spatula

This spatula has a flat blade that is used to create attractive designs on soft foods, such as cream cheese, butter, and frosting.

8. Paring Knife

The paring knife has a sharp, V-shaped blade. You can use this tool to carve fruits and vegetables.

9. Fluting Knife

Because this knife is small and very sharp, you can use it to do detail work that requires a lot of control. A fluting knife has a triangular blade that is about 2 inches long.

SECTION 18-1 Knowledge Check

1. What items must a garde manger consider when selecting foods?
2. What kinds of foods are prepared in the garde-manger department?
3. What is a garnish?

MINI LAB

Prepare garnishes using the following foods: cucumbers, carrots, tomatoes, leeks, melons, and radishes. Be sure to follow safe knife handling and garnishing tool techniques.

Salads & Salad Dressings

KEY TERMS

- kale
- radicchio
- mesclun
- croutons
- dressing

OBJECTIVES

After reading this section, you will be able to:

- Prepare salads made from a variety of greens.
- List the main types of salads served during a meal.
- Identify the four main parts of a salad.
- Prepare salad dressings.

WHAT comes to your mind when you hear the word salad? A bowl of lettuce with a few carrots and tomatoes mixed in? These ingredients may make up a common salad, but they're just the beginning. Salad really means a mixture of one or several ingredients with a dressing. Vegetables, leafy greens, meat, fish, cheese, pasta, fruits, nuts, and grains can all be used in salads.

✖ GREEN SALADS

Salads can include many different kinds of ingredients, from vegetables to meat. Chefs often include fresh herbs, nuts, or even edible flower petals. By carefully combining leafy greens, you can make your salad mild or spicy. By mixing different greens, you can make salads with interesting, unusual flavors and textures. Three main types of greens and leafy vegetables are used in tossed salads:

- Traditional greens.
- Flavor-adding greens.
- Herbs and other specialty items.

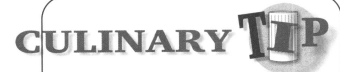

CULINARY TIP

NUTRIENTS IN SALAD GREENS—A mixture of darker greens increases nutrients such as vitamins A and C, and minerals such as potassium. This will also increase the amount of folic acid in the salad.

Traditional Greens

The traditional greens, which include mostly lettuces, have been used for years as the main ingredient in tossed salads. Because they have a mild flavor, they can be used by themselves or combined with other more flavorful greens. The romaine and butterhead lettuces add flavor and texture. Iceberg lettuce has less flavor, but it stays crisp longer than other greens.

Spinach is not a lettuce like the other members of the traditional greens group. This dark green, leafy vegetable is full of calcium and adds color and flavor to salads. Try to select small, young leaves for a delicate, distinctive flavor and texture. Spinach must be thoroughly washed and have its stems removed before serving.

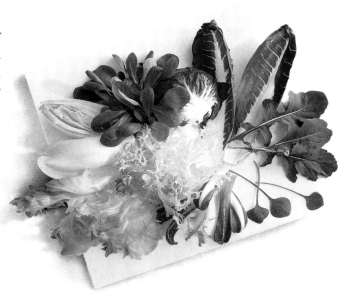

Fig. 18-7. Lettuce varieties add a wide range of textures and flavors to salads.

Flavor-Adding Greens

In recent years, many flavor-adding greens—some spicy, some bitter, and some with a distinct yet delicate flavor—have made their way into salads. These greens include arugula (ah-ROO-guh-luh), mizuna (mih-ZOO-nuh), and chicory (CHIH-kuh-ree). They are classified as greens, although they may be red, yellow, brown, or white. They add interesting new flavors, textures, and colors too. See Fig. 18-7.

Other flavor-adding greens that are more familiar as cooked vegetables are also being added to salads as raw leafy greens. These greens include **kale**, a cabbage with curly green or multicolored leaves, and Chinese cabbage.

Herbs & Other Specialty Items

Sprigs of fresh herbs, such as oregano and basil, can be included in green salads to add flavor and complement other dishes. Parsley, dill, mint, sage, chives, and cilantro all make flavorful additions. Only a small amount of an herb is needed. Leaves can be either torn or chopped.

There are two specialty items to consider including in salads. **Radicchio** (rah-DEE-kee-oh) is a cabbagelike plant with a slightly bitter, red leaf. In small quantities, radicchio adds color and

flavor to fresh salads. **Mesclun** (MEHS-kluhn) is a popular mix of baby leaves of lettuces and other more flavorful greens, such as arugula. The benefits of using mesclun are its tender texture and subtle flavors.

■ **Edible Flowers.** With new ingredients being added to salads, it shouldn't come as a surprise that some flowers are tailor-made for salads. They add unusual flavors, dashes of bright color, and interesting textures. Edible flowers should be purchased from a grower that doesn't use pesticides.

Nasturtiums (nuh-STUHR-shuhmz), with their tangy blossoms, are one of the more popular floral additions. Pansy, primrose, rose, and violet petals are also popular. Flowering herbs, such as oregano, rosemary, chives, and thyme, can be used as well.

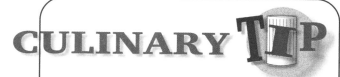

USING EDIBLE FLOWERS—When adding flower petals, be sure to clean them well. Dirt and insects can hide deep down in the petals and slip unnoticed into the salad.

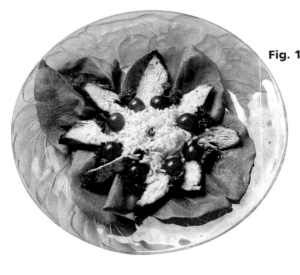

Fig. 18-8. Appetizer salad.

ing than by cutting. However, in a large foodservice setting, it may not be practical to tear all the greens. Cutting is faster, and if done quickly with a well-sharpened blade, will produce perfectly acceptable salad greens.

■ **Storing greens.** It's best to use up greens every day. Be sure to keep them in their original packaging. Store them three to four degrees above freezing away from ripening fruits, such as tomatoes and apples.

✖ SALAD PREPARATION TECHNIQUES

Selecting good, healthful greens for salads can make the difference between a flavorful salad with lots of texture, and a limp, tasteless dish. Here are some things to keep in mind when you're working with salad greens.

■ **Choosing quality greens.** Whenever possible, purchase salad greens daily, selecting ones that appear fresh and undamaged. Slightly wilted greens can be revived if they're submerged in ice water for 30–60 minutes. Remove the greens from their packing cartons and wash them just before preparing the salad.

■ **Preparing greens.** Leafy greens, which grow close to the ground and easily pick up dirt, dust, insects, and sand, need to be thoroughly cleaned before preparation. To ensure proper cleaning of salad greens, separate the leaves and submerge them in cold water several times to rinse off all dirt and grit. Never clean greens under running water or you'll bruise the greens. Change the water several times if necessary. Lift greens out of the water. Don't drain the water from the bottom. Be sure to dry the leaves thoroughly with paper towels.

Once the greens have been well cleaned, cut or tear them into bite-size pieces. Many culinary experts believe greens are less damaged by tear-

✖ TYPES OF SALADS

There are five main types of salads—appetizer salads, accompaniment salads, main-course salads, separate-course salads, and dessert salads. Each is served at a different time during the meal.

■ **Appetizer salads.** An attractively arranged salad served before the main course is designed to whet the appetite. Depending on the meal and setting, it might be quite simple, such as a salad of all greens, a garnish, and a vinaigrette (vihn-uh-GREHT) dressing. It might also be a more elaborate salad with poultry, fish, beans, or seafood as the main ingredient. See Fig. 18-8.

■ **Accompaniment salads.** An accompaniment salad is one that is served with, and complements, the main dish. If the main course is light, the accompaniment salad might be a heavier pasta, bean, or potato salad. If the main dish is heavy, a lighter tossed green salad is appropriate. The accompaniment salad should not include food items served with the main course.

■ **Main-course salads.** A main-course salad replaces the regular main course. This salad should function as a balanced meal, with a variety of vegetables and a protein serving, such as fish, chicken, beans, or a chicken or egg salad. Fruit can also be included. All ingredients should be attractively arranged. See Fig. 18-9.

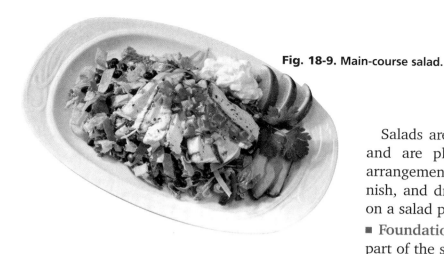

Fig. 18-9. Main-course salad.

■ **Separate-course salads.** A light salad served after the main course to refresh the appetite, a separate-course salad is served before dessert. This type of salad should be simple. For example, it may be just a small portion of mixed greens with a light vinaigrette dressing or a small salad of fresh citrus fruits or asparagus.

■ **Dessert salads.** A dessert salad made from fruits, nuts, gelatin, or a combination of similar ingredients can be served with a sweetened dressing. This dressing often has a whipped cream base.

✖ SALAD STRUCTURE & ARRANGEMENT

Since salads can be served before, during, or after the main course depending upon the type of meal service used, salad-making can be a challenging, creative task. To plan and prepare appealing salads that go with an overall menu, follow these guidelines:

• Combine colors, textures, and flavors that look and taste good together.

• Don't repeat ingredients in salads that appear in other dishes. For example, if chicken is the main dish, don't plan chicken salad as an appetizer.

• Match the type of dressing used with the salad ingredients. Select salad ingredients that complement the rest of the meal. For example, if the main course is heavy, end the meal with a light salad of seasonal fruit.

Salads are made from a variety of ingredients and are plated in a particular order. Salad arrangements consist of a foundation, body, garnish, and dressing that are arranged attractively on a salad plate.

■ **Foundation.** The foundation, or base, is the part of the salad on which the rest of the salad is built. This foundation may be a bed of lettuce leaves or another type of vegetable or fruit. See Fig. 18-10A below.

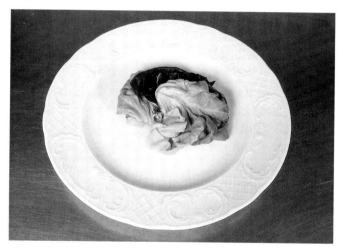

■ **Body.** The body of the salad features the main ingredients. These ingredients range from lettuce to vegetables to pasta to meat, poultry, or fish. See Fig. 18-10B below.

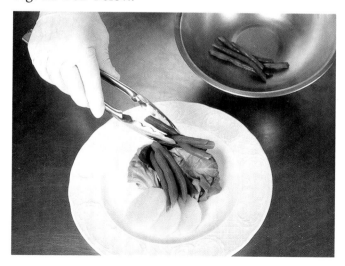

- **Garnish.** The salad garnish, like other garnishes, is a colorful element that adds eye appeal to the plate. Although a garnish such as an herb or a lemon wedge may be used, the garnish might also be hard-cooked egg wedges or black olives. See Fig. 18-10C below.

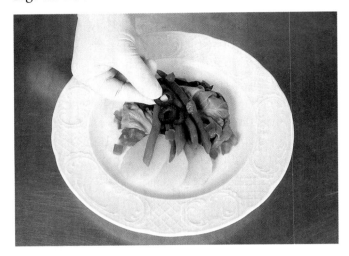

Other common salad garnishes include fruits, cheese, and nuts. **Croutons** (KROO-tawnz), or small pieces of bread that have been grilled, toasted, or fried and sometimes seasoned, are another popular garnish.

- **Dressing.** The salad **dressing** is a sauce that holds the salad together. Many types of dressing are available. See Fig. 18-10D below.

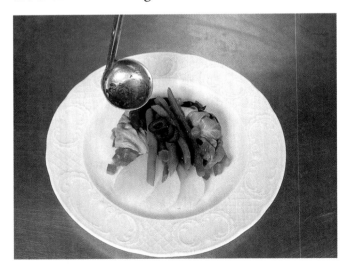

◼ SALAD DRESSINGS

Dressings are added to salads to give them flavor and to help hold the ingredients together. When planning dressings, pick ones that go well with the flavors in the salad but do not overwhelm them. Check the greens to make sure they are dry. Otherwise, the dressing will not stick to the greens.

There are many different types of salad dressings. Most dressings, however, fall under four main categories: vinaigrette, fatty (or creamy), cooked, and fruit dressings.

- **Vinaigrette dressings.** A mixture of vinegar and oil, most vinaigrette salad dressings have a ratio of three parts oil to one part vinegar. For interesting flavors, try different vinegars, such as balsamic or herbed, and different oils. Olive oil and nut oils are especially flavorful. Also, consider adding chopped fresh herbs if they complement the greens or other dishes in the menu. Pasteurized eggs can be added to any vinaigrette. When the eggs are well beaten with the other ingredients, the vinaigrette doesn't separate and clings well to the greens.

- **Fatty dressings.** Dressings made from mayonnaise or other dairy products can be used on green salads, fruit salads, and potato or pasta salads. As the name suggests, however, these fatty dressings have a high fat content and should be used in moderation. Some of the most common are creamy French, Thousand Island, Russian, ranch, bleu cheese, and creamy Italian.

- **Cooked dressings.** These dressings have a cooked ingredient as well as a thickening agent, such as cornstarch. Some cooked dressings use vinaigrette as a base. For example, you may add hot bacon or hot Dijon mustard to a vinaigrette dressing. Others use little or no oil. Most cooked dressings generally have a more tart flavor than mayonnaise-based dressings.

- **Fruit dressings.** Depending on what they accompany, these dressings may be sweet, tart, or spicy. They may be made with puréed fruit or fruit juice.

EMULSIONS

An emulsion is a mixture of two liquids that typically do not blend with each other. In food, an emulsion is a liquid fat and a water-based liquid held together. Vinaigrette is an example of a short-lived emulsion. Because of surface tension, the oil pulls away from the vinegar and the vinegar pulls away from the oil. Only when shaken will the oil and vinegar emulsify.

When an emulsifier is added to an oil and vinegar mixture or an oil and water mixture, a major change takes place. An emulsifier helps liquids, such as vinegar and oil, combine uniformly and remain combined without separating. Egg yolk is a natural emulsifier.

Basically, an emulsifier changes the surface tension of the two liquids. For example, egg yolk sticks to the surface of the oil droplets, keeping them separated and evenly dispersed throughout the vinegar or the water. In this particular case, it forms a common condiment known as mayonnaise.

APPLY IT!

Complete the following procedure to see the differences between a short-lived emulsion and a more permanent emulsion. You will need the following: ⅓ c. vinegar; ⅔ c. cooking oil; 1 pasteurized egg yolk; and a small bowl or bottle with a lid.

1. Place ⅓ c. vinegar and ⅔ c. oil into the small bowl. Record your observations.

2. Place the lid on the bowl and shake it for 10 seconds. Record your observations.

3. Let the bowl sit for 10 minutes. Record your observations.

4. How do your observations differ? Is this an example of a short-lived or permanent emulsion?

5. Now add the pasteurized egg yolk to the bowl. Replace the lid and shake the bowl again. Let the mixture sit for a few minutes. Record your observations.

6. How does adding the egg yolk change the mixture?

7. Does the mixture appear to be a short-lived emulsion or a permanent emulsion? Why?

Making Vinaigrette Dressings

Vinaigrette dressings are easy to prepare. They should sit at room temperature for several hours before being served. They also need to be stirred well right before use. Use these steps to make a vinaigrette dressing:

1. Combine the vinegar and herbs or spices in a bowl. Select an appropriate vinegar and add complementary herbs, spices, or mustard.

2. Slowly add the oil to the vinegar with a whisk. Blend well. Generally, the ratio of oil to vinegar is three to one.

3. If pasteurized eggs are added, whisk them thoroughly until the dressing is well blended.

Making Fatty Dressings

Mayonnaise is often the key ingredient in a fatty dressing. Even though most commercial kitchens buy ready-made mayonnaise, it's important to know how to make your own. Mayonnaise is made by whipping oil, lemon juice, pasteurized egg yolk, and flavorings. The following steps tell how to make a fatty dressing:

1. Whisk together dairy products to make the base of the dressing. Mayonnaise and dairy products, such as buttermilk, provide a good dressing base.

2. Blend lemon juice into the creamy base.

3. Add herbs, spices, condiments, and chopped eggs or vegetables for variety. See Fig. 18-11.

Making Cooked Dressings

Cooked dressings often have little or no oil and include a thickener. These dressings may be savory or sweet. Sweet cooked dressings may include fruit or fruit juice. To prepare a cooked dressing:

1. Mix the sugar, starch, and flavorings in a stainless steel bowl.

2. Add the eggs as directed by the recipe and beat until smooth.

3. Place the milk or fruit juice in a saucepan and bring it to a simmer, being careful not to scorch it.

4. Gradually beat the milk or fruit juice into the egg mixture.

5. Cook the mixture until no starch flavor remains. Stir constantly.

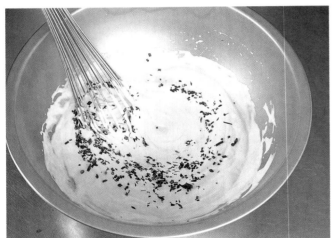

Fig. 18-11. Fatty dressing can be modified with herbs and condiments to go well with many types of salads.

SECTION 18-2   Knowledge Check

1. What categories of leafy greens are used in tossed green salads? Give two examples of specific greens in each category.

2. Describe the five main types of salads and when they are served.

3. Choose one of the main types of dressings and describe how it's made.

MINI LAB

In teams, prepare one of the following dressings: vinaigrette, fatty, cooked, or fruit. Evaluate the dressing. Serve the dressing on mixed salad greens to another team in your class.

Cheese

OBJECTIVES

After reading this section, you will be able to:

- Describe the five main types of cheese.

- Identify cheeses from each of the five main types.

- Explain how to store cheese so it is sanitary and well preserved.

CHEESE is one of the most varied foods available today. There are hard cheeses, such as Cheddar and Colby Jack, that can be sliced for sandwiches or grated and baked in hot dishes. There are soft cheeses for spreading on bread and crackers and crumbly cheeses that taste great in salads. Each cheese has its own distinct flavor and texture. Cheese is also nutritious, with plenty of protein and calcium.

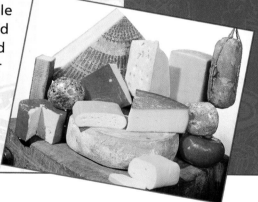

☒ TYPES OF CHEESE

Because there are so many types of cheese, you can always find one that will go well with other foods you're serving. To select cheeses that will go well with the menu, it helps to be able to identify the different types of cheese.

Hard Cheeses

The hard cheeses include Cheddar and Colby (KOHL-bee). These cheeses are made by a process called **cheddaring**, in which slabs of the cheese are stacked and turned. This process squeezes out the **whey**—the liquid portion of coagulated milk—and gives the cheese its special texture.

Cheeses with holes in them, including Gruyère (groo-YAIR), Jarlsberg (YAHRLZ-behrg), and Swiss, are also hard cheeses. The holes come from healthful bacteria growing inside the cheese that release gases during the ripening process. These cheeses are excellent for cheese trays, fancy open-face sandwiches, or with desserts.

■ **Ripening cheese.** The texture and flavor of most cheeses are affected by a process called ripening. During **ripening**, healthful bacteria and mold are at work in the cheese, changing its texture and flavor. As cheeses are ripened, they are stored in a temperature- and humidity-controlled environment. Ripening can occur from the surface of the cheese to the inside. Or, it can occur from the inside of the cheese outward.

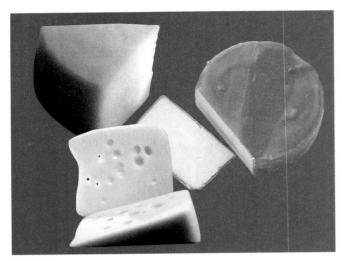

Fig. 18-12A. White cheddar, Romano, and Swiss cheese are hard cheeses.

Hard cheeses have been carefully ripened for a long time. The extra aging enhances their flavor and makes them dry and hard. Parmesan and Romano (roh-MAH-noh) are two other popular hard cheeses. Each has its own special flavor and is available in many market forms. See Fig. 18-12A.

Try adding Parmesan, with its deep, spicy flavor, to pasta salads for a buffet luncheon. Romano and Asiago (ah-SYAH-goh) have a sharp flavor that goes well with many salads. Include small chunks in main-course salads to add flavor and to make them more filling. You can also sprinkle finely grated hard cheeses on one of the tossed green salads featured in a buffet line.

Firm Cheeses

Firm cheeses are not brittle, hard, or soft. Some are flaky and others are dense. Provolone (proh-voh-LOH-nee) is a firm cheese with a mild flavor, smooth texture, and light ivory color. It's good on cold sandwiches as well as cooked dishes, such as pizza and pasta.

When ripened for several months, Gouda (GOO-dah), a Dutch cheese made from cow's milk, has a firm texture. It has a mild, nutty flavor that's popular for snacks and for dipping. Gouda is often sold in wheels of varying sizes that are covered with yellow or red wax.

Edam (EE-duhm) is another Dutch cheese made from cow's milk that is firm when aged. It is light yellow in color and has a slightly salty taste. See Fig. 18-12B.

Semisoft Cheeses

Semisoft cheeses are smooth and easy to slice. They come in two types. One type features the buttery cheeses that slice well. The other includes the softer, pungent cheeses, often called "veined" cheeses because they have veins of mold running through them. The mold in these cheeses is put into the cheese during ripening. It is beneficial, not harmful. In fact, it is this mold that gives the cheese its unique flavor.

■ **Buttery Semisoft Cheeses.** The texture of the buttery semisoft cheeses comes from the way the **rind**, the outer surface of the cheese, is made. These rinds vary in texture, color, and thickness. Cheeses such as Port du Salut (pohr doo suh-LOO) and Havarti (hah-VAHR-tee) are sealed in wax before they're ripened. Other semisoft cheeses, including Bel Paese (bel pah-AYZ-eh), form their own rind as they ripen. All these cheeses are excellent for making canapés and serving on cheese trays. The king of pizza, Mozzarella cheese, is also a semisoft cheese. See Fig. 18-12C.

Fig. 18-12B. Firm cheeses include Provolone, Edam, and Gouda.

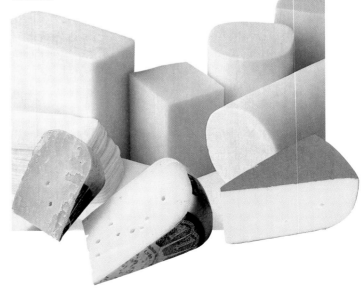

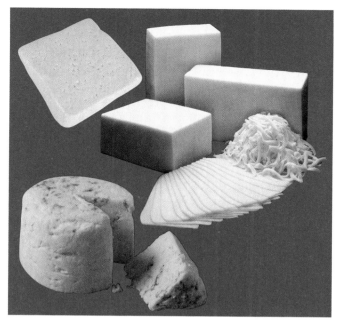

Fig. 18-12C. Havarti, Mozzarella, and Roquefort cheese are semi-soft cheeses.

■ **Veined Semisoft Cheeses.** The semisoft cheeses that have blue veins running through them have strong, distinctive flavors and aromas. The flavor comes from the type of beneficial mold allowed to grow in each one. The aging process also affects the flavor. All the veined cheeses are ripened in caves or in rooms that have the same moisture and temperature as caves.

Gorgonzola (gohr-guhn-ZOH-lah), Roquefort (ROHK-fuhr), and Stilton (STIHL-tuhn) are some of the most popular veined cheeses. They are named after the places where they are made. They are excellent cheeses to spread on crackers for appetizers. They can also be crumbled and added to tossed salads and salad dressings.

Soft Cheeses

Soft cheeses have a thin skin and a creamy center. This category includes many different kinds of cheeses. Fresh, creamy Ricotta (rih-COH-ta) is a soft cheese, as is runny, pungent Camembert (ka-muhm-BAIR). Farmer's cheese is made from whole or partly skimmed cow's milk. It has a slightly tangy flavor and is milky white. Another soft cheese similar to cottage cheese is baker's cheese. It's used to make baked goods, such as pastries and cheesecakes. The difference between these soft cheeses is that some have been ripened while others have not. During the ripening process, the bacteria and mold in an unripened cheese alter its flavor and texture.

Fresh Soft Cheeses

Another word used to describe unripened soft cheese is "fresh." Fresh cheeses are not ripened, or aged, after they're formed into a final shape. Cream cheese, cottage cheese, and Mascarpone (mas-kahr-POHN-ay) are popular unripened soft cheeses. Ricotta and Mascarpone have a sweet flavor and are often used in baking desserts. Cream cheese is also used in baking desserts, such as cheesecake. See Fig. 18-12D.

Feta (FEH-tah) is another popular unripened soft cheese. A sharp-flavored cheese made from sheep's or cow's milk, it can be crumbled and added to tossed salads and breads, such as focaccia (foh-KAH-chee-ah).

Fig. 18-12D. Ricotta, Brie, and cream cheese are soft cheeses.

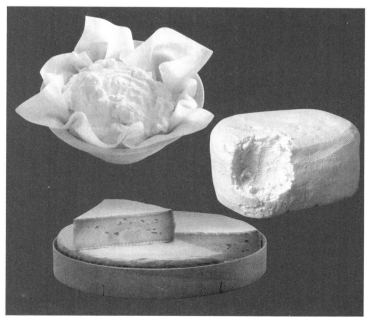

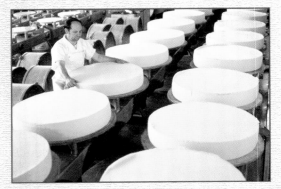
Ripened Soft Cheeses

Ripened soft cheeses have very different flavors and textures from unripened cheeses. High in butterfat, they have richer flavors and are runny and creamy when completely ripe. They are surrounded by a rind that bulges out when the cheese is ripe and ready to cut. If cut before they're ripe, these kinds of cheeses will have very little flavor and a dry texture. It's important to cut them only when they are really ripe, because they will not ripen once they've been cut. To test for ripeness, press firmly and gently in the cheese's middle before you cut it. If it's ripe, you'll feel some softness in the middle. If it's overripe, you'll smell an ammonia odor.

Camembert and Brie (bree) are the most well known ripened soft cheeses. Served ripe and at room temperature, they make excellent appetizers served with crackers. They are also good dessert cheeses, served with toasted bread rounds and fruit.

Specialty Cheeses

Specialty cheeses include pasteurized processed cheese and cold-pack cheese. **Processed cheese** is a combination of ripened and unripened cheese. These cheeses are pasteurized with flavorings and emulsifiers and poured into molds. An **emulsifier** is an additive, such as egg yolk, that allows unmixable liquids, such as oil and water, to combine uniformly. Once the cheeses have gone through this process, they do not continue to ripen. Since it does not continue to age the way other cheeses do, its flavor and texture remain the same for a long time. Even though pasteurized cheese is not as flavorful as other kinds of cheese, its long shelf life and consistency make it a good choice.

Cold-pack cheese, also known as club cheese, is another specialty cheese. It's a cheese product made from one or more varieties of cheese, especially Cheddar or Roquefort cheeses. The cheese is finely ground and mixed until it is spreadable. No heating is used to make cold-pack cheese.

✕ STORING CHEESE

Cheese needs special care. It is a moist substance with living organisms in it. To prevent it from drying out and to prevent harmful bacteria or mold from growing in it, it should be well wrapped and stored in the refrigerator. Cheeses that are not adequately wrapped will dry out and pick up flavors of other foods in the refrigerator. Loosely wrap soft cheeses with greaseproof or waxed paper.

✕ SERVING CHEESE

Because cheese is so versatile and comes in so many interesting flavors and textures, it can be served at breakfast, lunch, or dinner, and at any point during a meal. Cheese appetizers take the edge off a hungry crowd's appetite. Cheeses in main-course salads add flavor, substance, and nutrition. Some menus offer ripened cheeses, crackers, bread rounds, and fruit in place of dessert. See Fig. 18-13.

All ripened cheeses should be served at room temperature. To bring out their full flavor, take them out of the refrigerator 30–60 minutes before serving. Unripened, fresh cheeses should always be refrigerated until just before they're served. If you're preparing cheese boards or trays:

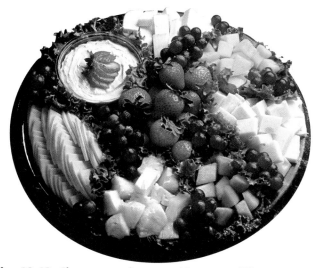

Fig. 18-13. Cheeses can be served in many different ways.

- Select cheeses with contrasting shapes and colors so the tray will look appealing.
- Choose cheeses that are easy to cut, such as the firm cheeses, the semisoft cheeses, and the ripened soft cheeses.
- Include a different knife with each type of cheese.
- Do not preslice the cheese. It will dry out and lose its special texture.
- Provide bread rounds, crackers, or sliced fruit with the cheese tray.

SECTION 18-3   Knowledge Check

1. How does aging affect cheese?
2. List the five main categories of cheese. Give an example of each.
3. Name at least three guidelines for serving cheese.

> **MINI LAB**
>
> Taste and identify different types of cheese. Give an example of how each type of cheese could be used in food service.

Cold Platters

- single-food hors d'oeuvre
- hors d'oeuvre variés
- finger foods
- canapé
- liner
- crudité
- antipasto

OBJECTIVES

After reading this section, you will be able to:

- Explain when hors d'oeuvres are served.
- List the main types of hors d'oeuvres.
- Prepare fancy sandwiches, fruit and cheese trays, and cold hors d'oeuvre platters.
- Describe a relish tray and the kinds of dips that accompany it.

COLD platters are an ideal way to offer guests many different kinds of interesting foods. They also work well in a variety of settings. At informal gatherings where people will be coming and going during the event, they are very convenient. In more formal settings, they bring people together and whet the appetite before the meal is served.

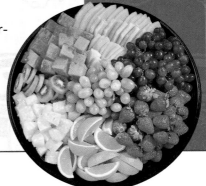

◩ COLD HORS D'OEUVRES

An hors d'oeuvre is a bite-size, tasty food that is served before the meal. Hors d'oeuvres can be very simple. They might just be a tray of olives, sliced vegetables, and dips. In other cases, they might be quite fancy, perhaps a tray of small seafood tarts. There are three main types of hors d'oeuvres.

■ **Single-food hors d'oeuvre.** Consisting of one item, a **single-food hors d'oeuvre** might be a jumbo shrimp.

■ **Hors d'oeuvre variés.** A combination of plated items with enough hors d'oeuvres for one person, **hors d'oeuvre variés** include about ten small food items.

■ **Finger foods.** Hors d'oeuvres presented on platters from which each guest serves him- or herself are called **finger foods**. Stuffed mushrooms, sliced vegetables often called crudités, small tarts, and canapés are examples of common finger foods.

In recent years, exactly when and how hors d'oeuvres are served has changed. People are loosening up a bit and looking for creative ways to make their meals and receptions interesting. When preparing and serving hors d'oeuvres as a traditional pre-meal food or as a complete meal, keep in mind these guidelines:

- Keep each food item small—one to two bites.

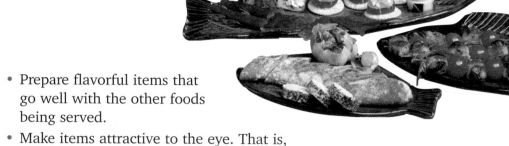

Fig. 18-14. Cold hors d'oeuvres can be served in a variety of ways to meet the needs of the event and the people attending.

- Prepare flavorful items that go well with the other foods being served.
- Make items attractive to the eye. That is, they should look good alone as well as with the other foods being served.

There are many different kinds of cold hors d'oeuvres. This section will focus on canapés and fancy sandwiches. See Chapter 21 for information on hot hors d'oeuvres.

Canapés

Have you ever eaten tiny, open-face sandwiches at a party or reception? Those flavorful, little sandwiches are called canapés (KAN-uh-pays). From the French word for "sofa," a **canapé** consists of a platform, or base, and a cushion, or topping.

- The base can be a cracker, toasted crustless bread, a thin slice of fried or fresh bread, sliced vegetables, or small pastry shells.
- The topping, sometimes called the nourishing element, can be anything from sliced meat, shrimp, and cheese to vegetable spreads.
- A spread, such as a flavored butter, mustard, cream cheese, or mayonnaise, to add flavor and prevent the base from getting soggy.

In addition to the base and the topping, a canapé might also have:

- A **liner** is an ingredient, such as a small lettuce leaf, that adds visual interest and texture.
- A garnish, such as an olive; pimiento (pih-MYEHN-toh); a sweet red pepper; onion slice; peas; or parsley sprig, to add visual interest and flavor.

The words creative and canapé go together. All kinds of meats, seafoods, cheeses, and vegetable spreads can be used alone or in combination. When selecting spreads, don't forget things like hummus (HOOM-uhs), a Middle-Eastern dish made from mashed chickpeas, lemon juice, garlic, and tahini (ta-HEE-nee), a sesame seed paste. Don't think that you have to stick with traditional breads, such as white, rye, and wheat. Although these can be used to make tasty canapés, try using herb breads and specialty breads that have chopped nuts or olives kneaded into the dough before baking.

If you're using vegetables as the base, consider using tomatoes, sliced cucumbers, mushroom caps, sliced zucchini, small Romaine lettuce leaves from the heart, and endive leaves. Vegetable spreads make excellent toppings for these vegetable bases. Follow these simple steps to make canapés.

1. Cut bread into basic geometric shapes and toast lightly. Let it cool. See Fig. 18-15.
2. Cover each piece of bread with a spread, if desired, to prevent bread from getting soggy. Add a liner such as a lettuce leaf.
3. Add toppings, from simple slices of meat to decorative vegetable spreads.
4. Add garnishes for flavor and visual interest.

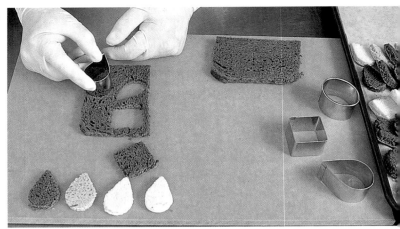

Fig. 18-15. Breads are cut into small geometric shapes, such as triangles, squares, rectangles, and circles, and then toasted lightly before other elements are added.

Fancy Sandwiches

The garde manger may be asked to prepare fancy sandwiches for many different occasions. These occasions may be as casual as a picnic or as formal as a reception. To prepare fancy sandwiches for more formal events, the garde manger must consider not just the breads and fillings but also the way the sandwiches are cut and presented.

One of the most eye-catching types of fancy sandwiches is a rolled sandwich filled with a spread and vegetables or cheese strips. See Fig. 18-16. To prepare these sandwiches, use the following five steps:

1. Cut several day-old loaves of bread into slices lengthwise. White, wheat, rye, and herb breads work well. Breads that contain nuts are not a good choice. A slicing machine will be needed for this step.

2. Cut the crust from all the slices using a serrated bread knife and roll each piece flat with a rolling pin. The bread should be less than ⅛ of an inch thick when you've finished rolling.

3. Cover each piece with a thin layer of a flavorful spread. Good fancy sandwich spreads include flavored butters, flavored and plain cream cheese, and vegetable spreads. You may also use softened blue-veined cheeses. If the main spread does not have a lot of fat, spread the bread with soft butter before adding the flavored spread. This will prevent the bread from getting soggy. All butters and spreads should be very soft to keep from tearing the bread.

4. Place the interior items at one end of the bread, and roll it up tightly. These items should be both tasty and colorful, such as cheese sticks, pimientos, green or black olives, pickles, and other pickled vegetables. Wrap the roll in plastic wrap and refrigerate for several hours.

5. When the roll is quite cold, unwrap it and cut the log into ½-inch slices with a slicer.

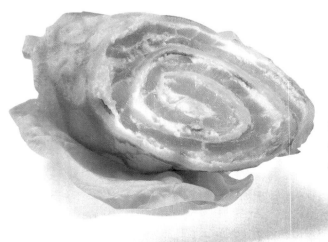

Fig. 18-16. A rolled fancy sandwich is an eye-catching way to combine interesting spreads and vegetables.

PREPARING COLD PLATTERS

Cold platters can be very simple or very complex. Here are some examples of typical foods that might be served on cold platters as part of a buffet, at a reception, or before a formal dinner:

- Platters of raw sliced vegetables served with dips. **Crudité** (kroo-dee-TAY) is the French word for "raw," or in this case, raw vegetables.
- Platters of specially prepared food items, such as canapés, salads on croutons, pinwheel sandwiches, or melon slices and prosciutto (proh-SHOO-toh).
- Platters of cheese, meat, fruit, or a combination can be served with dips, breads, sliced fruit, and crackers. Items can be combined to fit individual tastes.

Cold platters are a convenient way to offer guests tasty, nutritious foods in an informal format. In addition, cheese and meat trays provide high-quality protein. The breads and crackers that accompany them are full of energy-producing carbohydrates. When whole-grain breads are included, fiber, minerals, and other nutrients are also present. Fruits, as a base for cheese or served alone, add vitamins and minerals.

Cold platters give culinary professionals the chance to use their creative talents. A cold platter buffet consists of three main elements. See Fig. 18-17.

■ **Centerpiece.** This could be an uncut part of the main dish. The centerpiece for a cold meat platter, for example, may be a roast. It could also be a large, attractive bowl with a sauce or condiment. Not all centerpieces are meant to be eaten. They should, however, be made of edible items. For example, the centerpiece for a fruit platter could be a hollowed-out watermelon bowl filled with cantaloupe, honeydew, and watermelon balls.

■ **Serving portions.** These portions come from the main dish, such as slices of meat from a roast or sliced cheese. Portion sizes for meats average about 3 oz. For cheeses, portion sizes average about 1 oz. Display these servings artistically.

■ **Garnish.** This item should add both eye appeal and nutritive value. A garnish for a meat platter,

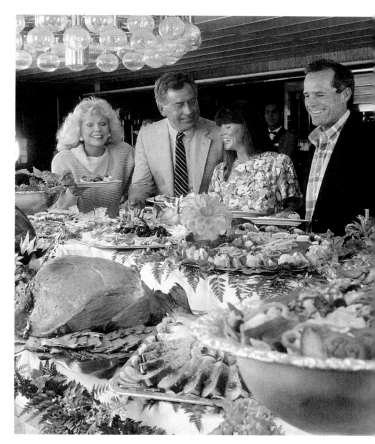

Fig. 18-17. A cold platter buffet.

for example, may be flower-shaped vegetables cut in sizes that are in proportion to the meat and cheese slices.

Here are some other things to keep in mind when preparing a visually appealing buffet:

1. Be sure the food is easy to pick up. Guests should be able to get individual servings without ruining the overall presentation of the buffet.

2. Keep it simple. No-frills displays hold up better than overdone ones.

3. Use attractive, durable platters that are suitable for what you're serving. Choices include mirrors, plastic, china, and silver or other metals. Because some metals discolor or leave a metallic taste, make sure they are covered with a liner or aspic (AS-pihk) before foods are added to the platter. Aspic is a savory jelly made from meat or vegetable stock and gelatin.

4. Don't remove a food item once you've placed it on the tray. Rearranging items on silver or mirrored platters will leave smudges. You must have a specific plan in mind before you begin arranging the platter. The best way to do this is to draw out a plan on paper. The plan should include shapes, sizes, color, number of items, and appropriate garnishes.

5. The platter must complement the overall buffet display. It should be visually appealing both on its own and as a part of the whole.

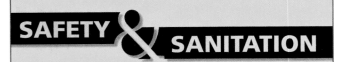

SAFETY & SANITATION

COLD PLATTERS—Since cold platters may sit out for several hours, it's important to keep them refrigerated until you serve them.

Fruit & Cheese Trays

You may prepare fruit and cheese trays as a main course for a lunch buffet or as a dessert course for a dinner buffet. Fruit is paired with cheese for two reasons. First, their flavors complement each other. Sweet, juicy fruits go well with earthy, rich cheeses. Second, cheese has more eye appeal when paired with fruit. The muted colors of cheese are enhanced by the vibrant colors of fruits, such as grapes, melons, apples, and pears.

There are many ways to prepare fruit and cheese trays. These trays are not always arranged with individual portions the way other buffet items are. Often, the trays are displayed with whole cheeses or large pieces of cheese. This arrangement is done partly because cheese dries out when it's cut. Cheese is also more attractive as a whole. Fruits, too, are not always displayed as individual portions. Many fruits become discolored when they are cut.

Choose cheeses based on their color, texture, shape, and flavor. Cheeses of varying colors and shapes make an attractive visual display, especially when combined with colorful fruits.

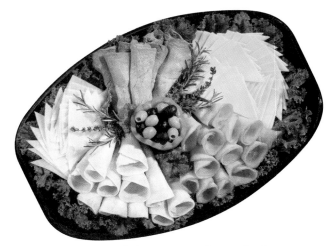

Fig. 18-18. Meats and cheeses are often paired on a combination tray.

Combination Trays

Combination trays may include meat with fruit, meat with cheese, or meat with fruit and cheese. See Fig. 18-18. Some combination trays also include raw or marinated vegetables.

An example of a combination tray is **antipasto** (ahn-tee-PAHS-toh)—the Italian word for "before pasta." A typical antipasto tray includes cold meats, such as Genoa salami and various hams, assorted cheeses, olives, and marinated vegetables. Fruits, such as cantaloupe and other melons, may also appear on an antipasto tray.

Relish Trays

Relish trays are attractive arrangements of raw, blanched, or marinated vegetables. Sometimes relishes are called crudités. The kinds of vegetables used and the way they are arranged is only as limited as the creativity of the chef.

You may arrange an assortment of carrots, cucumbers, mushrooms, radishes, zucchini, squash, peppers, jicama, cauliflower, broccoli, olives, cherry tomatoes, and endive with a special sauce for dipping. You can also use marinated vegetables. These vegetables have been soaked in a liquid, typically made of vinegar, oil, herbs, and spices. Relish vegetables should be attractively cut and served on a platter.

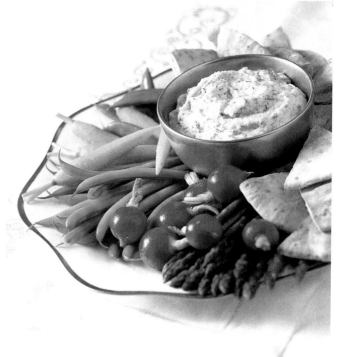

Fig. 18-19. Relish trays can be nutritious, tasty, and attractive.

- **Dips.** Relish trays are usually served with a dip that complements the vegetables featured. See Fig. 18-19. Creamy dips, made from a base of mayonnaise, sour cream, or cream cheese, are an especially good choice. Dips can be flavored with herbs, spices, clams, garlic, and chopped hard-cooked eggs. Dips can be served inside carved vegetables or breads.

Cold Hors d'Oeuvre Platters

Mixed hors d'oeuvres or a single type of hors d'oeuvre can be served as a cold platter. When served in this way, they should be artistically arranged. The arrangement should also make it easy for people to pick up an individual hors d'oeuvre without having to touch or move others.

Here are some other important things to keep in mind when preparing cold hors d'oeuvre platters:

- Season each hors d'oeuvre carefully. Since hors d'oeuvres are supposed to whet the appetite, seasonings are especially important. They should complement the flavor—not overpower it.

- Slice, shape, and portion the items carefully. The platter should offer a variety, but not overwhelming array of choices.

- Consider the overall color, shape, and look of the platter. There shouldn't be too much unused space, and the items should look good together.

- Include the proper sauces and utensils. Provide separate utensils for each item on a cold platter. For example, you could provide a spoon for a dip and small tongs for crudités.

SECTION 18-4 Knowledge Check

1. What is an hors d'oeuvre?
2. What are three things to keep in mind when preparing cold platters?
3. What kinds of dips are usually served with relish trays?

MINI LAB

In teams, create a cold platter that would be appropriate for a graduation party. Present your team's platter for evaluation before sampling it.

SECTION SUMMARIES

18-1 The garde manger and brigade specialize in the preparation of cold foods.

18-1 The garde manger must consider the variety of ingredients, the color and texture of dishes, and the cost to prepare and serve them.

18-1 The garde manger prepares hors d'oeuvres, salads, canapés, fancy sandwiches, and a variety of cold platters.

18-2 A garnish should complement the food it accompanies, adding nutrition and appeal.

18-2 There are many tools for garnish preparation, including a peeler, a cutter, a zester, and an assortment of knives.

18-3 All ingredients for a green salad need to be carefully chosen and prepared for a quality presentation.

18-3 The main types of salads can be served at a variety of times ranging from before the meal, during the meal, or at its conclusion.

18-3 There are four main parts to an arranged salad.

18-3 Within the four categories of salad dressings, there is a wide variety.

18-4 There are five main categories of cheese that contain many varieties.

18-4 Properly stored cheeses can last for varying lengths of time.

18-4 There are many kinds of cold hors d'oeuvres, including canapés and fancy finger sandwiches.

18-4 Cold platters featuring cheese, meat, or fruit may be simple or complex.

18-4 Relish trays are often accompanied by a dip that enhances the flavor of the vegetables.

CHECK YOUR KNOWLEDGE

1. Where might a garde manger find employment?

2. List four dishes that might be prepared by a garde manger and his or her brigade.

3. Name four garnish tools and describe their uses.

4. Identify the parts of an arranged salad. Give an example of foods that can be used for each part.

5. Contrast radicchio and mesclun.

6. Explain why vinaigrette salad dressing works well on salads.

7. Contrast hard and semisoft cheeses.

8. What are the three main elements of a cold buffet?

9. List vegetables that could be included on a relish tray.

CRITICAL-THINKING ACTIVITIES

1. Assume you have been asked to prepare an hors d'oeuvre tray that will be served prior to the main meal. What factors will impact your choice of hors d'oeuvre?

2. Imagine that you've been asked to prepare an accompaniment salad to go with a main course featuring baked fish. Describe the type of salad you'll prepare and explain why.

WORKPLACE KNOW-HOW

Decision making. You are to create a cheese tray to serve 100 people on a buffet table. Describe how you will choose the cheeses, the tray's presentation, and when you will serve it.

LAB-BASED ACTIVITY: Creating Garnishes

STEP 1 You will need five garnish tools to create a garnish. Determine which tool you will use on each food. Suggestions are provided below, but creativity is encouraged.

STEP 2 Use the vegetable peeler to shave a food item. You might try a carrot, chocolate, or butter.

STEP 3 Use the zester to remove small strips of the colored parts of citrus peel. You might try the orange and the lemon.

STEP 4 Use the butter cutter on the chilled butter. Is there another food item on which the butter cutter might work?

STEP 5 Use the melon baller to make cantaloupe balls. Name the different kinds of melons you could also use with this tool.

STEP 6 Use the channel knife to cut pieces of rind from the orange. Curl the rinds in a circle to create a "rose." Try this with another food item.

STEP 7 Use the pastry bag to spread cream cheese on the crackers or bread. What else could you spread with the pastry bag?

STEP 8 Use the egg wedger to slice the hard-cooked egg.

STEP 9 Determine the food item each garnish would best accompany.

STEP 10 After you've finished making the garnishes and chosen appropriate accompaniments, work with a partner to evaluate your work. What could you have done differently? What are some other possibilities that you didn't consider?

Tools & Food Choices

Tools
- ✔ Vegetable peeler
- ✔ Zester
- ✔ Butter cutter
- ✔ Parisienne scoop
- ✔ Channel knife
- ✔ Egg wedger
- ✔ Offset spatulas
- ✔ Pastry bags and tips
- ✔ Individual molds

Food Choices
- ✔ Lemon
- ✔ Chilled butter
- ✔ Cantaloupe
- ✔ Carrot, orange
- ✔ Leeks
- ✔ Cucumber
- ✔ Potato
- ✔ Jicama
- ✔ Star fruit

- ✔ Radish
- ✔ Cream cheese
- ✔ Crackers or various breads of different shapes and sizes
- ✔ Hard-cooked eggs
- ✔ Olives, herbs

Hot & Cold Sandwiches

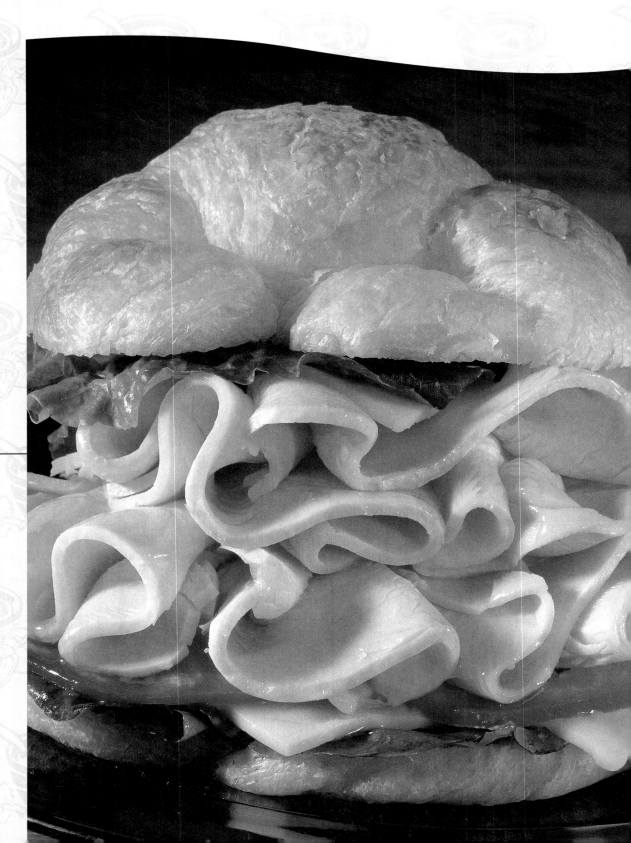

Sandwich Making Basics

OBJECTIVES

After reading this section, you will be able to:

• Describe different types of sandwiches, spreads, fillings, and cheeses.

• Identify common types of sandwich accompaniments.

• List the tools needed at a sandwich preparation workstation.

• Prepare sandwiches efficiently.

A L L it takes to make a sandwich is bread, a spread, and fillings. But from this simple set of ingredients, you can make a wide variety of tasty sandwiches. Depending on its ingredients, a sandwich can be a nutritional powerhouse or a high-fat meal. The vast array of ingredients also increases the skill level needed by foodservice workers. Through organization and practice, you can learn to make fresh, flavorful sandwiches.

✖ SANDWICH TYPES

Types of hot and cold sandwiches include closed, open-face, triple-decker, finger, and wraps.

■ **Closed sandwiches.** These sandwiches have two pieces of bread with the filling in between.

■ **Open-face sandwiches.** With two pieces of bread plated side by side, the spread and fillings are added to the top of one or both pieces of bread.

■ **Triple-decker sandwiches.** These sandwiches include three pieces of bread stacked with fillings between each layer.

■ **Finger sandwiches.** These small, fancy closed sandwiches with the crusts removed are often cut into various shapes.

■ **Wraps.** These easy-to-eat sandwiches are made with soft, flat breads that are folded, or "wrapped," around the fillings. A wide variety of fillings can be used in these sandwiches.

✖ BREADS & SPREADS

Bread provides the base to a sandwich and adds to the look and taste of the final product. If you choose a fresh and tasty bread, you'll be building a sandwich on a solid foundation. The spread acts as a barrier, preventing moist fillings from soaking into the bread.

Types of Bread

As shown in Fig. 19-1, there is a vast array of tasty and nutritional sandwich breads. These range from bagels to buns to **Pullman** breads, or rectangular loaves of sandwich bread with flat tops and even texture. Croissants (kruh-SAHNTS) and fruit breads can also be used to make flavorful sandwiches. Use the following guidelines when choosing breads:

- Choose breads that aren't too hard or crusty.
- Select breads that don't overpower the filling.
- Choose breads that are thick enough to hold the filling without tearing.

White, rye, and wheat bread are typical cold sandwich choices. Today, however, many types of flatbreads are also used. One popular flatbread is **focaccia** (foh-KAH-chee-ah), an Italian bread flavored with olive oil and herbs.

Flat loaves of white or rye bread are also used for finger sandwiches. These breads can be sliced thinly and still hold a circle, diamond, or triangle shape. Some breads crumble easily when sliced. Avoid using these breads for thin-sliced sandwiches unless they have been frozen before being sliced.

In addition to traditional hot dog and hamburger rolls, there are many other types of rolls. These rolls include hard, kaiser (KIGH-zerr), onion, and torpedo (tour-PEE-dough), a crusty, chewy Italian roll.

Pita (PEE-tah), a round-shaped bread cut open to form a pocket, makes whole-meal sandwiches. Tortilla (tohr-TEE-yuh), a flattened, round bread baked on a griddle or deep-fried, can be cut into pinwheel sections. Tortillas; chapati (chah-PAH-tee), which is a whole wheat flat bread; or **phyllo** (FEE-loh), a type of pastry can also be used to create sandwich wraps. Another option is **crêpes** (KRAYPS), small, thin pancakes made with egg batter.

Fig. 19-1.

Specialty Breads

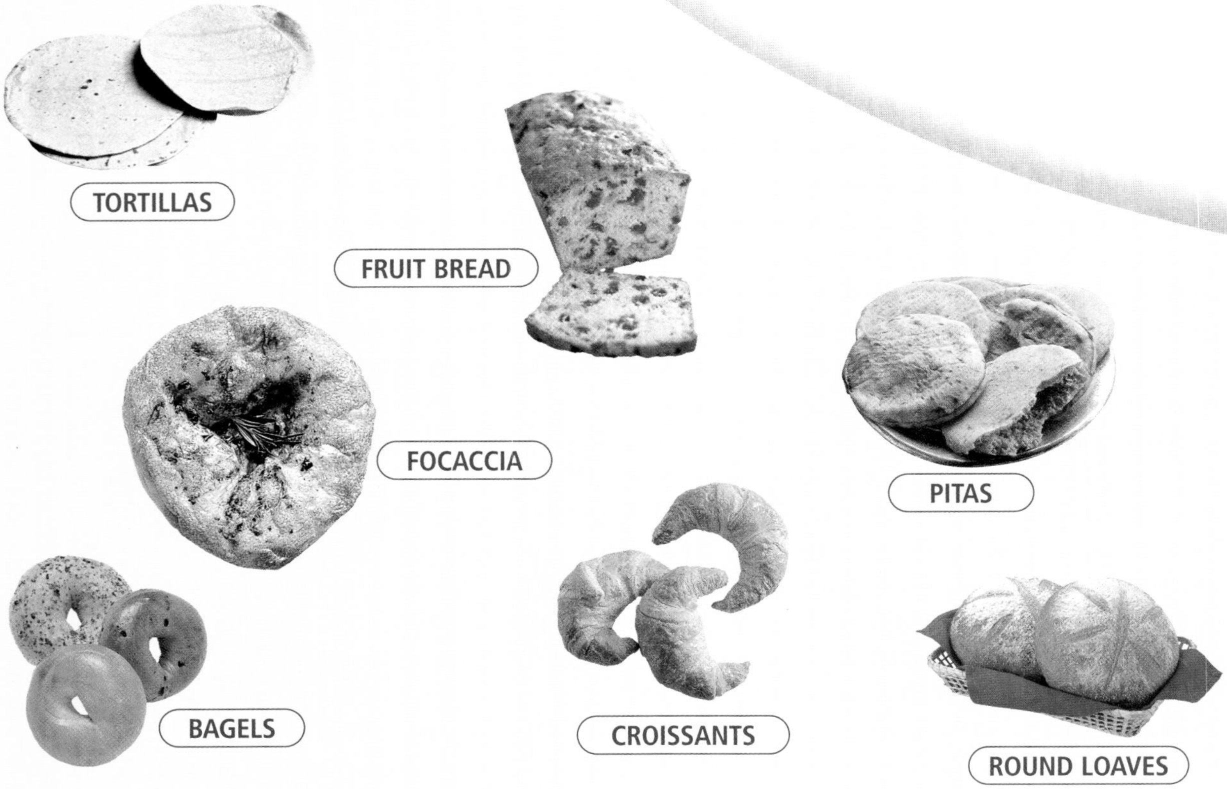

TORTILLAS

FRUIT BREAD

FOCACCIA

PITAS

BAGELS

CROISSANTS

ROUND LOAVES

Types of Spreads

There are three main types of sandwich spreads: butter, mayonnaise, and vegetable purées (pyuh-RAYS). Butter and mayonnaise keep wet fillings from soaking into the bread as well as falling off of the bread.

Butter adds a smooth, rich flavor to a sandwich. Flavored butters, such as red chili butter or garlic butter, can add zip to a blackened fish or pork sandwich. Be sure to whip or soften butter to increase its volume and softness for easy spreading. That way it won't tear the bread when it is spread. This will also cut food costs.

Mayonnaise has been the spread of choice of sandwich makers for generations. It's hard to imagine a BLT without mayonnaise. Even mayonnaise, however, can be flavored with herbs, fruits, pesto, and condiments such as mustard. **Pesto** (PEH-stoh) is a sauce made by combining olive oil, pine nuts or walnuts, a hard cheese such as parmesan, and fresh basil, garlic, salt, and pepper.

Vegetable purées made with chopped olives, avocados, or eggplant are an alternative spread. Purées add interesting flavors, but usually do not provide a moisture barrier for the filling.

❎ SANDWICH FILLINGS

Sandwich fillings may include hot or cold meats, poultry, fish, cheeses, vegetables, or a combination of items. The filling is the "main act," so prepare each item carefully. For example, a chicken breast must be carefully cooked and sliced. The lettuce must be crisp and completely rinsed and dried. Tomatoes and onions should be evenly sliced.

Vegetables that are grilled or marinated, such as red and yellow peppers, make elegant fillings. A pita filled with vegetables and a flavorful dressing is packed with nutrition. Finger sandwiches often contain cream cheese topped with finely chopped vegetables like zucchini, olives, or peppers. See Fig. 19-2.

Meats, Poultry, Fish & Seafood

Chicken, turkey, beef, pork, eggs, and tuna are common sandwich fillings. They can also be combined with other fillings to create a hearty sandwich. Corned beef and sauerkraut (SOW-uhr-krowt), spicy chicken sausage and red pepper, and broiled crab and cheese are good examples of combined fillings.

Cheese

Cheese plays an important part in many sandwiches. It is high in protein, vitamin A, calcium, and phosphorus. Cheese is also higher in fat, although low-fat and nonfat processed cheeses are available. Keep in mind, however, that low-fat and nonfat cheeses do not melt as easily as regular cheese.

Fig. 19-2. Vegetables are a common pita sandwich filling.

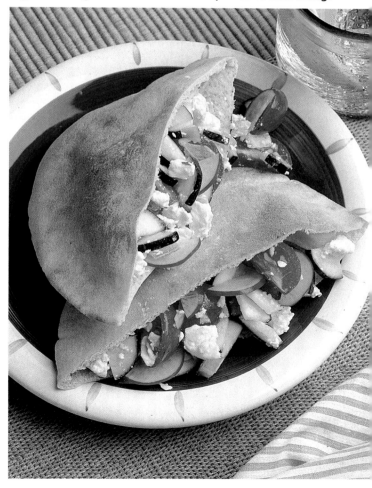

HANDLING CHEESE—Use the following guidelines when handling cheese:
- Wash your hands well to avoid contaminating the cheese.
- Keep your workspace, cutting equipment, and other utensils clean and sanitized to prevent cross-contamination.
- Keep cheese tightly covered in plastic wrap in the refrigerator. Cheese dries out quickly when unwrapped and sliced.

■ **Types of cheese.** Many types of soft, semisoft, and hard cheeses make good sandwich fillings. Sliced cheese may be added to closed sandwiches or melted on top of an open-face sandwich. Flavored, spreadable cream cheeses are often used for finger sandwiches made with fruit breads. For more information on cheese, see Chapter 18, Section 4.

■ **Selecting cheese.** Knowing the types and characteristics of cheeses will help you select the best cheese for a particular sandwich. Some popular sandwich cheeses are shown in Fig. 19-3.

Sandwich Accompaniments

Sandwich accompaniments may include one or more of the following. See Fig. 19-4 on page 439.
- Whole vegetables, such as small radishes, baby carrots, green onions, or cherry tomatoes.
- Sticks of carrots, celery, or summer squash.
- Lettuce leaves or baby spinach leaves.
- Sliced cucumbers or tomatoes.
- Grilled, marinated vegetables.
- Pickle spears or green or black olives.
- Sliced fruits.

Fig. 19-3.

Sandwich Cheeses

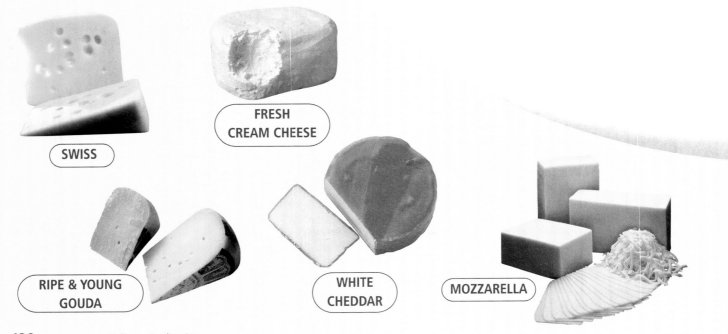

SWISS

FRESH CREAM CHEESE

RIPE & YOUNG GOUDA

WHITE CHEDDAR

MOZZARELLA

DETERMINING AMOUNTS

Suppose you need to prepare chicken salad sandwiches for 115 guests. How will you determine how much of each ingredient to purchase? To prevent overbuying or under-buying, use your knowledge of multiplication and division. Use the following information to determine how much bread, filling, and topping to buy. Each guest will be served 2 chicken salad sandwiches.

- The sandwiches will consist of 3 oz. of chicken salad with two tomato slices on a croissant.
- Chicken salad comes in 32-oz. containers.
- Croissants are sold 12 in a package.
- One tomato can be cut into 8 slices.

Step 1

Determine the number of sandwiches you need to make.

115 people × 2 sandwiches per person
115 × 2 = 230 sandwiches

Step 2

Determine the amount of chicken salad you need.

230 sandwiches × 3 oz. of chicken salad per sandwich

230 × 3 = 690 oz. of chicken salad
690 ounces ÷ 32 oz. per container
690 ÷ 32 = 21.56 containers

Round 21.56 up to 22 containers of chicken salad.

Step 3

Find the number of packages of croissants you need.

230 sandwiches × 1 croissant per sandwich
230 × 1 = 230 croissants
230 croissants ÷ 12 croissants per package
230 ÷ 12 = 19.17 packages of croissants

Round 19.17 up to 20 packages of croissants.

Step 4

Determine the number of tomatoes you need.

230 sandwiches × 2 tomato slices
230 × 2 = 460 tomato slices
460 tomato slices ÷ 8 slices per tomato
460 ÷ 8 = 57.5 tomatoes

Round 57.5 up to 58 tomatoes.

TRY IT!

You've been asked to prepare 50 egg and cheese sandwiches for a breakfast meeting. Determine how many packages of bread and cheese and how many dozens of eggs you need to buy.

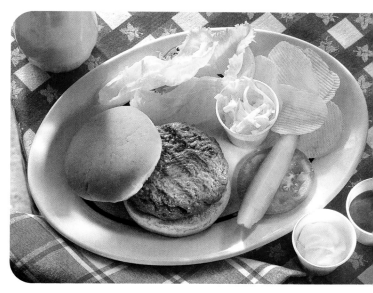

Fig. 19-4. Cooks can use different accompaniments to enhance the taste of a sandwich. What three foods could be used as sandwich accompaniments?

X NUTRITION

Sandwiches contain all of the food groups, providing protein, carbohydrates, vitamins, minerals, and fats. Carefully combining ingredients can make sandwiches hearty, healthful creations.

In the past, people relied on two slices of white bread in every sandwich. Today, the choices are more varied. Lighter alternatives include small tortillas, mini-pitas, or thin pizza crust. Whole wheat breads increase the nutritional value of sandwiches.

Sandwich fillings usually contain the main protein source. It is important to use high-quality protein foods. When menu planning, remember that many customers want low-fat sandwiches. Items such as broiled chicken breast or vegetarian sandwiches can meet this need.

X SANDWICH-MAKING TECHNIQUES

Keeping your work space organized will allow you to make many sandwiches at once. You will also need an organized work space and techniques that will keep you and your customers safe.

When setting up a sandwich work station, remember to have these utensils close at hand:

- Sharp knives, including a chef's knife and a bread knife.

SAFETY & SANITATION

GUARDING AGAINST BACTERIA GROWTH—
Sandwiches often combine hot and cold items. This is a perfect environment for the growth of bacteria. Avoid cross-contamination by:

- Keeping hot foods hot and cold foods cold.
- Washing your hands well and often.
- Minimizing the cross-use of utensils.
- Frequently cleaning <u>and</u> sanitizing all work surfaces and utensils.

- Serving spoons or scoops, for controlling portions of spreads and fillings.
- Spatula, for spreading or lifting fillings and spreads.
- Toaster, for toasting bread.
- Tongs, for moving food items.
- Cutting board, for cutting food items.

Quantity Sandwich Preparation

When preparing large quantities of sandwiches, an organized system will allow you to work safely and efficiently. Here is a 10-step method for making quantities of sandwiches:

1. Set up your work station so all necessary utensils and ingredients are close at hand. Items should be within your range of motion to avoid unnecessary movements that cause fatigue.

2. Use a sheet pan, lined with parchment paper, as the centerpiece of your work area.

3. Place bread loaves on your left if you are right-handed and on your right if you are left-handed. Bread dries out quickly. You must have everything ready to go before laying out the bread.

4. Arrange slices of bread in four equal rows on the sheet pan.

5. Use a spatula to apply a spread to each slice of bread. This seals the bread before the filling is added. It helps prevent sandwiches from getting soggy.

6. Arrange any vegetables such as lettuce or tomatoes on top of the spread. See Fig. 19-5A below.

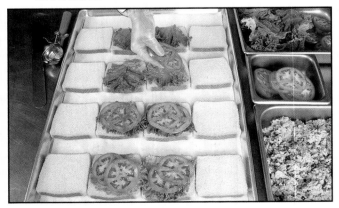

7. Add fillings to the two middle rows of bread. Use a portion scoop for fillings such as tuna or chicken salad. Carefully place fillings on top of the tomatoes. Make sure that the bread is covered well. See Fig. 19-5B below.

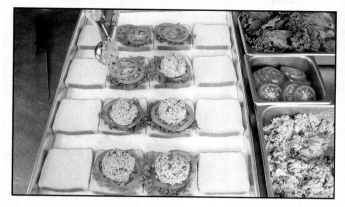

8. Use a spatula to spread the filling evenly. See Fig. 19-5C below.

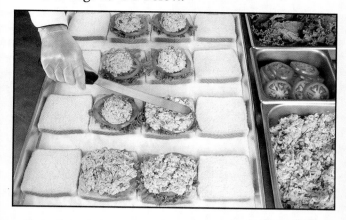

9. Using both hands, cover the two middle rows with the remaining slices of bread. See Fig. 19-5D below.

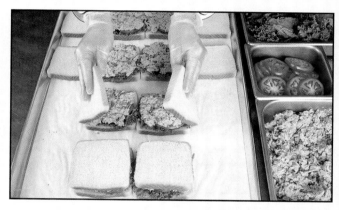

10. You should either plate the sandwiches immediately or wrap them in plastic wrap and refrigerate until they are served.

CULINARY TIP

CUTTING SANDWICHES—The way a sandwich is cut adds to its visual appeal. The arrangement of sandwich sections on a plate also gives the customer a hint of the filling inside. Avoid pushing down on a sandwich before or during cutting. This prevents the sandwich filling from flattening or oozing out the sides of the sandwich. Cut sandwiches into neat, uniform shapes as close to serving time as possible. Decorative toothpicks can be used to hold sandwiches together when needed.

SECTION 19-1   Knowledge Check

1. Name four different types of sandwiches and give an example of each one.
2. Identify three sandwich accompaniments.
3. Why does the process for making large quantities of sandwiches save time?

MINI LAB

In teams, prepare 15 sandwiches. Choose one of the following types of sandwiches to prepare: (a) one meat and one cheese; (b) tuna, chicken, or ham salad; (c) more than one meat. Use a variety of breads and spreads.

Preparing Hot & Cold Sandwiches

OBJECTIVES

After reading this section, you will be able to:

• Describe different types of hot and cold sandwiches.

• Explain guidelines for preparing and plating hot and cold sandwiches.

• Prepare sandwiches.

• List several garnishes and accompaniments for hot and cold sandwiches.

FROM the all-American hot dog to the elegant Monte Cristo, hot sandwiches are popular with customers of all ages. Likewise, cold sandwiches, such as tuna salad, are ordered by customers every day. Many of the same types of ingredients can be used in hot and cold sandwiches.

✖ TYPES OF HOT SANDWICHES

Examples of closed hot sandwiches include grilled ham and cheese and hot barbecued chicken. Popular open-face sandwiches are hot turkey and hot beef sandwiches, usually served with mashed potatoes and gravy. Hot crab with cheese and avocado is another example of a hot open-face sandwich.

One of the most popular hot open-face sandwiches is pizza, made with either thin or thick crust. There are many pizza topping combinations, such as pepperoni and mushroom. Many restaurants regularly offer individual-size pizzas. See Fig. 19-6.

Basic Sandwiches

Basic sandwiches contain at least one hot filling. The filling may be sandwiched between two slices of bread as a closed sandwich or served open-face. Basic closed sandwiches include the standard hamburger and hot dog. Tortillas are used to make burritos or tacos, with a hot filling of chicken, beef, or seafood inside. These fillings are often combined with cold vegetables such as lettuce, tomatoes, onions, or avocado.

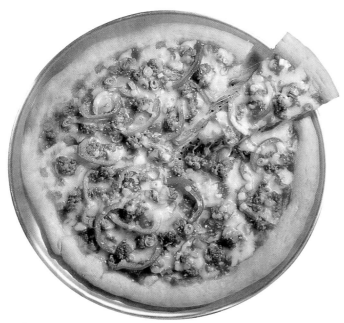

Fig. 19-6. Gourmet pizzas are a specialty of some restaurants. What might you serve with this hot, open-face sandwich?

Grilled Sandwiches

To make a grilled sandwich, butter and then brown the outside of each slice of bread on the griddle. Grilled cheese sandwiches are a traditional favorite. However, you can also create interesting varieties, such as grilled cheese and avocado or grilled tuna and cheese.

Fried Sandwiches

Have you ever heard of a Monte Cristo sandwich? There are many varieties of this elegant sandwich. Some old, elegant hotel dining rooms built their reputations on their own special versions of the Monte Cristo.

Monte Cristos are closed, shallow-fried or deep-fried sandwiches. Some chefs make Monte Cristos with thin slices of ham and Swiss cheese and Dijon mustard. Others include turkey or chicken breast and use butter or mayonnaise between the layers. Some chefs also add a layer of strawberry or raspberry jam. The sandwich is then dipped in egg batter and either deep-fried or shallow-fried. See Fig. 19-7.

a LINK to the Past

The History of the Sandwich

The sandwich is named after Sir John Montagu of England (1718–1792), the Fourth Earl of Sandwich. To satisfy his appetite, his servants brought him bread and meat. Sir John combined the two so he could eat with one hand. This combination became known as the sandwich.

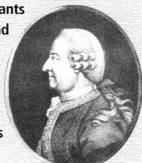

One of America's most popular sandwiches—the hamburger—was originally called a Hamburg steak after its city of origin, Hamburg, Germany. German immigrants introduced the hamburger to the United States.

The Earl of Sandwich's idea of not letting a meal interrupt other activities became a popular concept in the twentieth century. People wanted food in a hurry that could be eaten on the run. In 1954, Ray Kroc founded the McDonald's franchise, based on the concept of fast service at a low price. Fast food sandwiches as we know them today were born.

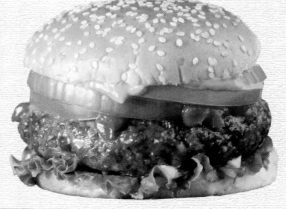

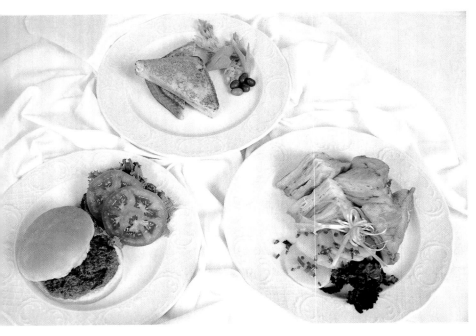

Fig. 19-7. The three types of hot sandwiches are basic, grilled, and fried.

Grilled Ham and Cheese Sandwich

YIELD: 50 SERVINGS   SERVING SIZE: 1 SANDWICH

INGREDIENTS

5 loaves	Sliced sandwich bread
4 lbs.	Ham, boneless, cooked, cut into 1-ounce slices
3 lbs.	American cheese, sliced
1½ lbs.	Clarified butter

METHOD OF PREPARATION

1. Lay out the bread slices on a clean, dry table.

2. Place one slice of ham and cheese on each second slice of bread.

3. Cover with the first slice of bread, and cut on an angle to create two triangle sandwiches.

4. Lightly coat with clarified butter.

5. Grill until golden brown on both sides.

6. Serve hot.

PREPARING HOT SANDWICHES

Here are some tips to keep in mind when preparing hot sandwiches:

- When grilling sandwiches, the filling is only heated. Make sure all hot meat fillings are thoroughly cooked before grilling them.
- Completely assemble the sandwiches before grilling. Since most of them contain cheese, they cannot be pulled apart to add other fillings after heating.
- Make sure that cold fillings, such as lettuce, are crisp and cold. If they are placed under hot fillings such as cheese, they may be "cooked."
- Some cooks place cold fillings on the side for the customer to add to the sandwich when it is served. This is almost always done with hamburgers: the lettuce, tomato, and onion are placed to the side.
- Don't overload hot wraps or they will become messy to eat. If one ingredient is too chunky, it can break the wrap or cause everything to fall out.
- Make sure that hot sandwiches are served on warm plates.

PLATING HOT SANDWICHES

Hot sandwiches may be served either open-face or closed. Grilled cheese sandwiches, for example, are always served closed. Hamburgers may be served either open or closed. Hot turkey or crab sandwiches are always served open-face with gravy or sauce spooned over the top.

Hot sandwiches are often served with a side salad or a cup of soup. Potatoes, such as French fries, are another popular accompaniment.

Tips for Hot Open-Face Sandwiches

Here are some tips to keep in mind when serving hot open-face sandwiches:

- If the sandwich has gravy, sauce, or melted cheese on top, don't let the sauce run onto any cold items on the plate. No one wants to eat carrots covered in gravy or lettuce drowning in barbecue sauce. See Fig. 19-8.
- Don't oversauce items.
- Make sure the sauce is not too thin or too thick.
- Make a nest for the lettuce or put cold relishes in a seashell for an elegant presentation.

■ **Garnishing.** Hot sandwich garnishes include lettuce, tomato, onion, and different condiments. Customers often appreciate sandwich garnishes being served on the side. That way they can add the ones they want and leave the rest off.

Open-face sandwiches are sometimes served **au jus** (oh ZHEW), or accompanied by the juices obtained from roasting meat. A barbecued chicken sandwich might be accompanied by a cup of barbecue sauce.

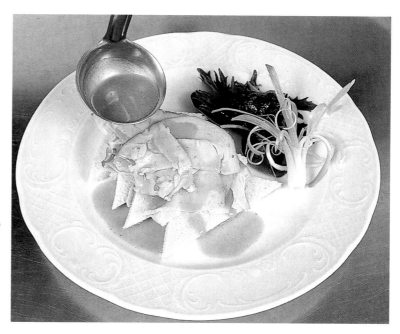

Fig. 19-8. Do not let a sandwich's gravy or sauce touch any cold foods on the plate.

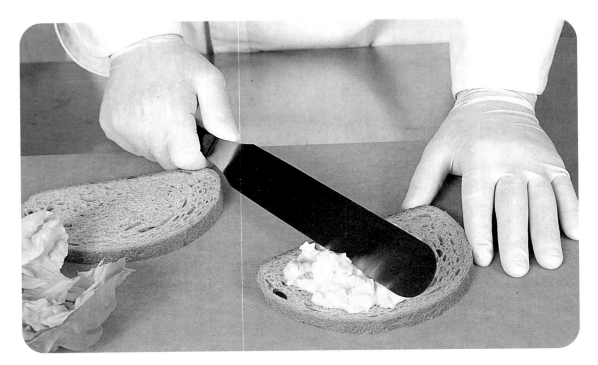

Fig. 19-9. Prepare salad sandwiches such as this egg salad sandwich immediately before serving, or the bread will become soggy.

TYPES OF COLD SANDWICHES

Some cold sandwiches are made with pre-cooked poultry, fish, or meat. Roast beef, pastrami (puh-STRAH-mee), or turkey deli sandwiches, for example, are typically served cold. The vegetables added to cold sandwiches, such as onions or pickles, are also served cold.

Some cold sandwiches are a full meal, such as a spicy lentil pita sandwich with yogurt sauce. Even sandwich wraps may contain cold fillings, such as cold turkey salad with cold cooked rice.

Cold sandwiches are rarely served open face. Usually, they are made from two or three pieces of bread, or a split soft or multigrain roll. A triple-decker sandwich that features cold, sliced cooked turkey and ham, or bacon, is called a **club sandwich**. Club sandwiches also contain cheese, tomato, and lettuce. The ingredients are layered between three slices of toasted bread and cut into four triangles.

PREPARING COLD SANDWICHES

When preparing cold sandwiches, keep in mind the following guidelines:

- Use the freshest bread possible. There is nothing worse than a cold sandwich prepared with tough, stale bread. If the bread is toasted, you can use day-old bread. However, butter it quickly after toasting. This preserves the moisture and keeps it from drying too quickly.
- Do not prepare salad sandwiches in advance. The moisture from chicken or egg salad will soak into the bread. The sandwich will be soggy by the time it is served. Use moisture barriers such as lettuce to help keep the bread dry. See Fig. 19-9.
- Make sure that cold sandwiches are served on cold plates.

PLATING COLD SANDWICHES

Cold sandwiches are usually cut into halves or thirds. Triple-decker sandwiches are often cut into fourths. Each section is held together by a frilled toothpick.

HACCP:
Keep all ingredients chilled to 41°F or below.

HAZARDOUS FOODS:
Mayonnaise
Ham
Salami
Turkey
Provolone and American cheese

NUTRITION:
Calories: 937
Fat: 44.5 g
Protein: 47.6 g

CHEF NOTES:
1. Serve with crosscut, seasoned French fries and cole slaw.
2. In quantity food production, the mayonnaise should be served on the side.

American Grinder

YIELD: 50 SERVINGS   SERVING SIZE: 1 SANDWICH

INGREDIENTS

50 each	Submarine rolls, split
1½ pts.	Mayonnaise
2 heads	Iceberg lettuce, cleaned and washed, cut **chiffonade**
7 lbs.	Tomatoes, washed, cored, and sliced
6 lbs.	Ham, sliced thin
3 lbs.	Salami, sliced thin
6 lbs.	Turkey, sliced thin
3 lbs.	Provolone cheese, sliced
3 lbs.	American cheese, sliced
50 each	Pickle spears

METHOD OF PREPARATION

1. Split the submarine roll, spread with mayonnaise, and fill with shredded lettuce and tomato slices.

2. Fill with meats, alternating ham, salami, and turkey.

3. Top with sliced cheeses, cut in half, and serve with a pickle.

Sandwiches are often served with such accompaniments as potato chips, French fries, or soup. Salads such as cole slaw, fruit, green, potato, macaroni, and three-bean are also popular choices. Many restaurants offer a combination of a half sandwich with salad or soup as a daily special.

■ **Garnishing.** Cold sandwich garnishes should be selected carefully, as they impact the appearance of the plate. Choose items whose shape, color, and texture add interest to the dish. Some popular garnishes include fruit, radishes, and parsley.

SECTION 19-2 Knowledge Check

1. Name three types of hot sandwiches and three types of cold sandwiches.

2. What special considerations must be followed when preparing grilled and other hot closed sandwiches?

3. List three possible accompaniments for cold sandwiches.

MINI LAB

Prepare a hot sandwich with the given ingredients and equipment in your lab. List possible garnishes and accompaniments for your sandwich. Sample each other's hot sandwich creation.

SECTION SUMMARIES

19-1 There are five types of sandwiches: closed, open-face, triple-decker, finger, and sandwich wraps. Common spreads include butter, mayonnaise, and vegetable purées. Fillings include meat, vegetables, cheeses, and poultry.

19-1 Fruit and vegetable accompaniments should be selected, prepared, and stored correctly.

19-1 Utensils needed at a sandwich work station include sharp knives, serving spoons or scoops, and a toaster.

19-1 Making large quantities of sandwiches involves several steps, including keeping all relevant ingredients and utensils close at hand.

19-2 There are many different kinds of hot and cold sandwiches, including hamburgers and tuna salad sandwiches.

19-2 Guidelines for preparing hot sandwiches include completely assembling grilled sandwiches before cooking. Guidelines for preparing cold sandwiches include using the freshest bread possible.

19-2 Hot and cold sandwiches are often served with a salad, soup, or type of potato, such as French fries.

19-2 Common garnishes for hot and cold sandwiches include pickles, lettuce, onion, and tomatoes.

CHECK YOUR KNOWLEDGE

1. Describe five types of hot and cold sandwiches.
2. Describe Pullman, focaccia, pita, and tortilla breads.
3. How is butter used as a sandwich spread?
4. What nutritional elements does cheese bring to a sandwich?
5. Briefly list the steps for making large quantities of sandwiches.
6. In what two ways can a basic sandwich be served?
7. How do you cook a grilled sandwich?
8. Can cold salad sandwiches be prepared in advance? Explain why or why not.
9. What are the advantages of placing garnishes on the side?

CRITICAL-THINKING ACTIVITIES

1. What factors do you think influence the type of bread used for a sandwich?
2. How are cost control and portion control techniques used in sandwich-making?
3. Suppose you are training a new employee to make large quantities of sandwiches. The employee wants to know why it is so important to follow an organized system. How would you respond?

WORKPLACE KNOW-HOW

System analysis. Imagine that you are the manager of the sandwich work station. Complaints have been made about soggy ham sandwiches being served at lunch. List steps you could take to correct the problem.

LAB-BASED ACTIVITY: Quantity Sandwich Production

STEP ❶ Imagine your class received an order to cater an outdoor company picnic. You need 160 cold meat sandwiches using whole-wheat, rye, sourdough, and white bread.

STEP ❷ In teams, choose a type of sandwich to make.

STEP ❸ Once you've chosen the sandwich type, answer the following questions:

- What type of bread, filling, spread, cheese, and garnishes will you use?
- What accompaniments will you include with the sandwiches?
- How will you determine what ingredients to order and how much?
- How will you determine the cost?
- How will you organize the task of preparing the sandwiches?
- What utensils and/or equipment will you need?
- How will you arrange the ingredients and utensils on a 5-ft. work space?

STEP ❹ Create a chart like the one below and record your team's sandwich production information.

STEP ❺ Draw a diagram of your work space with all the ingredients and utensils in place.

STEP ❻ Write out detailed guidelines for each step of the sandwich-making process.

STEP ❼ Share your team's sandwich production plan with the other teams. Discuss how each team's plan would impact the sandwich-making process.

STEP ❽ As a class, choose the best team plan for sandwich production.

STEP ❾ Prepare all the sandwiches according to the winning team's plan.

STEP ❿ Discuss what you learned about sandwich production from this experience.

	Team A	Team B	Team C	Team D
Sandwich Type				
Bread				
Filling				
Spread				
Cheese				
Garnish				
Accompaniment(s)				

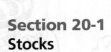
Stocks & Sauces

Stocks

KEY TERMS

• **stocks**

• **base**

• **mirepoix**

• **fumet**

• **glaze**

• **reduction**

OBJECTIVES

After reading this section, you will be able to:

• Describe the characteristics of the basic types of stocks.

• Explain how to prepare stock.

• Prepare a vegetable stock.

THE French word for stock is *fond*, meaning bottom, ground, or base. Since the sixteenth century, the quality of soups and sauces has depended upon the stocks on which they are based. Learning the skill of making animal- and plant-based stocks will allow you to build soups and sauces on a strong foundation.

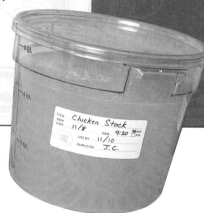

❎ WHAT ARE STOCKS?

Stocks are the liquids that form the foundation of sauces and soups. Simmering various combinations of bones, vegetables, and herbs extracts their flavors to create this foundation. Although it takes time to simmer stocks, you'll find that a good stock makes wonderful sauces and soups.

■ **Commercial stock bases.** Stocks can be purchased in a powdered or concentrated form, called a **base**. Using a commercial base saves time and money. However, what many bases add in convenience, they lose in the quality of their flavor.

When choosing a commercial base, check the list of ingredients. Remember that the ingredients are listed in order from highest amount to lowest

amount. A better-quality base will list fish, meat, or poultry extracts rather than salt or sodium first. You can give commercial bases a fresher taste by simmering them for a few hours with bones and **mirepoix** (meer-PWA), a mix of coarsely chopped vegetables and herbs. Then strain the mixture and use it like a stock.

Some chefs use bases to give sauces and soups a stronger flavor. Bases can also be added as a supplement when there is not enough stock available. Recipes must be adjusted when using bases because of the high amount of salt they contain.

WHAT MAKES UP A STOCK?

A stock is composed of four ingredients: the nourishing element, mirepoix, bouquet garni, and liquid. These ingredients are usually mixed in the following proportions to make most stocks:

- 50% nourishing element.
- 10% mirepoix.
- bouquet garni.
- 100% liquid.

■ **Nourishing element.** The most important ingredient in a stock is the nourishing element. Nourishing elements include any one or a combination of the following:

- Fresh bones (beef, lamb, chicken, fish, veal, or game).
- Meat trimmings.
- Fish trimmings for fish stock.
- Vegetables for vegetable stock.

The nourishing element provides flavor, nutrients, and color. Some nourishing elements may bring other benefits to the stock, such as bones, which add gelatin.

■ **Mirepoix.** Mirepoix is a mix of coarsely chopped vegetables that is used in a stock to add flavor, nutrients, and color. The ingredients vary with each recipe but usually include two parts onions, one part celery, and one part carrots. See Fig. 20-1.

■ **Bouquet garni.** A bouquet garni is a combination of fresh herbs and vegetables, such as carrots, leeks, celery, thyme, and parsley stems, that are tied in a bundle with butcher's twine. This bundle is added directly to the liquid and is allowed to simmer. The bouquet garni is removed before the stock is used in other foods.

■ **Liquid.** Liquid—almost always in the form of water—makes up the largest portion of stock. The liquid used to make stock should be cold when you begin cooking. This brings out the maximum flavor of the ingredients and prevents the stock from turning cloudy. When all the ingredients are prepared, the ratio of liquid to the nourishing element should be 2 to 1.

TYPES OF STOCKS

White, brown, fish, and vegetable stocks are the main types of stocks. They are sometimes referred to by their French names. See Fig. 20-2.

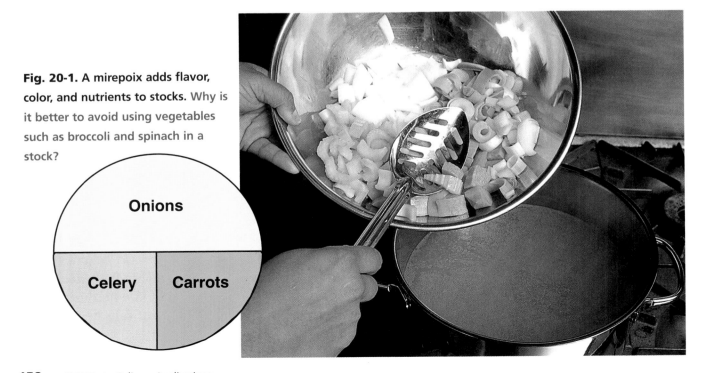

Fig. 20-1. A mirepoix adds flavor, color, and nutrients to stocks. Why is it better to avoid using vegetables such as broccoli and spinach in a stock?

Onions

Celery

Carrots

Fig. 20-2.

FRENCH NAME	ENGLISH TRANSLATION
Fond de boeuf (fahn duh buhf)	Beef stock
Fond de veau (fahn duh voh)	Veal stock
Fond de volaille (fahn duh vohl-YAY)	Poultry stock
Fond de légume (fahn duh lay-GEWM)	Vegetable stock
Fond d'agneau (fahn dahn-YOH)	Lamb stock
Fond de poisson (fahn duh pwah-SAWNG)	Fish stock
Fond de gibier (fahn duh jhee-BYAY)	Game stock

Preparing White Stock

White stocks are made from chicken, beef, veal, or fish bones simmered with vegetables. White stock is generally colorless while it is cooking. To keep the stock as clear as possible, you may blanch the bones before adding them. However, some chefs think doing so causes flavor to be lost.

1. Cut bones into 3- to 4-in. pieces, using a meat saw for thick, heavy bones. Chicken and fish bones do not need to be cut.

2. Rinse the bones in cold water to remove any impurities. You can blanch the bones, if desired.

3. Place the bones in a stockpot.

4. Add cold water until the bones are completely covered. Cold water dissolves impurities (ihm-PYUR-uh-teez) and blood in the bones it covers. These impurities will clump and rise to the surface when the water heats, where they can be skimmed off the top. Using hot water will cause the impurities to clump too rapidly. This prevents them from rising to the top and results in a cloudy stock.

5. Bring water to a boil; then reduce it to a simmer to slowly release the full flavor of the ingredients.

6. To keep the stock clear, use a skimmer or ladle to remove any impurities and fat from the surface. Continue skimming as needed throughout cooking.

7. Add the mirepoix. Boiling makes the stock cloudy, so keep the water at a simmer. Allowing the stock to boil for even a few minutes will cause the fats and impurities to blend into the rest of the liquid, turning it cloudy.

8. Make sure liquid is still completely covering the bones. Bones will not release their flavor unless they're under water, so add water if necessary. Bones will also darken if exposed to air.

9. For the best flavor, simmer stock for the recommended amount of time:

Fish bones	30–45 minutes
Chicken bones	3–4 hours
Beef or veal bones	6–8 hours

10. Add a small amount of cold water to bring impurities to the top; then skim the surface.

11. Strain the stock through a china cap lined with cheesecloth.

12. Cool the stock quickly, as discussed later in this section.

Preparing Brown Stock

Brown stock is made from either beef, veal, chicken, or game. It gets its color from roasting the ingredients without water, in a hot oven. The browned bones, mirepoix, and tomatoes or tomato product combine to give a brown stock its color. This mixture is then transferred to a stockpot and simmered along with water and herbs.

The procedures for making white stocks and brown stocks are essentially the same. The main difference is that for brown stocks, the bones and mirepoix are browned by roasting.

1. Cut the beef or veal bones into 3- to 4-in. pieces.

2. Browning is hindered by moisture, so don't wash or blanch the bones.

3. Place the bones one layer deep in a roasting pan.

4. Roast bones in the oven at 375°F or higher for over an hour, stirring occasionally. Some chefs lightly oil the bones before browning. See Fig. 20-3.

5. Place the browned bones in a stockpot and cover with water. Bring the water to a simmer.

6. Reserve the excess fat from the roasting pan.

7. Deglaze the pan with water. To deglaze means to add a liquid and stir over heat until the drippings are dissolved.

8. Add the deglazed mixture to the stockpot.

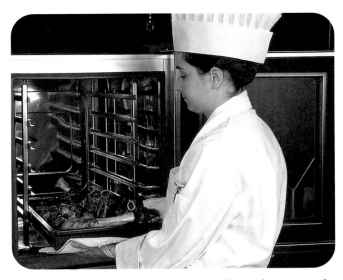

Fig. 20-3. The difference between making a brown stock and a white stock is that the bones and mirepoix are browned for a brown stock.

9. Combine the mirepoix and reserved fat in a pan, while the bones are beginning to simmer. Brown in the oven or on top of the range.

10. Skim impurities and fat from the stock as it begins to simmer.

11. Add the tomatoes or tomato product and caramelized vegetables to the stockpot, up to 3 or 4 hours before the end of cooking. Do not stir the stock or it will become cloudy. Continue following the steps for making white stocks.

Preparing Fish Stock

Fish stock is made by slowly cooking the bones of lean fish or shellfish. See Fig. 20-4. The procedure for making fish stock is the same as for making a white stock, although the cooking time for fish stock is shorter. If lemon juice or other acids are added to the water, the result is a flavorful liquid called a **fumet** (fyoo-MAY). A fumet is more strongly flavored than regular fish stock since it is reduced by 50%.

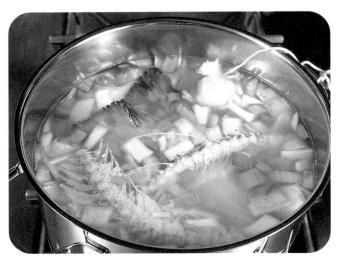

Fig. 20-4. A fish stock is made with the bones of lean fish or shellfish. What other ingredients can be added to a fish stock?

Preparing Vegetable Stock

Vegetable stocks, which do not include meat products, are an important addition to many healthful dishes. The basic ingredients are vegetables, herbs, spices, and water. Proportions and kinds of vegetables will vary with different recipes. Vegetable stock needs to be simmered only 30–45 minutes.

If you want a particular flavor of vegetable stock, use more of that vegetable. Then add neutral vegetables such as celery and onions to round out the flavor. All-purpose vegetable stock does not include strongly flavored vegetables, such as artichokes, Brussels sprouts, or cauliflower. These vegetables tend to be overpowering in flavor. Some dark green, leafy vegetables, such as spinach, develop an unpleasant odor when cooked too long.

Preparing Glazes

A **glaze** is a stock that is reduced and concentrated. This results in a flavorful, thick, and syrupy liquid that turns solid when refrigerated. Glazes are created through **reduction**, the process of evaporating part of a stock's water through simmering or boiling. Small amounts of glaze can be used to flavor sauces, vegetables, meat, poultry, and fish.

1. Place a large quantity of stock in a heavy pan.

2. Bring the stock to a simmer.

3. Skim the surface as needed.

4. Clean the sides of the pan with a moistened, natural-bristle brush as the stock reduces and becomes syrupy.

5. Transfer the stock to a smaller pan when reduced by half to two-thirds.

6. Continue to reduce until the stock coats a spoon.

7. Strain the stock through a chinois, or china cap, and pour into containers.

8. Follow recommended procedures for cooling stock; then label and refrigerate or freeze the containers.

a LINK to the Past

The History of the Tomato

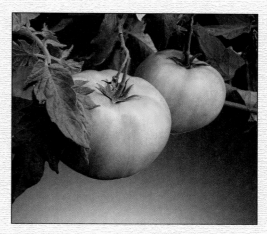

It's hard to imagine Italian sauces without tomatoes as a main ingredient. Tomatoes are also an important part of sauce espagnole and demi-glace sauces. Yet, the tomato wasn't introduced to Italy until the sixteenth century. It's a little-known fact that tomatoes are native to Central America—and not to Europe.

Sixteenth-century Spanish explorers discovered tomatoes during their travels to Mexico and Peru. The Indians told the explorers that tomatoes made an excellent sauce, especially when flavored with chile peppers.

Tomatoes didn't gain widespread popularity until after the Civil War. As late as 1900, tomatoes were little used except in sauces and purées.

Today, the United States is the world's leading producer of tomatoes. Most tomatoes are processed for use in products such as ketchup, tomato soup, tomato juice, tomato paste, and tomato sauce.

COOLING & STORING STOCKS

Always cool stock before storing it. There are three ways to cool stock. You can use Rapid Kool™ which is a container that has been filled with water and then frozen. This frozen container is then put into the stock to speed up the cooling process. Another method is to pour the stock into a container that is less than 4 in. deep and place it in the refrigerator. A third method is explained below. See Fig. 20-5.

1. First, place the stockpot on a rack or on blocks in an empty sink. Make sure the stockpot is balanced and will not spill. This is called venting. It will allow cold water to move beneath and around the pot as the sink fills with water.

2. Insert an overflow pipe over the drain to allow the water to circulate.

3. Next, turn on the cold water tap.

4. Continue to run cold water into the sink, forcing the extra water to drain out the overflow pipe as it becomes warm from the stockpot.

When the stock is cool, transfer it to a plastic container with a tight-fitting lid and label it. Never place hot stock in a refrigerator to cool it. The steam and heat may damage other foods. Stock can be stored for several days in a walk-in or reach-in refrigerator. However, stock that has not been cooled correctly can spoil within 6–8 hours.

Remove the layer of fat before using the stock. Fat rises to the surface and becomes solid when a stock chills. This fat layer acts as a preservative. However, it must be scraped or lifted off before reheating the stock. See Fig. 20-6.

Fig. 20-5. Use one of these methods to cool stock properly before storing it.

Overflow Pipe

Blocks

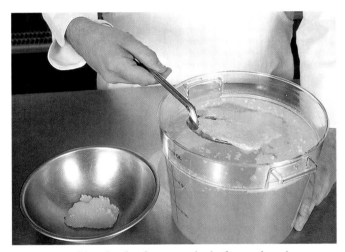

Fig. 20-6. Skim the fat from stocks before reheating them.

SECTION 20-1 · Knowledge Check

1. List the four main ingredients of stocks.
2. Identify the steps you would take to prepare a brown stock.
3. Compare the characteristics of a white stock, brown stock, fish stock, and vegetable stock.

MINI LAB

Working in teams, compare commercial bases to fresh white, brown, fish, or vegetable stock. Describe the differences in color, flavor, texture, and nutritional value.

Sauces

KEY TERMS

- sauces
- thickening agent
- gelatinization
- purée
- coulis
- mother sauces
- roux

OBJECTIVES

After reading this section, you will be able to:

- Describe the types of sauces.
- Explain the uses of sauces.
- Use thickening agents properly.
- Make a variety of sauces.

O N E of the best ways to add flavor and excitement to any dish is with a good sauce. In fact, a good sauce can turn a mediocre dish into a memorable one. People enjoy sauces with a variety of foods from chicken to vegetable dishes. Learning to make a good sauce is a basic step toward becoming a great cook.

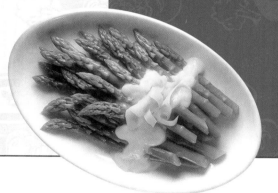

WHAT ARE SAUCES?

Most **sauces** are flavored, thickened liquids. They're usually formed by adding seasonings, flavorings, and a thickening agent to stock. A **thickening agent** is an ingredient, such as cornstarch, that adds body to the sauce. Two sauces that are not made this way are Béchamel (BAY-chuh-MEHL), a basic French white sauce made with milk and a thickener, and hollandaise sauce. Hollandaise sauce is made from lemon juice, butter, and eggs.

Sauces are meant to complement the foods they accompany. They should never overpower or detract from the food. Making a good sauce requires a lot of time. As discussed in Section 1, many restaurants use condensed or powdered commercial bases mixed with water to create stocks. The stocks and sauces then do not need to be reduced, since there is no gelatin in these commercial bases. Although quality may be a concern, these bases do guarantee a consistent flavor and texture.

SAUCE INGREDIENTS

Sauces are made of liquid ingredients, thickening agents, seasonings, and flavorings. Classic sauces rely on combinations of a few basic ingredients.

Liquid Ingredients

The liquid ingredient in most sauces serves as the base or body. You will commonly use some type of stock as the base for a sauce. You may use white stock made from chicken, veal, or fish. Other sauces call for brown stock.

Vinegar or tomato products may be added to sauces for acidity. Sometimes milk is used as a base. Clarified or drawn butter is another liquid ingredient in sauces.

Seasonings & Flavorings

The liquid ingredients may make up the basic flavor of most sauces, but the seasonings and flavorings you include will add the finishing touches to your sauce. You can change the character of your sauce simply by varying an ingredient or two.

You already know that seasonings and flavorings can be used to enhance the flavors of a dish. Salt, pepper, mustard, vinegar, spices, and herbs can all change the flavor of a sauce.

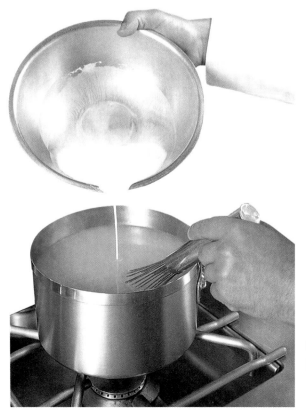

Thickening Agents

A major difference between stocks and sauces is that a sauce must be thickened. Most thickening agents are forms of starch. See Fig. 20-7. Starch granules will absorb moisture when placed in a liquid, a process called **gelatinization** (juh-la-tuhn-uh-ZAY-shuhn). Most sauces use this process in thickening. A good sauce will have these four characteristics:

- No lumps.
- A flavor that is not floury or pasty.
- Sticks to the back of a spoon.
- Will not break apart when it cooks down.

Thickening agents include flour, cornstarch, arrowroot, instant starches, bread crumbs, and vegetable purées.

■ **Flour.** Bread or all-purpose flour is most often used to thicken the fat from the pan in which the entrée has been sautéed. Flour may also be combined with butter that has just been melted as a quick way to thicken a sauce or soup.

■ **Cornstarch.** Cornstarch is a powdery, dense flour with almost twice the thickening power of flour. It is often used in desserts and sweet sauces. A sauce made with cornstarch will be almost clear in appearance and have a glossy texture.

■ **Arrowroot.** Arrowroot is similar to cornstarch but more expensive. It is made from the roots of several tropical plants. Arrowroot creates a clearer sauce than cornstarch does. It is also used in frozen foods because the sauce won't break down when frozen.

■ **Instant starches.** Instant starches have been dried after being cooked. They can thicken a liquid without being heated. They are used more commonly in baking than in sauce making.

■ **Bread crumbs.** Because they have already been cooked, bread crumbs can thicken a liquid quickly. Keep in mind, however, that a sauce made with bread crumbs will not be smooth.

Fig. 20-7. Thickening agents such as cornstarch are used in sauce making. Name some other thickening agents.

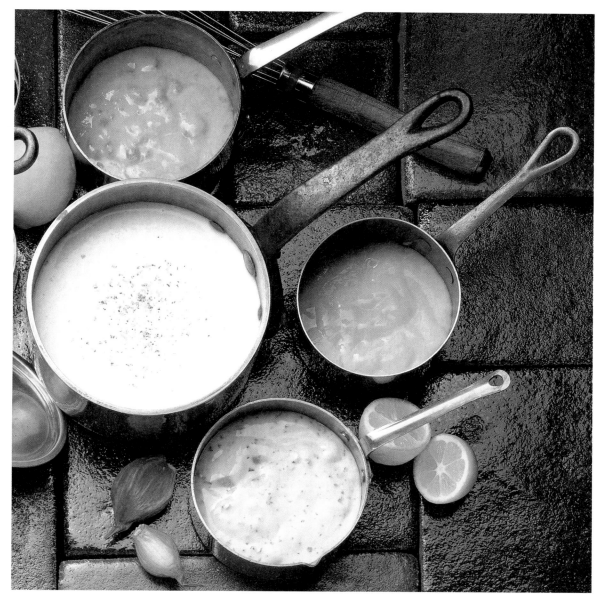

Fig. 20-8. Many sauces are thickened with a form of starch. How can you tell these sauces have been sitting too long?

■ **Vegetable purées.** A **purée** (pyuh-RAY) is a food that has been mashed, strained, or finely chopped into a smooth pulp. Purées can be used to thicken sauces. A vegetable, such as potatoes, or a combination of vegetables may be cooked with herbs, spices, and other flavorings and then puréed. If you need to thin a purée, add water, cream, or stock. A **coulis** (koo-LEE) is a sauce made from a fruit or vegetable purée. Vegetable purées and coulis are healthful choices because they do not rely on the fat content of the heavier sauces. See Fig. 20-8.

⊠ MOTHER SAUCES

The five basic sauces are known as mother sauces, or leading sauces. These sauces are all made by combining a liquid with a thickening agent. Compound sauces are made from these mother sauces. For example, a mother sauce such as Béchamel (BAY-chuh-MEHL) forms the basis for an additional five sauces. The five mother sauces are listed on page 461.

THE SCIENCE OF THICKENING

Starches, such as flour and cornstarch, are often used to thicken sauces. What is a starch, though, and how does the thickening process work?

A starch is made up of many glucose molecules that are bonded together. Although starch may look like a finely powdered solid, it is really made up of granules. Due to the large structure of a starch molecule, it normally doesn't dissolve in cold water. As the water is heated, however, the molecules that make up the starch begin to get more active, thus weakening the bonds between the starch molecules. This causes the starch granules to absorb the water. The hotter the water gets, the more the granules absorb. As the granules absorb the water, they begin to swell. This process is called **gelatinization**. Near the boiling point of the liquid (between 160°F–180°F), the granules have absorbed so much water that each granule finally pops. Starch rushes into the sauce and the sauce finally thickens.

One problem with using starch to thicken sauces is its tendency to form lumps. It helps to disperse the starch in some cold water before you apply it directly into the hot sauce.

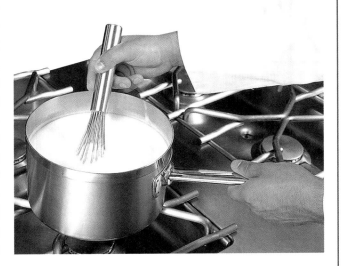

APPLY IT!

Complete the following experiment to observe what happens when you add a starch to a hot liquid. You will need 2 pts. of chicken broth, two small sauce pots, 4 tbsp. bread flour, and a ½-cup container with a cover.

1. Pour one pint of chicken broth into a pot and heat it until it becomes very hot.

2. Add 2 tbsp. of bread flour to the broth. Stir and continue heating. Observe and record what you notice about the broth.

3. Pour the remaining pint of broth into a pot and heat it until it becomes very hot.

4. Place remaining 2 tbsp. of bread flour into a small cup and add ¼ cup of water. Cover and shake well.

5. Pour this mixture into the broth, stir, and continue heating. Observe and record what you notice about this broth.

6. Explain what you observed in each pot of broth.

7. Why do you think it is a good idea to disperse the starch in a small amount of cold liquid before you add it to your soup or sauce?

■ **Sauce espagnole.** Made from thickened brown stock, sauce espagnole (ehs-pahn-YOHL)—French for "Spanish sauce"—also contains some type of tomato product. In general, this type of sauce has few added seasonings. Demi-glace (DEHM-ee-glahs) is made from sauce espagnole. It is half espagnole sauce and half brown stock that has been reduced by half. Demi-glace comes from the French for "half-glaze."

■ **Tomato sauce.** This sauce is made by simmering a tomato product with flavorings, seasonings, and stock or another liquid. Although basic tomato sauce is made with vegetables only, some variations add meat.

■ **Béchamel sauce.** Also known as a cream sauce or a white sauce, this mother sauce is made by thickening milk with a white roux (roo), seasonings, and flavorings. A **roux** is a cooked mixture made from equal parts of fat and flour by weight.

■ **Velouté.** From the French word for "velvety," Velouté (veh-loo-TAY) sauce, also known as blond sauce, is made by thickening a light-colored stock with a light-colored roux. The sauce is named after the type of stock it contains. For example,

chicken velouté is made with a white chicken stock.

■ **Hollandaise sauce.** From the French word for "Dutch," hollandaise (HOL-uhn-dayz) sauce is made from emulsified egg yolks, clarified butter, seasonings, and often lemon juice. Emulsifying takes place when substances, such as water and oil, are mixed with an emulsifier like egg yolks. Once mixed, these substances will not separate. See Fig. 20-9.

Other Sauces

From the five basic mother sauces come hundreds of different compound sauces. For example, adding olive oil and spices to a basic tomato sauce creates a marinara sauce.

Not all sauces, however, come from these mother sauces. Some sauces are made from a purée of fruits or vegetables. Other sauces are made from meat juices or butter. These familiar sauces include salsa, relishes, gravy, compound butters, and independent sauces.

Fig. 20-9. The five mother sauces.

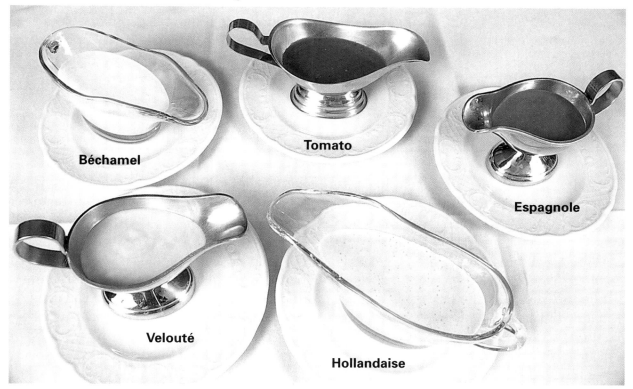

Béchamel

Tomato

Espagnole

Velouté

Hollandaise

Simmer:
1. Heat the cooking liquid to the proper temperature.
2. Submerge the food product completely.
3. Keep the cooked product moist and warm.

GLOSSARY:
Clouté: studded with cloves
Chinois: cone-shaped strainer
Bain-marie: hot-water bath

HACCP:
Hold at 135°F or above or cool to an internal temperature of 41°F or below.

HAZARDOUS FOOD:
Milk

NUTRITION:
Calories: 67.2
Fat: 4.23 g
Protein: 2.34 g

CHEF NOTES:
1. Béchamel sauce is a basic white cream sauce consisting simply of thickened, seasoned milk. Béchamel is often used as a binding agent or to make compound sauces.
2. The sauce is ready when the proper thickness has been achieved and the "floury" taste is cooked away.
3. To prevent a dried surface (skin) from forming while holding the sauce in a **bain marie**, cover the surface with plastic wrap.

Béchamel Sauce

YIELD: 1 GAL.   SERVING SIZE: 2 OZ.

INGREDIENTS

4 qts.	Milk
1 each	Onion **clouté**, cut in half
6 oz.	Clarified butter
6 oz.	All-purpose flour, sifted
	Salt and ground white pepper, to taste
	Nutmeg, to taste

METHOD OF PREPARATION

1. In a saucepan, heat the milk with the onion **clouté**, and simmer for 10 minutes.

2. In another saucepan, heat the clarified butter over moderate heat.

3. Gradually add flour to make a blonde roux. Using a spoon, mix the roux thoroughly, and cook it approximately 5–6 minutes. Remove from the heat, and cool slightly.

4. Remove the onion clouté from the milk.

5. Gradually add the hot milk to the roux, whisking constantly. Heat to a boil; reduce to a simmer. Simmer for 20 minutes or until the proper flavor and consistency are achieved.

6. Season to taste.

7. Strain through a fine **chinois** into a suitable container. Hold at 135°F or above, or cool to an internal temperature of 41°F or below. Label, date, and refrigerate.

8. Reheat to 165°F for 15 seconds.

■ **Salsa.** Salsa means "sauce" in Spanish. Salsas can include a combination of raw vegetables or fruits, spices, onions, and chiles. They can be used for more than dipping vegetables or chips, however. Salsas can also be used as sauces for potatoes, poultry, meat, or fish entrées. See Fig. 20-10.

■ **Relishes.** Relishes are another type of sauce. Often made with fruits or vegetables, this sauce may be used as a condiment or a sauce for meat, poultry, and fish. The sauce may be cooked or pickled—preserved in a seasoned solution of vinegar or brine (BRYN). Relishes may be sweet, savory, or spicy. They also vary in texture from smooth to chunky.

■ **Gravy.** Gravy is a type of sauce made from meat or poultry juices; a liquid such as milk, cream, or broth; and a thickening agent such as a roux. Pan gravy is made from the deglazed pan drippings of roasted meat or poultry. The pan gravy is served with the meat. You may also serve gravy with a side dish such as mashed potatoes.

Fig. 20-10. Salsa is a colorful and tasty addition to many foods.

■ **Compound butters.** By adding seasonings to softened butter, you can make compound butters. You may have eaten at a restaurant where herbs, such as basil, chives, or parsley, have been blended into the butter served with the bread. Sometimes a compound butter is placed on top of a piece of fish or meat just before serving. As it melts, the butter flavors the food.

■ **Independent sauces.** Applesauce, cocktail, sweet and sour, and barbecue sauce are four common examples of independent sauces. These sauces may be served hot or cold.

✖ PREPARING ROUX

Many sauces are formed from a stock and roux. A roux is the most commonly used thickening agent. Many chefs use 60% flour and 40% fat to decrease the calories and fat in sauces. Being able to make a good roux is a very important skill.

Roux Ingredients

Equal parts of fat and flour by weight form a paste when cooked together. Roux can be white, blond, or brown, depending in part on how long it is cooked.

Fat

The following cooking fats can be used to make roux.

■ **Clarified butter.** Also known as drawn butter, clarified butter is purified butterfat. This means that the butter is melted with the water and milk solids removed. Clarified butter is preferred for making roux because the water in unclarified butter changes the consistency of the roux. One pound of clarified butter results from 1¼ lbs. of butter. See Fig. 20-11.

■ **Margarine.** Because of its low cost, margarine is often used instead of butter. Although the quality of margarine varies, it does not generally make as good a sauce as butter.

Fig. 20-11. Water and milk solids have been removed from clarified butter. Why is clarified butter preferred for making roux?

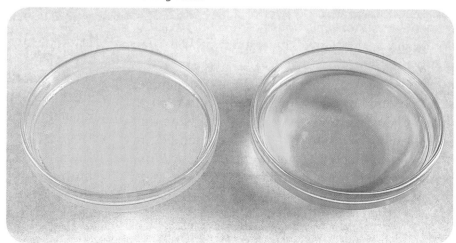

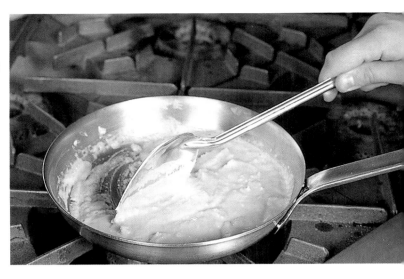

- **Animal fats.** These fats include lard, butter, and the fats that come directly from an animal, such as chicken fat. Use these fats to flavor sauces. For example, use veal fat in veal velouté and chicken drippings in chicken gravy.
- **Vegetable oil.** These oils include those specific oils that come from plants as well as blends of different vegetable oils, including corn, safflower, and soybean. Because these oils don't add flavor to a sauce, they are not recommended.
- **Shortening.** This white, solid fat has no flavor and a high melting point, which make it better for frying or baking than for sauce making.

Flour

Starch content plays an important role in the thickening power of flour. Because bread flour contains less starch than cake flour, 10 oz. of bread flour has the same thickening power as 8 oz. of cake flour.

Bread flour is used to thicken sauces in most commercial kitchens. That's why the recipes for most sauces are based on bread flour or all-purpose flour, which has about the same thickening power as bread flour. If you use a different kind of flour, be sure to adjust the ratio of roux to liquid. For example, Cajun (KAY-juhn) recipes may call for browned flour. This flour has been browned in an oven. It has less thickening power than unbrowned flour.

- **Proportions of roux ingredients.** Remember that you must use equal parts of fat and flour to make a good roux. Test this by making sure that there's enough fat to coat all the granules of starch. If too much fat is used, the excess will rise to the top and must be skimmed off. The right consistency for a roux is stiff, not runny.

Steps in Making Roux

Regardless of the color of roux desired, you'll follow these basic steps:

1. Heat the fat, usually clarified butter, in a heavy saucepan so that the fat will not scorch.
2. Make a paste by adding all of the bread flour and stirring.
3. Using medium heat, cook the paste until it is the consistency of sand and the right color.
4. Stir roux often to keep it from burning. See Fig. 20-12. Burnt roux will add an unpleasant flavor and dark spots to the liquid. It will not thicken properly. When finished, the roux should be stiff.

Keep the following in mind when preparing roux:

- DO NOT use aluminum cookware. It will give the roux a metallic taste and make light-colored sauces gray. Instead, use heavy stainless steel pots. They will keep the sauces from burning or scorching.
- DO NOT use very high or very low temperatures. A roux that is very hot can spatter and burn someone as it's mixed in a liquid. A roux that is colder than room temperature will cause the fat to solidify. An ice-cold roux will solidify.

Fig. 20-13.

ROUX COLOR	COOKING TIME
White	4–6 min.
Blond	6–8 min.
Brown	15–20 min.

- DO NOT overthicken. A sauce must almost reach the boiling point before the roux begins to thicken it. Add 1 lb. roux per gallon of sauce for a medium consistency.

The color of a sauce depends upon the length of time a roux is cooked. To achieve a white, blond, or brown roux, use the cooking times in Fig. 20-13.

To avoid creating lumps when mixing roux and the liquid base together, use one of the following methods:

- **Method A**: Add cold stock to the hot roux, using a whisk to stir briskly.
- **Method B**: Dissolve the cold roux with warm or hot liquid before adding it to a hot stock. This will prevent lumps from forming. Stir briskly.

Cook the sauce mixture at least 20 minutes after it begins to boil. The final cooking will take away any floury taste.

Thickening by Reduction

Sauces are also thickened by reduction, the process of simmering down a liquid. A liquid can be cooked down to one-half or one-fourth of its original amount. This concentrates the flavor even more, since the amount of water is reduced.

Use several layers of cheesecloth and a china cap to strain the sauce for the greatest smoothness. Straining will also remove the stems and leaves of any spices, herbs, or other seasonings. This will not remove the flavor.

Sauces will be judged by their quality in the following categories:

- Appearance, for shine and color.
- Flavor.
- Texture, or smoothness.
- Thickness, as appropriate to the type of sauce.
- Clarity (KLAIR-uh-tee), or how clear it is.

STORAGE

Sauces are generally prepared to be used the same day. If a sauce must be stored, pour melted butter on top or cover the sauce with oiled parchment paper before storing. This will reduce the amount of fat that will come to the surface of the sauce. Sauces should be kept refrigerated. Place the sauce in a plastic storage container with a tight-fitting lid.

SECTION 20-2 Knowledge Check

1. Contrast a béchamel and a velouté sauce.
2. What happens during gelatinization?
3. Explain how to avoid creating lumps when mixing a roux and a liquid base together.

MINI LAB

Working in teams, make a mother sauce or a compound sauce. Compare results by tasting each team's sauce.

SECTION SUMMARIES

20-1 The four basic types of stocks are white, brown, fish, and vegetable.

20-1 The steps in preparing white stock include: covering bones with cold water in a stock pot, skimming impurities from the surface, and straining the stock through a china cap lined with cheesecloth.

20-1 Brown stocks are prepared in the same way as white stocks except that the bones and mirepoix are browned in a brown stock.

20-1 Vegetable stocks, which do not include meat products, use a variety of vegetables with different recipes.

20-2 There are five basic sauces called mother, or leading sauces. Other sauces include compound sauces, which come from mother sauces; independent sauces; and those made from purées, meat juices, or butter.

20-2 Sauces should complement, not overpower, the foods they accompany and can be served directly with the food, on the side, or as a dip.

20-2 Thickening agents such as flour and cornstarch are used to thicken sauces.

20-2 Although all sauces are made by adding a thickening agent to stock or another liquid, you can change the sauce by carefully choosing seasonings and flavorings.

CHECK YOUR KNOWLEDGE

1. Name one advantage and one disadvantage of using commercial bases for stock.
2. Describe the four main ingredients found in all types of stocks.
3. Compare the characteristics of a white stock versus a brown stock.
4. Explain why it is important to begin with cold water when making a stock.
5. Describe how you cool a stock.
6. What is a glaze, and how is it made?
7. Contrast an espagnole and a demi-glace sauce.
8. What is a compound butter?
9. Contrast the use of flour and cornstarch as thickening agents.
10. Explain why most chefs prefer to use clarified butter in a sauce.

CRITICAL-THINKING ACTIVITIES

1. Beef stock and veal stock need to be cooked for up to 8 hours. Why do you think it takes so long to make these stocks? What could happen if you cut the cooking time in half?
2. The white stock you've made has turned out cloudy. List three reasons why this may have happened. How could you prevent this from happening the next time?

WORKPLACE KNOW-HOW

Problem solving. Suppose there is not enough stock to make the amount of sauce needed for the daily special. You don't have time to make another batch from scratch. How can you fill orders without sacrificing the quality and taste of the sauce?

LAB-BASED ACTIVITY: Making a Béchamel Sauce

STEP ❶ Working in teams, prepare a Béchamel sauce. The sauce will be judged by its taste, texture, and appearance. Before you make the roux, think about what type of fat and flour you'll use to make it and the specific procedures you'll follow.

STEP ❷ Keep in mind the characteristics of a good Béchamel sauce:
- Color of heavy cream.
- Shiny.
- Rich.
- Creamy.
- Completely smooth.
- Thick enough to coat.
- Creamy flavor not overpowered by onions or cloves.
- No floury taste.

STEP ❸ Here are some important things to remember while making your sauce:
- Clarified butter is preferred for making roux.
- Be sure to adjust the ratio of roux to liquid.
- You must use equal parts of fat and flour by weight to make a good roux. Make sure there's enough fat to coat all the starch granules with no excess fat left over.

- Use a heavy saucepan so the fat won't scorch. Don't use aluminum cookware. It will give the roux a metallic taste.
- To keep the roux from burning, use medium heat and stir often.
- Cook until the roux is the right color. The cooking time for a white roux is 4–6 minutes.
- Gradually add the hot milk to the roux. Stir constantly with a whisk to avoid creating lumps when mixing the roux and milk together.
- Continue cooking the sauce mixture at least 20 minutes after it boils to remove the floury taste.
- Strain the sauce through a china cap lined with cheesecloth.
- Serve immediately or hold at 135°F or above for less than 2 hours, stirring often.
- If you're holding the sauce, cover its surface with plastic wrap to keep a skin from forming.

STEP ❹ Prepare the Béchamel Sauce Recipe on page 462.

STEP ❺ After you've prepared the sauce, have another team evaluate its characteristics. Be sure to include comments about what could be done to improve the sauce.

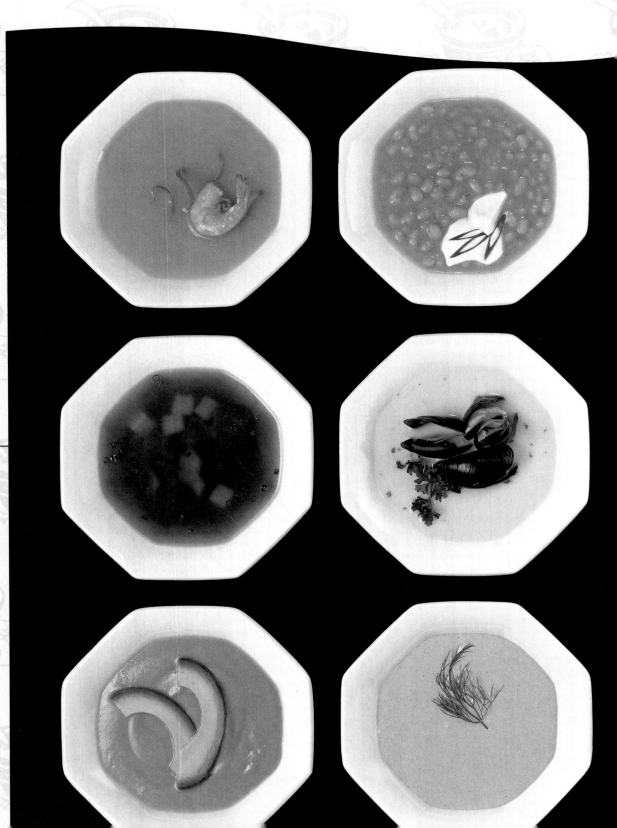

21 Soups & Appetizers

CHAPTER

Making Soups

KEY TERMS

- **consommé**

- **bisque**

- **chowder**

- **sweating**

- **clarify**

- **raft**

- **vichyssoise**

OBJECTIVES

After reading this section, you will be able to:

- Identify the various classes of soups.

- Describe how to prepare various soups, using commercial bases or stock.

- Present soups attractively garnished.

- Store soups safely for future use.

S O U P is a popular menu choice. As an appetizer or as the main course, customers like the variety of flavors and nutrition that different soups provide. This section introduces you to the skills involved in making soups. Once you understand the basic procedures for preparing soups, you will be able to make a wide variety of nourishing meals. You may even create some interesting new soups.

☒ TYPES OF SOUPS

Soups are frequently served at lunch and dinner. A lunch special may include a combination of soup and salad, soup and potato, or soup and sandwich. Likewise, a hearty minestrone (mee-nuh-STROH-nay) or French onion soup can satisfy your hunger at dinner when served with a chunk of crusty bread. Menus most often offer the choice of either a cup or a bowl of soup.

Soups are usually classified as clear or unthickened soups, thick soups, and specialty soups. Most soups begin with a stock. See Chapter 20 to learn how stock is made.

Clear Soups

They are made from clear stock or broth. Clear soups are not thickened. Broth is made from simmered meat and vegetables. Vegetable soup is made from a clear stock or broth that has been seasoned and may include meat, vegetables, and a starch such as potatoes. A concentrated, clear soup made from a rich broth is called a **consommé** (KON-suh-may).

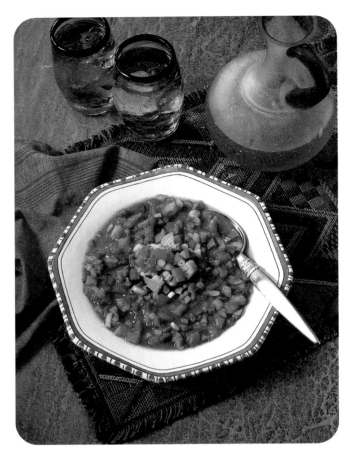

Fig. 21-1. International soups such as gazpacho have become commonplace on many restaurant menus.

Specialty Soups

Specialty soups highlight a specific region or reflect the use of special ingredients or techniques. Some examples of specialty soups are bisques, chowders, cold soups, and international soups. See Fig. 21-1.

■ **Bisques.** Specialty soups that are usually made from shellfish and contain cream are called **bisques** (bihsks). For example, lobster bisque is prepared like a cream soup.

■ **Chowders.** Specialty soups made from fish, seafood, or vegetables are called **chowders**. They usually contain potatoes and are often made with milk.

■ **Cold soups.** Cold soups are specialty soups that may be cooked or uncooked and then chilled. It depends on the ingredients. Yogurt, cream, or puréed fruit is often used as a thickener.

■ **International soups.** International soups are linked to different nations or cultures. For example, Borscht (BOHR-sht) is a beet soup originally from Russia, and gazpacho (gahz-PAH-choh) is a cold Spanish soup.

Thick Soups

Thick soups are not clear or transparent. Thick soups include a thickening agent, such as roux; milk; cream; or a vegetable purée. Thick soups such as cream of chicken or cream of mushroom are examples.

■ **Purée soups.** Soups that are thickened by grinding the soup's main ingredient in a food processor are called purées (pyuh-RAYS). Split pea, navy bean, and butternut squash soup are examples. These hearty soups are filling and are sometimes offered as a main course. Purées may contain milk or cream.

■ **Cream soups.** Cream soups are velvety-smooth thick soups. They are made with cooked vegetables that are sometimes puréed. They may also be made with rich chicken broth.

Fig. 21-2. Clear soups are fairly simple to prepare and, when garnished, are appealing to the eye. What would you serve alongside this soup?

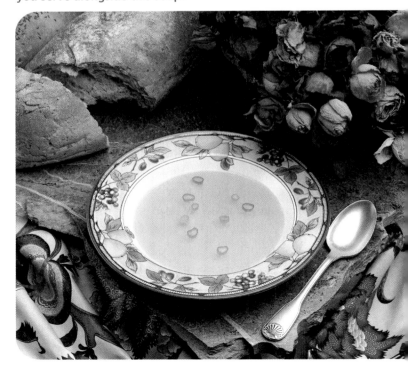

MAKING CLEAR SOUPS

Clear soups are made primarily of broths that can stand alone as a dish. See Fig. 21-2. Broths are more flavorful than stocks because the meat, not merely the bone, is simmered with the other ingredients. In addition, broth has even more flavor when stock, rather than water, is used as the liquid ingredient.

Clear soups are fairly simple to prepare. It is important that the ingredients are of the highest quality available. Follow these steps to make a clear soup.

1. Simmer or brown meats and sweat vegetables that will flavor the soup. **Sweating** vegetables in fat over low heat is a process that allows them to release moisture. This helps vegetables release their flavors more quickly when combined with other ingredients. Be sure not to let the vegetables brown. See Fig. 21-3.

2. Add simmering stock to the vegetables.

3. Continue to simmer the soup.

4. Skim off the impurities and fats as they rise to the surface while the mixture is simmering.

5. Season the soup to taste before serving.

Fig. 21-3. These vegetables are being "sweated" to add flavor to a clear soup.

Consommé

Consommé is made from stock or broth. The broth is reduced to evaporate some of the water. This makes the liquid more concentrated. A consommé's strong flavor is its most important characteristic. Second to its richness, however, is the clarity of the consommé. To **clarify** a consommé means to remove the particles as they float to the top. This way the particles don't cloud the consommé, and it remains clear.

Since a consommé must be completely clear, starting with the best broth is very important. The steps below explain how to make a consommé.

1. Combine ground poultry or beef, lightly beaten egg white, and other ingredients such as a tomato product.

2. Add cold broth and stir. If the broth has a weak flavor, heat it in a separate pan and reduce it until it is concentrated. Then add it to the other ingredients.

3. Stir the mixture occasionally as you bring it to a simmer over medium heat.

4. The egg white and meat proteins coagulate as they cook, forming a raft. The **raft** is a floating mass that forms from the mixture of meat and eggs. The raft traps the impurities that rise to the top of the broth. Do not stir the mixture after this point, and do not cover. See Fig. 21-4.

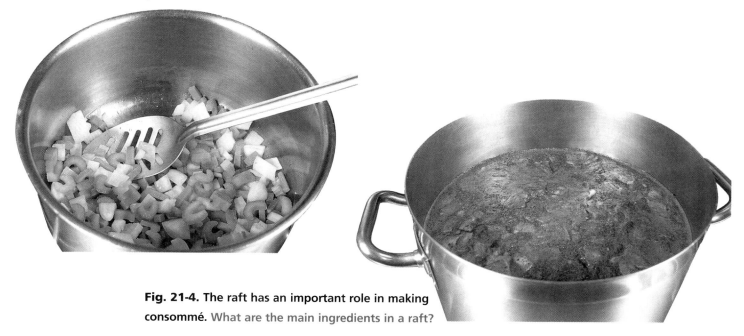

Fig. 21-4. The raft has an important role in making consommé. What are the main ingredients in a raft?

5. Lower the heat and simmer slowly for 1–1½ hours to extract flavor and clarify.

6. Use several layers of cheesecloth or coffee filters and a china cap to strain the consommé. Taste and adjust seasonings as needed.

7. Cool and refrigerate if the consommé is not going to be used immediately.

8. Remove any fat from the surface when the consommé is completely cooled.

9. When you reheat the consommé, remove any dots of remaining fat on the surface by blotting with a paper towel.

Vegetable Soups

Vegetable soup is one of the easiest clear soups to prepare, but attention to detail is still necessary. Meat-based stock or broth is used most often. For vegetarian soup, use a vegetable-based stock or broth. Make sure you cut all the vegetables approximately the same size so they will cook evenly. Pasta or grains, such as rice or barley, may be added for a heartier version.

CULINARY TIP

COOKING VEGETABLES—When making a vegetable soup, be sure to add the vegetables based on how long they will need to cook. For example, carrots take longer to soften than spinach does, so add the carrots first. If all of the vegetables are added at the same time, the softer vegetables will become overcooked.

KEY Science SKILLS

CLARIFYING STOCK

When stock is clarified for consommé, ground meat, egg whites, finely chopped mirepoix, and often a tomato product are added to the stock. The egg whites dissolve in the stock. They dissolve because they are almost completely made of albumin, which is a water-soluble protein.

The egg whites begin to coagulate when the albumin reaches about 120°–130°F. You can see this happen when whitish sticky strands begin to appear at the sides of the pot. As the egg whites coagulate, they capture the ground meat, and vegetable matter, along with other impurities that cloud the liquid. This makes a raft, or mat of cooked egg whites, ground meat and vegetables. Because the meat is lighter than the stock, it rises to the surface with vegetables and egg, clarifying the liquid as it rises. It is important not to let the stock boil through the raft and break it.

After the raft has risen to the top of the pot, and the consommé has simmered, you will need to drain off the clear consommé without breaking the raft. If the raft breaks, cloudy particles will disperse throughout the liquid. The clear liquid should be strained through a fine chinois lined with several layers of moistened cheese cloth. A stock pot with a spigot allows the consommé to be strained from the bottom without breaking the raft. The raft can be carefully cut and the liquid removed with a ladle.

APPLY IT!

Prepare a consommé from scratch. Then prepare a commercial liquid consommé base. Compare the final products for taste, clarity, and ease of preparation. What is the benefit of using each product?

Simmer & Poach:
1. Heat the cooking liquid to the proper temperature.
2. Submerge the food product completely.
3. Keep the cooked product moist and warm.

Boil: (at sea level)
1. Bring the cooking liquid to a rapid boil.
2. Stir the contents, and cook the food product throughout.
3. Serve hot.

GLOSSARY:
Mirepoix: roughly chopped vegetables
Brunoise: ⅛-in. dice
Marmite: stockpot
Chinois: fine, cone-shaped strainer

HACCP:
Hold at 135°F or above.
Cool to 41°F or below.

HAZARDOUS FOODS:
Egg whites
Ground beef

NUTRITION:
Calories: 116
Fat: 4.34 g
Protein: 13.8 g

CHEF NOTES:
1. There are many types of consommé. To create a chicken consommé, add ground chicken and use cold chicken stock. To create a fish consommé, use cold fish stock and lean white fish, omit the carrots and black peppercorns, use white peppercorns, and replace the onions with leeks; the tomato purée is optional. To create a vegetable consommé, use the vegetable stock, increase the egg whites, and replace the onions with leeks.
2. If the stock is gelatinous, allow it to liquify before using.

Beef Consommé

YIELD: 50 SERVINGS

SERVING SIZE: 8 OZ.

INGREDIENTS

5 gal.	Cold brown beef stock or strong beef broth
10 each	Egg whites, slightly whipped
3 lbs.	Ground beef, lean
16 each	Black peppercorns
6 each	Bay leaves
3 oz.	Parsley stems
1½ tsp.	Thyme leaves

MIREPOIX:

12 oz.	Onion, peeled, cut **brunoise**
2 lbs.	Carrots, washed, peeled, cut brunoise
4 stalks	Celery, washed, trimmed, cut brunoise
2 pts.	Tomato purée

METHOD OF PREPARATION

1. In a mixing bowl, combine the lean ground beef, mirepoix, tomato purée, herbs, spices, salt, and white pepper to taste. Mix the egg whites and meat mixture until blended. Refrigerate.

2. In a **marmite**, blend the cold beef stock with the above clarifying ingredients.

3. Place on moderate heat. Carefully watch the clarifying ingredients to make sure they do not scorch. Stir occasionally, until a raft forms. Then stop stirring.

4. Simmer the soup for 1½ hours or to the desired strength, making sure the raft does not break or sink. Remove the first cup of consommé through the spigot, and discard.

5. In a **chinois** lined with four to five layers of wet cheesecloth, slowly strain the liquid into a soup insert, separating the clarifying ingredients from the liquid. Hold at 135°F or above.

6. Adjust the seasonings. Remove all of the fat from the consommé, and serve very hot with the appropriate garnish.

7. Cool to an internal temperature of 41°F or below.

8. Reheat to 165°F for 15 seconds.

✖ MAKING THICK SOUPS

Thick soups differ from thin soups because of the thickening agents that are added to them. Cream soups, which are the most common thick soups, are often thickened with roux and finished with cream or milk. Milk thins the soup. Cream adds richness without thinning. Cream soups can be made from leafy or soft vegetables such as broccoli, asparagus, or spinach. Hard vegetables, including squash or roasted red peppers, may also be used.

Making Purée Soups

Purée soups are also thick soups. Though cream is occasionally used to thicken a purée soup, the main ingredient of the soup itself is puréed for thickness. Purée soups have a coarser texture than do cream soups. The coarse texture comes from legumes or starchy vegetables such as peas or potatoes. These ingredients form the basis of the soup. Because the soup is made from such ingredients, it is usually very thick and hearty. Making purée soups is simple, as the following steps show. See Fig. 21-5.

1. Cut up fresh vegetables and sweat them in fat over low heat.
2. Add the liquid, such as stock, that has been simmering in a separate pan.
3. Add starchy or dried vegetables.
4. Simmer the soup until all vegetables are cooked but not overcooked.
5. Purée the soup, using a food processor.
6. Simmer again, and check that the soup has the desired thickness.
7. Add a thickening agent or more liquid to adjust the thickness.
8. Add final seasonings and serve.

Making Cream Soups

One way cream soups get their velvety texture is by being puréed. Puréeing soup requires the vegetables to be cooked to a tender consistency so that they are easily folded into the soup. Follow these steps to make a cream soup:

1. Sweat hard vegetables, such as carrots or celery, in butter or oil by slowly cooking them over low heat.
2. Thicken the soup by adding flour to make a roux.
3. Add hot stock or milk to the roux and vegetables. Simmer, being careful that the soup doesn't brown.

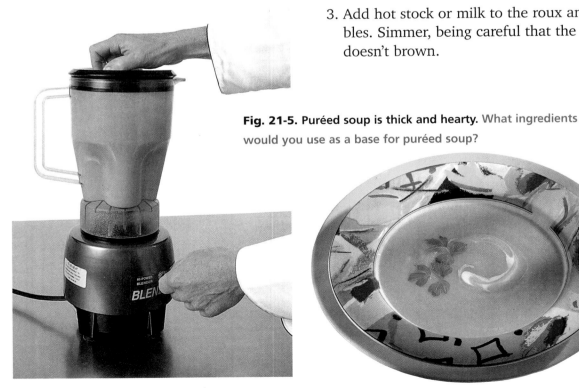
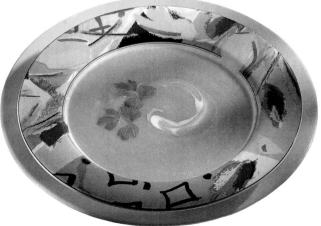

Fig. 21-5. Puréed soup is thick and hearty. What ingredients would you use as a base for puréed soup?

4. Add a spice sachet or bouquet garni if desired, along with any soft vegetables such as asparagus or broccoli. Cook the vegetables until just soft.

5. Skim impurities and fat from the soup as it simmers.

6. Purée the soup until it is very smooth.

7. Add hot Béchamel sauce or cream to finish the soup.

8. Adjust the seasonings before serving.

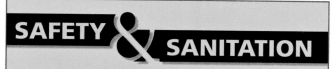

MAINTAINING TEMPERATURE—Since bacteria growth only slows down in cold food, it is important to reheat foods to safe temperatures at 165°F or above. Before placing cream soups on a steamtable, heat them to the proper temperature.

Making Bisques and Chowders

A bisque is made with a concentrated stock of shellfish, such as lobster or shrimp, cream, and roux. Even the shells are added for flavor before the bisque is strained.

Chowders may be compared to stews, because they are hearty, chunky soups. Most are based on vegetables, shellfish, or fish. They are thickened with roux, usually include potatoes, and use cream or milk for the liquid ingredient. See Fig. 21-6.

Because bisques and chowders generally include milk or cream, it is best not to leave them on the serving line too long. The milk may curdle or spoil the batch. Ideally, make small batches of these soups.

Making Cold Soups

Cold soups are either cooked and then chilled, or not cooked. This vague description is due to the many varied ways there are to prepare a cold soup. It is also important to note that adding dairy products to cold soups reduces their shelf life.

■ **Cooked cold soups.** A large number of hot soups may be chilled and served cold. One of the most popular cold cooked soups is **vichyssoise** (vih-shee-SWAHZ), a cold version of potato-leek soup. Cold cream soups are different from hot cream soups in the following ways:

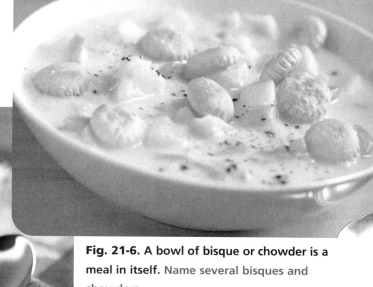

Fig. 21-6. A bowl of bisque or chowder is a meal in itself. Name several bisques and chowders.

- Cream is added to a cold soup just before serving, after it has already chilled. This process increases the soup's shelf life since the cold soup is not stored with the cream already added.
- Taste a cold cream soup just before serving to ensure that it is flavorful enough because cold dulls the flavor.
- The consistency of the cold cream soup should be thinner than the hot cream soup. Use either less thickener or more liquid.

■ **Uncooked cold soups.** Uncooked cold soups are fairly simple to prepare. The majority of the work comes from chopping the ingredients. Fresh fruit or vegetables are often puréed for thickness, and occasionally cream or yogurt is added, too. It is best to make uncooked cold soups in small batches.

✖ INTERNATIONAL SOUPS

There has been a steady increase in the number of ethnic restaurants in the United States in the last few years. It is not uncommon to find authentic Indian and Thai soups offered as specialties. Soup is almost always offered on both lunch and dinner menus in ethnic restaurants, highlighting ingredients associated with a culture's cuisine.

Certain international soups, such as French onion and gazpacho, have become mainstream. These soups are often found in restaurants with mostly American-style cuisine. Minestrone is one of the many international soups that can easily stand alone as a meal. It includes not only a wide array of vegetables, but pasta and beans, too.

Fig. 21-7. These four soups are presented in bread bowls. Name each soup.

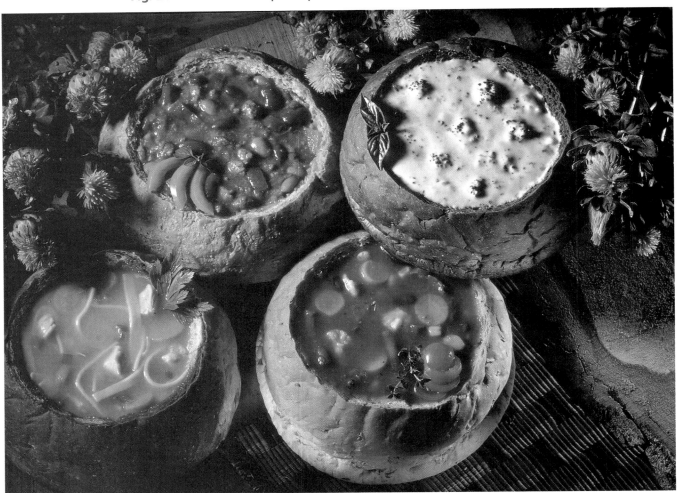

✕ PRESENTING SOUPS

Whether as an appetizer or a meal, a soup's presentation is important. The size and type of the cup or bowl is usually determined by the type of soup, the meal at which it is served, and when during the meal it is to be eaten—as an appetizer or an entrée. The soup portion served as an appetizer should be 6–8 oz., and 10–12 oz. for a main course portion.

The temperature of the bowl or cup will influence the presentation of the soup, too. See Fig. 21-7. The bowl should be heated for serving a hot soup and cold for serving a cold soup. Most importantly, when serving the soup, make sure the soup itself is the proper temperature. Serve cold soups at 41°F or below. Serve hot soups at 165°F or above.

Garnishing Soups

Since soups can be plain in appearance, their presentation should be enhanced with a garnish. Each hot consommé is named according to its garnish. For example, consommé Célestine (suh-LEHS-teen) is garnished with small, thin, savory pancakes cut into julienne strips. The soup's name was that of the chef to Napoleon III.

Garnishes such as parsley or sour cream often make the difference between an appetizing appearance and a dull one, and may be placed in the soup itself. An artistically cut vegetable that is a main ingredient in a puréed soup, for example, may be placed on top of the soup. Toppings other than the main ingredient, such as grated cheese, croutons, or fresh herbs, add contrast to a soup that is all one color, such as puréed soup. Garnishes must be applied just before they are served.

■ **Accompaniment suggestions.** Soups are often served with an accompaniment. Here are some alternatives:

- Whole-grain wafers.
- Corn chips.
- Saltine or oyster crackers.
- Melba toast.
- Bread sticks.

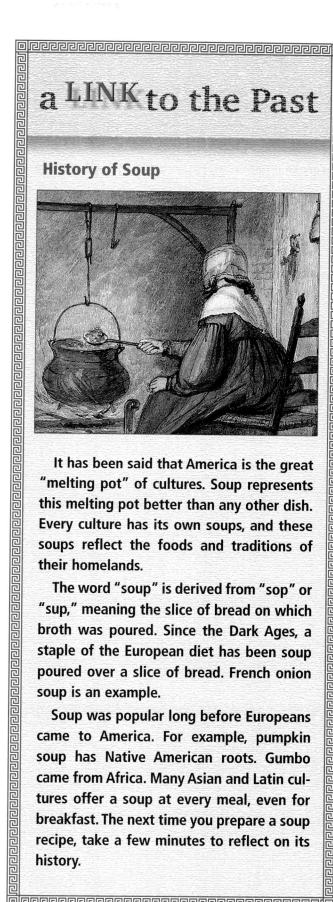

a LINK to the Past

History of Soup

It has been said that America is the great "melting pot" of cultures. Soup represents this melting pot better than any other dish. Every culture has its own soups, and these soups reflect the foods and traditions of their homelands.

The word "soup" is derived from "sop" or "sup," meaning the slice of bread on which broth was poured. Since the Dark Ages, a staple of the European diet has been soup poured over a slice of bread. French onion soup is an example.

Soup was popular long before Europeans came to America. For example, pumpkin soup has Native American roots. Gumbo came from Africa. Many Asian and Latin cultures offer a soup at every meal, even for breakfast. The next time you prepare a soup recipe, take a few minutes to reflect on its history.

■ **Guidelines for garnishing.** Use the following suggestions for garnishing soups.

• Garnishes should be attractively arranged.

• Vegetables or meats used as a garnish should be cut about the same size and shape. This is especially important for garnishing a consommé, because the clear soup will highlight any uneven cuts.

• The flavor and texture of the garnish should complement the soup.

• If you are using vegetables or starches as garnishes, cook them separately so they will not cloud the soup.

• Do not overcook garnishes. Vegetables should not be mushy; meat or poultry should not fall apart; rice and pasta should hold their shape. To keep from overcooking, prepare these garnishes separately and hold them on the side until just before serving.

✖ STORING SOUPS

When making large batches of thick soup, cool and refrigerate the soup before adding the milk or cream. See Fig. 21-8. It is best to heat only small batches of soup if holding the soup in a steam-table, and replenish when necessary. Soups will continue to thicken while in the steam table. Be sure to check the consistency before serving. Heat the base over low heat, then add the milk or cream. To keep the soup from scorching, stir it often. Taste the soup to see if the seasonings need to be adjusted before serving.

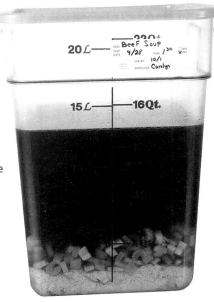

Fig. 21-8. Soup must be stored in tightly sealed containers. How fast should soup be cooled?

SECTION 21-1   Knowledge Check

1. Identify three classifications of soup.
2. List the key differences in preparing clear and thick soups.
3. Explain the difference between a broth and a consommé.

MINI LAB

Working in teams, prepare a clear soup, a thick soup, or a specialty soup. Taste each team's soup and evaluate it.

Hot Appetizers

OBJECTIVES

After reading this section, you will be able to:

- Prepare a variety of appetizers.

- Arrange appetizers in an appealing manner.

APPETIZERS probably could be called "appeteasers," since they are designed to stimulate the appetite. Ingredients in appetizers can come from every food group. Appetizers require a variety of advanced food preparation techniques. In this section, you will learn how to prepare and arrange hot appetizers.

⊠ TYPES OF HOT APPETIZERS

Appetizers are small portions of food served as the first course of a meal. Hors d'oeuvres are served separately from the meal. Appetizers can be hot or cold. Hot appetizers will be emphasized in this section. See Chapter 18 for more information on cold appetizers and hors d'oeuvres.

Appetizers can be passed, plated, or buffet line items such as Swedish meatballs or cocktail sausages. When selecting appetizers, it is important to include a variety of foods and flavors on the menu. Make sure they complement—not duplicate—the taste of the main dish.

Presentation is key in serving appetizers. They must be visually appealing and neatly organized. If appetizers are served buffet-style, arrange them so they seem to flow toward guests. If plated, use plates and trays with interesting shapes and sizes. Notice how the appetizers look on the plate. Do

not pack them in. Be sure to leave some open space on the plate. Adding a small garnish will improve the presentation. See Fig. 21-9.

⊠ MAKING HOT APPETIZERS

Hot appetizers are most often served at dinner, instead of or following the soup. Hot appetizers can be created from almost any ingredient, resulting in a range of flavors.

■ **Brochettes.** Combinations of meat, poultry, fish, and vegetables served on small skewers are called **brochettes**. The items are marinated, then baked, broiled, or grilled. Brochettes (broh-SHEHTS), sometimes called kebabs (kuh-BOBS), often come with a dipping sauce, such as teriyaki or peanut.

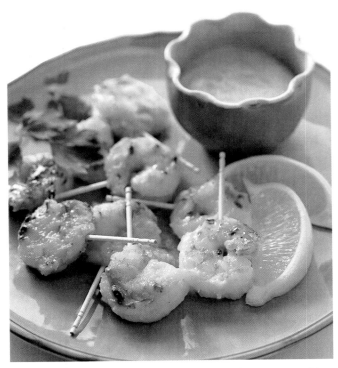

Fig. 21-9. Appetizers such as shrimp can be presented in many attractive ways. **What other garnishes could be used to present this appetizer?**

To make brochettes, cut all items into consistent shapes and sizes so that they are proportional when skewered. Before assembling, soak the bamboo skewers in water to help keep them from burning.

■ **Filled pastry shells.** This appetizer uses shells made from puff pastry, called bouchées (boo-SHAYZ), or from dough, called barquettes (bahr-KEHTS) or tartlets. The shells are baked ahead of time, then filled before serving so that they don't become soggy. Fillings can include cheeses, stews, meat, poultry, and vegetables. Phyllo (FEE-loh), a type of pastry, can also be used to hold fillings. See Fig. 21-10.

■ **Meatballs.** Meatballs can be made from ground beef, poultry, veal, or pork. They are usually served with a sweet and sour, mushroom, tomato, or cream sauce. Swedish meatballs are always a crowd pleaser.

■ **Rumaki.** Appetizers that consist of blanched bacon wrapped around vegetables, seafood, chicken liver, meat, poultry, or fruits are called **rumaki** (ruh-MAH-kee). Sometimes rumaki are brushed with a marinade or sauce before cooking. The rumaki are then fried, baked, or broiled.

■ **Stuffed potato skins.** Stuffed potato skins are made from hollowed out potatoes filled with a combination of cheese, bacon, and chives. They are then baked or broiled. Sour cream and onion are often added before serving.

■ **Chicken wings.** Chicken wings are dipped in a spicy coating of seasonings and then deep-fried. Their spicy flavor ranges from mild to extra hot. Chicken wings can also be served sweet, baked, or roasted in a honey barbecue or deviled sauce.

✖ PLATING & SERVING HOT APPETIZERS

An attractive and functional presentation of appetizers is necessary for their success. Appetizers served at the table, in a buffet, or at a cocktail party provide an opportunity for creative plating and service.

■ **Table service.** The art of serving hot appetizers to each individual at the table depends on the appetizer. For example, brochettes could be served on a small plate atop a drizzle of sauce, with a garnish to the side. Chicken wings may be served on a plate with a small ramekin, or container of sauce for dipping. When serving appetizers at the table, take the opportunity to make each plate or bowl a special presentation. See Fig. 21-11.

Fig. 21-10. Phyllo can also be filled with a variety of ingredients.

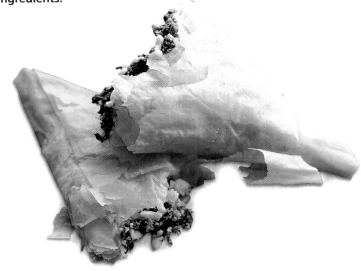

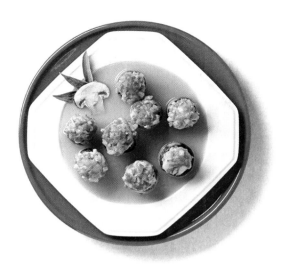

Fig. 21-11. The presentation of hot appetizers adds to their appeal.

called **butler service**. When appetizers are passed, people must be able to choose them and eat them easily while standing. Remember to allow sufficient space on the plate and arrange the items so they flow toward the customer. Be sure each item is small enough to eat in one or two bites and without a knife and fork. Customers should be able to eat with their fingers or a toothpick, and should be given a napkin on which to hold the appetizer.

■ **Buffet service.** For buffet service, food is presented all together on one or more tables. The individual presentation depends on how the appetizers are grouped on each serving plate. It is customary to place a garnish on each plate that holds appetizers. Regardless of which appetizer and garnish you use, arrange them in a manner that is pleasing to the eye. Do not pack them in tightly. Allow space between each one so that they can be picked up easily.

■ **Butler service.** Appetizers that are carried on a serving plate at a standing event, such as a party or reception, are passed according to what is

✕ HOLDING & STORING HOT APPETIZERS

For hot appetizers to taste their best, they should be served hot. This often means cooking and assembling them just prior to serving.

Some appetizers, such as Swedish meatballs, may be baked and then kept warm for a short period of time. Other appetizers, such as bouchées, need to be assembled just before serving because they do not keep well. Chafing dishes are the best option for holding appetizers on a buffet line.

Polysulfone (pah-lee-suhl-phohn) containers can be used to hold appetizers on the steam table or to store appetizers in the refrigerator. These containers range in size from 6"×12" to 12"×20". They can be as deep as six inches. In other words, they can hold a large supply of food.

SECTION 21-2   Knowledge Check

1. What is an hors d'oeuvre?
2. Name two guidelines for preparing hot appetizers.
3. Explain the different types of appetizer service: table, buffet, and butler.

MINI LAB

Suppose your catering company has been hired to provide appetizers for 100 people. Work together in teams to prepare a display of hot appetizers you would serve at the event.

SECTION SUMMARIES

21-1 The types of soups are clear, thick, and specialty.

21-1 Consommé is a type of clear soup; purée, cream, bisque, chowder, and cold are types of specialty soups; French onion, gazpacho, and minestrone are types of national soups.

21-1 Presenting and garnishing soups varies according to their type and includes toppings and bread choices.

21-1 Store soups in tightly sealed containers. Make cold cream soups in small batches so they don't spoil, and keep small batches of hot cream soups on the steamtable and replenish when necessary.

21-2 Appetizers are sometimes prepared ahead of time and then assembled just before serving. They may also be prepared and cooked just prior to serving.

21-2 Appetizer service depends on what, where, and when the appetizers are being served. The type of appetizer; buffet, butler, or table service; and the occasion determine the presentation of appetizers.

CHECK YOUR KNOWLEDGE

1. Explain how to clarify a consommé, and the reason behind doing it.

2. How is a purée soup thickened?

3. Describe the process of cooking vegetables for soup.

4. Why should you heat a hot cream soup to proper temperature, after it has chilled, before placing it on a steamtable?

5. How do cold cream soups differ from hot cream soups?

6. Explain why soup garnishes are important.

7. What is an appetizer? Contrast the different types of appetizers.

8. Why is the arrangement of appetizers on the plate important?

9. What is the best method for holding hot appetizers on a buffet line?

CRITICAL-THINKING ACTIVITIES

1. If you wanted to make a thick soup and realized that you had about ⅓ of the cream needed, how would you thicken the soup?

2. Which type of soup do you think has more nutritional value: vegetable soup or a cold, uncooked soup such as gazpacho? Why?

WORKPLACE KNOW-HOW

Problem solving. Imagine you are preparing appetizers for a small, last-minute celebration. Which appetizers would you prepare if you had the following items on hand: large potatoes, firm fish, bacon, bell peppers, onions, and various cheeses?

LAB-BASED ACTIVITY: Making Thick Soups

STEP ❶ Working in teams, develop a thick soup that has not been mentioned in this chapter. Choose either a purée or cream soup.

STEP ❷ When choosing the soup, also consider how appropriate the soup is for the current season. Rich, heavy soups are usually more appropriate for winter months, and lighter soups are often best eaten during summer months. Be careful—just because purée soup is thick and hearty, it may be delicious in the summer because of the fresh ingredients available.

STEP ❸ Use the chart below to help your team decide which type of soup to make.

STEP ❹ Prepare the soup.

STEP ❺ Taste each team's soup and rate the flavor, texture, and appearance. Use the following scale to rate each soup:

1=Poor; 2=Fair; 3=Good; 4=Great

STEP ❻ Answer the following questions:
- Why did your team choose a particular type of soup?
- Did your team experience any difficulties while preparing the soup?
- What would you do differently if you made this soup again?

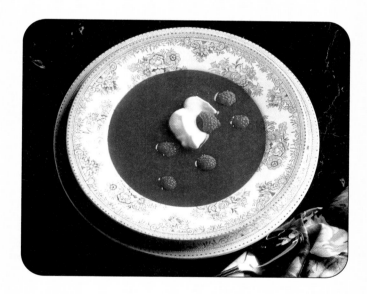

Soup Type	Consistency	Thickening Agent	Main Ingredient
Purée	Very thick.	Purée main ingredient or add cream.	Starchy vegetables; legumes.
Cream	Thick.	Béchamel sauce or cream.	Leafy, soft, or hard vegetables.
Cold	Thick, but thinner than cream soup.	Purée main ingredient or add yogurt or cream.	Fresh fruit or vegetables.

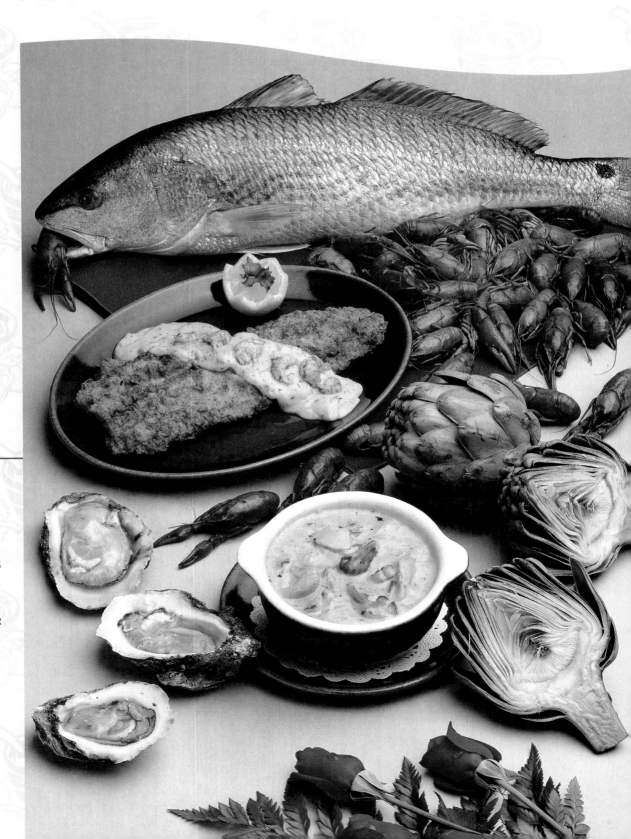

Fish & Shellfish

Section 22-1
Fish Basics

Section 22-2
Shellfish Basics

Section 22-3
**Cooking Fish &
Shellfish**

Fish Basics

KEY TERMS

- fillets
- drawn
- dressed
- butterflied
- freezer burn
- drip loss
- vacuum packed

OBJECTIVES

After reading this section, you will be able to:

- Describe the composition and structure of fish.
- Identify several varieties of saltwater and freshwater fish.
- Identify common market forms of fish.
- Describe how to purchase and store fish.

OVER 30,000 species of fish live in oceans or freshwater sources. These cold-blooded animals are becoming more important to the foodservice industry. Approximately 75% of all the fish consumed in the U.S. is eaten in restaurants. Customers looking for a tasty, low-fat, healthful alternative to meat often choose fish. Knowing how to select, purchase, and store fish will allow a foodservice operation to serve fish of the highest quality.

☒ STRUCTURE OF FISH

Like poultry and meat, fish is made up of protein, fat, and water, as well as vitamins and minerals. Some fish, called fatty fish, have a relatively large amount of fat. Salmon is a popular type of fatty fish. Fish with little fat, such as haddock, are known as lean fish. A major difference between fish and meat is that fish has very little connective tissue. Because of this, fish:

- Are naturally tender.
- Cook rapidly, requiring low heat.
- Can be cooked using moist cooking techniques to keep its natural moistness.
- Will fall apart when cooked, if not handled carefully.

Fish have backbones, an internal skeleton of cartilage and bones, gills for breathing, and fins for swimming. Fish may be divided into three categories, based on skeletal type.

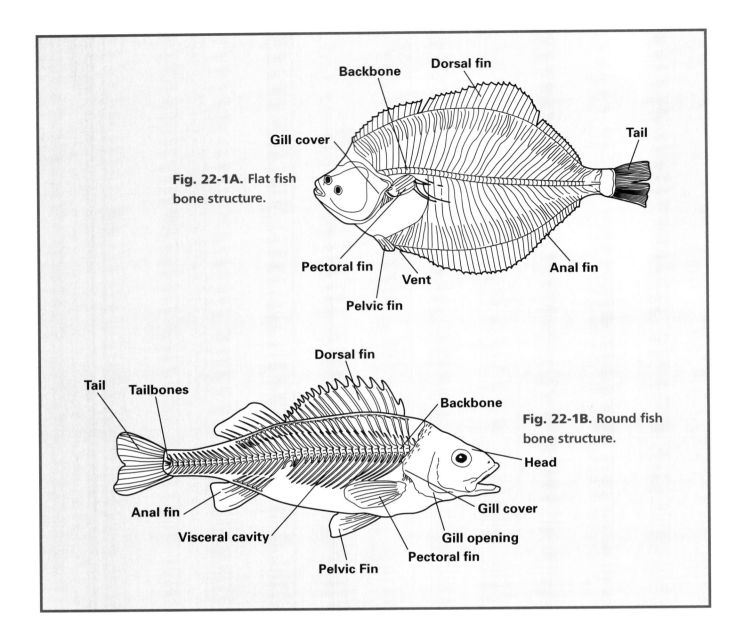

Backbone
Dorsal fin

Gill cover

Tail

Fig. 22-1A. Flat fish
bone structure.

Pectoral fin

Vent

Anal fin

Pelvic fin

Dorsal fin

Tail Tailbones

Backbone

Fig. 22-1B. Round fish
bone structure.

Head

Anal fin

Gill cover

Visceral cavity

Gill opening

Pelvic Fin

Pectoral fin

■ **Flat fish.** Flat fish have a backbone running horizontally through the center of the fish. They swim horizontally and have both eyes on the top of their heads. Flat fish, such as flounder and halibut, have dark skin on the upper side to hide from predators. See Fig. 22-1A.

■ **Round fish.** Round fish have a backbone on the upper edge of their bodies. They have an eye on each side of their heads, and they swim vertically. Trout and cod are common types of round fish. See Fig. 22-1B.

■ **Boneless fish.** Boneless fish, such as sharks, have cartilage instead of bones. Many boneless fish also have smooth skin instead of scales. Sometimes boneless fish are classified with round fish.

⊠ VARIETIES OF FISH

Most foodservice operations serve only a small portion of the fish varieties that exist worldwide. Fig. 22-2 shows examples of some of the most commonly used varieties of fish.

Fig. 22-2.

Types of Fish

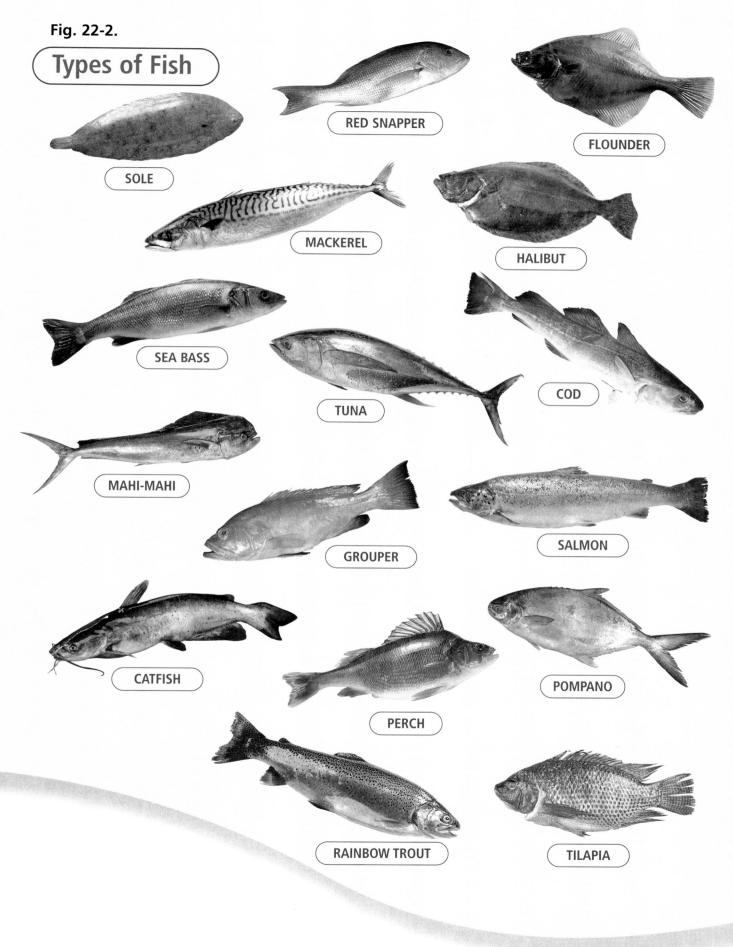

SOLE

RED SNAPPER

FLOUNDER

MACKEREL

HALIBUT

SEA BASS

TUNA

COD

MAHI-MAHI

GROUPER

SALMON

CATFISH

PERCH

POMPANO

RAINBOW TROUT

TILAPIA

✖ MARKET FORMS OF FISH

As the demand for fish has increased and the supply has decreased, fish have become more expensive. Once available only to those living along the coasts or near freshwater sources, fish can now be preserved and shipped to any location quickly and safely. However, the names used for different fish may vary from one region of the country to another.

Fish may be purchased whole or in the form in which it will be cooked and served. Generally, restaurant owners find it less expensive to buy fish already processed.

Inspection and grading of fish is not required like it is for meat and poultry. See Section 2 for more information on inspection and grading of fish.

Fresh Fish

Before most fresh fish is made available for purchase, it is usually processed in some way. The undesirable parts of the fish, such as heads and fins, are often removed. There are eight forms of fish that can be purchased. Fig. 22-3 shows six of them.

■ **Whole.** Whole fish refers to the entire fish as it comes out of the water. Because the internal organs are not removed, this form has the shortest shelf life.

■ **Drawn.** Fish that have had their gills and entrails removed are called **drawn** fish. This form has the longest shelf life. Whole fish are often purchased drawn.

■ **Dressed.** Drawn fish that have had their fins, scales, and sometimes their head removed are called **dressed** fish.

Fig. 22-3. Market Forms of Fish.

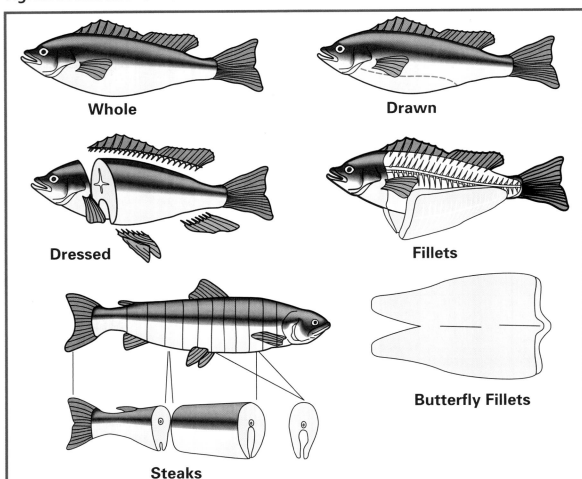

Whole

Drawn

Dressed

Fillets

Steaks

Butterfly Fillets

- **Fillets.** The sides of fish, **fillets**, are the most common cut offered in restaurants. Fillets can be cut with or without bones and skin. Round fish produce two fillets, one from each side. Flat fish produce four fillets. Two large fillets are cut from the top and two are cut from the bottom of the fish.

- **Butterflied.** A **butterflied** fish resembles an open book. The fish is dressed, then cut so the two sides lay open, yet are attached by skin.

- **Steaks.** Cross-section cuts of dressed fish are called steaks. The backbone and skin may still be attached. When the cuts are from a large fish, such as swordfish, they are boneless.

- **Cubes.** Leftover pieces from large fish are called cubes. They are often used in stir-fries, stews, or kebabs.

- **Sticks.** Small, leftover pieces of fish that are pressed together form fish sticks. They are breaded or battered and sold frozen.

Frozen Fish

Some people believe that frozen fish is not as good as fresh fish. However, modern processing methods often mean that frozen fish is less likely to be contaminated. More frozen fish is served in restaurants than fresh fish.

- **Quality characteristics.** Use the following quality checks when purchasing and receiving frozen fish.

- Frozen fish should not be thawed.

- Fish should not have **freezer burn**, the discoloration and dehydration caused by moisture loss as a food freezes. Fish also should be kept well-wrapped.

- Fish should have a thin layer of ice as a glaze. This glaze should not have evaporated or melted.

- Fish should not have a "fishy" smell. A fishy smell results from improper handling.

- **Thawing and handling frozen fish.** Frozen fish products are usually raw or battered and breaded. Follow these guidelines for safe handling:

- Never thaw fish at room temperature. Always thaw fish in the refrigerator. Allow 18–36 hours for frozen fish to thaw in the refrigerator. If you are in a hurry, keep fish in its packaging, and run it under cold water.

- You can cook small pieces of fish while they are frozen. This makes for easier handling and less drip loss. **Drip loss** is the loss of moisture that occurs as the fish thaws.

- Fish may be partially thawed, then prepped and cooked. Partially thawed fish will handle more easily than completely thawed fish.

- If frozen fish is already breaded or prepared in some way, be sure to follow the package directions for cooking.

- Do not refreeze fish.

Because fish spoils quickly, it is important to store and use it carefully. If a fish tastes strong, it has already begun to decompose. Always check for quality before preparing fish.

Canned Fish

The main varieties of canned fish are tuna and salmon. Tuna is packed in oil or water in solid form, chunk style, or flaked.

Do not purchase cans that are dented or damaged. As with other canned goods, store canned fish on shelves in a cool, dry place. When opened, transfer any unused fish to a covered container. Label the container and refrigerate. The fish will keep for two to three days.

✖ PURCHASING & STORING FRESH FISH

Since fresh fish is not usually graded, the person receiving a shipment of fish must check for freshness. This quality check should be done using the three tests described in Fig. 22-4.

Fresh fish spoils more quickly than fresh poultry or meat. Whole fish should be stored on ice, while fillets should be kept on ice in watertight containers. From the time fish is caught, to the time it is cooked and served, maintaining proper storage temperatures is critical to the quality and safety of fish. The shelf life of fish decreases one day for every day it is stored above 32°F.

Fig. 22-4.
Quality Tests for Fresh Fish

LOOK	FEEL	SMELL
• Does the meat separate when the fillet is bent? This is a sign of deteriorated connective tissue between the muscles.	• When the fish is pressed, is there a fingerprint left? Fish should be firm. If a dent is visible after the fish is pressed, the fish has begun to decay.	• Does the fish smell bad? Fresh fish should smell like seaweed or the ocean. If the fish smells like ammonia, it has gone bad and should not be used.
• Are there blood spots in the flesh? Is the fish dry? Fish should be moist and free of blood.	• Is the fish slimy? This can be a good sign in whole fish, but a bad sign in fillets.	
• If the gills are still attached, are they pink or grayish brown? Fresh fish will have red gills.		
• Are the eyes sunken or cloudy? Fresh fish generally have round, clear eyes.		

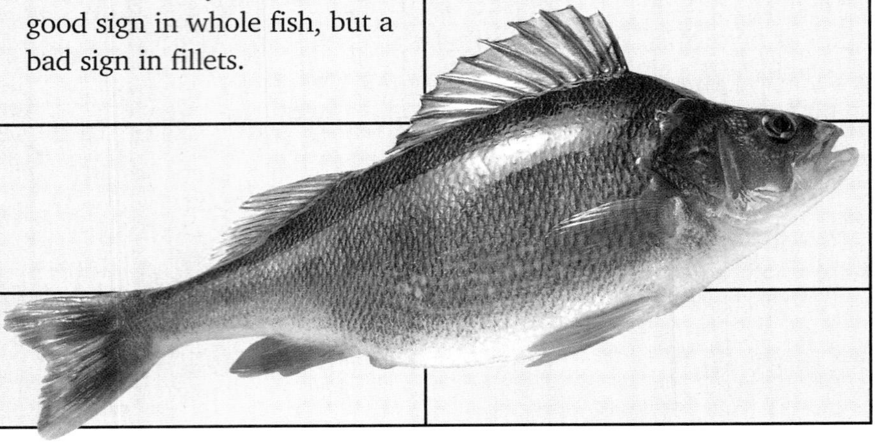

⊠ PURCHASING & STORING FROZEN FISH

When buying frozen fish, look for ice inside the fish. This shows that the fish was partially thawed and then refrozen. Be sure that there are no white spots or dry spots, which are signs of freezer burn.

Frozen fish can be kept safely frozen for up to six months, if stored at 0°F. To prevent freezer burn, keep fish vacuum packed or wrapped tightly in plastic. **Vacuum packed** fish have been placed in airtight containers from which the air has been removed to prevent the growth of bacteria.

SECTION 22-1   Knowledge Check

1. Name two varieties of freshwater fish and two varieties of saltwater fish.
2. Describe four market forms of fresh fish.
3. What three general tests can be done when checking the quality of fresh fish?

MINI LAB

Choose three of the fish shown on page 489. Use print or Internet resources to find out how it is commonly cooked. Obtain a recipe for preparing one of these fish. Share your recipe with the class.

Shellfish Basics

KEY TERMS

- **mollusks**
- **univalve**
- **bivalve**
- **cephalopod**
- **shucked**
- **crustaceans**
- **devein**
- **calamari**
- **escargot**
- **surimi**

OBJECTIVES

After reading this chapter, you will be able to:

- Explain how fish and shellfish are inspected and graded.
- Describe the structure and composition of shellfish.
- Identify market forms of shellfish.
- Describe proper handling procedures for shellfish.

SHELLFISH are often considered a luxury food. Because much of the body is not used in preparing special dishes, shellfish meat is expensive. However, shellfish appear in many places on the menu: as appetizers, in soups, and as entrées. Knowing how to prepare shellfish is an important skill for every foodservice professional.

✖ INSPECTION & GRADING OF FISH & SHELLFISH

The inspection of fish and shellfish is required, just like it is for meat and poultry. Although grading is not required, the U.S. Department of Commerce (USDC) will inspect and grade fresh fish and shellfish for a fee. The inspection of frozen and canned fish is mandatory.

Fish are inspected for accurate labeling, safety and cleanliness in preparation, and wholesomeness. Grading is done to be sure that the fish meet standards for flavor and appearance. Because there are so many kinds of fish, the USDC has set criteria for only the most common types of fish.

Inspection

The USDC inspects fish and shellfish in one of the following three ways:

- **Type 1** inspection covers processing methods and the processing plant itself. The product receives a PUFI mark—Packed Under Federal Inspection—if it is safe, clean, accurately labeled, and has a good flavor and odor. See Fig. 22-5.
- **Type 2** inspection covers criteria such as labeling, weight, and packaging.
- **Type 3** inspection is for sanitary conditions only.

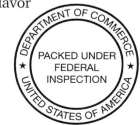

Fig. 22-5.

Grading

Fish are graded based on standards for flavor and appearance. Only fish inspected under Type 1 criteria can be graded. Fish may be judged A, B, or C. Processed or canned products are either B or C quality.

- **Grade A**—Highest quality, no physical defects, good odor and flavor.
- **Grade B**—Good quality.
- **Grade C**—Fairly good quality.

✖ STRUCTURE OF SHELLFISH

Unlike fish, shellfish have no bones. They have hard shells covering their bodies. Shellfish are found in both freshwater and saltwater. Two types of shellfish are mollusks (MAH-luhsks) and crustaceans (CRUS-tae-shuns).

Fig. 22-6. Cephalopods and bivalves are two forms of shellfish. Contrast their differences.

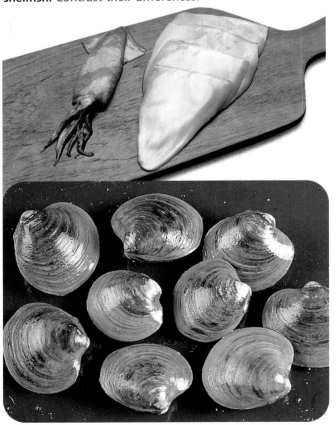

People eat many different parts of shellfish. Muscles, legs, tails, claws, and tentacles are all used in various dishes. Sometimes the shellfish are eaten whole, with or without the shell. Most shellfish are lean and composed primarily of water, vitamins, minerals, protein, and fats.

Learning to prepare shellfish takes time and practice. Each species has special physical characteristics that must be taken into account. For example, some need to be removed from the shell before cooking, while others are cooked in the shell.

✖ MOLLUSKS

Mollusks have no internal skeletal structure. They have shells covering their soft bodies. Mollusks are classified in three major groups. The groups are divided according to the kind of shell the mollusk has.

Univalves (YOO-nih-valvs), such as conch, have a single shell. **Bivalves** (BY-valvs), such as mussels, oysters, and clams, have two shells that are hinged together. Instead of an outer shell, **cephalopods** (SEHF-uh-luh-pods), such as squid or octopus, have a thin internal shell. Cephalopods have tentacles, or false legs, attached to the head near the mouth. See Fig. 22-6.

Oysters

Oysters can be purchased any time during the year, but they are best to eat in fall, winter, and spring. Oyster meat is very delicate with a high percentage of water. Because the salts, nutrients, and minerals of the water flavor the meat, oysters within the same species may taste different, depending on where each was harvested.

■ **Market forms.** Oysters may be purchased live, shucked, or canned. Whole oysters are often served "on-the-half-shell." A **shucked** oyster has had the meat removed from the shell. Shucked oysters, either fresh or frozen, range from very small to extra large. They are graded by size, as shown in Fig. 22-7. Canned oysters are rarely used in commercial kitchens.

Fig. 22-7.

GRADE OF OYSTERS	NUMBER PER GALLON
Very Small	over 500
Small or Standards	301-500
Medium or Selects	211-300
Large or Extra Selects	161-210
Extra Large or Counts	160 or fewer

Clams

Clams from the East Coast are known by their shells—soft shell or hard shell. Soft-shell clams may be called steamers or longnecks. Hard-shell clams are also called quahogs (KWAH-hahgs) and are classified according to size. Chowders are the largest clams, then cherrystones, which are most common. The smallest clams are called littlenecks. See Fig. 22-8:

■ **Market forms.** Like oysters, clams should be purchased live for greatest freshness. They should smell fresh and sweet. Clams may be purchased in three forms:

• Whole, in the shell.

• Shucked, either frozen or fresh.

• Canned, either chopped or whole.

■ **Handling and Storage.** Treat clams carefully so their shells do not break. Store live clams in cardboard containers in the refrigerator for up to one week. Like oysters, they must be kept damp.

Scrub clams before opening them. If a clam is sandy inside, put cornmeal in water and refrigerate the clams for 24 hours. After the clams eat the cornmeal, they will expel the sand. Be sure to rinse the clams with fresh water before using them.

■ **Handling and Storage.** When purchasing live oysters, check that the shells are tightly closed or that they close quickly when tapped. They should have a clear appearance and be plump. Both shucked and live oysters should have a sweet, mild smell.

Store live oysters in cardboard containers in the cooler. They should be draped with seaweed or damp towels. Check oysters daily, and throw out any dead ones. If the oysters have already been shucked, treat them like fish fillets and keep them in containers surrounded by ice on all sides. Fresh oysters should keep a week in the refrigerator.

Before opening oysters, scrub the shells. Then place them on a sheet pan in a hot oven until the shells open. The oysters can be removed from the shell and prepared for serving. If a shell does not open, throw the oyster away.

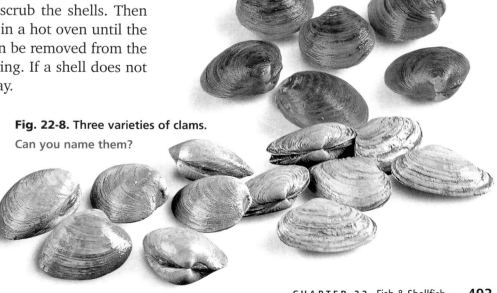

Fig. 22-8. Three varieties of clams.
Can you name them?

SAVING IN BULK

Items such as shellfish are typically sold in bulk. Before placing an order to buy large quantities of shellfish, check if the vendor offers quantity discounts. A quantity discount is used to encourage purchasers to buy in large quantities. For example, a discount of 5% off the total price may be given if a purchaser buys at least 10 gallons of oysters, 10% for 15 gallons, 20% for 20 gallons, and so on.

For instance, one gallon of medium oysters sells for $75.00. You need to buy 15 gallons. Determine the cost with and without the quantity discount.

$75/gallon $\times$ 15 gallons = $1125.00

$75/gallon $\times$ 15 gallons $\times$ 0.10 discount = $112.50

Math Tip: To change the percent to a decimal, write the number without the percentage sign, and move the decimal point two places to the left.

Without the quantity discount, your cost is $1125.00. With the 10% discount, your cost is $1125.00 − $112.50 = $1012.50. So you save $112.50 by taking advantage of the quantity discount.

TRY IT!

1. A seafood vendor offers a 20% discount off the total price if you purchase 25 gallons of oysters. Each gallon sells for $70.00. If you bought 25 gallons of oysters, what would be your price without the discount?

2. What would be your price with the discount?

Mussels

Mussels are farmed and harvested around the world. Mussels look like small, dark blue or black clams. Their meat ranges from yellow to orange in color and is tender but firm when cooked. Mussels from Southeast Asia and New Zealand are green, with a green edge to their tan or light gray shells. These mussels are generally more expensive. See Fig. 22-9.

■ **Market forms.** Mussels may be sold live, shucked, vacuum packed, or frozen in the shell. The shells of live mussels should be closed or should close when tapped lightly. Throw out any mussels that seem hollow or are very lightweight. If the mussels are too heavy, they are most likely filled with sand, and should also be thrown away. If mussels have been shucked, they are generally packed in brine to preserve them.

■ **Handling and storage.** When preparing mussels, scrub the shells under cold running water. Use a clam knife to scrape off any barnacles (BAR-ni-kuhls) that have attached themselves to the shells. Just before cooking, pull off the mussel's "beard," which sticks out between the two shells. If the mussel is sandy, treat it as you would a clam by soaking it in water and cornmeal to get rid of the sand.

Keep mussels in the refrigerator and away from light. Store them in the paper sack or cardboard box they arrive in, and keep the container damp.

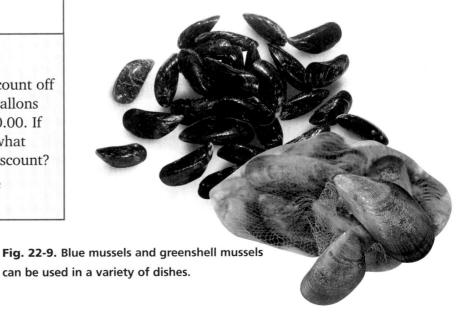

Fig. 22-9. Blue mussels and greenshell mussels can be used in a variety of dishes.

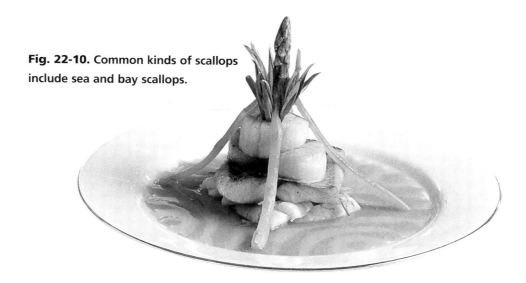

Fig. 22-10. Common kinds of scallops include sea and bay scallops.

Scallops

Scallops are available year-round and are sweet in flavor and white in color. They generally are sold already shucked. The muscle that closes the shell is the only edible part. If scallops smell fishy or strong, they have spoiled or aged. Scallops should smell clean and sweet.

Sea scallops and bay scallops are the two most common kinds of scallops. Sea scallops are the largest, with about 10–15 per pound. Bay scallops are small and more delicately flavored, with about 32–40 per pound. See Fig. 22-10.

■ **Market forms.** Scallops are sold fresh and shucked by the pound or the gallon. They may also be sold frozen, in 5-pound blocks, or IQF (individually quick frozen).

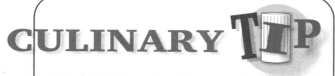

CULINARY TIP

IQF—IQF fish or shellfish have been quickly frozen piece by piece. Because the freezing happens so fast, few ice crystals form, which improves the quality.

■ **Handling and storage.** Remove the tough adductor muscle on the sides of scallops. This is the muscle that opens and closes the valves on a bivalve mollusk. Although scallops can be prepared with this muscle attached, they will taste better without it. Cover and refrigerate scallops.

Do not place them directly on ice or they will become watery and lose their flavor. Sometimes large sea scallops are cut into smaller pieces before cooking.

✖ CRUSTACEANS

Crustaceans have a hard outer shell and jointed skeletons. Examples include lobster, shrimp, crab, and crayfish. Crustaceans tend to be expensive because so much work is needed to produce a small amount of meat. Restaurants often purchase these animals already processed to save preparation time. Crustaceans can be prepared in almost any fashion, as long as they are not overcooked. Overcooking makes them tough.

Lobsters

Northern lobsters may be considered the most valued seafood delicacy. This animal has two large claws, four pairs of legs, and a flexible, large tail. The lobster shell, which turns red when cooked, is actually bluish green or dark green. Lobster meat from the tail, legs, and claws is sweet and white. Lobsters can weigh up to about 20 pounds. Rock, or spiny, lobsters are warm-water lobsters. They are only sold as IQF lobster tails.

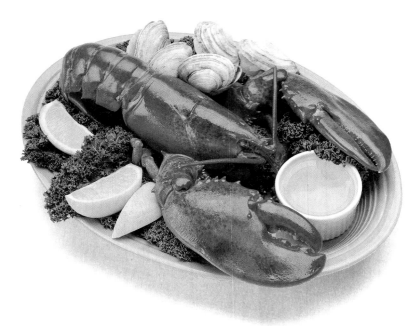

Fig. 22-11. Lobsters are a seafood delicacy. Name three ways lobster can be served to customers.

Cooked lobster meat smells sweet and fresh. If the lobsters are in the process of dying, they are called "sleepers." Sleepers should be cooked at once so the meat will still be good. Once lobster meat has been cooked, cover and refrigerate it. The meat will only keep a day or two. See Fig. 22-11.

■ **Market forms.** Lobsters are sold live, frozen, or as fresh-cooked meat. Uncooked lobster tails are also available IQF.

■ **Handling and storage.** The lobster must be split and cut for certain food preparations, such as broiling or cubing for use in stews or sautés. When cooking lobster live, plunge it head first into boiling water.

Live lobsters should be stored in special saltwater tanks. They can also be kept in a cool location, wrapped in seaweed or heavy, wet paper.

Shrimp

Shrimp are classified by the count per pound—the smaller the shrimp, the higher the count. It takes less work to peel and devein large shrimp, but they are more expensive. To **devein** (dee-VANE) a shrimp means to remove its intestinal tract, located along the back. Deveined shrimp cost more and are sold either raw or cooked. It takes about a pound of raw shrimp to make a half pound of peeled and cooked shrimp.

Here are the steps to use in peeling and deveining shrimp:

1. First, use your forefinger to remove the legs.

2. Peel and remove the shell.

3. Leave the tail on if the shrimp will be broiled or deep-fried. Remove the tail for most other preparations.

4. Cut down the back of the shrimp with a paring knife and remove the vein just below the surface.

5. Make the cut deeper to butterfly the shrimp.

■ **Market forms.** Shrimp may be purchased raw in the shell, either fresh or frozen. These are called "green" shrimp. They may also be P/D, an abbreviation for peeled and deveined. The third form available is PDC—peeled, deveined, and cooked. Both P/D and PDC shrimp are usually individually quick frozen (IQF) with a glaze of ice on them.

■ **Handling and storage.** Keep already frozen shrimp frozen until they need to be used. To thaw shrimp, place them in the refrigerator. Keep thawed or fresh shrimp wrapped and on crushed ice, as unwrapped shrimp will lose flavor and nutrients.

If shrimp are being served cold, they can be peeled after they are cooked. If shrimp are to be served hot, they should be peeled and deveined before cooking. Shrimp can also be butterflied to make them seem larger and reduce their thickness so they cook faster.

Crab

Popular in casseroles, curries, and chowders, crab are plentiful along North America's coasts. Crab may be shipped canned, fresh, or frozen. See Fig. 22-12. The following types of crab are used in restaurants:

- **Blue crab.** A small, 4–6 oz. crab from the East Coast. Most frozen crabmeat comes from this type.
- **Soft-shell crab.** A blue crab that has just molted, or shed its shell. Because the shell hasn't had time to harden, it is eaten as well as the meat. Only the head and the gills must be removed before frying or sautéing the crab.
- **Alaskan king crab.** The largest crab. They can weigh between 6 and 20 pounds. Even though they are expensive, this type is popular in restaurants because large chunks of meat can be removed.
- **Alaskan snow crab.** Also called spider crab. Snow crab can be used as a less expensive substitute for king crab.

- **Dungeness (duhn-juh-nes) crab.** Found along the West Coast, they range from 1½–4 lbs. and have very sweet meat.
- **Stone crab.** The claws of stone crab are popular in the southeast. To protect the species, people fishing can harvest only one claw per stone crab. They twist off the claw and put the crab back in the sea. The crab will grow a new claw within 18 months.

■ **Market forms.** Although crab taste best fresh, picking the meat is an involved and lengthy process. Most crab are purchased in the shell, already cooked and frozen. Soft-shell crab are sold whole, while king crab legs are sold both split and whole. Snow and stone crab claws are also sold whole.

■ **Handling and storage.** Frozen crabmeat spoils rapidly when defrosted. It should be kept frozen until ready to be used. Keep live crab cool and packed in damp seaweed until ready to be cooked.

Fig. 22-12.

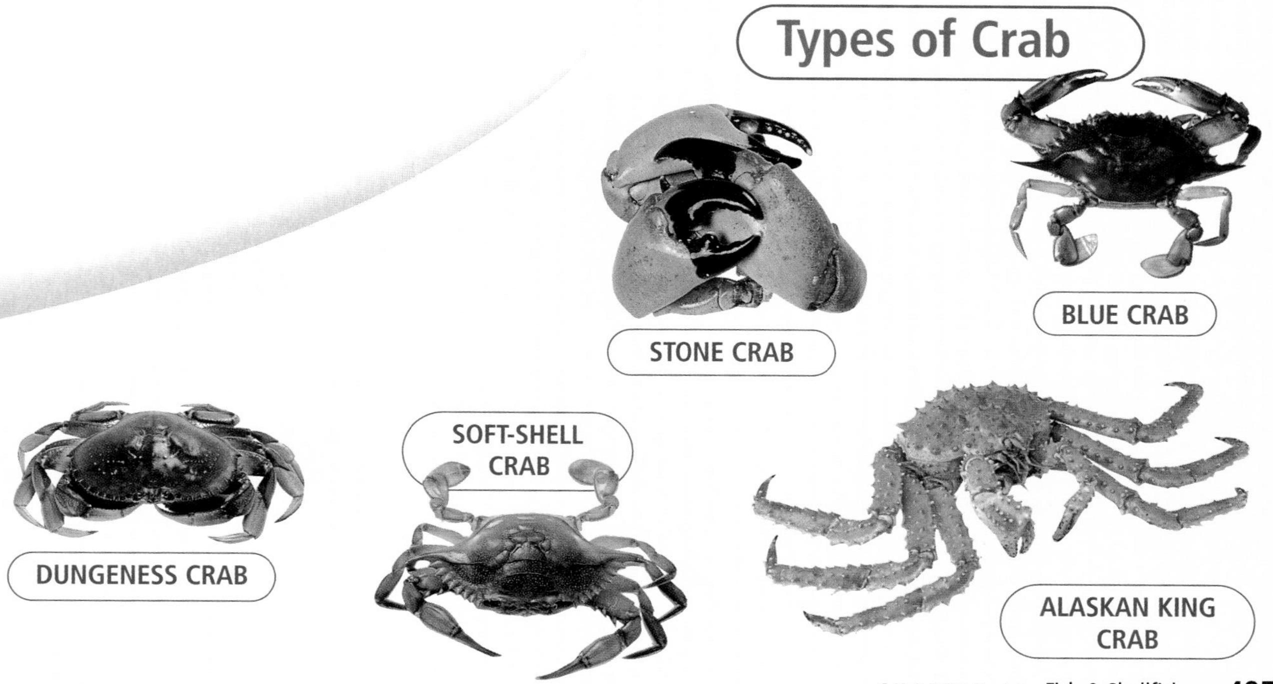

Types of Crab

STONE CRAB

BLUE CRAB

DUNGENESS CRAB

SOFT-SHELL CRAB

ALASKAN KING CRAB

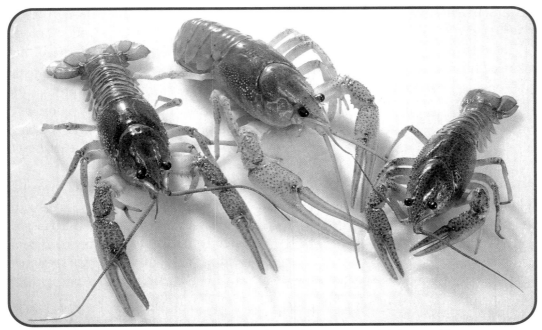

Fig. 22-13. Crayfish are commonly used in Creole and Cajun cooking.

Crayfish

Crayfish are freshwater crustaceans that look like miniature lobsters from 3½–7 inches in length. Crayfish are called crawfish and crawdads in the Southern U.S. Their tail meat is lean, sweet, and tender. Whole crayfish and peeled tail meat are both marketed live and frozen. They are available year round. See Fig. 22-13.

Crayfish are served in French restaurants and used in Cajun and Creole cooking. Whole crayfish are often boiled and served on top of rice. Crayfish tail meat is usually deep-fried and used in soups and sauces.

✗ OTHER SEAFOOD

Some types of seafood, such as frogs and snails, spend part of their lives on land, but are still classified as seafood. These seafood products are often sold smoked, pickled, or in brine. The processing preserves, but more importantly, it adds flavor. These products need to be refrigerated. See Fig. 22-14.

Squid

On some menus, squid goes by its Italian name, **calamari** (kah-lah-MAH-ree). Squid have ten tentacles and look somewhat like an octopus. It is these tentacles and the hollowed-out body that are eaten. Squid is cut into small pieces, which may be either simmered in a seasoned sauce or liquid, or quickly fried.

Frog Legs

Frog legs are from frogs that are farm raised. Frog legs are only sold in pairs. Foodservice operations use only the rear legs. They can be served poached with a sauce, deep-fried, or sautéed.

Escargot

Imported from France, where they are called **escargot** (ess-kahr-go), snails are generally served as appetizers in the shell, with a garlic butter. It takes about 32 snails to make a pound of meat. Commercial farming of snails in the United States is becoming more popular, since fresh snails taste better than canned snails.

Fig. 22-14.

Other Seafood

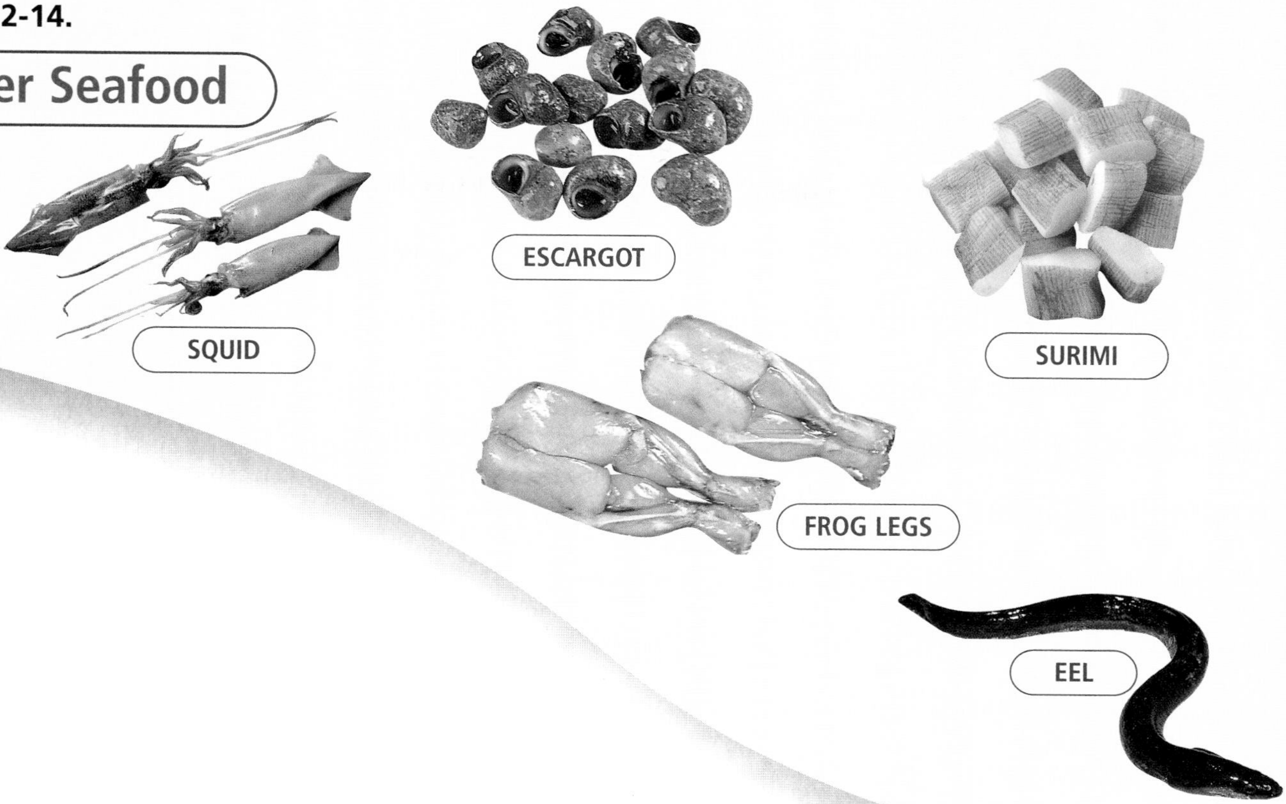

SQUID

ESCARGOT

SURIMI

FROG LEGS

EEL

Surimi

Surimi (soo-REE-mee) is a combination of different kinds of white fish and flavoring, formed into different shapes. Crab and lobster are two popular forms. To make these imitations seem more real, color is added. Surimi is a widely used substitute for lobster and crab in North America due to its lower cost.

Eel

Eels are long, thin fish with a sweet, mild flavor. They are very popular in Europe and in some ethnic communities in the United States. They are sold fresh, smoked, and pickled.

SECTION 22-2 Knowledge Check

1. Explain Type 1 inspection and the grading procedures for fish and shellfish.
2. Compare mollusks and crustaceans. How are they different?
3. Explain how live oysters, clams, and mussels are stored.

MINI LAB

Working in teams, prepare different forms of shellfish to serve as appetizers. For example, one team might peel, devein, and cook shrimp. Another team could prepare oysters or clams. Be sure to follow safety and sanitation guidelines.

SECTION 22-3

Cooking Fish & Shellfish

KEY TERMS

- sushi
- en papillote

OBJECTIVES

After reading this section, you will be able to:

- Explain how cooking affects fish and shellfish.
- Cook fish and shellfish.
- Demonstrate ways to garnish fish and shellfish.

YOU have many methods to choose from when cooking fish and shellfish. Dishes may be simple or elaborate, low-fat or rich. Moist cooking methods and deep-frying, as well as baking and sautéing, offer a number of ways to prepare seafood.

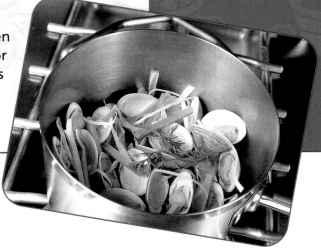

✖ FISH & SHELLFISH COOKERY

Fish has little connective tissue, so a long cooking time is not needed to tenderize the flesh. When cooking fish, the chef must pay attention to time, temperature, and the cooking process. Cook fish until the internal temperature is 145°F or above for 15 seconds.

Fish is also usually low in fat and can quickly dry out when overcooked. To prevent this, chefs sometimes use moist cooking techniques, such as steaming or poaching. Fish flesh flakes, or breaks away in small layers, when it is done. Remember that fish retains heat, even when removed from a heat source. Therefore, it continues cooking and can easily overcook.

Like fish, shellfish can easily be overcooked. Overcooking and excessively high heat will cause shellfish to dry up and shrink or become rubbery and tough. Clams or mussels cooked in the shell will open as they cook. Discard any shells that do not open, since the meat will not be good to eat. To prevent dryness, moist cooking methods are often used.

✖ BAKING FISH & SHELLFISH

Fish steaks and fillets, as well as small fish and shellfish, can be baked in an oven. Combination cooking methods are sometimes used to bake fish. For example, fish may be initially browned in a small amount of oil in a sauté pan to give it color and flavor, then baked to finish cooking. When baking lean fish, baste it frequently with oil or butter to prevent the fish from drying out.

Fish or shellfish may also be baked in a sauce, such as curry or tomato. Baking in a sauce also helps prevent the meat from becoming dry.

Baking Guidelines

Since fatty fish, such as pompano or salmon, are not as likely to dry out, they are the best fish for baking. Generally, fish and shellfish are baked between 350°F and 400°F. Large fish will bake more evenly at the lower temperature. Cook fish until the internal temperature of the thickest part is 145°F or above for 15 seconds.

■ **Moist baking.** Adding vegetables and liquid to a large piece of fish or a whole fish is called moist baking. Other moist cooking techniques used for fish and shellfish include simmering, poaching, and steaming. Liquids from moist cooking are often turned into sauces that accompany the fish or shellfish. Wrapping fish or shellfish in parchment paper with vegetables, herbs, and sauces or butters is a method of steaming called **en papillote** (ahn pah-pee-yoa). These cooking methods do not add fat and keep the meat from becoming dry. They also preserve nutrients and natural flavors.

Use the following steps to steam en papillote:

1. Cut the parchment paper into the desired shape and size to prepare the fish. Fold the parchment in half and crease the folded edge.

2. Butter the parchment paper on one side. Place the buttered side down on the baking dish.

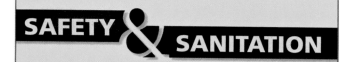

SERVING RAW FISH & SHELLFISH—Many restaurants offer raw fish or shellfish on the menu, such as sushi or raw oysters. **Sushi** (SOO-shee) is a Japanese dish of raw, fresh fish or seafood wrapped in cooked and cooled rice, often with a layer of seaweed to hold it together. See Fig. 22-15 below.

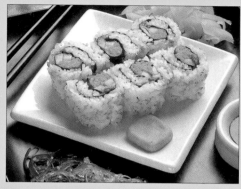

Many health officials advise against serving raw fish or shellfish because of the danger of parasites and contamination from polluted water. However, if you do serve these items, follow these guidelines:

• Buy fish from reputable vendors.
• Choose only the highest quality fish since it will not be cooked.
• Handle the fish as little as possible.
• Follow state-mandated guidelines concerning the serving of raw fish and shellfish.

3. Add the fish, vegetables, and butter to one side of the parchment paper. Fold the parchment over the fish.

4. Seal the edges of the paper by crimping, or pinching and pressing them together around the entire paper.

5. Bake when completely sealed.

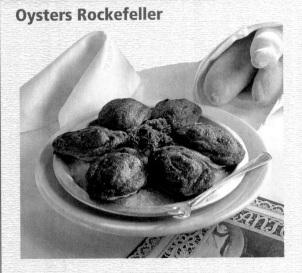

a LINK to the Past

Oysters Rockefeller

Oysters have been cultivated worldwide for over two thousand years and have long been a popular food in America. Cookbooks from the eighteenth century contain recipes for dishes such as oyster pie and pickled oysters. New England oyster stew is still popular today and is prepared much the same way it was centuries ago.

New Orleans is the birthplace for a number of famous oyster dishes, including Oysters Rockefeller. A shortage of snails from Europe in 1899 prompted Jules Alciatore to choose oysters as a main dish for Antoine's, his father's restaurant. Named after business tycoon John D. Rockefeller, Oysters Rockefeller consists of baked oysters on the half shell topped with a rich sauce and served on a bed of rock salt. To this day, the recipe for the sauce is a closely guarded secret, although it is known to include a puréed green vegetable.

✕ BROILING & GRILLING FISH & SHELLFISH

Because of the high heat used, broiled and grilled seafood dishes can be prepared quickly. Many diners view broiled and grilled dishes as more healthful than dishes cooked with other methods.

The appearance of broiled or grilled fish or shellfish may be enhanced by a relish or side sauce. Grilled vegetables are also a natural accompaniment. Citrus garnishes, such as lemon, lime, or orange, are generally served with broiled or grilled seafood. Sometimes lemon and herb butters are served instead.

Broiling & Grilling Guidelines

The high heat of broiling or grilling gives fish and shellfish a smoky flavor. Brush butter or oil over the fish before broiling. This keeps the meat from sticking, and it keeps lean fish moist.

To cook a thicker cut of fish or shellfish evenly, turn it once during broiling. Thin pieces of fish and lobster are broiled on one side only.

Fatty fish, such as swordfish or trout, are a good choice for broiling. Many types of shellfish are broiled on the half shell or on skewers for ease of handling.

■ **Lean versus fat.** All varieties of fish may be broiled. However, fatty fish is the best choice, since lean fish can become dry very quickly. Before broiling both lean and fatty fish, you may wish to coat them with butter, oil, or a vegetable oil spray. See Fig. 22-16.

■ **Use small fish steaks or fillets for broiling.** Thick fish steaks and whole fish are not good choices for broiling. The high heat used in broiling will finish cooking the outside of thick fish before the interior is done. Use fillets or small fish steaks for best results.

■ **Avoid overcooking.** Broiling and grilling require high temperatures, which cook fish and shellfish quickly. Overcooking will make fish dry and shellfish tough.

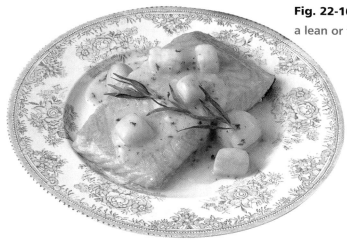

Fig. 22-16. This is baked salmon. Is salmon a lean or fatty fish?

SAUTÉING & PAN-FRYING

The terms sauté and pan-fry are often mistaken as the same thing. Sautéing adds flavor to the food because the surface is lightly browned. Pan-frying uses more fat than sautéing does, and the food to be pan-fried is coated with seasoned batters, flour, or breading before cooking. This coating creates a flavorful crust that protects the fish during cooking.

Be sure the pan and the cooking fat are both hot before adding fish or shellfish. Since only a short cooking time is needed, use high heat to brown the surface when sautéing thin slices of fish or small pieces of shellfish. Thicker pieces may require lower heat so they don't get too brown. Adding too much fish or shellfish to the pan at the same time causes the fat to cool, and the food will then simmer in its own juices.

Sautéing & Pan-Frying Guidelines

Since both sautéing and pan-frying use oil or clarified butter, these cooking methods work well for lean fish. Usually just enough fat to cover the bottom of the pan is sufficient for sautéing. Pan-frying requires more fat.

To keep fish from sticking, use flour or breading to form a crust. For better appearance, brown the presentation side, which is generally the thicker side of a fillet, first. Turn pan-fried fish or shellfish only once during cooking to help prevent fillets

from breaking. Sautéed or pan-fried items will cook quickly over a high heat.

■ **Dredging and breading.** To dredge a food is to evenly coat it with a bit of flour or cornmeal. Make small batches if there are several pounds of fish to prepare. For a better crust, soak fish in milk and drain before breading to prevent a pasty, heavy coating. Dredge the fish or use large shakers with handles to sprinkle the breading. See Fig. 22-17.

DEEP-FRYING

Deep-frying is the most common method used to fry fish in the U.S. Although the foodservice industry often uses frozen, breaded fish for deep-frying, fresh fish or shellfish may also be deep-fried. To protect both the fat and the fish, coat the item with batter or breading. This provides an attractive coating and a crispy texture. The best shellfish to deep-fry are scallops, oysters, shrimp, and clams. Lean fish, usually in sticks or small fillets, are also a good choice.

Fig. 22-17. Coat fish evenly and be sure to shake off excess breading before cooking.

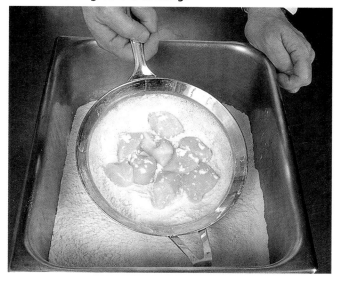

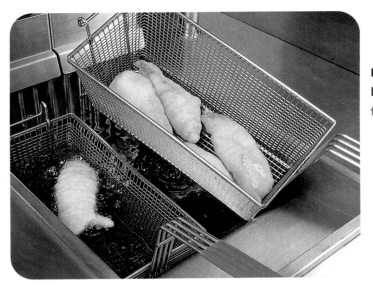

Fig. 22-18. Many types of fish and shellfish can be deep-fried. Why is it important to serve deep-fried fish and shellfish immediately after cooking?

Deep-Frying Guidelines

When preparing frozen breaded fish, cook the fish without first thawing it. If the portion thaws, the fish will be soggy. Review the guidelines for breading and frying in Chapter 15. Batter recipes for vegetables can also be used for fish or shellfish. See Fig. 22-18.

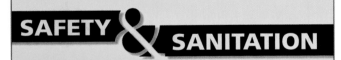

FRYING FAT—Always take special care when working with hot fat, which can easily spatter and burn. Drain and serve deep-fried foods immediately after cooking.

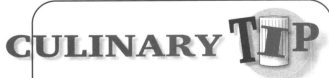

FAT QUALITY—To maintain the quality of frying fat, only heat oil to the temperature needed. Once a day, filter all the oil through a strainer and replace 20% of it with fresh oil.

✖ DETERMINING DONENESS

Because fish and shellfish are naturally tender, it is critical to avoid overcooking. Using the following guidelines will help you determine when fish and shellfish are done cooking:

- Fish starts flaking. When fish cooks, the muscle fibers begin to separate from each other.
- Flesh pulls away from the bones or shell easily.
- Flesh springs back when pressed. Uncooked seafood is soft and mushy instead.
- Flesh becomes opaque. Light cannot be seen through the flesh.

In addition, use these guidelines with each specific cooking technique.

■ **Baking.** Bake fish until the internal temperature is 145°F or above for fifteen seconds. Also check that the flesh flakes, pulls away from the bones or shell, springs back when pressed, and is opaque.

■ **Broiling and grilling.** When broiled or grilled, the outside of fish and shellfish should be slightly browned and crispy. The inside should be juicy and tender.

■ **Sautéing and pan-frying.** Sautéed and pan-fried fish and shellfish are done cooking when their surfaces are slightly browned or crispy. As in broiling and grilling, the insides should be juicy and tender.

■ **Deep-frying.** If the oil has reached the proper temperature, deep-fried fish and shellfish are done when their batter is a rich golden brown. When using prepackaged frozen items, follow the package guidelines. These generally give a range of times and temperatures.

PLATING FISH & SHELLFISH

Serving seafood attractively is an important part of preparation. Since seafood tends to be pale, color is a must in side dishes. The contrasting color and texture make the overall meal appealing. For example:

- A mix of steamed carrots and broccoli brightens the plate and is low in fat.
- A well-garnished rice, pasta, or potato makes a good choice for a side dish.
- If shellfish is served chilled, a cocktail sauce and fresh lemon slices usually accompany it.
- Some seafood dishes are served on beds of sautéed leeks or seaweed.
- Colorful sauces can be plated under seafood to add color and flavor.

Garnishing Fish & Shellfish

Tartar sauce may be the most familiar sauce accompanying seafood. However, other sauces, such as hollandaise or a caper sauce, work just as well for steamed or poached items.

Citrus wedges often accompany grilled or broiled seafood items. If an item has been broiled with a seasoned butter, an additional serving of the butter may be used for garnish. See Fig. 22-19.

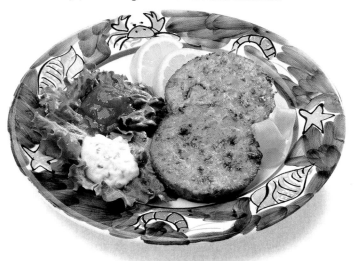

Fig. 22-19. Garnishes are an important step in attractively presenting cooked fish and shellfish.

SECTION 22-3 Knowledge Check

1. Explain three ways that cooking affects fish and shellfish.
2. What are two signs that fish is done cooking?
3. Name three garnishes that are commonly used with different types of fish and shellfish.

MINI LAB

Working in teams, prepare a garnished fish or seafood dish. Exchange dishes with another team and evaluate the quality of the dish. Discuss your findings as a class.

SECTION SUMMARIES

22-1 Fish is similar to poultry and meat in that it has protein, fats, and water. Fish have very little connective tissue.

22-1 Fresh, frozen, or canned fish are available whole or in the form in which they will be cooked, such as fillets or cubes.

22-1 Some popular varieties of fish are cod, orange roughy, salmon, catfish, and trout.

22-1 Since only canned and frozen fish are federally inspected, carefully check these forms of fish for freshness.

22-2 Inspect fresh fish closely before purchasing. Store fresh fish on ice and use quickly. Keep frozen fish well-wrapped and in the freezer.

22-2 Shellfish have outer shell coverings and no bones. They are composed of water, vitamins, minerals, proteins, and fat.

22-2 Most types of shellfish can be purchased canned, fresh, or frozen. Oysters and clams are also available shucked.

22-2 Foodservice employers need to know the different handling and storage methods for each type of shellfish. For example, live lobsters must be stored in saltwater tanks, and shrimp must be peeled and deveined before serving.

22-3 To retain moisture and tenderness while cooking fish and shellfish, closely monitor time, temperature, and the cooking process.

22-3 Cooking fish and shellfish provides a variety of options, including grilling and moist cooking techniques.

22-3 Garnishes for fish and seafood might include sauce, citrus wedges, or seasoned butter.

CHECK YOUR KNOWLEDGE

1. Define fatty and lean fish and give an example of each.
2. Describe the market forms of fish: fillets, whole, drawn, dressed, steaks, cross-section, butterflied, cubes.
3. Describe how the look, feel, and smell of fish can be used to determine its freshness.
4. Name and compare the two main types of shellfish. Give an example of each.
5. How do you clean the sand out of a clam or mussel?
6. Describe the steps needed to peel and devein shrimp.
7. Define calamari, escargot, and surimi.
8. How does cooking affect the tenderness and moistness of fish and shellfish?
9. List the advantages of using moist cooking techniques to cook fish and shellfish.
10. Name two ways to make a plated meal of fish or shellfish more visually appealing.

CRITICAL-THINKING ACTIVITIES

1. Draw some conclusions about how to retain nutrients in fish and shellfish.
2. How can a foodservice operation offer customers sushi that is free of contamination?

WORKPLACE KNOW-HOW

Decision making. As the manager of a hotel food operation, it is your decision to order either fresh fish or frozen fish to be served fried. Which will you choose and why?

LAB-BASED ACTIVITY: Preparing Fish Dishes

STEP ❶ In teams, practice processing fish into the following forms: drawn, dressed, fillets, steaks, butterflied, and cubes. Refer to pages 488-489 for information on market forms of fish. Follow safety guidelines and use safe knife handling techniques.

STEP ❷ After processing the fish, choose one of the following cooking techniques to use to prepare the fish.
- Baking
- Broiling
- Grilling
- Sautéing
- Pan-frying
- Deep-frying

STEP ❸ Determine the doneness of your fish using the chart below.

STEP ❹ Plate and garnish your fish. Share your creation with the other teams.

STEP ❺ Taste each team's fish and answer the following questions:
- Was the form of each team's fish recognizable even after cooking? Why or why not?
- Was the cooking method for each team's fish appropriate to the market form? Why or why not?
- How would you rate the visual appeal and flavor of each team's fish? Use the following scale:

  1 = Poor; 2 = Fair; 3 = Good; 4 = Great

Cooking Technique	Determining Doneness of Fish
Baking	• Internal temperature is 145°F or above for 15 seconds.
Broiling or Grilling	• Outside of fish is slightly browned and crispy. • The interior is juicy and tender.
Sautéing or Pan-Frying	• Outside of fish is slightly browned and crispy. • The interior is juicy and tender.
Deep-Frying	• The batter is a rich golden brown. • The interior is juicy and tender.

Poultry Cookery

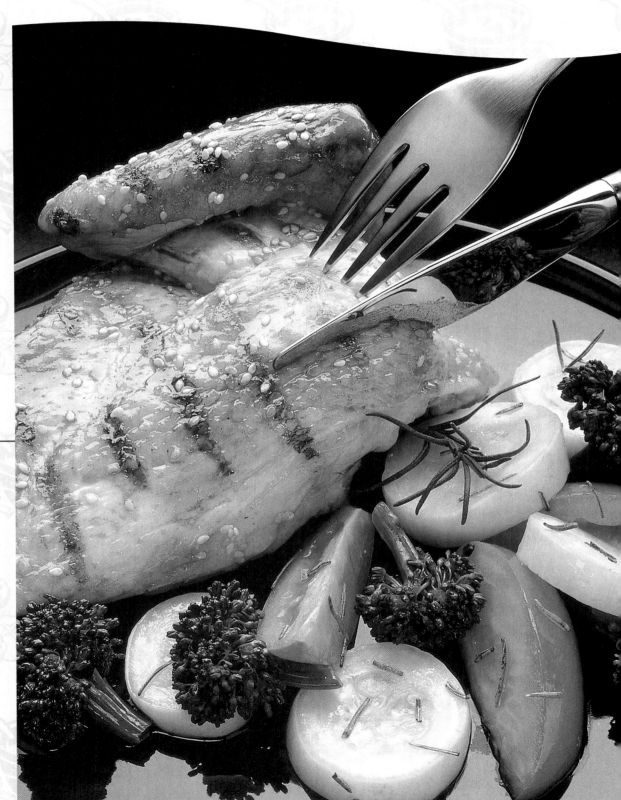

Poultry Basics

KEY TERMS

- connective tissue
- market form
- RTC
- trussing

OBJECTIVES

After reading this section, you will be able to:

- Identify different kinds, classes, and market forms of poultry.

- Explain how poultry is inspected and graded.

- Handle, store, and prepare poultry for cooking.

POULTRY refers to domestic birds that are raised for human consumption, such as chicken, turkey, ducks, and geese. Poultry products are less expensive than many meat products and may be adapted to a wide variety of dishes. Before you cook poultry dishes, you need to know how to identify, classify, and prepare poultry.

WHAT IS POULTRY?

The USDA categorizes poultry according to species, or kind. The kinds of poultry include chicken, turkey, duck, goose, guinea, and pigeon. Within the kinds of poultry, there are different classes, which are based on the age and gender of the bird.

Poultry is similar to meat in structure. It is made up of muscle, connective tissue, fat, and bone. Poultry flesh is made up of protein, water, and fat. The fat in poultry is found just under the skin.

Maturity & Tenderness

The older the poultry, the tougher the bird. This age factor is commonly called a bird's maturity. If you want tender poultry, you should select a younger, less mature bird.

In addition to age, tenderness is also affected by the amount of exercise a bird gets. For example, the more a bird exercises a muscle, the stronger and tougher that muscle becomes. This happens because with exercise, more connective tissue is created in muscles. **Connective tissue** is the tissue that holds muscle fiber together. A bird with more connective tissue will have tougher flesh.

Light or Dark Meat

Birds that rarely fly, such as turkeys and chickens, have much lighter-colored wing and breast meat, commonly called light meat. Light meat has less fat and cooks faster than dark meat.

The parts of a bird that have more muscle and connective tissue are darker in color. For example, the flesh of a bird's thighs and legs has more muscle and connective tissue because it is exercised more often. Dark meat has more fat and generally takes longer to cook. Duck and goose are composed of mostly dark meat.

Fig. 23-1.
Poultry Classification Chart

CHICKEN	DESCRIPTION
• Cornish hen	Young bird (5—6 weeks); very tender.
• Fryer or broiler	Young bird (9—12 weeks) of either gender; tender.
• Roaster	Young bird (3–5 months) of either gender; tender.
• Capon	Male chicken, under 10 months; very tender.
• Stewer	Mature female, over 10 months; tough.
DUCK	**DESCRIPTION**
• Broiler or fryer duckling	Young, tender duck with soft windpipe.
• Roasting duckling	Young, tender duck with hardening windpipe.
• Mature duck	Old duck with tough flesh.
GOOSE	**DESCRIPTION**
• Young goose	Under 6 months; tender.
• Mature goose	Over 6 months; tough.
GUINEA	**DESCRIPTION**
• Young guinea	Under 6 months; tender.
• Old guinea	Up to 12 months; tough.
PIGEON	**DESCRIPTION**
• Squab	3–4 weeks; light, tender meat.
• Pigeon	Over 4 weeks; dark, tough meat.
TURKEY	**DESCRIPTION**
• Fryer-roaster	Young bird of either gender; tender.
• Young turkey	Hen or tom with tender flesh but firmer cartilage.
• Yearling turkey	Fully mature yet still tender.
• Mature or old turkey	Hen or tom with tough flesh and coarse skin.

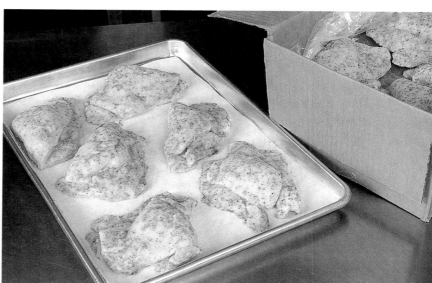
✗ PURCHASING POULTRY

Poultry is available in a variety of market forms, classes, and styles. **Market form** is the form poultry is in when purchased. The market form, class, or style of poultry purchased by a foodservice establishment will depend upon the type of establishment and the menu. See Fig. 23-1.

■ **Market forms.** Poultry can be purchased in different market forms, including fresh, frozen, or fully cooked.

• Fresh poultry works well when poultry is to be cooked within 24 hours.

• Frozen poultry may be kept up to six months.

• Many establishments find fully cooked poultry convenient for soups, salads, and casserole dishes. It can be purchased frozen and canned.

■ **Class.** The two classes of poultry are age and gender. Both classes affect the tenderness of the bird. Older birds are tougher than young birds and male birds are tougher than female birds.

■ **Style.** Poultry is also classified by style. Style refers to the condition or state the bird is in when it is received at a foodservice operation. It also reflects the amount of processing that was done to the product. Poultry is sold whole or in parts, bone-in or boneless, or ground.

Foodservice operations purchase poultry either whole or in parts. Poultry that has been prepared and packaged is called ready-to-cook, or **RTC** poultry. See Fig. 23-2. Whole, fresh poultry is usually less expensive than cut poultry.

Foodservice professionals who purchase whole poultry can cut it into pieces themselves. The type of poultry purchased is determined by the:

• Menu.
• Skill level of the kitchen staff.
• Preparation schedules.
• Available storage facilities.

Judging Quality

As a foodservice professional, you need to be familiar with what makes a poultry product acceptable.

■ **Color.** First, check the color of the poultry. It should vary from cream to yellow. It should not be purple or green from bruising or spoiling. Poultry shouldn't have dark wing tips. This is an indication of spoilage.

■ **Odor.** Poultry should not have a strong odor or feel sticky under the wings or around the joints. A strong odor and sticky feel indicate the poultry is spoiled.

To judge quality, you also need to check the poultry for the appropriate government inspection stamps.

Fig. 23-2. RTC poultry is ready-to-cook. What are the advantages of using RTC poultry?

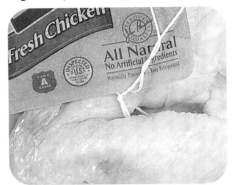
Inspection & Grading

All poultry must be federally inspected by the United States Department of Agriculture (USDA). Inspectors check samples of poultry to see that it is processed in sanitary conditions and is safe to be eaten. Poultry that passes inspection receives the USDA Inspection Stamp of approval.

Foodservice professionals check the poultry they use to ensure it has this stamp. With the USDA stamp, you can be assured that the poultry is free from visible signs of disease at the time of inspection. However, poultry must be properly handled and stored to maintain this level of safety.

Most poultry should also be graded. Unlike USDA inspection, which is mandatory for poultry, grading is voluntary. The poultry grading system is a way to judge quality.

The poultry grading system assigns a letter to indicate the level of quality. The highest grade poultry can receive is an "A." Only the best poultry is labeled "Grade A." Using Grade A poultry allows a foodservice establishment to provide a better quality and more consistent product. See Fig. 23-4.

For a bird to earn top poultry marks and receive Grade A, it must:

- Be plump and meaty.
- Have clean skin with no blemishes, tears, cuts, or bruises.
- Have no broken bones.
- Have all feathers plucked and removed, including pinfeathers.

Fig. 23-4.

Birds that do not meet these standards receive lower grades such as a "B" or "C." Lower-quality birds are used to make processed poultry products, such as chicken fingers or turkey pot pies.

✖ HANDLING & STORAGE

Fresh and frozen poultry must be handled very carefully. Fresh poultry is highly perishable, which means that it can quickly spoil if not handled properly. Make sure that any unfrozen poultry you receive is packed in ice until it is used. Poultry should be frozen immediately if it will not be used within 2–3 days. Once you receive poultry, repackage it immediately. Then place the poultry in cold storage until you are ready to prepare it.

Store frozen poultry at or below 0°F in its original packaging. You can store frozen poultry for up to six months. When you remove it from the freezer to thaw, keep it in its packaging. Thawing should be done under refrigeration. Never refreeze poultry.

✖ CUTTING UP POULTRY

The way you cut up poultry depends on how it will be cooked. In general, the first thing you'll want to do is cut the bird in half.

1. Place the bird on its breast, and grasp the chicken firmly. Cut through the skin and straight down the left or right side of the backbone using a wide-blade boning knife or a French knife. See Fig. 23-5A below.

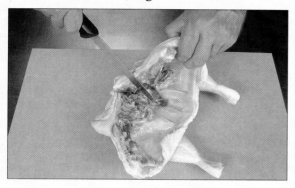

2. Split the bird open and lay it flat on the cutting board. See Fig. 23-5B below.

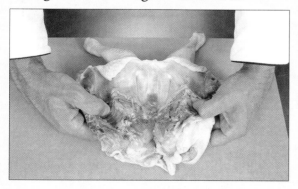

3. Cut the ribs that connect the backbone to the breast and remove the backbone. See Fig. 23-5C below.

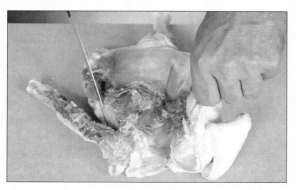

4. Bend the sides of the bird backward to break the breastbone; then remove the bone. Make sure to remove any cartilage along the bone. See Fig. 23-5D below.

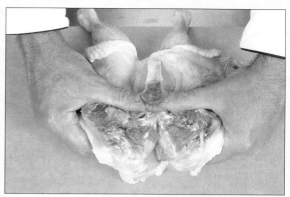

5. Cut the bird completely in half. See Fig. 23-5E below.

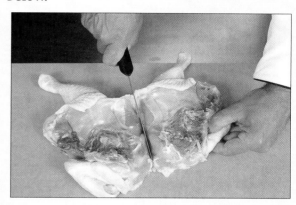

6. Cut the legs off each half of the bird by using a boning knife to cut through the skin between the thigh and the breast. See Fig. 23-5F below.

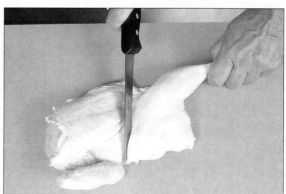

SALMONELLA BACTERIA

Salmonella bacteria causes much of the food poisoning in the world. Most persons infected with salmonella develop diarrhea, fever, and abdominal cramps within 12–72 hours. The illness usually lasts 5–7 days, and often does not require treatment unless severe dehydration occurs or the infection spreads from the intestines.

Keep these guidelines in mind to prevent salmonella food poisoning:

- Do not serve undercooked poultry.
- Cross-contamination of foods should also be avoided. Uncooked meats should be kept separate from produce, cooked foods, and ready-to-eat foods.
- Hands, cutting boards, counters, knives, and other utensils must be washed thoroughly after they have come in contact with uncooked foods.
- Salmonella may live dormant for a year or more inside a cutting board and then resurface when food is present.

APPLY IT!

Select three different types of cutting boards to be cultured. Place the cultures in a growing medium in a petri dish and examine the results. Which cutting boards were contaminated? Discuss how to thoroughly clean different types of cutting boards.

7. Cut off the drumstick portion of the leg from the thigh at the joint. See Fig. 23-5G below.

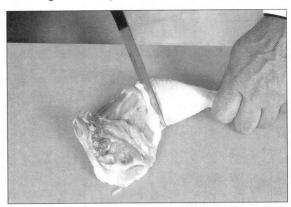

8. Separate the breast and wing into two parts by cutting at the joint. See Fig. 23-5H below.

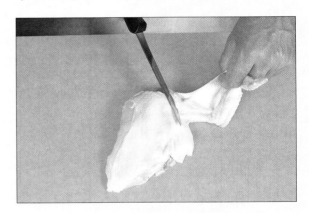

Trussing Whole Birds

If you'll be preparing and serving a whole bird, you will want to truss the bird. **Trussing** involves tying the legs and wings against the bird's body. It allows for even cooking and creates an attractive final product when served. Follow these steps for trussing poultry.

1. Place the poultry on a cutting board with the breastbone facing up. Make sure the neck is facing you.
2. Cut a piece of butcher's twine about three times the bird's length.
3. Tuck the wings behind the back.

4. Press the legs against the body by moving them forward and then down. See Fig. 23-6A below.

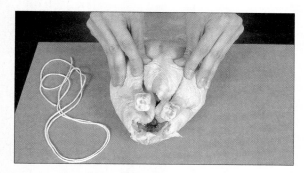

5. Pass twine under the hip, above the tail. See Fig. 23-6B below.

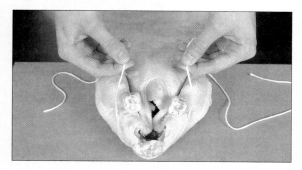

6. Pull the twine up and across the legs. See Fig. 23-6C below.

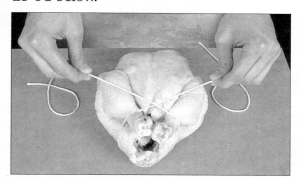

7. Firmly pull the ends of the twine toward the neck. See Fig. 23-6D below.

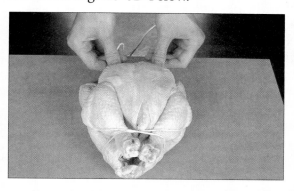

8. Press your thumbs into the breast and tie the twine tightly around the neck. See Fig. 23-6E below.

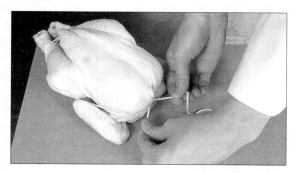

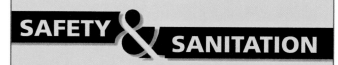

SAFETY & SANITATION

THAWING POULTRY—When thawing poultry, never defrost any poultry product at room temperature. Thaw poultry in the refrigerator. Once raw poultry thaws, it should be used within 2–3 days.

SECTION 23-1 Knowledge Check

1. Name the species, or kinds, of poultry as categorized by the USDA.
2. List the characteristics poultry must have to be labeled "Grade A" by the USDA.
3. Explain what a "class of poultry" refers to.

MINI LAB

Imagine that your restaurant received a shipment of whole chickens a week early. Describe the procedures you would follow to check the chickens for quality. Explain how you would store them.

Cooking Poultry

KEY TERMS

• **baste**

• **pressure-frying**

OBJECTIVES

After reading this section, you will be able to:

• Prepare poultry using various dry and moist cooking techniques.

• Present a properly cooked and plated poultry product.

• Demonstrate how to carve roasted or baked poultry.

Y O U can use a variety of techniques to cook poultry. For example, you could use a dry or moist cooking technique when preparing a young, tender chicken or turkey. To cook a more mature bird, you will want to use a moist cooking technique. There are many different ways to prepare poultry, making it one of the most versatile food products served.

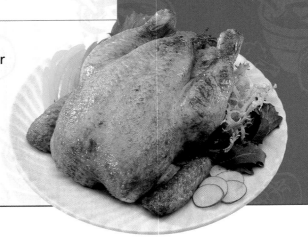

✖ POULTRY COOKING PRINCIPLES

Most poultry products are low in fat and can quickly become dry during cooking. Learning how to best apply proper cooking methods will help you create a successful final product. Overcooking is a common problem when cooking poultry. Using lower temperatures and slower cooking times can produce better results. Cooking with low heat, however, has its disadvantages. Low heat doesn't brown the surface of poultry well. High heat creates a crispy, golden surface. Because skin contains fat, cooking at high temperatures causes the fat to render, creating a well-browned and crispy skin that seals in the juices.

The presence or absence of bones influences moisture content and flavor during the cooking process. Bones actually help the bird retain some

of its moisture. For example, when cooking a boneless chicken breast you'll need to be especially attentive during the cooking process to avoid overcooking and drying out the meat.

✖ ROASTING & BAKING

Roasting and baking poultry are essentially the same process. Many chefs use the term roasting when they cook whole birds and baking when they cook parts of a bird. Roasted or baked poultry should be golden brown on the outside and tender and juicy on the inside. Using the proper cooking temperature makes all the difference when using these cooking methods. See Fig. 23-7. The goal is to make the skin crispy and brown without drying out the meat.

Fig. 23-7.

ROASTING & BAKING POULTRY	
• **Chicken**	375°F–400°F
• **Turkey**	Start at 400°F–425°F to brown skin. Reduce to 325°F to finish.
• **Duck & Goose**	375°F–425°F
• **Squab**	400°F
• **Game Hen**	375°F–400°F

Often a poultry recipe will direct you to start the cooking process using a high temperature. Then you will be directed to lower the temperature to complete the cooking process. This technique helps promote even cooking and seals in juices that prevent the meat from drying out.

To help whole poultry retain moisture during the roasting process, you should baste it during the last stage of cooking. To **baste**, spoon the fat drippings that have collected in the pan over the bird every 15–20 minutes. Only baste larger birds, such as turkey.

You don't have to baste a duck or goose. These birds have a high fat content. Basting will make them too juicy and possibly cause the bird to taste greasy. Make sure to roast them on a rack so the fat will drip into the pan. Some kinds of poultry, such as guineas and squabs, benefit from barding before cooking. These kinds of poultry have very little fat. Barding, or wrapping poultry in a layer of fat before cooking, will help the bird retain moisture while it cooks.

Another way to help poultry maintain its juiciness is to oil the skin prior to the cooking process. This will help prevent the skin from drying out and will lock in moisture.

Searing

Your recipe may call for you to sear the poultry product before it is roasted or baked. Searing means to brown the surface quickly over high heat, usually in a hot pan. This is commonly done with chicken parts. For example, the chicken is first cooked at 450°F for 15 minutes. This allows the outside to brown. The heat source is then reduced to 325°F. Searing helps seal in the juices that otherwise might escape during baking. Searing is also done by dredging poultry parts in seasoned flour and browning them in a skillet. Then the chicken is allowed to finish cooking in a 325°F–350°F oven.

✖ CARVING POULTRY

Once the roasted or baked poultry product is done, it will need to be carved. A variety of different carving methods exist. The method you use depends on the size of the bird. Turkey has the most meat in proportion to the bone. Here are the basic steps for carving a turkey:

1. Place the cooked turkey on a clean and sanitary cutting surface. Allow the turkey to stand for 20 minutes.

2. Remove the legs and thighs. To do this, pull the leg away from the body with a fork. Use a boning knife to cut through the joint. See Fig. 23-8A below.

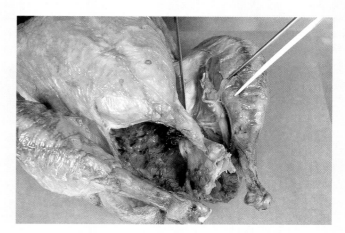

3. Separate the thigh from the leg and cut through the joint. See Fig. 23-8B below.

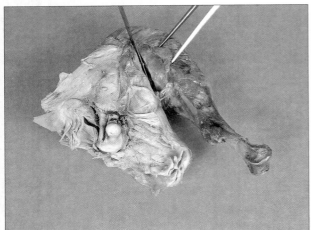

4. Slice the meat off the thigh parallel to the bone. See Fig. 23-8C below.

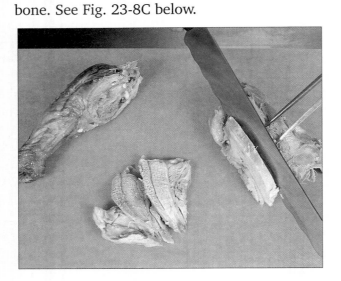

5. Carve the bird along one side of its breastbone to remove a breast. See Fig. 23-8D below.

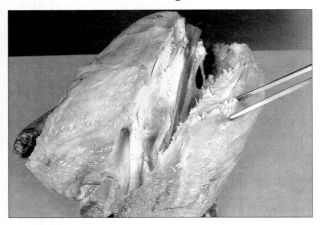

6. Cut the breast meat into slices at an angle across the grain of the flesh. See Fig. 23-8E below.

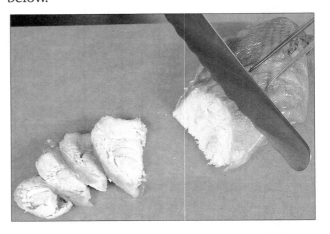

7. The breast can also be carved without removing it from the bird. Make a horizontal cut just above the wing toward the rib bones. See Fig. 23-8F below.

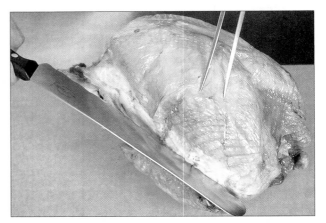

8. Slice the breast meat at an angle. See Fig. 23-8G below.

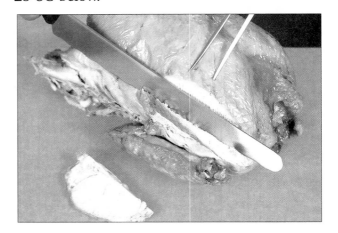

✖ BROILING & GRILLING

Broiled or grilled poultry can make a very attractive dinner plate. The food should have a well-browned surface and crosshatch grill marks. Smaller birds or poultry pieces are ideal for broiling or grilling. Follow these general steps to broil or grill poultry:

1. Preheat the broiler or grill.

2. Prepare the poultry. It can be marinated, seasoned, or simply brushed lightly with oil. See Fig. 23-9A below.

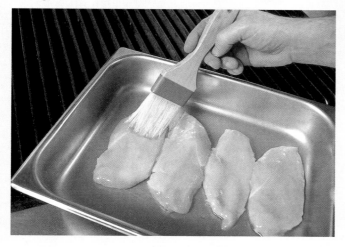

3. Place the poultry with its presentation side down on a grid or rack in a broiler. See Fig. 23-9B below.

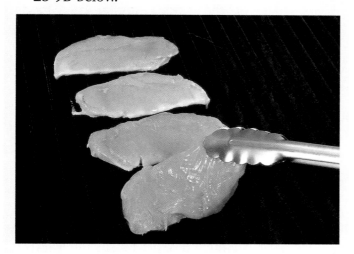

4. Turn the poultry 90° midway through cooking to create grill marks. See Fig. 23-9C below.

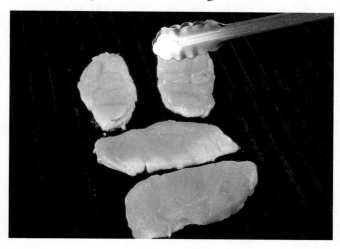

5. Periodically brush the poultry with oil or marinade to help keep it moist.

6. Carefully turn the poultry over using tongs so it can cook on the opposite side. If the poultry has skin, use a spatula and tongs to avoid breaking the skin while turning.

7. Poultry is done when it reaches an internal temperature of 165°F or above for 15 seconds.

✖ FRYING POULTRY

Fried chicken is a popular food item, especially in fast-food restaurants. There are three ways to fry poultry: pan-frying, deep-frying, and pressure-frying. All three usually require that the food first be coated with a seasoned flour mixture or batter.

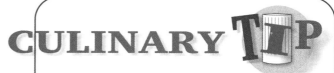

CHANGING THE OIL—To keep deep-fried products tasting their best, the oil in the fryer must be changed on a regular basis. The time frame depends on the type of fryer and the amount of frying done at the foodservice establishment.

Pan-Frying

Like the final product for other poultry cooking methods, poultry should emerge from the pan juicy and flavorful. In pan-frying, the poultry is dipped in a batter or seasoned flour mixture that will turn golden brown and crispy when the food is done. The challenge is to avoid making fried poultry taste oily or greasy. When pan-frying, the fat or oil should be under the smoking point, which is 400°F. Cooking at the proper temperature will help avoid an oily taste. Always brown the presentation side first. See Fig. 23-10.

Deep-Frying

Many times poultry, especially chicken, is deep-fried in fat. The poultry pieces are coated prior to frying. Common coatings for deep-frying include batter, flour, egg, and cracker or cereal crumbs.

Deep-fried chicken should be cooked at 325°F–350°F. The actual time will depend on the size of the chicken pieces and the color of the meat. Dark meat, for example, takes longer to fry than light meat, and should be cooked separately. There should never be more than one layer of chicken in a basket. If too many pieces are added to the fryer, it will cool down and result in a greasy product.

Fig. 23-10. Pan-frying is a common method of preparing poultry. Why is chicken dipped in batter or seasoned flour prior to frying?

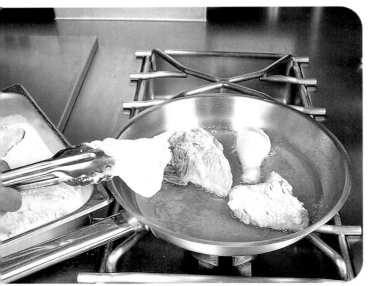

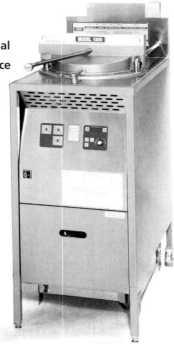

Fig. 23-11. Commercial pressure fryers produce foods that are crispy and moist, but not greasy.

Pressure-Frying

Similar to other frying methods, pressure-frying uses the same frying principles as other frying methods but uses a commercial pressure fryer. Using a pressure fryer cooks foods more quickly and at lower temperatures than other frying methods. **Pressure-frying** makes foods that are extra crispy on the outside, with their natural juices sealed on the inside. Pressure-fried foods are less greasy than other fried foods. You can pressure-fry any food that you would deep-fry. Kentucky Fried Chicken® and Broasted® Chicken are examples of this type of frying. See Fig. 23-11.

✖ SAUTÉING

Sautéing is a way of cooking poultry in an open pan until it is brown and juicy. Sautéing requires little fat. To sauté poultry:

1. Prepare the poultry product by cutting it into thin slices. You may also flatten the poultry with a meat mallet prior to cooking.

2. Heat a small amount of fat in a pan. Make sure the fat is hot before adding the poultry.

3. Dredge the poultry in seasoned flour if desired and lay it into the hot fat, presentation side down. See Fig. 23-12A below.

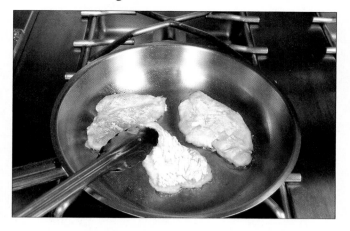

4. Cook until the presentation side is golden brown. Then turn the poultry over and cook until the product is fully cooked. Check the internal temperature. See Fig. 23-12B below.

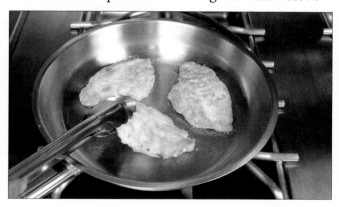

5. Finish some sautéed dishes by deglazing the pan with liquid to make a flavorful pan juice or sauce. See Fig. 23-12C below.

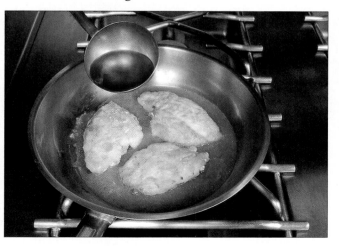

a LINK to the Past

Colonel Harland Sanders

Imagine creating a chicken recipe that would evenutally earn you $2 million! Born September 9, 1890, young Harland Sanders began cooking at the age of six after his father died and his mother had to work outside the home. In the early 1930s, Sanders owned a service station in Corbin, Kentucky, and served meals to travelers on his own dining table. His food became so popular that he moved his business across the street to a motel and restaurant that seated 142.

Over the years, Sanders perfected his blend of 11 herbs and spices and basic cooking technique. He found that cooking chicken in a pressure cooker produced an especially tender product. In 1935, Kentucky Governor Ruby Laffoon made Sanders a Kentucky Colonel in recognition of his contribution to the state's cuisine.

By 1964, Colonel Sanders sold the business, over 600 franchise outlets, for $2 million. He stayed on as a paid spokesperson for Kentucky Fried Chicken until he retired at the age of 81.

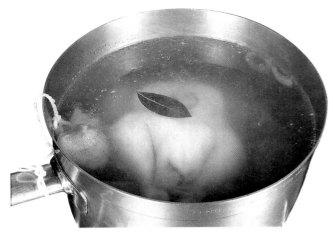

Fig. 23-13. Poaching poultry creates a flavorful liquid.

SIMMERING & POACHING

Unlike many other methods of preparing poultry, simmering and poaching produce a delicately flavored final product. Poaching is commonly used to cook whole, young, tender birds, while simmering is used for older, tougher birds. For simmering, poultry is cut into pieces.

Because these two cooking methods do not create strong flavors, it is important that the poultry be seasoned when it is cooked. One way to accomplish this is to use well-seasoned stock as the cooking liquid. A mirepoix or bouquet garni can also be added to enhance the flavor.

In both simmering and poaching, the liquid should completely cover the poultry. The broth created during cooking can be especially flavorful. You can reserve some of the liquid for later use with other recipes such as gravies or sauces. See Fig. 23-13.

BRAISING

Braising is a combination technique that starts with a dry-heat cooking method and ends with a moist-heat cooking method. When you serve braised poultry, it should always be accompanied by the liquid in which it was prepared. Some examples include chicken paprika (pa-PREE-kuh), coq au vin (kohk-oh-VAHN), and chicken fricassee (FRIHK-uh-see).

Like poultry that is simmered or poached, braised poultry gets a boost of flavor from its cooking liquid. Seasonings can be added to the liquid during cooking.

Follow these general steps to braise poultry:

1. Brown and sear the poultry in a small amount of fat in a rondeau or braising pan. See Fig. 23-14A below.

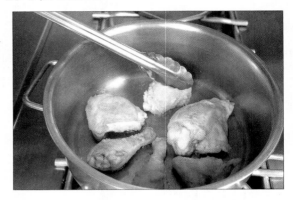

2. Add liquid, and bring to a simmer. The liquid should cover two-thirds of the poultry. See Fig. 23-14B below.

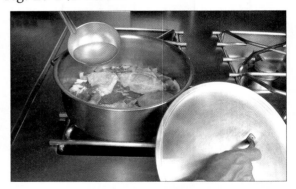

3. Cover the pan and continue to simmer on the rangetop or in the oven until the poultry is done. To test for doneness, use a fork to see that the meat is tender and cuts easily without falling apart. The meat must hold an internal temperature of 165°F for at least 15 seconds.

Determining Doneness of Poultry

Cook poultry until the meat is well done. Any type of poultry should be cooked to a minimum internal temperature of 165°F. The cooked poultry should hold this temperature for at least 15 seconds to be done safely. To properly measure this temperature, place a meat thermometer in the thigh of the bird at its thickest part, away from the bone. Keep in mind that no matter what method you use, the poultry must be fully cooked.

✖ STUFFINGS

Stuffing can be an excellent addition to a poultry dish. However, stuffing must be prepared and cooked separately from the poultry. Federal health codes mandate that poultry dishes sold in food-service establishments cannot be stuffed since stuffing poultry may pose health risks to the customer. This is because bacteria can quickly multiply in the stuffing inside the bird's cavity. Although the flesh of the bird may reach an adequate, safe temperature, the stuffing inside the bird may not reach a safe temperature in an adequate amount of time. To be safe, you should prepare the stuffing for poultry separately. Keep in mind that if you prepare the wet and dry stuffing ingredients ahead of time, they should be kept refrigerated in a shallow baking pan. Never store stuffing in the same container as poultry. Do not overmix or pack down stuffing ingredients.

✖ PLATING POULTRY DISHES

Like other food products, it's important to pay attention to how poultry is presented on the plate that you serve to a customer. Dishes can be prepared and garnished in the kitchen area, or poultry can be sliced and served at the table side.

Many recipes recommend serving stuffing with poultry. Don't ignore other possible accompaniments, such as gravies, sauces, soups, salsas, vegetables, casseroles, wild rice, potatoes, and pasta. Common garnishes for poultry include vegetables, fruits, and nuts. See Fig. 23-15.

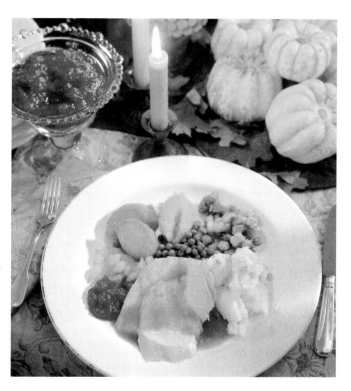

Fig. 23-15. Side dishes and presentation make poultry even more appealing.

SECTION 23-2 Knowledge Check

1. When should you use a dry or moist technique when cooking poultry?
2. Identify the various methods that can be used to cook poultry.
3. List food items that can accompany plated poultry.

MINI LAB

You have been asked to select side dishes to accompany the poultry dishes on a new menu. Select side dishes for the following: roasted turkey, fried chicken, grilled chicken breast. Prepare one of these three poultry dishes.

SECTION SUMMARIES

23-1 The USDA first classifies poultry according to species, then divides the birds into classes according to age and gender.

23-1 Poultry flesh is made of three main components: water, protein, and fat.

23-1 All poultry must be federally inspected by the USDA.

23-1 Poultry is highly perishable and must be handled carefully, with fresh poultry being used or frozen within 72 hours.

23-2 Since it easy to overcook poultry, take into consideration the presence of bones, light or dark meat, and the desired final result.

23-2 Follow individual cooking instructions so that the well done poultry product is tender and juicy.

23-2 The roasting and baking process for poultry involves cooking the bird in the oven using methods that help retain moisture.

23-2 Poultry may be prepared by a variety of dry heat methods including roasted, baked, broiled, grilled, sautéed, pan-fried, deep-fried, and pressure-fried.

23-2 Simmering, poaching, and braising are all moist heat cooking methods that involve liquids.

23-2 Stuffing can be an excellent addition to a poultry dish if prepared properly and stored separately from the bird.

CHECK YOUR KNOWLEDGE

1. How does the age and sex of the bird affect the tenderness of poultry?
2. Explain the differences between light and dark meat.
3. List the qualities the USDA uses to grade poultry.
4. List three uses for Grade B poultry.
5. Describe how to thaw poultry.
6. What do barding and basting have in common?
7. Why is it important to clean and sanitize any surface that comes into contact with raw poultry?
8. Explain how to carve a whole bird for serving.
9. Compare simmering and poaching.
10. Define mirepoix and its use.

CRITICAL-THINKING ACTIVITIES

1. You need to order chicken for your busy fried chicken restaurant. Whole chicken is less expensive than chicken parts, but requires more labor to prepare. Which type of chicken will you order? Why?
2. Create a recipe for a turkey sandwich. What qualities will make your sandwich healthful and flavorful? Draw some conclusions about how you could promote this heart-healthy sandwich with your customers.

WORKPLACE KNOW-HOW

Problem solving. Customers in your restaurant have been complaining that the roasted turkey is too dry. How can you make a more tender and moist product?

LAB-BASED ACTIVITY: Preparing Poultry

STEP ❶ **In teams, choose a cooking method to use in preparing poultry.** Each team should choose a different cooking method from the following:

- Roasted.
- Baked.
- Broiled.
- Grilled.
- Pan-fried.
- Deep-fried.
- Pressure-fried.
- Poached.
- Braised.

STEP ❷ **Find a recipe that uses the cooking method your team chose.**

STEP ❸ **Make a list of the cooking materials you will need to prepare your poultry dish.** Include oils, coatings, spices, and seasonings in addition to equipment.

STEP ❹ **Prepare and plate your poultry dish.**

STEP ❺ **Serve your poultry to another team and have that team evaluate it.**

STEP ❻ **Use the following rating scale to evaluate each team's poultry dish for appearance, flavor, and texture.** Use the following scale along with the chart below in your evaluation.

1 = Poor; 2 = Fair; 3 = Good; 4 = Great

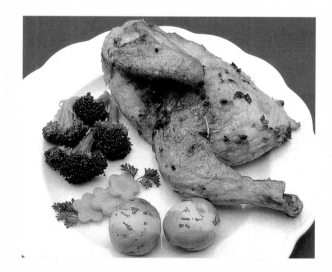

Cooked Poultry Evaluation

Appearance	• Cooked to appropriate doneness. Doesn't appear burned or undercooked. • Appropriately plated and garnished.
Flavor	• Flavor appropriate to preparation method and food product.
Texture	• Poultry is moist, tender, and juicy, not dry and tough.

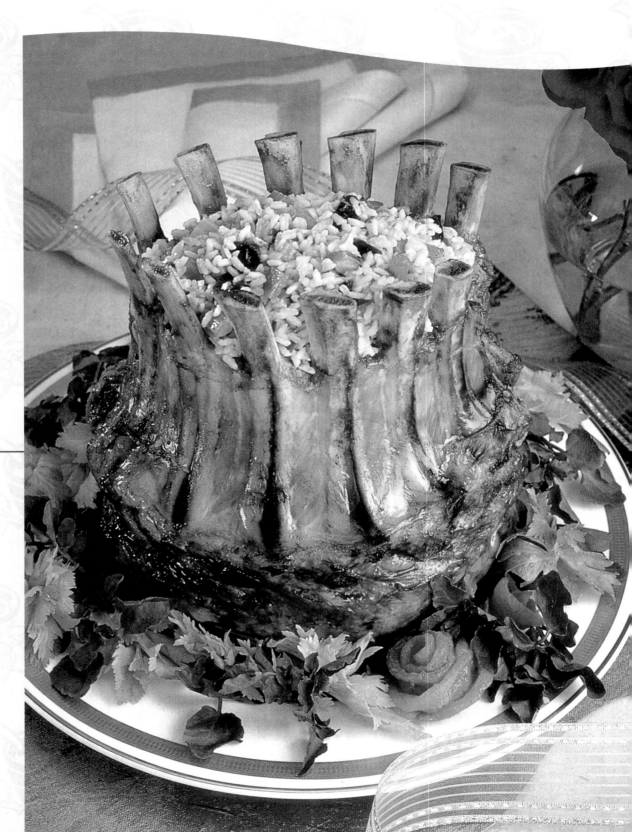

Meat Cookery

24

CHAPTER

Section 24-1
Meat Basics

Section 24-2
Meat Cuts

Section 24-3
Principles of
Cooking Meat

Meat Basics

OBJECTIVES

After reading this section, you will be able to:

- Describe the nutritional composition of meat.
- Describe the internal structure of meat.
- Describe the quality grades of meat.
- Describe the process of aging meat.

MEAT is an important part of many people's diets. It is also an essential part of most foodservice establishment menu offerings. Therefore, it is very important to learn about the different types of meats available. You will need to know how to purchase the best cuts of meat and how to safely store them.

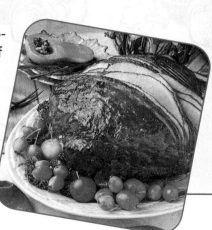

NUTRITIONAL COMPOSITION OF MEAT

Meat is the muscle of animals, such as cattle and hogs. In general, all meats contain four basic nutrients: water, protein, fat, and carbohydrates.

Meat has the following amount of nutrients:

- About 75% of muscle is water.
- About 20% of muscle is protein.
- About 5% of muscle is fat.

Water is a very important nutrient to keep in mind when preparing meat. Too much cooking will make meat dry. As meat cooks, it gets smaller due to shrinkage. **Shrinkage** occurs when the meat loses water as it cooks. So, the longer you cook meat, the less it weighs. Meats cooked at low temperatures don't lose as much water as meats cooked at high temperatures.

There are two types of fat in meat: marbling and fat cap. **Marbling** is fat within the muscle tissue. The amount of marbling affects the meat's tenderness, taste, and quality. In general, the more marbling in a piece of meat, the more tender and flavorful the meat will be. See Fig. 24-1.

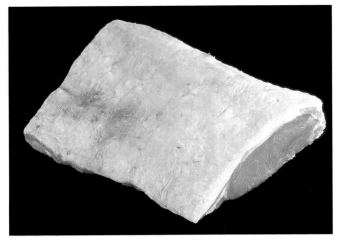

Fig. 24-1. Fat is a nutrient found in all meats. Why is fat essential to meat?

Fat cap is the fat that surrounds muscle tissue. An animal uses this layer of fat as an energy source and to keep itself warm. This layer of fat is frequently left on during cooking to keep meat moist and juicy. If there is not a fat cap, barding or larding is an alternative.

With **barding**, you wrap a lean meat with fat, such as bacon, before roasting. A few minutes before doneness, you remove the meat from the oven, unwrap the fat, put the meat back in the oven, and allow the surface of the meat to brown.

With **larding**, long, thin strips of fat or vegetables are inserted into the center of the lean meat. This adds moisture and can make the final product visually appealing.

⊠ THE STRUCTURE OF MEAT

Meat products have three components: muscle fibers, connective tissue, and bones.

■ **Muscle fibers.** You may have heard that leaner cuts of meat have fewer calories. That's because lean meat is almost completely composed of muscle fibers with little fat. These fibers determine meat's texture and contribute to its flavor. For example, coarsely textured meat such as ham has tough, large fibers. Smooth-textured meat such as beef tenderloin has tender, small fibers.

■ **Connective tissue.** Muscle fibers are bound together by connective tissue. Connective tissue connects muscles to bones and binds muscle fibers together. Connective tissue is tough. So, to cook meats properly, you need to understand how connective tissue functions. Connective tissue is composed of either collagen or elastin. **Collagen** is soft, white tissue that breaks down into gelatin and water during slow, moist cooking processes. **Elastin** is a hard, yellow tissue that doesn't break down during cooking. Elastin is the tissue some people refer to as "gristle." Older animals generally have a lot of elastin. To reduce the effects of elastin, cut it away from the meat.

To tenderize meat that has a lot of connective tissue, try the following techniques:

• Sear the meat and then use a long, slow, moist cooking method, such as braising.
• Tenderize meat. See Fig. 24-2.

Fig. 24-2. This veal is being tenderized.

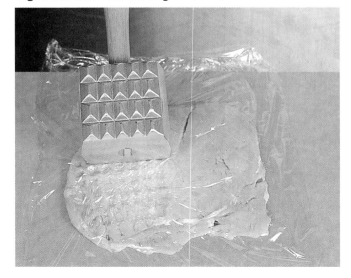

- Slice meat thinly, against the grain.
- Grind the meat.
- Break down collagen in connective tissue by adding a chemical tenderizer, such as those that are made from papaya and pineapple enzymes.

■ **Bones.** Bones make up the skeleton of the animal. An older animal has whiter bones, while a younger one has redder bones. Learning the bone structure of an animal will help you identify the different cuts of meat and how they are carved.

Primal Cuts

Primal cuts, sometimes called wholesale cuts, are large, primary pieces of meat separated from the animal. Primal cuts are the most popular forms of meat purchased by foodservice operations. Although primal cuts are large cuts of meat, they are easily handled and stored.

Fabricated Cuts

Fabricated cuts are smaller portions taken from primal cuts. That is, they are smaller, menu-sized portions of meat. You would likely purchase fabricated cuts if you were planning to serve roasts, stews, or steaks. Purchasing fabricated cuts as exact portions can limit waste.

Whole Carcass

The carcass is what is left of the whole animal after it has been slaughtered. The carcass does not usually include the head, feet, or hide. However, pork can be purchased with the feet and head still attached. Most foodservice establishments don't purchase meat in this form. The labor, equipment, and facilities needed to process a whole carcass are expensive.

■ **Cutting the carcass.** Beef carcasses are split into two sides called the forequarter and the hindquarter. In general, veal and lamb carcasses are divided between their ribs to create the fore-saddle and hindsaddle. See Fig. 24-3.

a LINK to the Past

History of the Butcher

The history of the butcher extends back to Ancient Rome. The Roman butcher slaughtered (SLAW-tuhrd) and sold meat according to regulations that governed the type of meat the butcher sold.

In the early Middle Ages in France, the King granted stalls to butchers from which they butchered and sold meat. By the late Middle Ages, open stalls in large meat markets were the sites for butchering and selling meat. At this same time, butchers also maintained open shops. Here people would choose a cut of meat that the butcher had just prepared. In both cases, butchers were restricted to slaughtering and selling meat in specified areas in the towns and cities.

Today, slaughtering animals for meat most often takes place at the meat packer rather than by the butcher. In large-scale meat packing operations, lasers are often used to fabricate the carcasses. Then the meat is sold to purveyors after it has been approved according to USDA standards.

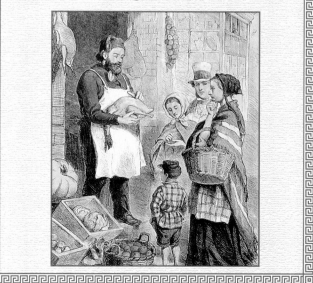

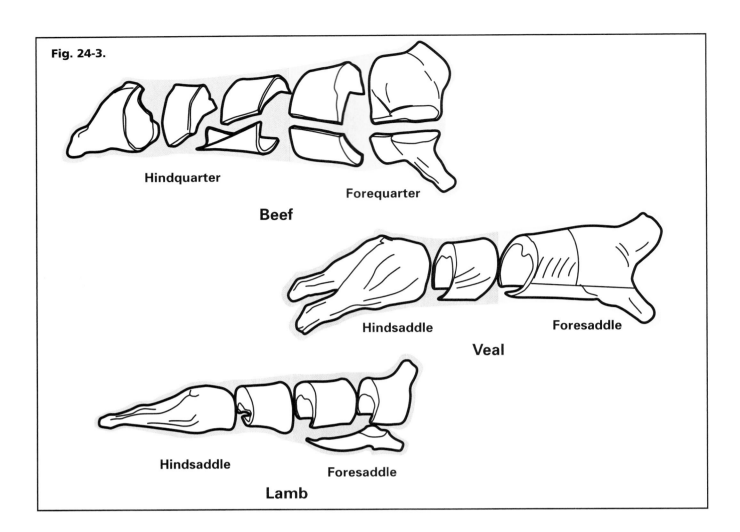

Fig. 24-3.

Hindquarter

Forequarter

Beef

Hindsaddle

Foresaddle

Veal

Hindsaddle

Foresaddle

Lamb

☒ MEAT INSPECTION

In 1906, the federal government passed the Meat Inspection Act. This law requires the inspection of all meats transported across state lines. It guarantees that the meat is wholesome, and that the animal was not diseased.

The meat for foodservice operations must have a United States Department of Agriculture (USDA) Inspection Stamp. The USDA stamp will not reveal anything about the quality or tenderness of the meat, only that it is fit for human consumption. See Fig. 24-4.

Fig. 24-4. USDA Inspection stamps.

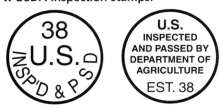

☒ GRADING MEAT

As with poultry, meat is graded to indicate its quality. The grading shield stamp indicates how tender and flavorful the meat will be when it is prepared. Meat is graded for both quality and yield.

■ **Quality Grades.** Quality grading is a means to measure differences in the quality of the meat you purchase. This type of grading reveals meat's tenderness, juiciness, and flavor. The quality grades are different for each type of meat. See Fig. 24-5.

USDA Prime meats are used in the very best foodservice establishments. These meats are also the most expensive. For a meat product to receive a USDA Prime grade, it must have excellent marbling and a thick layer of fat cap. See Fig. 24-6.

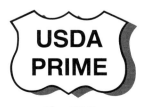

Fig. 24-6.

Fig. 24-5.

MEAT	QUALITY GRADES
Beef	USDA Prime, Choice, Select, Standard, Commercial, Utility, Cutter, Canner.
Pork	Pork is not quality graded since the quality is always uniform.
Veal	USDA Prime, Choice, Good, Standard, Utility.
Lamb	USDA Prime, Choice, Good, Utility.

The Choice grade is more widely accepted in the foodservice industry. It is the grade most preferred by consumers because of its flavor and tenderness. It is also a great value.

The Select grade has very little marbling. It is usually purchased by foodservice operations that are concerned about keeping costs down. Below the Select grade are the Utility, Cutter, and Canner grades. These are used primarily for processed meat products, such as hamburger patties and luncheon meats.

■ **Yield Grades.** Yield grades measure the amount of usable meat on beef and lamb. The best grade is Yield Grade 1, and the lowest is Yield Grade 5. If you purchase a piece of beef that is marked "Yield Grade 5," it probably has a large amount of fat and not much muscle. See Fig. 24-7.

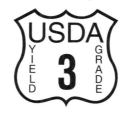

Fig. 24-7.

🗙 PURCHASING MEATS

Imagine you've been given the job of buying meat for your foodservice operation. Where would you begin? There are several factors to consider when purchasing meat.

- Consider the menu and then select meats that will fit those recipes.
- Consider the cooking methods to be used.

- Consider the price. For example, how much can your customers afford and how much is your foodservice operation willing to pay for top-quality meats.
- Always keep quality and value in mind.

To assist in making quality meat purchases, many foodservice operations use publications such as "The Meat Buyers Guide," which is put out by the North American Meat Processors Association. In this guide, you will find the Institutional Meat Purchase Specifications (IMPS) for quality meats along with photos of various meat cuts.

The storage facilities, the cooking techniques that a facility uses, and the speed with which food must be prepared all affect the selection of types and sizes of meat. See Fig. 24-8.

Fig. 24-8. Meats must be stored properly to prevent spoilage. Which standards or regulations guide proper storage of meats?

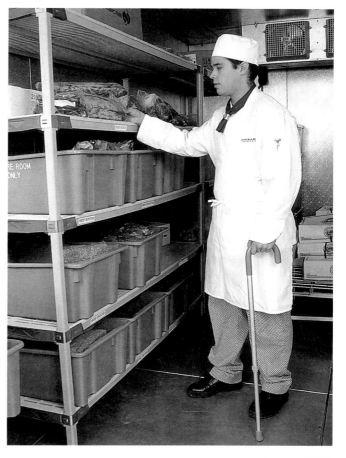

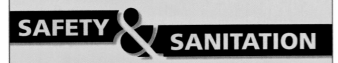

MEAT HANDLING & STORAGE

Meat storage requires careful attention. Meat can quickly spoil if it is not properly handled.

■ **Fresh meat.** Fresh meat should be stored in the refrigerator at 41°F or below. Wet-aged meat should remain sealed until the meat is ready for use. Ground meat, such as hamburger, must be wrapped air-tight. Place meat on trays so that juices from the meat will not contaminate other foods or the storage unit floors. Store uncooked meats on the lower shelves of the refrigerator, with ground meats shelved below other meats. Raw meats should always be placed on the lowest shelf.

■ **Frozen meats.** To freeze fresh meat, place it in a freezer at 0°F or below. Never freeze meat in containers. Always wrap the meat in air-tight, moisture-proof packaging to prevent freezer burn. Freezer burn causes meat to spoil. Labeling packages and following FIFO help avoid spoilage. Meats should always be thawed under refrigeration and never on the counter. See Fig. 24-9.

Fig. 24-9.

MEAT PRODUCTS	REFRIGERATOR	FREEZER
Beef, roasts & steaks	2–5 days	6–9 months
Lamb, roasts & steaks	2–5 days	6–9 months
Pork, roasts & chops	2–5 days	4–8 months
Beef & lamb, ground	1–2 days	3–4 months
Pork, sausage	1–2 days	2 months

SECTION 24-1 Knowledge Check

1. Explain how the size of muscle fibers in meat is related to the meat's texture, and give one example.
2. Why does meat develop more flavor as it ages?
3. List the guidelines for storing and handling frozen meats.

MINI LAB

Divide into teams and use one of the five methods on pages 528-529 to tenderize beef, pork, veal, or lamb. Cook the meat and have another team evaluate your team's product. Which tenderizing technique worked best?

Meat Cuts

- **processing**
- **curing**
- **irradiation**

OBJECTIVES

After reading this section, you will be able to:

- Identify primal and fabricated cuts of pork, lamb, veal, and beef.

- Identify the quality characteristics of pork, lamb, veal, and beef.

- Describe the techniques used to process meat.

- Demonstrate appropriate storage procedures for pork, lamb, veal, and beef.

BEFORE being shipped to foodservice operations, a meat carcass is usually divided into primal cuts and portioned. Primal cuts are easier for foodservice workers to handle. Standards have been established that specify how pork, lamb, veal, and beef should be divided into smaller fabricated cuts. These smaller pieces of meat can be prepared in a variety of ways. Learning the basic primal and fabricated cuts, the location and shape of the bones, and the characteristics and processes of each kind of meat will prepare you to handle and serve meat correctly.

CUTS OF PORK

Pork is the meat from hogs that are less than one year old. There are five different primal pork cuts: loin, shoulder, Boston butt, belly, and fresh ham. The largest primal cut is the loin. See Fig. 24-10 on page 534 (**Foodservice Cuts of Pork**).

■ **Loin.** The loin can be divided into several fabricated cuts, such as pork tenderloin, pork chops, and pork back ribs. Pork tenderloin is the most tender cut of pork. The pork chop is a favorite of many customers. The best pork chops are those that are center cut. All loin cuts can be cooked using a variety of cooking methods.

■ **Shoulder butt.** The shoulder is the lower part of the foreleg. It is sometimes called a picnic ham. This part of the ham has a higher fat content than other cuts, making it ideal for roasting. The shoulder cut can be cooked using any method. It can be fabricated into fresh and smoked picnic hams. The shoulder also may be boned and cut into smaller pieces, and then sautéed, braised, or stewed. Just above the shoulder is the Boston butt. This cut has a high fat content but is very meaty. The Boston butt can be divided into steaks and chops. It can be boned and smoked like a ham.

FOODSERVICE CUTS OF PORK

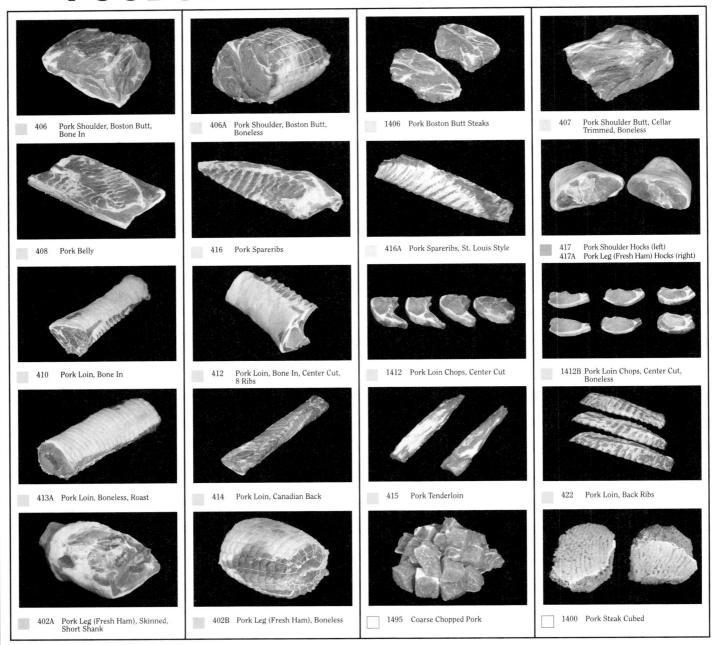

406 Pork Shoulder, Boston Butt, Bone In	406A Pork Shoulder, Boston Butt, Boneless	1406 Pork Boston Butt Steaks	407 Pork Shoulder Butt, Cellar Trimmed, Boneless
408 Pork Belly	416 Pork Spareribs	416A Pork Spareribs, St. Louis Style	417 Pork Shoulder Hocks (left) 417A Pork Leg (Fresh Ham) Hocks (right)
410 Pork Loin, Bone In	412 Pork Loin, Bone In, Center Cut, 8 Ribs	1412 Pork Loin Chops, Center Cut	1412B Pork Loin Chops, Center Cut, Boneless
413A Pork Loin, Boneless, Roast	414 Pork Loin, Canadian Back	415 Pork Tenderloin	422 Pork Loin, Back Ribs
402A Pork Leg (Fresh Ham), Skinned, Short Shank	402B Pork Leg (Fresh Ham), Boneless	1495 Coarse Chopped Pork	1400 Pork Steak Cubed

The above cuts are a partial representation of NAMP/IMPS items. For further representation and explanation of all cuts see *The Meat Buyers Guide* by the North American Meat Processors Association.

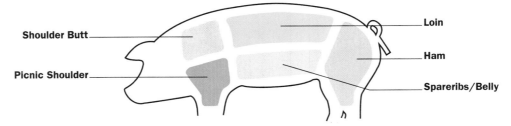

Shoulder Butt

Picnic Shoulder

Loin

Ham

Spareribs/Belly

NAMP/IMPS Number (North American Meat Processors Association/Institutional Meat Purchase Specifications)

©2002 North American Meat Processors Association

American Meat Science Association

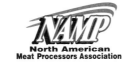

North American Meat Processors Association

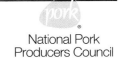

National Pork Producers Council

- **Spareribs belly.** The pork belly is a primal cut with a high percentage of fat and little lean meat. The fabricated cut is spareribs. Any left over meat is cut for bacon.
- **Ham.** The primal cut called the ham is actually a portion of the hind leg. This cut is very large and has lots of muscle and little connective tissue. Fresh ham can be cut with the bone in or boneless, or with the shank removed. The shank of the ham is sometimes called the ham hock.

Quality Characteristics of Pork

Today pork is much leaner than it once was. Pork can be nearly as lean as skinless chicken. Three ounces of pork tenderloin, the leanest cut, has about 1.4 g of fat, while a 3-oz. skinless chicken breast has about 0.9 g of fat.

Hogs are butchered before they are one year old. Therefore, they are more tender than older animals. There are many rules and regulations about how hogs are raised and slaughtered that protect both the animals and the public from disease, infection, and contamination.

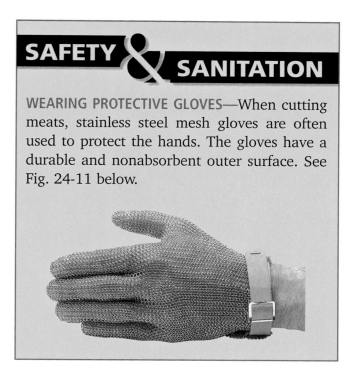

SAFETY & SANITATION

WEARING PROTECTIVE GLOVES—When cutting meats, stainless steel mesh gloves are often used to protect the hands. The gloves have a durable and nonabsorbent outer surface. See Fig. 24-11 below.

PROCESSING PORK

While some pork is purchased fresh, such as pork chops, most pork is processed. **Processing** is the act of changing pork by artificial means. When pork is processed and cut to make ham and bacon, it usually is cured, aged, or smoked. Processing may also involve a combination of these three processes. About 70% of the carcass is processed before it ever arrives at a foodservice operation.

Curing and smoking are types of processing. Processing not only changes the flavor of the food but also greatly improves its preservation.

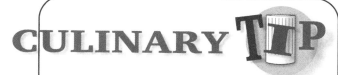

CULINARY TIP

AGING OF PORK—Cured and smoked pork are aged due to processing. Fresh pork is not aged because it is naturally tender.

Curing

Preserving pork with salt, sugar, spices, flavoring, and nitrites is called **curing**. Ham that has been cured, for example, has a pink color that makes it visually appealing. Cured pork resists spoilage better than fresh pork. It also retains a fresher flavor for a longer period of time.

Curing changes the color and flavor of the pork. The oldest form of curing is dry curing. In dry curing, the seasonings, such as salt, are rubbed on the surface of the pork. Usually the entire surface of the pork is covered and then stored until the seasoning is absorbed into the meat.

- **Pickle curing.** Pork is submerged in brine, or pickling liquid, until the mix completely penetrates the meat.
- **Injection curing.** Brine is injected directly into the meat.
- **Sugar curing.** Pork is covered with a seasoned, sweet brine that contains brown sugar or molasses.

Smoking

Aged hams are a popular variety of pork. These hams are cured and then smoked. Smoking involves exposing the pork to the smoke of fragrant hardwoods, such as hickory.

Irradiation

Outbreaks of foodborne illnesses have increased consumer awareness about environmental issues and potential health risks. Concerns over food safety have led to a change in how meat, particularly pork, is processed. **Irradiation** (ih-ray-dee-AY-shun) has proven to be an effective way to eliminate potentially harmful microorganisms and enhance food safety.

When pork is irradiated, it is exposed to medium doses of radiation. This process does not cook the meat, but it delays spoilage by destroying cells that cause it. It also greatly enhances food safety. However, it should never replace proper food handling and sanitation techniques.

⊗ CUTS OF LAMB

Lamb meat comes from sheep that are less than one year old. Meat from older sheep is called mutton, and it is usually tough. The carcass of a lamb is normally divided into the shoulder, shank/breast, rack or rib, foresaddle, hindsaddle, loin, and leg. See Fig. 24-12 on page 537 (**Foodservice Cuts of Lamb**).

- **Shoulder.** The shoulder is a large piece of primal-cut meat that contains rib bones, the arm, blade, neck bones, and muscles. It is difficult to divide the shoulder into fabricated cuts because of the large number of bones and muscles it contains. Either the shoulder is cut into pieces and used for stew, or the meat is ground.

- **Shank/breast.** This primal cut includes the breast and foreshank of the carcass. It is not used often in food service. If the breast is used, it is braised either as boneless or bone-in. The foreshank is meatier and can be served as an entrée.

- **Rack.** The rack is what results from cutting the rib tips in the breast. It is located between the shoulder and the loin and includes eight ribs and some of the backbone. The tender rib-eye muscle is a part of the rack. Fabricated cuts include the lamb rack and rib chops.

- **Loin.** The primal cut that comes from the area between the rib and leg is called the loin. It includes a rib and some of the backbone, tenderloin, loin-eye muscle, and flank. Loin meat is generally very tender. Fabricated cuts include boneless roasts and bone-in or boneless chops.

- **Leg.** The hind leg of the lamb contains some of the backbone, tail, hip, round, and shank bones. Usually the leg is split and boned before cooking. Sometimes a bone-in leg is roasted or braised. The fabricated cuts are steaks. The leg also can be diced and stewed or ground into patties.

Quality Characteristics of Lamb

The lamb meat purchased by a foodservice operation should have these characteristics:
- Pinkish to deep red color.
- Firm and finely textured.
- Some marbling in its lean areas.

Storing Lamb

Fresh lamb can spoil quickly even when kept in a cooler. Don't exceed these maximum refrigeration storage times:
- 2–5 days in the refrigerator at 41°F or below.
- 6–9 months in the freezer at 0°F or below.

FOODSERVICE CUTS OF LAMB

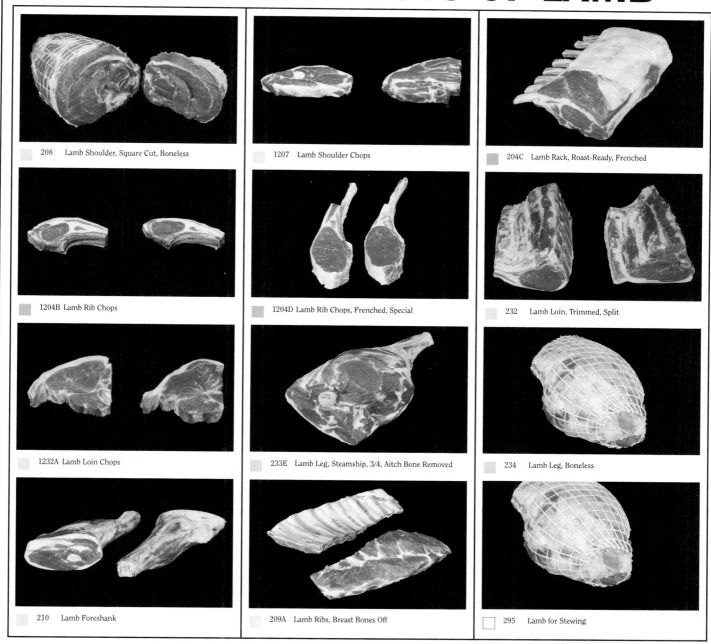

208   Lamb Shoulder, Square Cut, Boneless

1207   Lamb Shoulder Chops

204C   Lamb Rack, Roast-Ready, Frenched

1204B   Lamb Rib Chops

1204D   Lamb Rib Chops, Frenched, Special

232   Lamb Loin, Trimmed, Split

1232A   Lamb Loin Chops

233E   Lamb Leg, Steamship, 3/4, Aitch Bone Removed

234   Lamb Leg, Boneless

210   Lamb Foreshank

209A   Lamb Ribs, Breast Bones Off

295   Lamb for Stewing

The above cuts are a partial representation of NAMP/IMPS items. For further representation and explanation of all cuts see *The Meat Buyers Guide* by the North American Meat Processors Association.

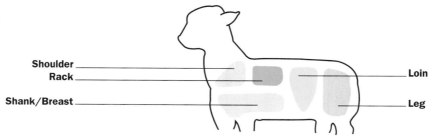

Shoulder
Rack
Shank/Breast
Loin
Leg

NAMP/IMPS Number (North American Meat Processors Association/Institutional Meat Purchase Specifications)

©2000 North American Meat Processors Association

American Meat Science
Association

NAMP
North American
Meat Processors Association

FOODSERVICE CUTS OF VEAL

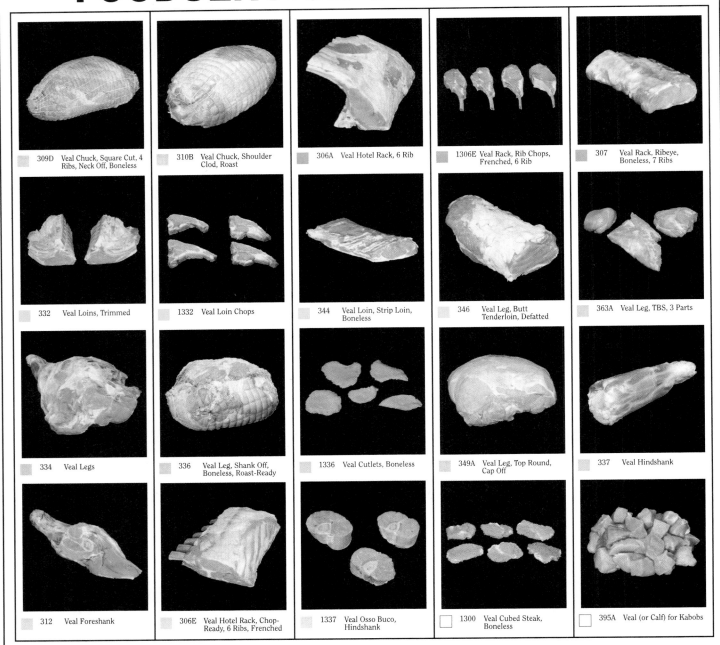

309D Veal Chuck, Square Cut, 4 Ribs, Neck Off, Boneless	310B Veal Chuck, Shoulder Clod, Roast	306A Veal Hotel Rack, 6 Rib	1306E Veal Rack, Rib Chops, Frenched, 6 Rib	307 Veal Rack, Ribeye, Boneless, 7 Ribs
332 Veal Loins, Trimmed	1332 Veal Loin Chops	344 Veal Loin, Strip Loin, Boneless	346 Veal Leg, Butt Tenderloin, Defatted	363A Veal Leg, TBS, 3 Parts
334 Veal Legs	336 Veal Leg, Shank Off, Boneless, Roast-Ready	1336 Veal Cutlets, Boneless	349A Veal Leg, Top Round, Cap Off	337 Veal Hindshank
312 Veal Foreshank	306E Veal Hotel Rack, Chop-Ready, 6 Ribs, Frenched	1337 Veal Osso Buco, Hindshank	1300 Veal Cubed Steak, Boneless	395A Veal (or Calf) for Kabobs

The above cuts are a partial representation of NAMP/IMPS items. For further representation and explanation of all cuts see *The Meat Buyers Guide* by the North American Meat Processors Association.

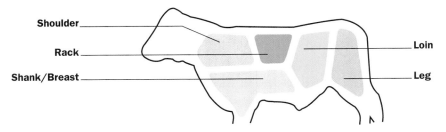

Shoulder

Rack

Shank/Breast

Loin

Leg

NAMP/IMPS Number (North American Meat Processors Association/Institutional Meat Purchase Specifications)

American Meat Science Association

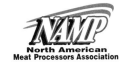

North American Meat Processors Association

BEEF
USA
National Cattlemen's Beef Association

⊠ CUTS OF VEAL

Veal is the meat from calves that are less than nine months old. Some veal is from calves that are only eight to sixteen weeks old. Veal primal cuts include the shoulder, foreshank/breast, rack, loin, and leg. See Fig. 24-13 on page 538 (**Foodservice Cuts of Veal**).

■ **Shoulder.** The primal shoulder cut includes four rib bones and some of the backbone, blade, and arm bones. Fabricated cuts include steaks and chops, but they are not as tender as those from the loin. Therefore, meat from the shoulder is usually braised or stewed.

■ **Shank/breast.** The shank and breast are one primal cut. It includes rib bones, cartilage, breastbones, and shank bones. The rib is very tender, which makes it a popular menu choice.

■ **Rack.** The double rib primal cut is very small, tender, and expensive. The rib cut consists of a double rack of ribs and part of the backbone. Fabricated cuts include whole or halved racks, rib-eye, and chops.

■ **Loin.** The primal loin cut is located behind the ribs. It consists of the loin eye, the top of the rib bones, and the tenderloin. Fabricated cuts include tenderloin, medallions, and chops.

■ **Leg.** The primal leg cut includes the leg and the sirloin. The leg is fabricated into scallops and cutlets. The leg also can be cooked whole.

Quality Characteristics of Veal

Veal is delicately flavored and tender. In general, veal should have the following characteristics:

• Firm texture.
• Light pink color.
• Little fat.

⊠ CUTS OF BEEF

Americans eat more beef than any other kind of meat. The carcass is divided into these primal cuts: chuck, brisket/plate/flank, rib, loin, and round. See Fig. 24-14 on page 540 (**Foodservice Cuts of Beef**).

■ **Chuck.** The chuck comes from the shoulder. The chuck contains part of the backbone, rib bones, blade bones, and arm bones. It has quite a bit of flavor but is tough. Fabricated cuts include ground chuck, stew meat, cube steak, short ribs, and rib pot roast. Chuck is best cooked using a moist heat or combination cooking method.

■ **Brisket/plate/flank.** Brisket is made up of the breast, breastbone, ribs, and arm. The brisket can be salt-cured to make corned beef. Salt curing is a method of preserving that uses corn-size pellets of salt. The brisket may also be cured to make pastrami. The shank is used in soups, stocks, and consommés.

The plate is located on the side of the beef. It contains rib bones and cartilage. Fabricated cuts include short ribs and skirt steak. Short ribs are meaty, but because of the large amount of connective tissue, they are tough. Skirt steak is often used in fajitas.

Located along the edge of the rib and loin, the flank is a tough, but flavorful, cut of beef. Fabricated cuts include London broil and flank steak. The flank can also be ground.

■ **Rib.** Rib is the primal cut of beef that consists of ribs and some of the backbone. Fabricated cuts include rib-eye roast, rib-eye steaks, rib roast, beef ribs, and beef short ribs. A popular dish with customers is prime rib.

■ **Loin.** The loin is the front portion of the beef loin that has a rib and some of the backbone. Short loin includes some of the most tender and expensive parts of the carcass. Fabricated cuts include club steaks, porterhouse steaks, T-bone steaks, filet mignon, and boneless strip loin. The sirloin contains the backbone and some of the hipbone. Fabricated cuts are sirloin roast and sirloin steaks, which are best prepared by broiling, roasting, or grilling.

■ **Round.** The round is the large, hind leg. Fabricated cuts include eye of round, outside round, top round, bottom round, knuckle, and shank. The bottom round includes the outside round and the eye of round. These tougher cuts are used for stew beef or braising. The top round is more tender than the bottom, and is usually prepared as a roast.

FOODSERVICE CUTS OF BEEF

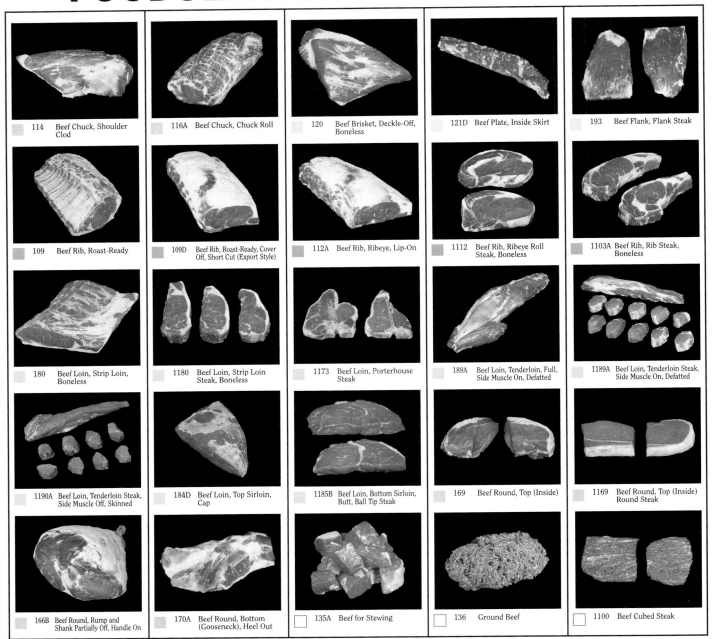

114 Beef Chuck, Shoulder Clod	116A Beef Chuck, Chuck Roll	120 Beef Brisket, Deckle-Off, Boneless
121D Beef Plate, Inside Skirt	193 Beef Flank, Flank Steak	
109 Beef Rib, Roast-Ready	109D Beef Rib, Roast-Ready, Cover Off, Short Cut (Export Style)	112A Beef Rib, Ribeye, Lip-On
1112 Beef Rib, Ribeye Roll Steak, Boneless	1103A Beef Rib, Rib Steak, Boneless	
180 Beef Loin, Strip Loin, Boneless	1180 Beef Loin, Strip Loin Steak, Boneless	1173 Beef Loin, Porterhouse Steak
189A Beef Loin, Tenderloin, Full, Side Muscle On, Defatted	1189A Beef Loin, Tenderloin Steak, Side Muscle On, Defatted	
1190A Beef Loin, Tenderloin Steak, Side Muscle Off, Skinned	184D Beef Loin, Top Sirloin, Cap	1185B Beef Loin, Bottom Sirloin, Butt, Ball Tip Steak
169 Beef Round, Top (Inside)	1169 Beef Round, Top (Inside) Round Steak	
166B Beef Round, Rump and Shank Partially Off, Handle On	170A Beef Round, Bottom (Gooseneck), Heel Out	135A Beef for Stewing
136 Ground Beef	1100 Beef Cubed Steak	

The above cuts are a partial representation of NAMP/IMPS items. For further representation and explanation of all cuts see *The Meat Buyers Guide* by the North American Meat Processors Association.

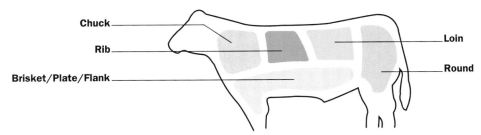

Chuck

Rib

Brisket/Plate/Flank

Loin

Round

NAMP/IMPS Number (North American Meat Processors Association/Institutional Meat Purchase Specifications)

©2000 North American Meat Processors Association

American Meat Science Association

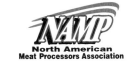

North American Meat Processors Association

BEEF
USA
National Cattlemen's Beef Association

Quality Characteristics of Beef

When purchasing beef for a foodservice operation, always check for the grade and inspection stamps. The best quality beef will have a bright red color. The meat purchaser will also need to decide on the desired fat thickness for the meat. Fat marbling in beef ranges from slight to moderately abundant.

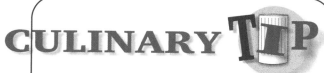

WHAT'S IN A BURGER—Hamburger meat is often labeled "ground beef." It should be ground from fresh beef and should not contain by-products or extenders. If it's labeled "hamburger," it might have beef fat and seasonings added. Hamburger, or ground beef, should not contain more than 22% fat.

⊠ PROCESSING BEEF

Like pork, beef can be processed in several different ways before it arrives at a foodservice operation. The method of processing greatly affects how the beef will taste.

■ **Curing.** Beef, like pork, also can be cured and smoked. These processes help increase the shelf life of beef and greatly affect its flavor. Smoking meat will also decrease its surface moisture, helping to prevent bacterial growth and spoilage.

■ **Aging.** Aging beef under refrigeration has long been known to increase its tenderness and enhance its flavor. Aging beef is hung in a controlled environment, such as a meat locker, with strict humidity and temperature conditions. Under these conditions, the meat fibers begin to break down, tenderizing and flavoring the meat.

■ **Irradiation.** Beef can also be irradiated to kill microorganisms. Although irradiated beef has far fewer microorganisms, such as E. coli bacteria, it still must be refrigerated and carefully stored to prevent cross-contamination. Irradiated beef also has a longer shelf life.

SECTION 24-2   Knowledge Check

1. Name the primal cuts of pork, lamb, veal, and beef.
2. Name the fabricated cuts of pork, lamb, veal, and beef.
3. Explain why irradiation is used to process meat.

MINI LAB

Research the pros and cons of irradiated or genetically-engineered meat. Prepare a presentation about the advantages and disadvantages of the process.

Principles of Cooking Meat

KEY TERMS

- high-heat cooking
- low-heat cooking
- demi glace
- grain

OBJECTIVES

After reading this section, you will be able to:

- Explain how cooking affects pork, veal, lamb, and beef.
- Determine the doneness of meat.
- Demonstrate different cooking methods used for meats.

MEAT is one of the highest expenses for foodservice operations. Selecting the right cuts of meat is just the first step. To get the most value for its purchasing dollars and to satisfy customers' appetites, a foodservice operation must fully understand meat-cooking techniques. Tender cuts of meat become tough when cooked improperly. Likewise, tough cuts of meat can become tender when cooked correctly. Meat can be delicious and nutritious, but only when it is properly prepared.

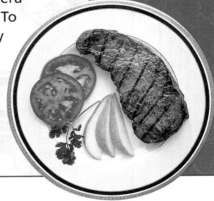

✖ COOKING IMPACTS TENDERNESS

If you've ever eaten a burned hamburger, you know what overcooking does to meat. Some dry cooking techniques firm proteins without breaking down connective tissue. You wouldn't want to use a dry cooking technique with a less-tender piece of meat that has a great deal of connective tissue. A better choice would be a moist cooking technique, which exposes the meat to moisture and heat during cooking. This helps to break down the connective tissue and tenderize the meat.

The type of cut will affect how much connective tissue there is, and, therefore, how tough the piece of meat will be prior to cooking. In general, the more tender the cut of meat, the drier the cooking technique can be. See Fig. 24-15.

High-Heat & Low-Heat Cooking

The temperature of the heat source has an important effect on how meat is cooked and how the final product will taste. **High-heat cooking** can toughen proteins and dry out meat over extended periods of time. However, high heat, when used correctly, can result in an excellent final product. High-heat cooking, such as broiling and grilling, is used for tender cuts of meat like tenderloins and strip steaks.

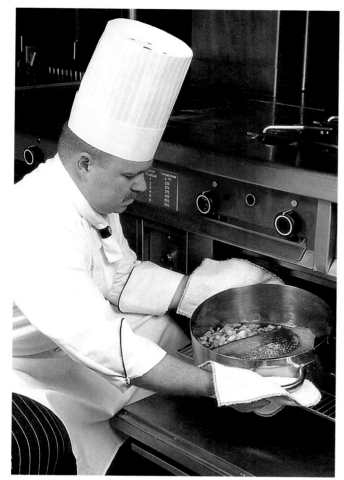

Fig. 24-15. Use the cooking technique that is right for the cut of meat you're preparing.

✖ DETERMINING DONENESS

Most people are particular about how they like their meat cooked. The difference between meat that's well done and rare can be considerable. See Fig. 24-16.

A meat's doneness depends on several factors:
* The cooking method.
* The type of meat.
* The internal temperature of the meat.
* The color of the meat.
* The size of the piece of meat.
* The amount of time the meat is cooked.

Fig. 24-16. The color of red meat is not enough to determine doneness. What should you do in order to determine doneness?

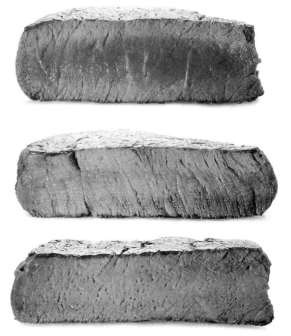

Low-heat cooking is the best method for preparing large cuts of meat, such as top round. Low-heat cooking does not shrink the meat because moist heat, in the form of steam or liquid, penetrates the meat more quickly than dry heat. However, many restaurants use cuts of meat that don't require long cooking times.

Pay close attention to how much fat a cut of meat has prior to cooking. A meat's fat content will affect the cooking technique. In general, if a meat is high in fat do not add additional fat while cooking. Adding fat, will make the final product oily or greasy.

Fat can be added for meats that are low in fat, such as veal. Veal roasts could be barded or larded. Marinades can also add fat to lower fat meats. You can also add a small amount of fat to the cooking pan. This will help prevent the meat from drying out.

Internal Temperature

The best way to test a meat's doneness is to test its internal temperature. This is the temperature below the meat's surface. It is usually taken at or near the center of the meat. To take the internal temperature, follow these rules:

- Insert the thermometer at an angle, into the thickest part of the meat.
- Avoid taking the temperature in fatty areas.
- Avoid touching or getting near bone.
- Meat is done when it reaches its proper internal temperature, and held at that temperature for at least 15 seconds.

Pork must be cooked to the correct internal temperature. To kill parasites, cook pork to an internal temperature of 145°F for 15 seconds. If pork is not cooked correctly, your customers could contract trichinosis (trick-i-NO-sis). Trichinosis can be a life-threatening disease.

Although many people enjoy eating beef and lamb rare, there is a risk of parasites surviving when meat is cooked at low internal temperatures. Steaks should be cooked to an internal temperature of 145°F and held at this temperature for at least 15 seconds. Ground beef should be cooked to 160°F and held at that temperature for 15 seconds.

Be sure to follow the safe temperature guidelines set by the Food Code published by the FDA and the U.S. Public Health Service. Many states require restaurants to warn their customers of the danger of eating undercooked meats by including a disclaimer on the menu. Check with your local and state health departments for further guidelines.

Color

The color of meat changes when it is cooked. Learning what the colors indicate helps to determine when a particular type of meat product is done. Red meat starts red and changes to gray as the product cooks. Light meat turns pink and changes to white and then to tan as it cooks. Pork and veal become white to tan in color when cooked.

Here are general guidelines for determining doneness of red meat by color:

- Rare meat is browned on the surface, with a red center. A thin outer layer of cooked meat appears gray.
- Medium-rare meat is browned on the surface with a thicker outer layer of gray.
- Medium meat is browned on the surface with an even thicker outer layer of gray and a pink center.
- Medium-well meat is browned on the surface with a thick outer layer of gray and a center that is barely pink.
- Well done meat is browned on the surface and gray on the inside.

ROASTING MEATS

Customers expect roasted meats to be tender and juicy. Remember that roasting is a dry technique that uses hot, dry air to cook the food. To roast meat, season it and then place it in a hot oven. Roasted meats do not use water or other liquids and are not generally covered during the cooking process. It is helpful to baste the meat with its natural juices or a flavorful seasoned stock. This keeps the meat from drying out.

Whether you use barding or the meat's own layer of fat, lay the meat fat side up when cooking. This way, the fat will naturally baste the meat and keep it moist. See Fig. 24-17.

■ **Barding.** To help enhance flavor and retain moisture, chefs often bard the meat when they roast it. Barding involves wrapping meat with fat, such as bacon, prior to cooking. Tie the fat to the meat with butcher's twine. A few minutes before the meat is done, remove the fat and allow the surface of the meat to brown.

■ **Seasoning.** Seasoning meats that will be roasted can be tricky. Salt cannot simply be added to the meat because the salt will not penetrate the meat during cooking. To season meat that will be roasted, follow these tips:

- Trim any heavy fat covering, leaving a thin fat layer. This will help the seasoning penetrate the meat.

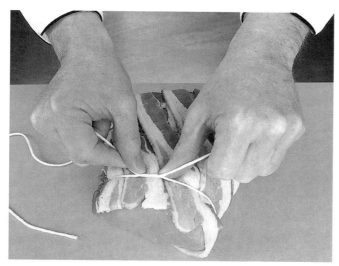

Fig. 24-17. Barding involves wrapping meat with fat before cooking. What cuts of meat would benefit most from barding?

- Season the meat several hours prior to roasting. This may mean adding seasonings to the surface of the meat, larding the meat with strips of fat, or inserting seasonings, such as garlic or cloves.
- Season the meat again after it is done.
- Season the meat's juices and serve them with the meat.

■ **Sauces and gravies.** Sauces and gravies add flavor and moisture to roasted meats. It is especially important to add sauce or gravy if the meat is well done. To make a rich gravy, deglaze the roasting pan and combine the drippings with a thickening agent and a **demi glace**, or a concentrated brown stock that has been reduced. For more on stocks and sauces, see Chapter 20.

Carving Roasted Meats

Carving roasted meats correctly is the important final step to serving an appetizing roast meat dish. Allow the meat to rest before carving. This makes it easier to slice the meat.

Always carve against the grain. **Grain** is the direction of muscle fibers, or treads, in meat. This means to cut against the tread structure of the meat. If the meat is sliced along the tread structure, it will be tough and stringy. Cut across muscle fibers.

THE MAILLARD REACTIONS

When meat is roasted, it is often browned beforehand in a skillet. The meat is then roasted at a much lower temperature. Browning kills surface bacteria and makes a flavorful crust. You have probably enjoyed the taste of a richly browned roast or steak due to the browning process.

The Maillard (may-YARD) reactions, named after Dr. L.C. Maillard, are a series of complex reactions between certain sugars and proteins. These reactions produce a deep brown color and sweet caramel crust on roasted meats.

When browning at a high temperature, there are three conditions necessary for a Maillard reaction to occur:

1. A nonacidic or base environment (pH higher than 7). An acidic environment prevents browning.

2. The more protein there is, the more amino acids are present to brown the meat.

3. Meat carbohydrates combined with the amino acid from a protein also help to brown the meat.

APPLY IT!

Prepare two pork chops. Grill or pan fry one pork chop to medium well, and braise the other to medium well.

1. Which pork chop is crispier?

2. Which pork chop has a darker color?

3. What conclusions can you draw about why the braised pork chop did not get crisp?

✕ BROILING & GRILLING MEATS

Two other dry cooking techniques, broiling and grilling, are popular ways to prepare meats. They both use high temperatures and relatively fast cooking times. Broiled and grilled meats are usually cooked to rare or medium with a browned, crusty surface and a tender, juicy interior. Restaurants that serve meat rare must have a warning on the menu. Remember these tips when broiling and grilling:

- The shorter the cooking time, the higher the heat needed.
- The thicker the cut, the longer the cooking time needed.
- Set the grill controls for different temperatures across the surface of the commercial grill. Vary the cooking temperature by moving the meat to different areas of the grill, depending upon the heat needed.
- When grilling red meats, make sure the heat is high enough so that the surface becomes brown and crispy.
- To create cross-hatch grill marks, or grill lines, place the presentation side of the meat down on the grill. Cook long enough for the grill lines to show. Then rotate the meat about 90 degrees to form the additional grill lines.

■ **Seasoning.** Seasoning meats that will be broiled or grilled rather than roasted is best done just prior to cooking them. Meats that tend to become dry when broiled or grilled, such as veal or pork, may be marinated or served with seasoned butter. Meats can be placed in marinades minutes or hours before cooking. Spice rubs can also be used to season meats.

■ **Sauces & accompaniments.** One of the best ways to serve broiled or grilled meats is with an accompaniment, such as a sauce. Butter sauces, such as Béarnaise, and brown sauces, such as mushroom, are excellent additions to meat dishes. Sauces are usually served in a separate bowl, next to the meat, under the meat, or drizzled over the meat on a dinner plate. Most sauces are made prior to broiling or grilling and do not use juices from the meat itself.

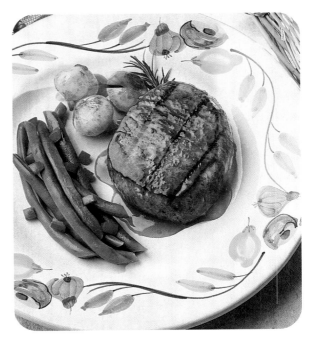

Fig. 24-18. Flavorful sauces and other accompaniments are usually served with broiled or grilled meat. Name some accompaniments that could be served with broiled or grilled meats.

Other accompaniments include vegetables, such as green beans and potatoes. These can be an excellent addition to the meal if they are grilled or broiled. See Fig. 24-18.

✕ SAUTÉING & PAN-FRYING MEATS

Tender cuts of meat and thin pieces of meat are usually sautéed. Meats containing bones or breaded meats are pan-fried. Both cooking techniques require you to pay attention to the amount of heat and fat used. Follow these tips to successfully sauté or pan-fry meat:

- Heat the pan before adding the fat.
- Use the correct amount of oil called for in the recipe. It should be enough to evenly cook all surfaces.
- Never overcrowd the pan.
- Turn or move the meat as little as possible.
- Avoid using unclarified butter because it burns easily.

■ **Seasoning.** The sauces that accompany sautéed or pan-fried meats will greatly enhance their flavor. A variety of sauces will bring out the flavors of meat cooked with these techniques.

You might also want to marinate the meat prior to cooking. If so, make sure to thoroughly pat the meat dry before cooking or it will not brown correctly.

■ **Use of fat.** The amount of fat used in sautéing and pan-frying differs. To sauté, use a small amount of fat and heat until very hot prior to adding meat. The amount of fat used depends on the amount of meat sautéed. The reason such a small amount is needed is that all surface areas of the meat will touch the pan.

To pan fry, use a moderate amount of fat in a pan, and heat until very hot prior to adding meat. To evenly brown the meat, use enough fat to conduct heat to the meat's surfaces. Flat meats do not require as much fat as unevenly-shaped meats.

⊠ BRAISING & STEWING MEATS

Braising and stewing are both combination techniques that begin by browning the food using dry heat. Braising involves partially covering the meat with liquid and cooking in a tightly-covered pan. When stewing, the liquid completely covers the meat. Both methods finish cooking by simmering in a liquid. The liquid used in both of these cooking methods is extremely important to the success of the final dish. Commonly used liquids include marinades, brown stock, demi glace, vegetable juices, fruit juices, and broth.

To begin the braising or stewing process, first season the meat. Avoid using large amounts of salt as this will slow the browning process. Many chefs marinate meat for several hours or a day prior to braising or stewing. Keep the following tips in mind when braising or stewing:

- Pat the meat dry prior to browning, especially if it has been marinated.
- Dredge the meat in flour just before cooking to improve browning.
- Do not use more liquid than is necessary.
- When meat is done, it should be fork tender.

⊠ PLATING MEATS

Meats are presented as the focal point of the plate. They may be placed on top of a sauce or a sauce may be drizzled over the meat. The accompaniments with which the meat is served help determine the presentation. For example, pork chops could be placed on top of mashed potatoes for a creative presentation.

SECTION 24-3 Knowledge Check

1. Compare how high-heat cooking and low-heat cooking affect meat.
2. Explain how to take the internal temperature of meat and why this is important.
3. Describe at least two cooking methods that can be used with meat.

MINI LAB

Divide into teams and either roast, broil, grill, sauté, pan-fry, or braise a pork loin. Set a goal for doneness and evaluate your team's product. Compare the results of each team's efforts.

SECTION SUMMARIES

24-1 All meats contain the four basic nutrients of water, protein, fat, and carbohydrates.

24-1 Meat fibers are bound together and to the bones by connective tissue.

24-1 Meats can be purchased in the form of primal cuts or fabricated cuts.

24-1 The two methods of aging meat are wet and dry. Aging helps to enhance the meat's flavor and tenderness.

24-2 Primal cuts of pork, lamb, veal, and beef are then divided into fabricated cuts for ease of handling and preparation.

24-2 To buy the highest quality of pork, lamb, veal, or beef, look for the quality characteristics for each type of meat.

24-2 The form in which pork, lamb, veal, and beef are purchased will determine the method of storage.

24-3 Using the correct method to cook meat can enhance its flavor and tenderize it.

24-3 The doneness of meat depends on the cooking method, the type and cut of meat, the internal color and temperature, and the customer's preferences.

24-3 Using different cooking methods allows you to take advantage of the flavors and textures of meats at various price levels.

CHECK YOUR KNOWLEDGE

1. Why does meat shrink when it is cooked?
2. Describe marbling and its effect on meat.
3. Compare collagen and elastin.
4. Why is meat graded according to quality?
5. What information does yield grade provide?
6. Compare primal and fabricated cuts of meat.
7. Describe the three types of dry-cured pork.
8. Explain irradiation and why it is used with meat.
9. Explain how knowing the fat content of a cut of meat helps determine the cooking method.
10. Compare doneness and color with the type of meat.

CRITICAL-THINKING ACTIVITIES

1. Suppose you discovered fresh meat was discoloring in the refrigerator. The meat was fresh when you purchased it, so what might have caused this change?

2. A sirloin steak weighed 16 oz. before it was cooked and weighed 14 oz. after it was cooked. Which cooking method do you think was used and why?

WORKPLACE KNOW-HOW

Decision making. A customer at your food-service operation has requested a low-fat meat dish. The menu includes pork, lamb, veal, and beef. What options might you suggest?

LAB-BASED ACTIVITY: Preparing Quality Meats

STEP 1 In teams, choose a beef dish to prepare.

STEP 2 Use the following criteria to choose the best cut of meat. It requires a well-trained eye to be able to judge quality meats by observing the characteristics of a portion of meat.

- **Marbling.** The more marbling, the more tender and flavorful the meat.
- **Fibers.** Small, tender fibers produce tender meat. Large fibers are likely to produce tough meat.
- **Color.** Fresh high-quality beef is red.

STEP 3 Choose a cooking method for your type of meat and prepare accordingly.

STEP 4 Cook the beef and share your finished product with the class. Explain why you chose a particular cooking method.

STEP 5 Evaluate each team's meat dish. Use the rating scale and the criteria in the chart below to judge the quality of each team's dish.

1 = Poor; 2 = Fair; 3 = Good; 4 = Great

STEP 5 Answer the following questions:

- How did the cut of meat chosen impact the final cooked meat dish for each team?
- How did the cut of meat impact the flavor and texture of each team's dish?

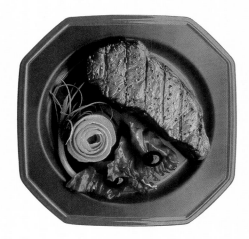

Cooked Meat Evaluation	
Appearance	• Cooked to appropriate doneness. Doesn't appear burned or undercooked. • Appropriately plated and garnished.
Flavor	• Flavor appropriate to preparation method and food product.
Texture	• Meat is moist, tender, and juicy, not dry and tough.

Pasta & Grains

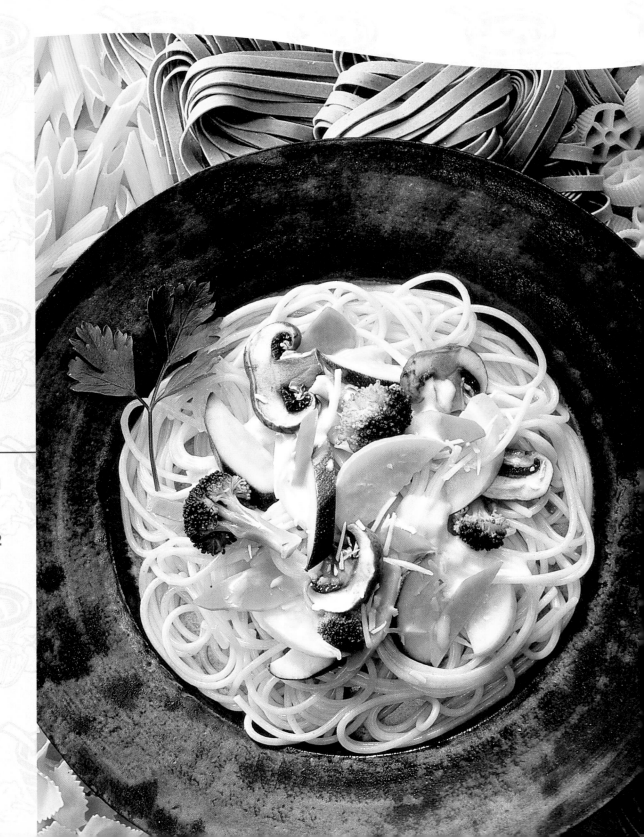

Pasta

OBJECTIVES

After reading this section, you will be able to:

• Identify various types of pasta.

• Describe the standards of quality for pasta.

• Explain how to purchase and store fresh and dry pasta.

• Demonstrate how to stuff, boil, and bake pasta.

PASTA is one of the easiest and most versatile food products used today. It is available in a variety of sizes, shapes, colors, and flavors. Pasta is a starchy food product that is made from grains. It is considered a staple in many commercial kitchens. Pasta increases in volume as it cooks and yields a high profit. Pasta is a very popular menu choice. To prepare pasta successfully, you need to become familiar with the varieties of pasta available and how to prepare them.

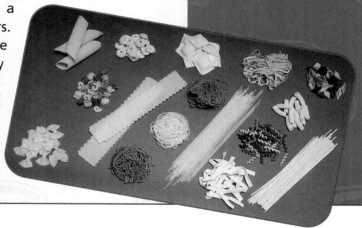

⊠ TYPES OF PASTA

Pasta is a product that can be used in place of other starchy foods in a meal. One of the main ingredients of pasta is flour, which is usually wheat flour. The other main ingredient in pasta is a liquid such as water or eggs. Oil is sometimes added to pasta dough to give it a richer texture.

Most commercial dried pastas are made from **semolina** (seh-muh-LEE-nuh) **flour**, a hard-grain wheat flour that is high in the proteins that form gluten. Semolina flour produces a smooth dough and creamy yellow color.

There are over 100 varieties of pasta. Pasta is available in a number of shapes, sizes, and flavors. The color of the pasta reflects its flavor. Pasta can be either dried or fresh. Fresh pasta cooks faster than dried pasta.

The shape of some pastas makes them ideal for certain sauces. For example, a thinner, tomato-based sauce like marinara is ideal for angel hair pasta, while Alfredo sauce adheres well to fettuci-ni (feh-TAH-chee-nee). Fig. 25-1 describes the characteristics of some of the different types of pasta and how each may be used.

Fig. 25-1.

PASTA	DESCRIPTION	USES
Elbow macaroni 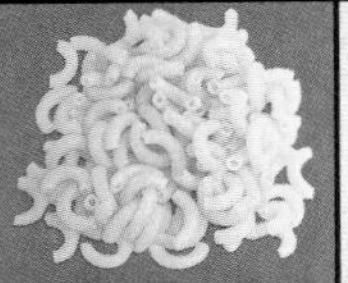	Narrow 1-inch tubes, short length, curved.	Baked; macaroni and cheese, macaroni salad, casseroles.
Spaghetti 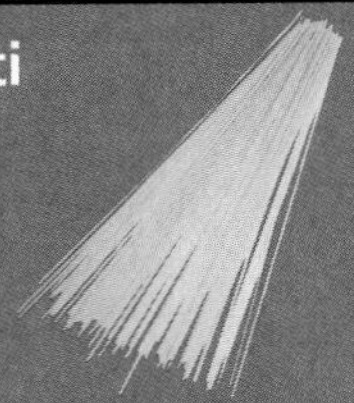	Thin, round strands; very thin spaghetti is called spaghettini.	Boiled; meat or tomato sauce, oil, butter, thin sauces.
Egg noodles 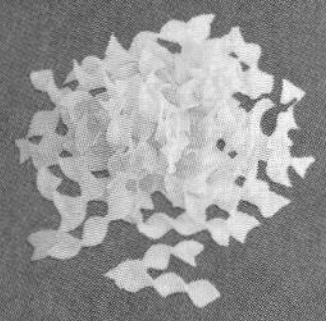	Long or short ribbons with spinach, tomato, or other flavorings.	Baked; casseroles, some sauces, puddings.
Lasagne (luh-ZAHN-yuh) 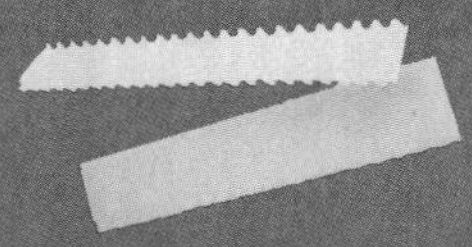	Wide, flat noodles with rippled edges.	Baked as a layered casserole with tomato sauce, cheese, and meat or seafood.
Capellini/Angel hair (cah-peh-LEAN-ee) 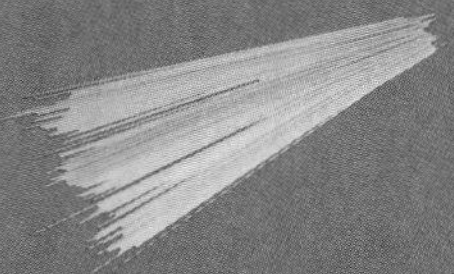	Fine, solid, strand-like pasta, thinner than spaghetti.	Boiled; use with thin sauces, seafood, tomatoes, garlic, or in soups.
Linguine (lyn-GWEE-nee) 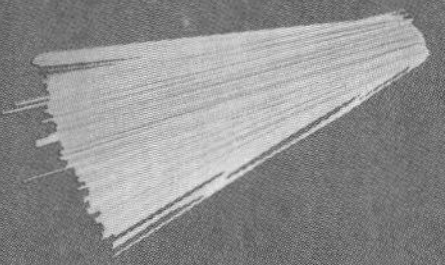	Thin, flattened spaghetti about ⅛-inch wide.	Boiled; clam sauce, marinara sauce, seafood.
Farfalle (fah-FALL-lay) 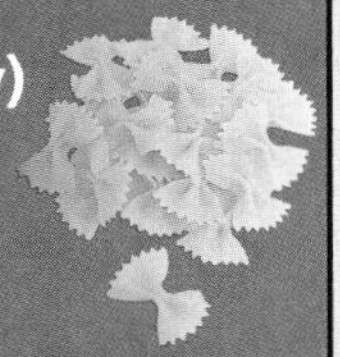	Flat, wide noodles that are squeezed in the center to resemble bow ties.	Boiled; baked with artichokes or seafood, medium or rich sauces with meat or vegetables.
Fettucini (feh-TAH-chee-nee) 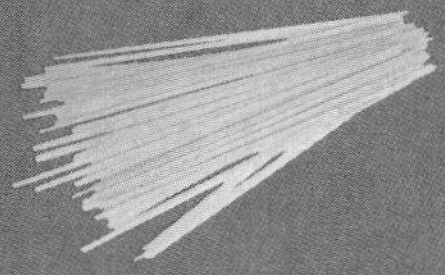	Flat, long, ¼-inch wide noodles.	Boiled; rich cream sauces, such as alfredo, or meat sauces adhere well to these ribbonlike noodles.

(Continued on next page)

Fig. 25-1 (Cont'd.).

PASTA	DESCRIPTION	USES
Orzo (OHR-zoh)	Small, rice-shaped pasta.	Pilaf, salads, soups.
Fusilli (foo-SEAL-lee)	Corkscrew-shaped twists.	Boiled; baked dishes with medium or thick, creamy sauces.
Manicotti (mah-nah-COT-tee)	Medium-sized hollow tubes, cut straight or angled.	Stuffed with cheese, meat, seafood, or vegetables and baked.
Soba (so-BAH)	Japanese noodles similar in appearance to egg pasta.	Asian foods, hot and cold dishes, salads.
Penne (PEN-nay)	Short to medium-sized hollow tubes cut diagonally; also called quills or pens.	Baked; hearty meat or tomato sauces, cheese.
Conchiglie (con-KEY-lyay)	Shaped like shells.	Stuffed; salads; meat or seafood sauces; filled with seafood, meat, or cheese and baked.

Quality Characteristics of Pasta

Imagine a 20-lb. case of pasta has been delivered to your establishment. Do you know if it meets the standards of quality? How can you tell? Here are two ways to determine the quality of the pasta used in foodservice operations.

- **Flour.** Semolina, a high-protein flour, produces the best dry pasta. Dry pasta should be made with 100% semolina flour.
- **Freshness.** Pasta should be hard and brittle. It should snap cleanly instead of bending easily.

a LINK to the Past

Pass the Pasta

The debate over where pasta originated is an old one. Many countries, including Italy, China, and Germany, claim to be its true home. Marco Polo is said to have discovered pasta in China in the 13th century. Some Italian historians, however, say that Marco Polo's documents were misinterpreted. They claim that the word "discovered" meant he discovered that the Chinese had pasta similar to theirs. The Italians were the first to appreciate pasta in the 14th century.

Wherever pasta truly originated, it was a far cry from how we know of it today. For example, in medieval Italy, macaroni was flat. It was tossed with butter and served with grated cheese on the side. Today, foodservice operations often serve macaroni smothered in melted cheese.

Italians kept devising new forms and varieties of pasta until they reached today's total of over 150 varieties. Pasta is a staple in many foodservice operations. It can be served a variety of ways—with traditional tomato and cream sauces, oils, herbs, vegetables, and seafood to name a few.

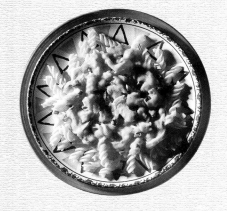

CULINARY TIP

NUTRIENTS IN PASTA—All pasta products are high in carbohydrates and the B vitamins thiamin and riboflavin. The protein in pasta varies based on the amount of semolina it contains. Semolina is high in protein, so the more semolina used, the more protein the pasta provides. On average, one serving of pasta (2 oz. dry) contains 1 gram of fiber, 1 gram of fat, 3 grams of protein, and .65 milligrams of iron.

PURCHASING PASTA

Both dried and fresh pasta usually are purchased by weight. Dried pasta is available in 1-, 5-, and 10-lb. bags and boxes. Twenty pound bulk cases are also common. Fresh pasta can be purchased from a pasta supplier in 1–2 lb. boxes or frozen in 10–20 lb. cases. Fresh pasta is also available in bags or cartons. Most foodservice operations, however, purchase more dried pasta than fresh pasta. See Fig. 25-2.

■ **Dried pasta.** Dried pastas, often purchased in bags or boxes, are available in tube, flat, and shaped forms. Tubes and shaped pastas are generally not available fresh. Dried pasta should be brittle and break easily. The surface should look dull or be marked by small pits or scars. Sauces cannot soak into smooth, shiny, dried pasta.

Dried pasta comes in a variety of interesting and unusual flavors. Besides the typical spinach, tomato, and plain pastas, you can also get a variety of combination flavors, such as tomato-dill, spinach-herb, or carrot-ginger.

■ **Fresh pasta.** Fresh pasta can be made in the kitchen. However, it is a labor-intensive process. It is also difficult to get a consistent product. Fresh pasta can also be purchased from a pasta supplier or purchased frozen. Fresh pasta also comes in a variety of flavors, such as spinach, tomato-garlic, and whole-wheat.

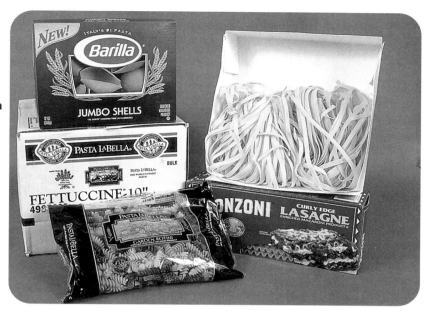

Fig. 25-2. Dried and fresh pasta are packaged differently.

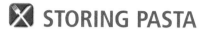 STORING PASTA

Dried pasta can be stored in a cool, dry place for several months. When storing dried pasta, temperatures in the storage area should be between 50°F–70°F.

Fresh pasta must be tightly wrapped and kept refrigerated. Fresh pasta should be used within a few days after it has been made. It can also be kept in the freezer to be used within a few weeks.

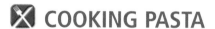 COOKING PASTA

Cooking pasta is a simple process. However, before you actually cook the pasta, you will need to complete the mise en place for everything you're going to use. You also will need to be familiar with the recipe. Some pasta dishes require the pasta to be fully cooked. Others require pasta to be partially cooked and added to a casserole with a variety of other ingredients.

Pasta can be cooked two ways: by boiling or by baking. Boiling pasta is a simple process. Both fresh and dried pastas can be boiled. Baked pasta is usually one of the main ingredients of a casserole dish, such as stuffed manicotti or lasagne. However, even when pasta is baked, the noodles are partly cooked first by boiling.

Boiling Pasta

When boiling pasta, you need to use enough water to cook it properly. In foodservice operations, pasta can be cooked when a customer orders it. It also can be cooked in large amounts ahead of time. Dried pasta is sometimes cooked ahead of time. Fresh pasta isn't because it cooks quickly and becomes too soft.

The general process for boiling pasta follows:

1. Use at least one gallon of water for each pound of pasta in a large enough stockpot for the pasta to move around freely.

2. Add about 1 oz. of salt per gallon of water. The pasta will absorb the water and salt during the cooking process.

3. Bring the water to a full boil and add the pasta. See Fig. 25-3A below.

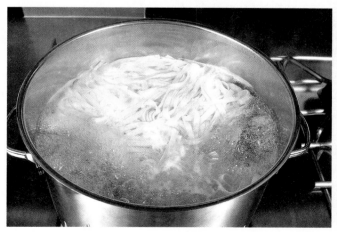

4. Stir the pasta with a large cooking spoon or braising fork occasionally as it continues to boil for the indicated time. The combination of rapid convection movement, the large

KEY Science SKILLS

INVESTIGATING STARCH

Have you ever noticed how pasta can be fluffy and separated, or a sticky lump? Have you ever wondered what makes pasta sticky? Sticky pasta is the result of improper cooking, and it can be avoided.

When pasta is added to a pot of boiling water, the starch contained within the noodles begins to dissolve. As the pasta is cooled down, the starch in the water turns into a sticky, glue-like substance. This substance attaches to the pasta and forms sticky clumps.

To avoid sticky pasta, it helps to boil the pasta in a large pot of water. The more water used, the more area the starch has to disperse. This minimizes its attachment to the noodles. You can also add oil to the water. The oil will absorb the starch molecules, and prevent the pasta from becoming sticky and clumping together. However, oil has a tendency to prevent the sauce from sticking to the pasta.

APPLY IT!

Cook 1½ lbs. of pasta in 2½ qts. of salted, boiling water. Cook another ½ lb. of pasta in 1 qt. of salted boiling water. Cook both pots of the pasta until they are done. Pour the contents of one pot into a strainer. Set the contents in one bowl. Repeat this procedure with the other pot, placing the pasta in a separate bowl. Describe the appearance, consistency, and taste of each bowl of pasta.

amount of water, the small amount of pasta, and the stirring motion will keep the pasta from sticking together.

5. Test the pasta for doneness. Put a few pieces of pasta on a plate and cut them with a fork. If it cuts easily, the pasta is done. See Fig. 25-3B below.

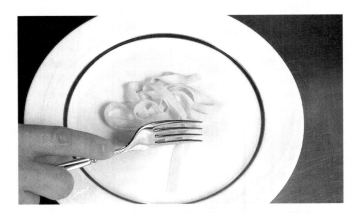

6. When the pasta is done, drain it into a **colander**, a container with small holes in the bottom for rinsing and draining food.

7. If serving immediately, don't cool or rinse the pasta. Just plate the pasta and serve it. If serving the pasta later, rinse it with cold, running tap water to halt the cooking process. This will help keep the pasta from sticking together. If serving pasta in a salad, let the pasta cool before mixing.

Baking Pasta

When pasta is baked with a filling and a sauce, or simply a sauce, the flavors blend during the baking process. This can't be achieved simply by adding a sauce to the top of plain cooked pasta.

Some types of pasta, such as lasagne noodles, are cooked and then layered in a casserole with other ingredients such as cheese, meat, spinach, and tomato sauce for a hearty baked dish. Other types of baked pasta include manicotti and cannelloni. These types of pasta are stuffed with a filling such as cheese and covered in sauce. Macaroni and cheese is also a baked pasta dish.

In most cases, the pasta is partially cooked before it is layered or stuffed. Then it is assembled

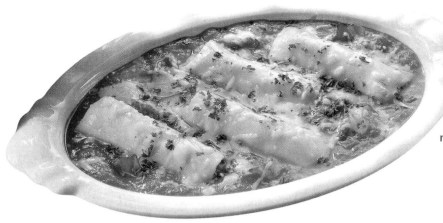

Fig. 25-4. Baked pasta is served hot from the oven. What accompaniments may be served with pasta dishes?

with other ingredients and baked. In many food-service operations, baked pasta dishes are served piping hot in individual baking dishes, along with fresh bread and a cold, crispy salad on a separate plate. See Fig. 25-4.

Determining Doneness

When cooking Italian-style pasta, it is important to cook it **al dente** (al-DEHN-tay), or "to the bite." If pasta is cooked past the stage at which it is tender but still firm when bitten into, it quickly becomes soft and mushy. This can make pasta very unappetizing.

Each type of pasta has a different cooking time. If pasta is overcooked or undercooked, the dish being prepared could be ruined. The amount of water, the altitude, and other factors can affect the cooking time, too. It is important to time pasta carefully in order to stop the cooking process at the al dente stage.

To check for doneness, you can bite into a piece of the pasta. If it is tender but still firm, remove the pasta from the heat and drain it carefully over the sink. Another alternative is to cut through a piece of pasta with a fork. If it cuts easily, it is done.

Stuffing Pasta

Some pasta can be stuffed with ingredients. Tubular pastas, such as manicotti or cannelloni, are usually stuffed. Ravioli are stuffed squares, rounds, or triangles. A variety of other pasta shapes can be stuffed, too. The filling ingredients may include cheese, meat, seafood, poultry, or vegetables.

The fillings, with the exception of meat, can be cooked or uncooked. Meat fillings, however, must be completely cooked before being stuffed into the pasta. This is because the time it takes the pasta to cook may not be sufficient to cook the meat safely.

Some large tubular pastas, such as cannelloni and manicotti, are often only partly cooked in boiling water. They are then stuffed with a filling and covered in a sauce. These dishes are baked as casseroles to finish the cooking process. When partially cooking pasta, make sure it is not over-cooked. It will continue to cook during baking. If it is too soft, it will not adequately hold the stuffing. Follow these guidelines to stuff pasta.

1. Determine the pasta to be used.
2. Prepare the pasta by cooking it in boiling salted water. You can use either dry or fresh pasta. The cooking time will depend on the form of pasta used. It will also depend on whether you will fully or partially cook the pasta.
3. Make the filling and chill in the refrigerator.
4. Drain the pasta and shock it in cold water to stop the cooking process. Drain and rinse.
5. Remove the filling from the refrigerator.

6. Ladle a small amount of sauce into the bottom of the baking dish or hotel pan. See Fig. 25-5A below.

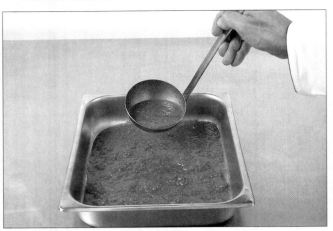

7. Use a pastry bag to pipe the filling into the cooked pasta. See Fig. 25-5B below.

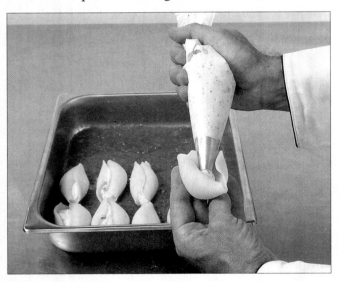

8. Place the stuffed pasta into the baking dish and ladle a small amount of sauce over the filled pasta. See Fig. 25-5C below.

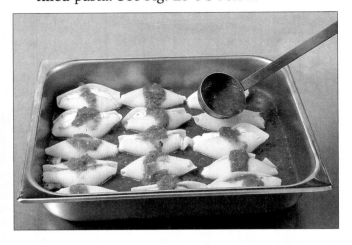

9. Bake as indicated on the standardized recipe.

✖ SERVING PASTA

When pasta is cooked to order, it is important to plate and serve it immediately. This means that whatever is to be plated and served with the pasta must be ready to go at the moment the pasta is done. The sauce and other ingredients must be added, and any side vegetables and garnishes must be ready to place on the plate and serve to the customer immediately.

Often, pasta with sauce is served alone on a plate. Some pasta dishes are served on soup plates, a shallow bowl-shaped plate. Others are served as side dishes in smaller portions.

SECTION 25-1 Knowledge Check

1. Identify 10 different types of pasta. Briefly describe each.
2. What standards of quality should be looked for when evaluating pasta?
3. Explain how to boil pasta.

MINI LAB

In teams, cook cannelloni, manicotti, penne, or conchiglie pasta to the al dente stage. Then stuff the pasta and bake it. Serve the finished product and evaluate the results.

Rice & Other Grains

KEY TERMS

- risotto
- brown rice
- enriched rice
- parboiled rice
- polenta
- hominy
- pilaf method
- risotto method

After reading this section, you will be able to:

- Describe different varieties of rice.
- Describe four common grains.
- Demonstrate various cooking methods used for rice and other grains.

GRAINS are a staple in the diets of people around the world. This is because of the variety of grains, and the fact that they store well and have high nutritional value. The seed, or grain, which is packed with nutrients, is the part of the plant people eat. The main nutrients in grains are in the form of carbohydrates and fat. Grains are usually dried for storage. Cooking grains with liquid adds water back to the dehydrated grains. This makes the grain tender and edible.

There is a wide variety of grains to choose from. Rice, wheat, and corn are three of the most common grains. Others include barley, oats, cornmeal, and hominy. By learning how to prepare rice and other grains, you will be able to prepare a variety of dishes.

▣ TYPES OF RICE

Rice is served around the world. Rice picks up the flavors of other foods so it is often served as part of a main dish. Rice increases in volume as it cooks and yields a high profit. All varieties of rice come in different grain types: short-grain, long-grain, and medium-grain. See Fig. 25-6.

■ **Short-grain.** Short grain rice contains the most starch. It becomes sticky when cooked, but is the most tender type of rice. Short-grain rice is used in risotto, for example. Risotto is a rice dish in which the grain has been sautéed in butter, and then simmered in a flavored cooking liquid, which

has been added gradually to the rice until it has finished cooking.

■ **Medium-grain.** Medium-grain rice is firm when it is hot. It becomes sticky, like short-grain rice, when it cools.

■ **Long-grain.** Like short-grain rice, long-grain rice remains slightly firm when cooked properly. However, it should not become sticky when cooked. The grains of rice separate easily after cooking. Long-grain rice can be used in just about any food dish.

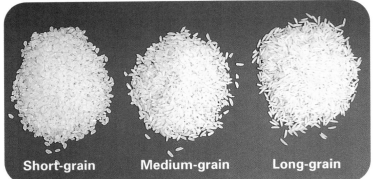

Fig. 25-6. Here are three grain types of rice. How do they differ?

Short-grain   Medium-grain   Long-grain

All three types of rice can be processed. Processing rice removes the hull, or outer covering, from the grain. If the grain is left whole, the rice is brown. If the grain is polished, the rice is white. White rice can be processed even further, producing converted rice and instant rice. Rice varieties are helpful in selecting rice for different menus.

Brown Rice

Rice that has had the hull, or outer covering, removed is called **brown rice**. Brown rice has a tan color, a chewy texture, and slightly nutty taste. Available in long-grain, short-grain, and medium-grain, brown rice takes longer to cook and needs more cooking liquid than white rice. See Fig. 25-7.

White Rice

White rice has had the outer layers of the grain removed. Without the outer layers, the rice grain is white and cooks more quickly with less water. White rice has a lighter texture, but is also lower in some vitamins and minerals. There are a number of varieties of white rice: long-grain rice, short-grain rice, hard rice, soft rice, and enriched rice. **Enriched rice** has a vitamin and mineral coating added to the grain. This makes up for nutrients lost when the outer coating is removed. All types of white rice can be enriched.

Converted Rice

Converted rice, sometimes called **parboiled rice**, has been partially cooked with steam and then dried. This process removes some of the surface starch and increases the nutrient value by forcing nutrients from the outer layer into the grain. After it's steamed, the rice is polished and milled. This results in a light white-grain rice that has more nutrients than regular white rice.

Converted rice can be used in the same way as regular white rice, except it takes longer to cook and requires slightly more liquid. It also is very fluffy. The grains don't clump together if they are served from a steam table.

Specialty Rices

Many interesting, flavorful rices have made their way into American menus from a variety of foreign foods. These rices, with their different textures and flavors, offer foodservice professionals interesting options for including rice in planning menus. Fig. 25-8 provides an overview of the most popular specialty rices.

Fig. 25-7. Brown rice gets it color from the bran.

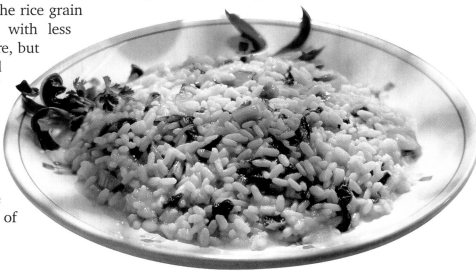

Fig. 25-8.

SPECIALTY RICE	DESCRIPTION	USES
Arborio (ar-BOH-ree-oh)	Short-grain, white rice; sticky when cooked; cook in 3 cups of water for every cup of rice.	Best rice for risotto-style preparation.
Basmati (bahs-MAT-tee)	Extra long-grain with polished, cream-colored grain; light, sweet flavor; aged before use, so should be well-rinsed; cook in 1½ cups of water for every cup of rice.	Delicate flavor best used in side dishes, including pilaf.
Jasmine (JAZ-muhn)	Long-grain white rice; similar to basmati, but more delicate flavor.	Side dishes.
Wild Rice	Not a true rice, but a wild water grass; brown and black grain with a nutty flavor; chewy texture; three grades, with the best having very long grain; cook in three times the amount of water as rice.	Served as a side dish and used in poultry stuffing; lower grades used in soups and baked goods.
Red Rice	A red rice, also called Wehani (we-HAN-i) rice; aromatic, earthy flavor.	Served with meat and bean dishes.

✖ HANDLING & STORING RICE

Uncooked rice should be stored in airtight containers at room temperature in a dry, dark room. White rice has a long shelf life if properly stored because the sprouting portion of the grain, which contains oil, has been removed with the hull.

Brown rice, even when properly stored, has a shorter shelf life because the oil in the grain can spoil.

After rice has been cooked, it should be used as soon as possible. Its high protein content and neutral pH mean it can spoil easily and be dangerous to eat if left at room temperature. Refrigerate any unused, cooked rice as soon as possible.

OTHER GRAINS

While rice is a very versatile and popular grain, there are many other grains that can add variety and nutrition to the menu. The high carbohydrate and protein content of traditional grains, such as oats, wheat, and barley, can add nutritional value and flavor to any meal. In addition, specialty grains, such as kasha (KAH-shuh), quinoa (KEEN-wah), and triticale (trih-tuh-KAY-lee), offer diverse flavors, textures, and colors.

Grains are also an important part of menu planning because they can be used from breakfast to dinner to prepare many different kinds of dishes. For example, kasha and oatmeal make excellent breakfast cereals. Cracked wheat can be used in cold salads.

Barley

Barley is a hardy, adaptable grain that can grow in both warm and cold climates. It is available unmilled, and in a form called pearled barley, which has been milled and polished.

Barley has a slightly sweet flavor and chewy texture. It is often added to soups and stews, giv-ing them a hearty consistency and rich texture. Barley is also used as a poultry stuffing and as a pilaf side dish. Its mild flavor makes it a good candidate for cooking with onions, garlic, herbs, and other seasonings. A ratio of three parts liquid to one part barley is used for cooking barley. See Fig. 25-9A.

Oats

Oats are the berries of oat grass. They can be purchased as oatmeal and as a whole grain, called groats or oat berries. See Fig. 25-9B. Oatmeal, a popular, but plain hot cereal, can be dressed up with fruits, berries, cream, maple syrup, and other similar toppings to make a simple breakfast something special. Oatmeal also makes an excellent addition to bread and cookies, adding flavor, nutrition, and texture. A ratio of two parts liquid to one part oats is used to cook oatmeal.

Oat berries, or groats, do not have the outer layer removed, so they are a whole grain, with all the texture and nutrients found in other whole grains. They can be cooked and served as a hot cereal, used to stuff poultry, and added to baked goods. A ratio of four parts liquid to one part oat groats is used for cooking groats.

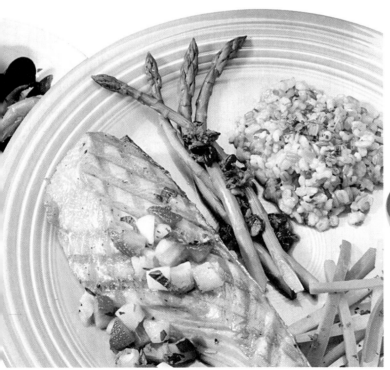

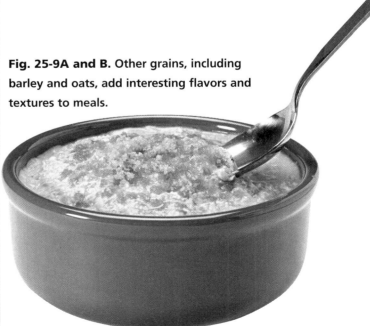

Fig. 25-9A and B. Other grains, including barley and oats, add interesting flavors and textures to meals.

Wheat Products

When you think of wheat, flour and bread are probably two of the first things that come to mind. Certainly wheat, in the form of flour, is a staple in bread-making and other kinds of baking. It is actually a very versatile grain that is also milled into semolina and cracked wheat. These two wheat products can be served as side dishes, and used in stuffings and casseroles. Couscous (KOOS-koos) is made from the semolina that is milled from wheat. Fig. 25-10, on pages 564-565, provides an overview of these grain products.

Corn Products

Corn is different from the other grains discussed in this section because it can be eaten fresh. It also can be eaten as a dried grain. When eaten fresh, it is served as a vegetable. As a dried grain, it comes in two main forms: cornmeal, used to make breads and polenta; and hominy, a dried corn kernel. See Fig. 25-11.

Polenta

Polenta (po-LEN-tah) is made from cornmeal that is gradually sprinkled into simmering water or stock and cooked until it becomes a thick paste. It is the right consistency when it pulls away from the pot when stirred. Polenta can be served with butter, cheese, or various sauces. It also can be poured into shaped containers or spread on a baking sheet to cool. When cool, it can be sliced or cut into interesting shapes that can be baked, fried, grilled, or broiled. A very versatile food, polenta can be served as a breakfast food with maple syrup, or as a side dish for dinner. Spices, dried tomatoes, cheese, herbs, and other ingredients can be added during the simmering process.

Hominy

Hominy is made by soaking dried corn in lye so that the kernels become swollen. As they swell, the outer layers loosen and are easily removed.

Hominy is often served as a side dish or added to soups. When cooking hominy, use 2–2½ times the amount of water as grain. Hominy also is made into other corn products, including grits and masa harina.

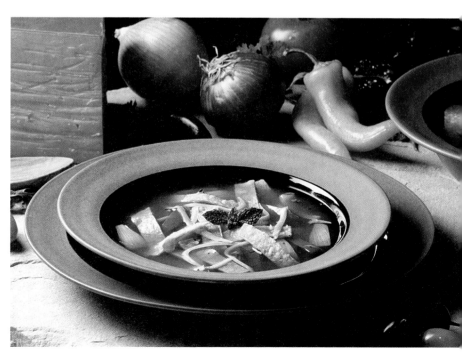

Fig. 25-11. Corn products may be used in a variety of ways, as in this tortilla soup.

Fig. 25-10.

GRAINS	DESCRIPTION	USES
Cracked wheat 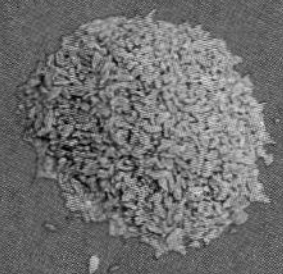	The whole wheat berry cracked into irregular pieces; cooks more quickly than whole berries; brown exterior, white interior; unmilled grain is high in nutrients; cook in twice as much water as wheat.	Side dishes, hot cereal.
Semolina (seh-muh-LEE-nuh) 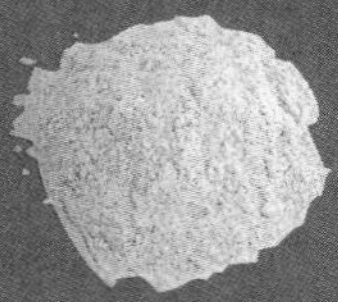	Bran and germ are removed from Durum wheat; cream-colored pellets; partially cooked; to cook, soak briefly in water, drain, and steam until tender.	Side dishes, hot cereal, dumplings, and sweet pudding.
Couscous (Koos-koos) 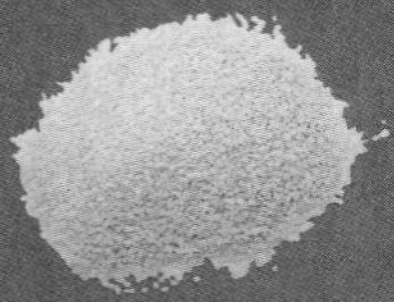	A granular form of semolina, to cook, soak in water, drain, and then steam. Packaged, precooked couscous is also available. Add precooked couscous to boiling water and let stand about 5 minutes.	Sweet and savory side dishes.
Kasha 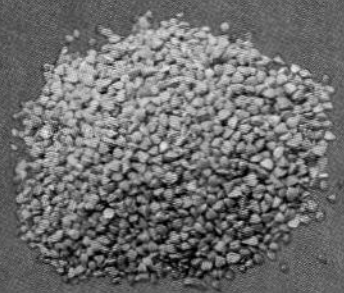	Hulled, roasted buckwheat groats; sometimes ground or cracked; strong nutty flavor; cook in 1 to 1½ times the water as groats.	Side dishes, cold salads.
Quinoa (KEEN-wah) 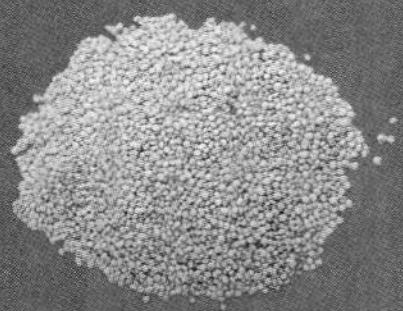	A small, bead-shaped grain; ivory color; neutral flavor; cooks fast and is high in protein.	Add to side dishes and soups.
Triticale (Triht-ih-KAY-lee) 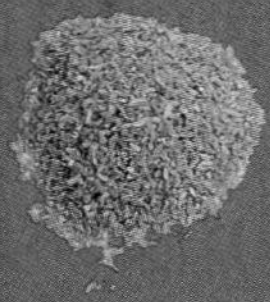	A type of wheat and rye that has more protein, a nutty-sweet flavor, and lower gluten content; comes as berries, flour, or flakes; cooked similarly to cracked wheat and semolina.	Side dishes, casseroles, cereal.

(Continued on next page)

Fig. 25-10 (Cont'd.).

GRAINS	DESCRIPTION	USES
Kamut (kah-MOOT) 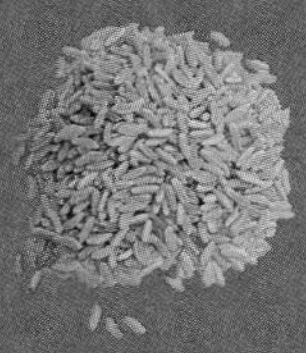	Brown, rice-like shape; earthy, nutty flavor.	Pastas.
Spelt (SPEHLT) 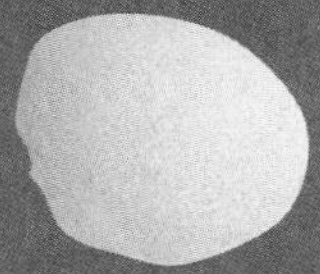	Wheat product available as a whole grain or ground; can be boiled or simmered; mild, nutty flavor.	Baked goods.
Amaranth 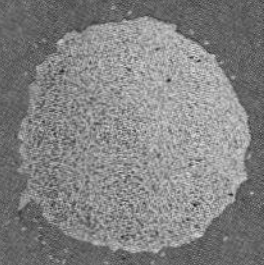	Very small, round grain; light brown in color.	Salads, baked goods, and in cooking.

■ **Grits.** Cracked hominy is served as a side dish or cereal called grits. Cook grits in four parts water to one part grits.

■ **Masa harina (MAH-sah ah-REE-nah).** This finely ground hominy is used for making tortillas and breads.

✗ COOKING RICE & OTHER GRAINS

Cooking rice and grains involves adding enough water to make the grain moist and tender. Depending upon the length of the rice or grain, the proportion of water to rice or grain, and the cooking method, the product can be light and fluffy or sticky. The degree of tenderness may vary, depending on the grain and the way in which it will be served. There are times when a very tender product may be needed, or when a chewier one is most desirable. There are four main methods of cooking grain: boiling, steaming, braising, and the risotto method.

Boiling

To boil grains, the grain is added to slightly salted boiling water and then simmered until tender. Boiling produces a good product that can be served as is—usually with the addition of seasonings—or incorporated into other dishes such as salads or casseroles. The proportion of water to grain is about the same as for cooking pasta.

Steaming

Steaming grains is different from steaming vegetables. To steam grains, add the appropriate amount of boiling liquid to the grain. Cover and cook the grain until the liquid is completely absorbed by the grain.

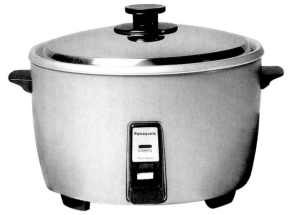

Fig. 25-12. A rice cooker is often used to steam rice.
What other equipment could be used to steam rice?

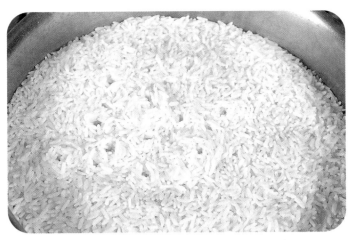

Fig. 25-13. Rice is considered done when the surface develops characteristic steam holes or tunnels that appear on the surface of the rice.

You can steam grains a number of ways. Grains can be steamed in a saucepan on the rangetop. They can also be steamed in the appropriate bakeware in the oven. Another way to steam grains is by using a convection steamer.

In addition, grains can be steamed in a rice cooker. This piece of equipment controls the cooking time by automatically shutting off when the cooking process is done. This prevents burning. See Fig. 25-12.

Braising

Braising, often called the **pilaf method**, involves sautéing the grain in oil or butter before adding the liquid. Often, onions, garlic, seasonings, and items such as red or green peppers may be added to the rice during the sautéing process. The coating of oil on each grain results in a fluffy product in which individual grains do not stick together.

Once the grain is sautéed, a seasoned liquid is added. The grain is then usually cooked on the range in a saucepan or baked in the oven in a hotel pan.

Generally, the grain is done when all the water has been absorbed and there are small, tube-like holes on the surface. See Fig. 25-13. Cooking can either be completed on the range, or the saucepan or stockpot can be removed from the heat for the last five or ten minutes of cooking and left to stand tightly covered.

Baking is the preferred method because the uniform heat results in a more flavorful product in which each grain remains separate from the others. Ethnic spices and a variety of chopped foods can be added after sautéing, before the liquid is added. Foods such as nuts, mushrooms, peas, carrots, raisins, diced ham, or bacon add flavor and texture. Pilaf can be made with rice, barley, cracked wheat, and other grains. See Fig. 25-14.

Fig. 25-14. Seasonings, nuts, and dried fruits can be added to couscous or barley for flavor. What herbs and spices would you use to flavor couscous?

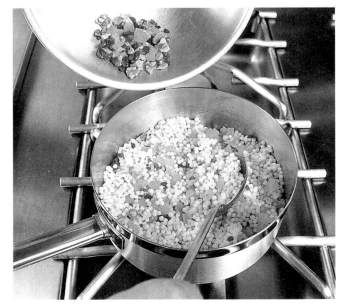

Risotto

The **risotto method** is a little like boiling and the pilaf method combined. First, the grain is sautéed, and then a small amount of hot liquid—often a soup stock—is added. The grain is stirred until all the liquid is absorbed. This process of adding liquid and stirring the grain is continued until the grain is completely cooked. When the grain is done, it will still be firm. Seasonings and chopped mushrooms can be added to risotto after the sautéing stage.

Grains cooked by the risotto method are creamy. Risotto should be served immediately after being cooked to maintain its texture and creamy consistency. Butter, olive oil, or cheese are often stirred in just before serving.

1. Simmer the seasoned liquid in a pot.

2. In a separate saucepan, heat the fat.

3. When the fat is melted, add onions, garlic, and seasonings. Sauté for 2 minutes.

4. Add the grains to the melted fat and other ingredients in the saucepan. Stir the grains into the fat so they are evenly coated. Do not scorch the grains. See Fig. 25-15.

5. Gradually add the simmering liquid to the grains in stages. Stir frequently to prevent scorching.

6. Test for doneness.

7. Remove saucepan from heat source.

8. Add butter, herbs, cheese. Mix and serve.

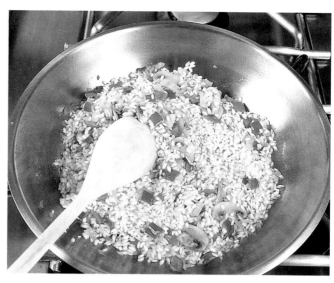

Fig. 25-15. Each grain must be evenly coated with melted fat to create a good risotto dish.

SERVING RICE & OTHER GRAINS

All grains should be served as soon as possible after being cooked. They lose their texture quickly and can become either clumped or dried out if they are held for a period of time. Any grains not used immediately after being cooked should be refrigerated in an airtight container.

SECTION 25-2 Knowledge Check

1. What are the three main types of rice grains?
2. Name four different specialty grains.
3. What are the four most common ways of cooking grains?

MINI LAB

In teams, boil, steam, or braise a grain. Each team's dish must be different. Serve your finished product to another team and have that team evaluate the results.

CHAPTER 25 Review & Activities

SECTION SUMMARIES

25-1 Pastas are available in a variety of shapes, sizes, colors, and flavors. Pastas can be fresh, frozen, or dried.

25-1 Quality pasta should be made with 100% semolina flour. It should be hard and brittle and snap cleanly.

25-1 Both dry and fresh pasta are purchased by weight with storage determined by the type of pasta purchased.

25-1 Most pasta dishes require pasta to be boiled, at least partially, prior to being stuffed or baked.

25-2 Short-grain, long-grain, and medium-grain are the three types of rice.

25-2 The four basic varieties of rice are brown, white, converted, and specialty rices.

25-2 Specialty rices, such as arborio, basmati, jasmine, and wild rice, offer foodservice professionals interesting options.

25-2 Rice, wheat, and corn are three of the most common grains, but barley, oats, cornmeal, and hominy are also used frequently by foodservice operations.

25-2 The four main methods of cooking grains are boiling, steaming, braising, and the risotto method.

CHECK YOUR KNOWLEDGE

1. Explain the benefits of using semolina flour when making pasta.
2. Describe the nutrients in pasta.
3. Explain how to prevent pasta from sticking together when it is cooked.
4. Describe the procedure for preparing stuffed pasta.
5. List some possible ingredients used to stuff pasta.
6. Define al dente and explain how it relates to cooking pasta.
7. Identify the part of the grain that provides nutritional value.
8. Describe brown rice and its cooking method.
9. Describe the source and use of wild rice.
10. Explain why water is needed to prepare rice.

CRITICAL-THINKING ACTIVITIES

1. A cannelloni dish did not come out as it should have. You followed the recipe and used the right ingredients. You partially cooked the pasta before stuffing it, and baked the dish as recommended. Why did the cannelloni fall apart? How can you prevent this in the future?

2. Use print or Internet resources to analyze the features of rice steamers. Draw conclusions about their effectiveness and efficiency.

WORKPLACE KNOW-HOW

Decision Making. Imagine that you have been asked to prepare rice for 150 people at an awards banquet. What equipment would you need and how would you make sure the rice is served hot?

LAB-BASED ACTIVITY: Preparing Polenta

STEP 1 Divide into four teams. Each team will be preparing a variation of the Polenta Recipe found at the bottom of this page.

- **Team A** will substitute 2 qts. vegetable stock in place of the water.
- **Team B** will substitute 1½ qts. chicken stock and 4 oz. of butter in place of the water.
- **Team C** will add 6 oz. of finely diced carrots, 8 oz. of diced Vidalia onions, and 1 green pepper that has been washed, seeded, and finely diced. These items should be sautéed and then added to the cornmeal mixture just before you perform Preparation Step 2.
- **Team D** will add ½ tsp. lemon pepper seasoning and 2 medium-size red peppers that have been washed, seeded, and finely diced. Do <u>not</u> sauté the peppers before adding them. These items should be added to the polenta mixture just before you perform Preparation Step 3. If a stronger lemon pepper flavor is desired, continue to add ½ tsp. until it suits your taste.

STEP 2 Make a list of the equipment and smallwares your team will need to prepare its version of the Polenta recipe.

STEP 3 Prepare your Polenta recipe.

STEP 4 Plate one serving of your team's Polenta. Cut the serving into four equal pieces. Give each team a serving.

STEP 5 Evaluate the polenta by answering each of the following questions.

- Which variation of the polenta recipe was the most time consuming to prepare? Why?
- Which variation of the polenta recipe was the most difficult to prepare? Why?
- Which variation of the polenta recipe made the best presentation? Why?
- Which variation of the polenta recipe tasted the best? Why?

Polenta

YIELD: 10 SERVINGS   SERVING SIZE: 4 OZ.

INGREDIENTS

2 qts.	Water
1½ tsp.	Salt
1 lb.	Cornmeal, medium-ground

METHOD OF PREPARATION

1. In a medium saucepot, heat the water to a boil; add the salt, and gradually add the cornmeal, stirring continuously with a wooden spoon.

2. When blended without lumps, lower the heat, and simmer until thickened, approximately 30 minutes. When done, the polenta will pull away from the side of the pot.

3. Pour the polenta into an oiled pan, and spread to a ½-in. thickness.

4. Allow it to rest a few minutes; then cut into portions. Hold at 135°F or above.

Fruits, Vegetables & Legumes

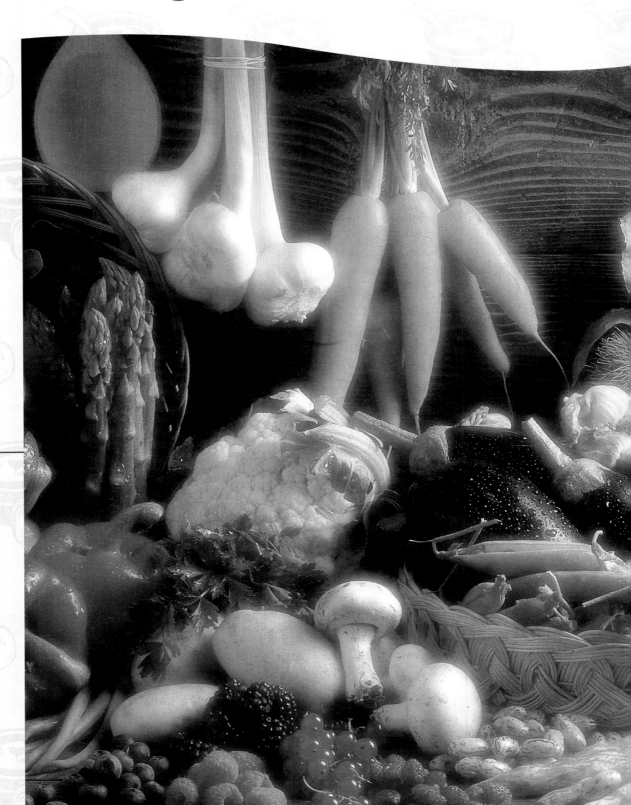

Fruits

OBJECTIVES

After reading this section, you will be able to:

- Identify the quality characteristics of fresh, frozen, canned, and dried fruits.

- Explain how to purchase and store varieties of fresh, frozen, canned, and dried fruits.

- Demonstrate dry and moist cooking of fruits.

FROM appetizers to desserts, fruits add texture, nutrition, color, and flavor to any meal. Fruits come from flowering plants. They contain at least one seed. Fruits are divided into eight categories: citrus fruits, melons, berries, drupes (DROOPS), pomes, grapes, tropical fruits, and exotic fruits. Drupes are fruits with stones, such as peaches. You need to understand the types and forms of fruits. You also need to know how to serve and store each of them.

✖ FRESH FRUIT

Fresh fruit, when in season, adds color and flavor to any meal. Fruits that are locally out of season can be shipped from other parts of the world where they are in season. Knowing what is in season in your area allows you to plan menus that take advantage of these fruits. This will also help keep purchasing costs down.

The type of fruit, its nutritional content, and the food product in which it will be used determine whether a foodservice operation purchases ripe or unripe fruit. These factors also determine the grade of fruit purchased.

■ **Grading.** The USDA has a voluntary grading program for fresh fruits. Grades are based on a variety of factors, including shape, size, texture, color, and defects. These grades are:

- U.S. Fancy—Premium quality.
- U.S. No. 1—Good, average quality.
- U.S. No. 2—Medium quality; represents most produce.
- U.S. No. 3—Lowest grade quality.

Most foodservice operations purchase U.S. Fancy grade products when serving fresh fruit. Lesser grades of fruits are typically made into jams, jellies, and sauces. See Fig. 26-1 (**Fruits**).

Fruits

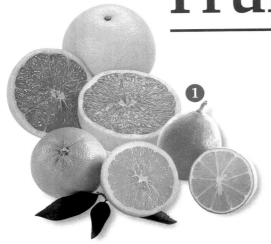

1. Citrus Fruits

Citrus fruits have a thick, firm rind covered by a thin layer of colored skin, called the zest. The soft, white layer between the zest and the flesh of the fruit is called the pith. The pith is slightly bitter. The flesh of citrus fruits is segmented and acidic. They grow on trees and shrubs and are harvested when ripe. Quality citrus fruits are not blemished, or soft and puffy. Citrus fruits will not continue to ripen after they are picked.

2. Melons

Sweet melons are fruits with a netted skin or a smooth rind that range in color from creamy to jade green. Sweet melons belong to the class of muskmelons (muhsk-meh-luhns). Quality melons are firm, heavy for their size, and have a good aroma. Watermelons are in a class of their own. Some melons are picked when they are ripe. Others ripen after being picked. Because they are 90% water, melons are usually served raw or puréed into soups or sorbets.

3. Berries

Berries are juicy, thin-skinned fruits with tiny seeds. They grow on bushes and vines and are picked when fully ripened. Berries will not continue to ripen after harvest. Quality berries are sweet, plump, and even in color.

4. Drupes

Drupes have soft flesh, thin skin, and one pit, or stone. Drupes can be picked ripe or they can ripen after they are picked. Quality drupes are firm and plump, without bruises or blemishes. These fragile fruits grow on shrubs and trees.

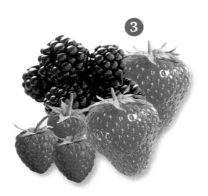

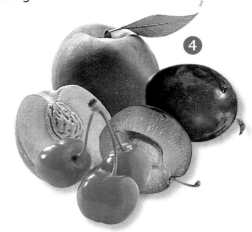

5. Pomes

Pomes are firm, thin-skinned fruits that grow on trees. They have a central core filled with tiny seeds. Pomes can be picked ripe or be ripened after they are picked. Quality pomes have smooth skin and no blemishes, bruises, or soft spots.

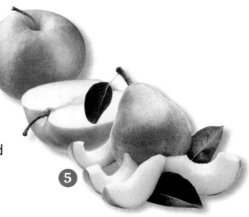

6. Grapes

Grapes grow in clusters on vines. Their flavor and color are found mostly in their skin. Grapes are almost always eaten raw. They can be picked ripe or ripen after they are picked. Quality grapes are plump and juicy, with rich color.

7. Tropical Fruits

Tropical fruits grow in hot, tropical regions of the world. These fruits ripen after they are picked. Because of quick transportation and distribution, these fruits are readily available in the United States. Quality tropical fruits are firm, plump, unblemished, and have good color.

8. Exotic Fruits

The exotic fruit category contains many types of unusual fruits. These fruits can be picked ripe or ripen after they are picked. Quality exotic fruits are semi-soft, slightly heavy, and have good color. The exotic fruits shown here are available in most areas of the United States.

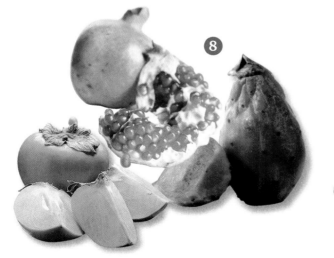

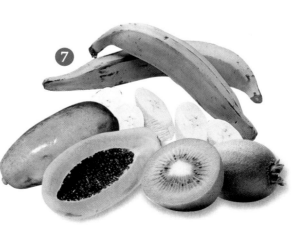

Purchasing Fresh Fruit

Fresh fruits may be purchased ripe or unripe. They are sold by count or weight and packed in flats, lugs, or cartons. **Lugs** are boxes, crates, or baskets in which produce is shipped to market. Lugs often hold 25–40 lbs. of produce. Flats are shallow boxes, crates, or baskets that are used to ship pints and quarts of produce such as strawberries. See Fig. 26-2. States have different weight requirements for each type of packaging.

Some fruits, such as melons, berries, and pineapples, are purchased cleaned, peeled, or cut. They may be purchased in bulk with sugar and preservatives added or packed in large containers of water. Although purchasing prepared fresh fruit may save time in trimming and cutting, the price is often greater. Also, the taste and freshness may diminish as a result of the processing.

Ripening & Storing Fresh Fruit

Fruits change in several ways as they ripen. They grow into their full size, and the color deepens and changes. The flesh becomes soft, juicy, and less tart, and the flavor and aroma intensify. Fresh fruits should be used at the height of their ripeness, as judged by taste and appearance.

Because ripening doesn't stop when a fruit is perfectly ripe, it is important to understand when a fruit is ripe and how much longer it will take until it turns bad. Some fruits, such as bananas, are often purchased unripened, since they continue to ripen after harvesting. Other fruits, such as pineapples, ripen only on the plant and must be rushed to market. They should never be purchased unripened.

Fresh fruits in season provide color and flavor to any meal. Fruits give off **ethylene** (eh-THE-lean) **gas**, an odorless, colorless gas that is emitted naturally as fruits ripen. Unripened fruits can be exposed to ethylene gas to encourage ripening. To stop fruits from ripening further, keep them chilled and isolated from other fruits.

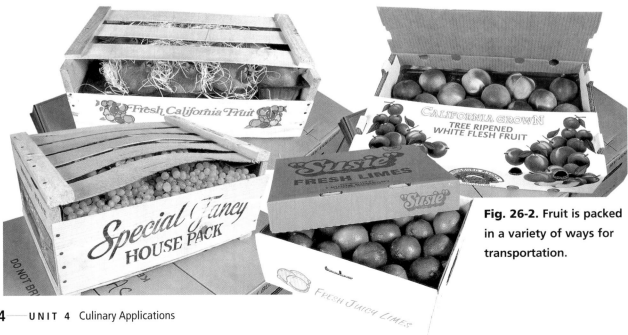

Fig. 26-2. Fruit is packed in a variety of ways for transportation.

Apples, melons, and bananas give off large amounts of ethylene gas. Store them separately from more delicate fruits and vegetables.

CANNED FRUIT

Most fruits can be successfully canned. Commonly canned fruits include pears, peaches, and pineapples. Fruits can be canned in heavy or light syrup, in water or fruit juice, or in solid pack cans that contain little or no water.

Fruits are exposed to high temperatures during canning. The heat destroys microorganisms and eliminates oxidation, both of which cause fruit to spoil. This sealed environment also slows the decomposition of the fruit. The heat required in canning softens fruit, but it doesn't affect the nutritional content.

Purchasing & Storing Canned Fruit

Canned fruits are available in different standard-size cans. Cooked fruit products, such as pie fillings, also come in cans. Store canned fruit on shelves in a cool, dry area. After opening a can, transfer any leftover fruit to a storage container and refrigerate.

Canned fruit has an extended shelf life as long as the can remains sealed and undamaged. Don't purchase dented cans. If a can has a bulge, throw it away immediately without opening it. Bulges are a sign that botulism, a foodborne illness, is present. People can become ill if they eat food from these damaged cans.

FROZEN FRUIT

Fresh fruit can be effectively preserved through freezing. Freezing stops the growth of microorganisms that cause food to spoil. Freezing doesn't affect the nutritional value, but it does change the texture of the fruit. Freezing breaks down the cell structure of fruit when the water in the fruit expands during freezing. Then, as fruit thaws, it

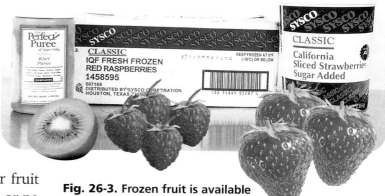

Fig. 26-3. Frozen fruit is available in many forms and packages. How else might frozen fruit be purchased?

loses shape because part of the cell structure has been broken down. This leaves the fruit mushy.

Many fruits, such as pears and berries, are individually quick frozen (IQF). This reduces the number of ice crystals that form, keeping the quality of the frozen product higher. It also helps the fruit retain its shape. You do not have to use, or thaw, the whole container at one time.

■ **Grading.** Frozen fruits are labeled U.S. Grade A—Fancy, U.S. Grade B—Choice or Extra Standard, or U.S. Grade C—Standard. The characteristics of each are as follows:

• U.S. Grade A—Premium quality.
• U.S. Grade B—Above average quality.
• U.S. Grade C—Medium quality.

Purchasing & Storing Frozen Fruit

Frozen fruits are available sliced; packed in sugar syrup; whole; or pitted, peeled, and sliced. Frozen purées are also available. All forms of frozen fruits should be sealed in moisture-proof bags or other containers. Frozen canned fruits are also available. They come in cans or large plastic containers and usually contain a large amount of sugar and water. See Fig. 26-3.

After frozen fruit is purchased, immediately transfer fruit that will not be used to a freezer so it doesn't thaw. Keep the temperature at a constant 0°F or below. If the temperature is allowed to vary, the fruit may develop freezer burn.

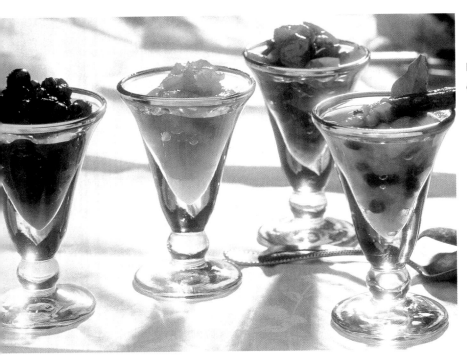

Fig. 26-4. Compotes and chutneys are often served with poultry and meats.

They are available in 1 lb. packages. They also come in 30 lb. bulk sizes.

Store dried fruits in airtight containers. Keep the containers in a cool place out of direct sunlight to prevent mold from forming. Dried fruits with low moisture, such as raisins, spoil more quickly than other types. Only purchase amounts that will be used within a month.

☒ DRIED FRUITS

Drying is another common technique for preserving fruits. Popular dried fruits include bananas, apples, apricots, grapes, plums, and figs. You can add dried fruits to biscuits and muffins, cakes, and pies.

Dried fruits are also used in compotes and chutneys. **Compotes** are fresh or dried fruits that have been cooked in a sugar syrup. **Chutney** is a condiment made of fruit, vinegar, sugar, and spices. It can be smooth or chunky, hot or mild. Chutneys are served cold, warm, or hot. See Fig. 26-4. Compotes and chutneys often accompany poultry and meats.

Rehydrate (ree-HI-drayt), or add water into, dried fruits before use. This is done by placing the fruit in boiling water for one-half to one minute. Fruit juices formed by soaking dried fruits in hot liquid until the liquid absorbs the flavor of the fruit can be used in fruit soups and smoothies.

Purchasing & Storing Dried Fruit

Dried fruits are **cryovaced** (cry-OH-vacked), or shrink-wrapped, for purchasing and shipping.

☒ COOKING FRUIT

Although fruits are usually served raw, they can also be cooked using a variety of methods. The most common cooking techniques include baking, poaching, simmering, deep-frying, sautéing, broiling, and grilling.

When cooking fruits, take care not to overcook them. If you do, they become mushy and lose their flavor. Adding sugar or acid, such as lemon juice, helps prevent overcooking. The fruit takes the sugar or acid into its cells, which helps keep it firm and retain its form.

Preparation of Fruit

Before preparing and cooking fruit, you need to gather your ingredients, smallwares, and utensils. You also need to complete the mise en place for the fruit. Each type of fruit will require different pre-preparation. For some fruits, such as bananas, mangoes, and papayas, your first step in pre-preparation would be to soften and ripen them at room temperature. In general, you can follow these guidelines:

1. Wash the fruit in cold water. Drain well.
   Remove any stems. If the fruits have skin that needs to be peeled or pulled, do so now.

2. Cut the fruit in halves, quarters, slices, or chunks.

3. Remove any seeds and pits. Some fruit may also need to be cored.

4. To prevent browning, dip the fruit in citrus juice. This step is not necessary for all fruit.

Cooking with Dry Heat

Dry cooking methods for fruit include broiling and grilling, baking, sautéing, and deep-frying. Take care not to dry out the fruit by overcooking.

■ **Broiling and grilling.** Bananas, apples, peaches, and pineapples are often broiled or grilled. The fruits must be quickly cooked so they don't become mushy and lose their shape. These fruits can be sliced or served as halves. Often they are coated with honey or sugar, or sprinkled with lemon juice, cinnamon, or nutmeg.

Place fruits to be broiled on a sheet pan. For grilling, place large fruits directly on the grill or thread them onto skewers. Rotate thick slices to make sure they cook all the way through.

1. Place prepared fruits on a sheet pan for broiling. The sheet pan must be clean and have a smooth surface. Some chefs use parchment paper to avoid sticking. See Fig. 26-5A.

2. Place the sheet pans in a broiler. Broil on high heat.

3. Broil fruit long enough to heat through. You want to make sure that each side is clearly marked. See Fig. 26-5B.

■ **Baking.** Many fruits can be baked into delicious desserts. For example, berries, peaches, and apples can be baked with a crust to make fruit cobblers. These can be served with whipped cream or vanilla ice cream. You can also bake sweet and tart fruits together to provide an interesting contrast of flavors. Or, try stuffing whole, cored apples or peach halves with raisins; then drizzle them with honey and bake. The fruit skins help hold in moisture and flavor.

Some fruits are added to meats and baked. For example, ham is often baked with pineapple. Other fruits, such as plums, can be cooked with poultry to make a flavorful sauce.

■ **Sautéing.** When fruits are sautéed in butter, sugar, and other spices, they develop a sweet, rich, syrupy flavor. You can serve bananas, cherries, pears, and apples this way for a scrumptious dessert. To sauté fruits, first peel and core them and remove any seeds. Cut them into neat, even slices, place them in a sauté pan, and cook over high heat. Sautéed fruits can be used in a main course and as desserts served with ice cream.

■ **Deep-frying.** A few fruits, such as bananas, pineapples, and apples, can be coated in batter and deep-fried. Peel, core, and slice the fruit into neat, even slices. If the fruit is too moist, dry it with a paper towel so the batter will stick to it. Then the fruit can be deep-fried as described in Chapter 15.

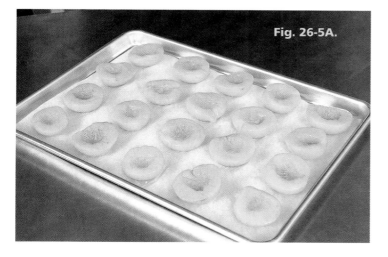
Fig. 26-5A.

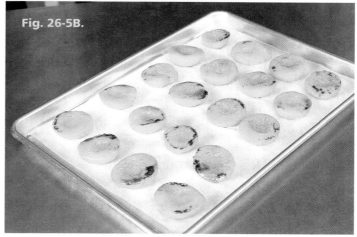
Fig. 26-5B.

■ **Fondue.** The term fondue (fahn-DOO) refers to cooking or dipping foods into a central heated pot. The word fondue comes from the French word meaning "to melt." In the case of fruit fondue, bite-size chunks of fresh fruits are often dipped into a chocolate sauce made of melted chocolate and cream.

Cooking with Moist Heat

Two moist cooking methods are poaching and simmering.

■ **Poaching.** In poaching, fruits are submerged in various liquids, such as water or sugar syrup. Apples, apricots, peaches, pears, and plums are often poached. See Fig. 26-6. Poaching is done at very low temperatures, so it takes some time to cook fruits using this method. The slow cooking time helps the fruit retain its shape and flavor and soften gradually.

■ **Simmering.** Simmering is used to make fruit compotes and stewed fruits. Fresh, frozen, canned, or dried fruits can be simmered successfully. Serve stewed or simmered fruits hot or cold, as appetizers, side dishes, or desserts.

To simmer fruit, first peel, core, and slice the fruit. Place it in a pan with cooking liquid, such as water, sugar, syrup, honey, and spices. Bring the liquid to a simmer. Cook until the fruit is done, and add a sweetener if desired.

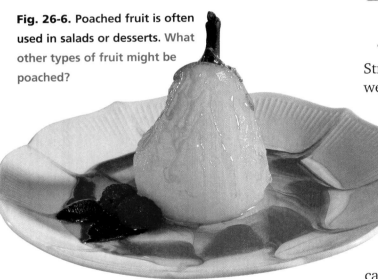

Fig. 26-6. Poached fruit is often used in salads or desserts. What other types of fruit might be poached?

✕ PLATING & GARNISHING FRUITS

The fundamentals of plating apply to all fruits. Strive for an attractive plate that's colorful and well balanced. It's important to use a variety of different fruits. This will provide better plate composition. Do not allow drippings to touch the rim of the plate. Avoid leaving thumbprints on the rim, too.

Fruits may be served on special serving ware. For example, compotes are served in a glass or crystal compotier (KAHM-poht-tee-ay). A **compotier** is a deep, stemmed dish used to serve compotes, candies, and nuts.

SECTION 26-1 Knowledge Check

1. List the eight categories of fruit.
2. Compare how canned, frozen, and dried fruits are purchased and stored.
3. How might you choose a moist or dry method of cooking fruit?

MINI LAB

In teams, choose a fruit to cook. Complete the necessary mise en place. Then prepare and serve your dish to each team.

Vegetables

KEY TERMS

- tuber
- mealy
- waxy
- solanine
- drained weight
- packing medium
- mandoline
- bouquetière

OBJECTIVES

After reading this section, you will be able to:

- Identify the quality characteristics of fresh, canned, frozen, and dried vegetables.

- Explain how to purchase and store varieties of fresh, canned, frozen, and dried vegetables.

- Demonstrate dry and moist cooking of vegetables.

LIKE fruits, vegetables are versatile foods that add color, flavor, and texture to any meal. Many commercial kitchens offer vegetable-based entrées to meet the demands of health-conscious customers. Becoming familiar with the types and flavors of vegetables and the best ways to prepare and store them is important for every foodservice employee.

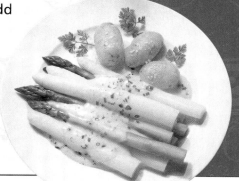

✖ IDENTIFYING VEGETABLES

Vegetables are edible plants. Different parts of vegetables are eaten, including the flowers, seeds, stems, leaves, roots, and **tubers**, or the short, fleshy underground stems of plants. The potato is an example of a tuber. Certain types of fruit are classified as vegetables by commercial kitchens because they are savory rather than sweet. These fruits, such as eggplants and tomatoes, are prepared and served like vegetables.

Classifying Vegetables

Commercial kitchens usually classify vegetables into the following categories: the squash family; roots and tubers; seeds and pods; the cabbage family; stems, stalks, and shoots; the onion family; fruit-vegetables; and leafy greens. These categories group vegetables by how they are used in the kitchen. For example, kale and cauliflower are members of the cabbage family, but from a culinary perspective they are used quite differently. Kale is a leafy green and cauliflower is a vegetable floret (FLOHR-uht). See Fig. 26-7 (**Vegetables**).

Vegetables

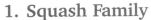

1. Squash Family

Members of the squash family have large root systems and trailing vines. Their flowers are often edible in addition to the main vegetable. Quality squash are firm, free of blemishes, and show no signs of mold.

2. Roots & Tubers

Roots grow deep into the soil, while tubers are large, round, underground stems that grow just below the surface of the soil. Both store and provide food to their plants, making them rich in nutrients. Quality roots and tubers are firm, unwrinkled, unblemished, and have good color.

3. Seeds & Pods

This category consists of vegetables with edible seeds. Some of the pods are also edible, but the seeds are more nutritious. Quality seeds and pods are firm, well-shaped, and without blemishes.

4. Cabbage Family

Vegetables in the cabbage family grow quickly in cool weather. Commercial kitchens use the flowers, leaves, and heads of these plants. They are served raw as well as cooked. Quality cauliflower, broccoli, and cabbage are firm, heavy for their size, and have good color.

5. Stems, Stalks & Shoots

Vegetables in this category produce edible stems, stalks, and shoots. They are picked when young and tender. Quality stems, stalks, and shoots are firm, unblemished, and have no browning.

6. Onion Family

Vegetables in the onion family are often used for seasoning and flavoring. Most have a strong taste and odor. Quality onions are firm, fresh-looking, and have good color.

7. Fruit-Vegetables

Vegetables that are often called fruit-vegetables come from flowering plants and contain at least one seed. Therefore, they are technically the fruit of the plant. For the purpose of commercial kitchens, however, they are categorized as vegetables since they are savory rather than sweet. Quality fruit-vegetables have smooth, unblemished skin.

8. Leafy Greens

Vegetables in this category can be served raw or cooked. They shrink when cooked because of their high water content. Flavors of leafy greens range from mild to spicy. Quality greens have crisp, bright leaves without any brown spots.

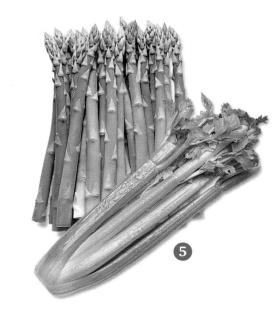

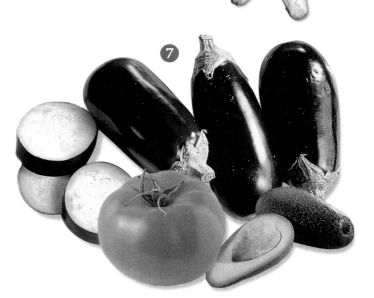

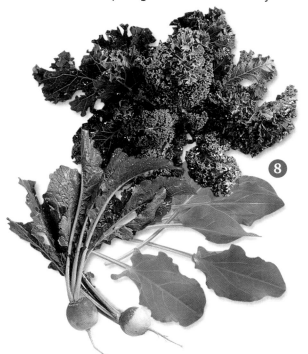

PURCHASING & STORING FRESH VEGETABLES

The quality of the ingredients you use to prepare dishes directly affects the outcome of the finished product. Vegetables are no exception. Understanding how to select fresh, high-quality vegetables and store them in a way that maintains this quality helps ensure fresh, flavorful dishes.

Grading

The USDA provides a voluntary grading system for vegetables that is used by almost all wholesalers. Grades are based on the appearance, quality, and condition of vegetables when they arrive on the market. Vegetables are graded as:

- U.S. Extra Fancy.
- U.S. Fancy.
- U.S. Extra No. 1.
- U.S. No. 1.

Premium quality is classified as U.S. Extra Fancy. When choosing vegetables to use in a food-service operation, look for the highest quality product. Some recipes, however, allow a lesser quality product to be used.

Some vegetables are graded differently for the retail market. Onions, potatoes, and carrots are graded by an alphabetical system, with Grade A being the best. See Fig. 26-8.

Ripening

Although many vegetables are fully ripe when purchased, they continue to ripen when exposed to oxygen in the air. The ripening rate depends on the type of vegetable and the way it is stored.

There are some vegetables you will want to continue to ripen. For example, tomatoes and other fruit-vegetables may be purchased unripe so they're damaged less in shipping. As with fruits, you can hasten ripening by exposing these fruit-vegetables to ethylene gas.

Storing

Different vegetables require different storage conditions. Starchy vegetables, such as potatoes, winter squash, and vegetables in the onion family, are best stored at 60°F–70°F in a dry location. If they are stored in a refrigerator, they will lose flavor and texture. Most other vegetables should be stored at refrigerator temperatures of 41°F or below. Store vegetables away from fruits that emit ethylene gas, such as bananas. The gas will cause continued ripening and possible decay.

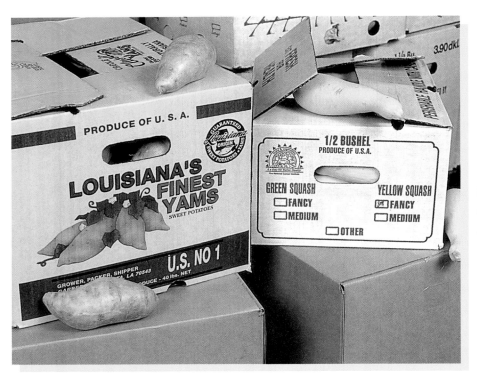

Fig. 26-8. USDA grades are used by wholesalers and buyers to ensure quality control.

X PURCHASING & STORING POTATOES

Potatoes are a versatile vegetable. Foodservice operations use potatoes in some form at each meal. Most foodservice operations purchase potatoes in 50-lb. cartons or bags. See Fig. 26-9. The number of potatoes in each carton varies depending on the size of the potatoes.

Store potatoes in a dry, dark area with temperatures of 60°F–70°F. Do not refrigerate potatoes. The cool temperature will convert some of the potato starch to sugar, making the potato too sweet.

Types of Potatoes

Potatoes are divided into two main types: mealy and waxy. **Mealy** potatoes have thick skin and starchy flesh. They are best for deep-frying, baking, whipping, and puréeing. **Waxy** potatoes have thin skin and contain less starch than mealy potatoes. They are best for boiling.

There are a wide variety of mealy and waxy potatoes. See Fig. 26-10.

■ **Russet.** A mealy potato also known as Idaho. Russets are a popular choice for baking and frying.

■ **Red.** A waxy, pink- to red-skinned potato. Red potatoes are good roasted and in salads, soups, and purées.

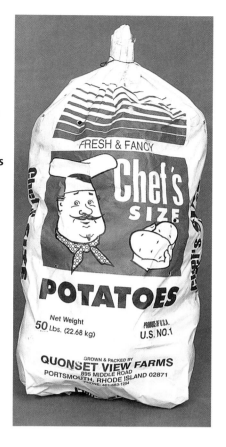

Fig. 26-9. Potatoes are purchased in 50-lb. cartons or bags.

Fig. 26-10.

Types of Potatoes

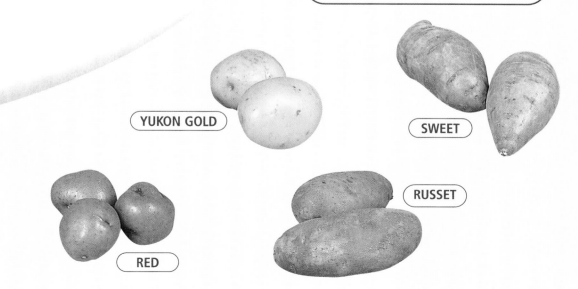

YUKON GOLD

SWEET

RED

RUSSET

a LINK to the Past

Potato Soup

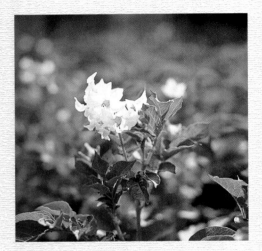

Many Europeans, especially the Irish, considered the potato an ideal staple food. However, the French were slow to accept the potato. It took an eighteenth-century French pharmacist named Antoine Augustin Parmentier (par-mawn-TYAY) to change their minds. Parmentier had eaten a diet mainly of potatoes while in prison in Prussia during the Seven Years War.

He believed potatoes would stop the starvation caused by the famine. Parmentier became a one-man promoter of the potato. He set up potato soup kitchens throughout Paris to assist the poor. Parmentier also presented a potato flower bouquet to Louis XVI in honor of his birthday. The potato flower became quite fashionable.

Louis XVI ordered that potatoes were to be planted on public grounds and protected by armed guards. As a result of Parmentier's efforts, the potato became an important part of French cuisine. Today, the term *Potage parmentier* means potato soup.

■ **Yukon.** A buttery-flavored mealy potato with golden flesh. Yukon potatoes can be baked, puréed, and made into salads and casseroles.

■ **Sweet.** This type comes in two varieties: white and red. White sweet potatoes have yellow flesh and a mealy texture. Red sweet potatoes have a darker orange flesh and a less mealy texture. Both types are used in soups and casseroles and can be boiled, roasted, and puréed.

Quality Characteristics

Use the following characteristics when selecting potatoes:

- All varieties of potatoes should be heavy and firm, without soft spots, green color, or sprouting eyes.
- Sweet potatoes should have dry-looking, orange and golden-orange skins.
- Avoid sweet potatoes with softened ends. This marks the beginning of spoilage.
- Other potatoes should have dry, tight skins, without wrinkles.

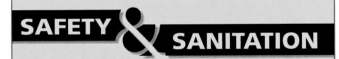

SAFETY & SANITATION

GREEN POTATOES—Discard potatoes with green skin or green spots on the skin. Potatoes tinged with green contain a toxin called **solanine** (SOH-luh-neen). Solanine is caused by prolonged exposure to light. Solanine is not destroyed by heat and doesn't dissolve in water. This toxin can cause gastrointestinal (gas-troh-in-TEHS-tuh-nuhl) problems and central nervous system problems.

Market Forms of Potatoes

Many market forms of potatoes can be used in the professional kitchen.

■ **Fresh.** Fresh potatoes are readily available year-round. They can be baked, fried, boiled, whipped, or puréed and served with sour cream, nonfat yogurt, or butter.

- **Canned.** Most types of potatoes are available in cans, already cooked, whole or sliced. Use of canned potatoes eliminates the risk of spoilage and can result in a high-quality dish. Keep in mind, however, that most canned sweet potatoes are packed in a sugary or spicy sauce.

- **Frozen.** Many foodservice operations purchase frozen potatoes that are precut for French fries. The French fries are blanched in deep-frying fat and then frozen. This product enables foodservice operations to quickly prepare French fries, without cleaning, peeling, and slicing fresh potatoes. Prepared potato dishes available frozen include hash browns and stuffed baked potatoes. These items can be heated, fried, or cooked in casseroles.

- **Dehydrated.** Dried potato flakes can be mixed with milk or hot water to make mashed potatoes, hash browns, scalloped potatoes, and other popular dishes. Some dehydrated potatoes may need soaking before cooking.

✖ PURCHASING & STORING PRESERVED VEGETABLES

Techniques like canning, freezing, and drying are used to lengthen the shelf life of vegetables. Cooked vegetables can also be preserved through canning and freezing. These techniques may affect the flavor and texture of vegetables.

Canned Vegetables

Almost every variety of vegetable is available canned, which brings many advantages to the commercial kitchen. Canned vegetables are already cleaned, peeled, cut into pieces, and cooked. Combinations of vegetables combined with seasonings and flavorings are also available canned. Additionally, they have been heat-treated to kill microorganisms.

Canning effectively preserves the flavor and texture of such vegetables as tomatoes, sweet potatoes, peas, corn, and beans. However, the heat used during canning softens most vegetables

Fig. 26-11.

CAN SIZE	WEIGHT	CANS PER CASE
No. 2	20 oz.	24
No. 2 ½	28 oz.	24
No. 300	14–15 oz.	36
No. 303	16–17 oz.	36
No. 5	46–51 oz.	12
No. 10	6 lb. 10 oz.	6

and can cause some nutrient loss. Using the liquid from the canned vegetables retains some of these nutrients. Canning can also dull the color of green vegetables.

The USDA grading system for canned vegetables is:

- U.S. Grade A or Fancy.
- U.S. Grade B or Extra-Select.
- U.S. Grade C or Standard.

The net weight of canned vegetables is the weight of the contents. **Drained weight** is the weight of the food product without the packing medium. A **packing medium** is a liquid used to protect the food product. It can be thin or thick. Canned vegetables come in a variety of commercial sizes. See Fig. 26-11.

SAFETY & SANITATION

CANNED VEGETABLES—The high heat used during the canning process kills microorganisms. However, occasionally, cans are not properly sealed, processed, or handled. Throw away any swollen or dented cans and cans that contain discolored food. People can become seriously ill if they eat food from these cans.

Frozen Vegetables

Frozen vegetables offer convenience similar to that found with canned vegetables, but the quality is higher. Most nutrients are retained during freezing. Vegetables also retain their bright colors and flavors due to the quickness with which they are precooked and frozen. As with fruits, some vegetables are individually quick frozen. This improves their texture and appearance.

Some frozen vegetables are frozen raw, while others are completely cooked and need only to be thawed and heated before serving. Do not refreeze unused portions. Instead, store them in the refrigerator as you would fresh vegetables.

The same grading system used for canned vegetables is used for frozen vegetables. The most common pack for frozen vegetables is a 20-lb. bulk bag in a cardboard case. Other packs include six 4-lb. bags and twelve 2.5-lb. bags or boxes. Keep all packages in a freezer at a steady temperature of 0°F or below.

Dried Vegetables

Dried vegetables are not as common in foodservice operations as canned and frozen vegetables. The drying process impacts the appearance, taste, and texture of vegetables. The advantage to using dehydrated vegetables is convenience. Essentially, everything is done in the processing plant instead of the commercial kitchen.

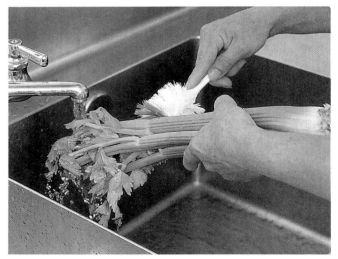

✖ COOKING VEGETABLES

Unlike fruits, most vegetables are served cooked. Cooking softens vegetables and intensifies their flavor. To maintain flavor and quality, cook vegetables in batches as close to serving time as possible. Improper cooking and holding techniques can cause a loss of nutrients and damage to the texture, color, and flavor of vegetables. For example, to help white and red vegetables retain their color, cook them in liquid that is slightly acidic (uh-SIH-dihk). Learning how to apply the right cooking techniques will help you serve tender vegetables packed with nutrition and flavor.

Determining Doneness

Every vegetable has slightly different characteristics when properly cooked, so there is no one rule of thumb to follow regarding cooking time. However, most vegetables are finished cooking when they are just tender enough to cut with a fork. Leafy vegetables should become brighter in color than when raw and be just slightly wilted. Instead of relying on a specific cooking time, pay attention to how vegetables look, taste, smell, and feel.

Pre-Preparation for Vegetables

Efficiently preparing and arranging vegetables is an important step in vegetable cookery. The number and types of vegetables you will need to prepare vary with each recipe.

■ **Washing.** Because vegetables grow outside and often close to the ground, they can pick up sand, dirt, grit, chemicals, and even insects. It is critical to clean them thoroughly just before preparation. Since water can leach nutrients from vegetables, clean the produce quickly under cold running water. See Fig. 26-12. Follow these other guidelines:

Fig. 26-12. Vegetables should be thoroughly cleaned before preparation.

Fig. 26-13.

VEGETABLE CUTS					

French Fry	½ × ½ × 3 inches		**Brunoise (broo-NWAHZ)**	⅛ × ⅛ × ⅛ inch (extra-small dice)
Stick	⅜ × ⅜ × 2 inches		**Mirepoix (mihr-PWAH)**	½ inch average rough cut
Baton	¼ × ¼ × 3 inches (small stick)		**Chips**	⅛ inch thick slice
Julienne (joo-lee-EHN)	⅛ × ⅛ × 2 inches (short, matchstick)		**Waffle**	⅛ inch thick slice; perforated
Fine Matchstick	1/16 × 1/16 × 2 inches		**Tourne (toor-nay)**	7-sided; 2 inch-long barrel
Large Dice	¾ × ¾ × ¾ inch		**Round**	Round disks of varying thickness
Medium Dice	½ × ½ × ½ inch		**Diagonal**	Bias-cut slices of variable thickness
Small Dice	¼ × ¼ × ¼ inch		**Chiffonade (shihf-uh-NAHD)**	Thin ribbons

- Scrub root vegetables with a strong-bristled brush.
- Soak cabbage family vegetables, such as broccoli, in salted water for a short amount of time. This will draw out any insects.
- Store cut vegetables, such as carrots, in the refrigerator until ready to be used.

Unlike other vegetables, leafy green vegetables are washed in a water bath. This allows debris and sand to settle to the bottom of the vegetable sink. To avoid further contact with the debris and sand, lift the greens out of the water.

■ **Peeling, cutting, and shaping.** Peeling, cutting, and shaping vegetables influence how they will cook and how they will look when served. Depending on how each vegetable will be used, its preparation will differ.

Always trim off and discard only inedible skins, leaves, stems, and stalks using the appropriate tools. For example, you could use a vegetable peeler to remove a thin layer of vegetable skin.

Cut vegetables into uniform pieces to ensure even cooking. Many foodservice operations use food processors to uniformly cut vegetables. Another hand-operated machine, called a **mandoline** (MAHN-duh-lihn), is used for slicing vegetables and fruits, such as potatoes and apples. In using a mandoline, food is held in a metal carriage while slicing to protect the fingers. See Fig. 26-13 for popular cuts and shapes used on vegetables and potatoes.

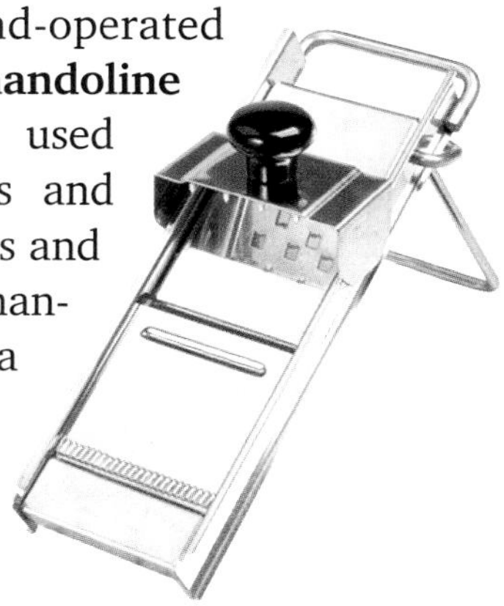

Cooking Vegetables with Dry Heat

Cooking vegetables with dry heat preserves flavors and nutrients. Since vegetables aren't submerged in water, the risk of nutrients leaching

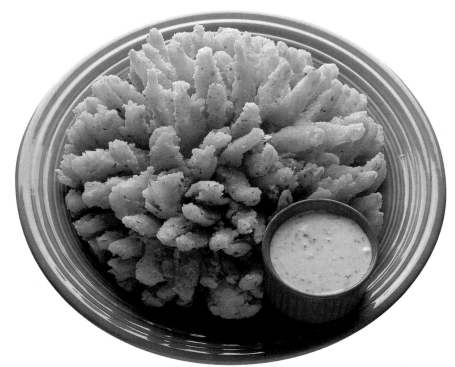

Fig. 26-14. This vegetable has been prepared using a dry cooking technique. What specific technique was used?

into liquid is eliminated. Dry cooking techniques such as grilling can also give vegetables interesting flavors.

You can brush butter, seasonings, flavorings, or flavored oils on vegetables before cooking for added flavor. Never use flavored oils for deep-frying. Evenly slice vegetables to ensure uniform cooking and add to the visual appeal of the final product. See Fig. 26-14.

■ **Broiling and grilling.** Broiling and grilling both cook vegetables quickly under relatively high heat. The heat caramelizes the vegetables, giving a pleasing flavor. Many kinds of vegetables can be grilled or broiled, including potatoes, tomatoes, peppers, squash, eggplant, zucchini, and corn.

You can thread small sliced vegetables, such as mushrooms and tomatoes, onto wooden or metal skewers for grilling. Be sure to cut larger vegetables, such as eggplant and squash, into slices and place them directly on the grill. For broiling, arrange slices or chunks of vegetables on a sheet pan. Broiling can also be used to reheat a vegetable that has already been cooked.

■ **Baking.** Baked vegetables are cooked at a lower temperature for a longer period of time than grilled or broiled vegetables. Squash, onions, potatoes, and other root vegetables are excellent

baked. They should be well cleaned, peeled, and unless baked whole, cut into uniform pieces.

■ **Sautéing.** Sautéing cooks vegetables in a small amount of butter or oil in a hot sauté pan. Sautéing happens quickly because the heat is high, so have all vegetables cut and ready to cook before you begin.

Many different kinds of vegetables can be sautéed, including mushrooms, summer squash, and onions. Firm vegetables such as broccoli, Brussels sprouts, carrots, beans, celery, and potatoes need to be blanched before sautéing. Sautéed vegetables should look brightly colored and still be slightly crisp.

■ **Deep-frying.** Deep-fried vegetables are usually coated in batter, then submerged in hot oil. Potatoes are popular deep-fried as French fries or potato chips. Other vegetables that can be deep-fried include onions, mushrooms, cauliflower, okra, and eggplant. Be sure to cut vegetables into even pieces and wipe off any excess moisture before deep-frying.

■ **Fondue.** When cooking fondue for vegetables, vegetable chunks such as cauliflower, mushrooms, and broccoli are cooked on skewers in hot oil. The cooked vegetables can then be dipped in a variety of flavorful sauces.

Cooking Vegetables with Moist Heat

Moist cooking methods used in vegetable cookery include blanching, parboiling, steaming, simmering, poaching, and braising. Before cooking with these techniques, clean vegetables thoroughly and cut them into uniform pieces. Add bouillon, herbs, spices, or butter to the cooking liquid for extra flavor. To retain nutrients, cook vegetables for the minimum amount of time needed and in a small amount of liquid. If possible, reuse this flavored liquid in the dish you're preparing, or in soups or stocks.

Green vegetables need to be cooked without a cover to let the acid escape. Red vegetables need to be cooked covered to keep the acid inside. They also may need to have an acid such as vinegar added to the water to replace lost acid. See Fig. 26-15.

■ **Blanching.** Often used to loosen the skins of vegetables, blanching involves plunging foods briefly into boiling water and then plunging them into cold water to stop the cooking process. Blanching is also used to increase the color and flavor of vegetables before freezing.

■ **Parboiling.** Parboiling is used to partially cook vegetables. Another method is then used to finish cooking the vegetables, such as grilling or sautéing. Parboiling is also helpful for removing strong flavors and loosening skins or peels. Winter squash, root vegetables, and members of the cabbage family are commonly parboiled.

■ **Steaming and simmering.** Steamed vegetables are cooked by being placed above boiling water in a perforated container. Today most commercial kitchens use combination or pressureless steamers. Simmered vegetables sit in a shallow layer of lightly boiling water. The end result of both techniques—soft, colorful, flavorful vegetables—is the same.

■ **Poaching and braising.** Poached vegetables cook in just enough simmering liquid to cover the food. Braising vegetables is achieved by simmering them in a seasoned brown sauce in the oven. Save this liquid and serve it with the vegetables for added flavor. Popular vegetables used for braising are cabbages, celery, leeks, onions, endive, and lettuces such as romaine. Refer to Chapter 15 for more information on poaching and braising.

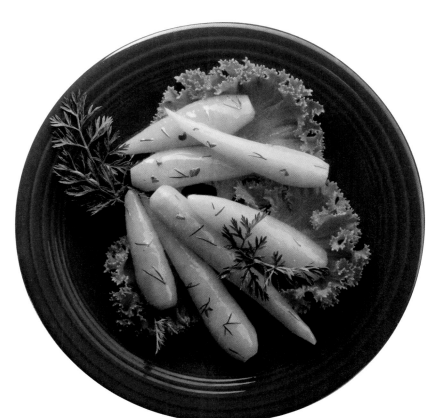

Fig. 26-15. Moist cooking techniques also offer many ways to prepare vegetables. Describe two ways to cook vegetables with moist heat.

PLATING & GARNISHING VEGETABLES

As with any other food, an important factor in vegetable cookery is its visual appeal on the plate. Uniform-size pieces arranged in an attractive pattern make the entire plate appealing. When plating vegetables, the following arrangements may be used:

• Place the main entrée to the front of the plate with the vegetables to the back.

• Place the main item in the center of the plate with vegetables placed randomly around the item. Vegetables could be arranged in a pattern instead.

• Place vegetables in the center of the plate with the main item leaning against it. The main item also could be sliced and placed around the vegetables.

• Put a **bouquetière** (boo-kuh-tyehr), or bouquet of three or more vegetables, arranged on a plate surrounded by other foods. See Fig. 26-16.

You can use a lot of creativity when plating vegetables. Simple garnishes, such as chopped scallions or minced lemon zest, add eye appeal, texture, and flavor. For example, to zest a lemon you pull the zester over the lemon to cut thin strips of the lemon zest.

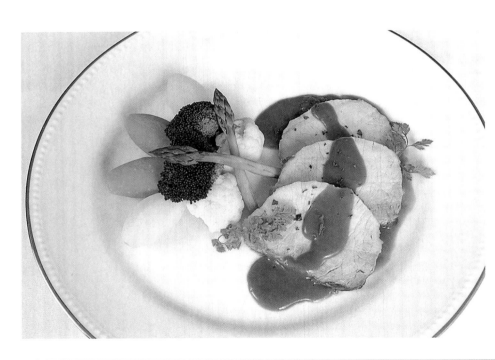

Fig. 26-16. A colorful combination of vegetables adds to the visual appeal of a plated dish. When presenting a plated dish to a customer, where should the vegetables be located?

SECTION 26-2 | Knowledge Check

1. List the eight groups into which vegetables are classified, and give two examples of each.

2. Explain the advantages of using canned, frozen, and dried vegetables in a foodservice operation.

3. Describe one dry and one moist cooking method that can be used to cook vegetables.

MINI LAB

You've been asked to add some vegetarian items to a café menu. The new menu items must include an appetizer, a soup, and two entrées. Describe how you would select, prepare, cook, and store the vegetables for each of these new menu items.

Legumes

KEY TERMS

- legumes
- pulses
- preprocessed
- quick soak

OBJECTIVES

After reading this section, you will be able to:

- Identify various types of legumes.
- Identify the quality characteristics of legumes.
- Explain how to purchase and store legumes.
- Prepare and cook legumes.

LEGUMES are considered vegetables, but are treated as a separate topic. **Legumes** (lehg-YOOMS) are a group of plants that have double-seamed pods containing a single row of seeds. Examples include peas, beans, lentils (LEHN-tuhls), soybeans, and peanuts. Cultures around the world have used legumes as a staple food for thousands of years—and for good reason. Legumes are nutritious, have a long shelf life, and contribute flavor and texture to any meal. As customers demand healthful foods with flavor, commercial kitchens are making legumes an important part of their menus.

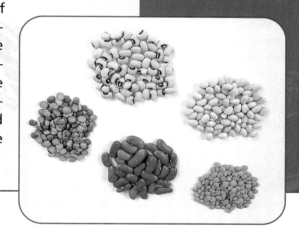

✖ TYPES OF LEGUMES

Legumes are not picked as fresh beans and peas. They are left on the vine until the bean or pea is plump and beginning to dry. At this point, the pods are harvested from the vine and the legumes are removed. When the seeds of a legume are dried, they are called **pulses**. Lentils and dried peas are examples of pulses.

Legumes come in different shapes, sizes, and colors. There are dozens of types of legumes, each with a different texture and flavor. The types pictured are most commonly used in commercial kitchens. See Fig. 26-17.

Legumes can be used in a variety of dishes and in many different ways. They are often added to soups and salads, and substituted for meat. For example, when making tacos, you could use legumes instead of ground beef as the main ingredient. Legumes can also be made into dips and spreads. They can be eaten as a snack item, or served as the main entrée.

Fig. 26-17.

LEGUME	DESCRIPTION	QUALITY CHARACTERISTICS
Baby Lima Beans 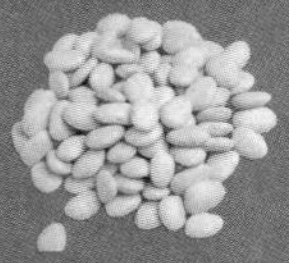	Flat-shaped bean.	Pale light green in color; smooth texture; sweet flavor.
Black-eyed Peas 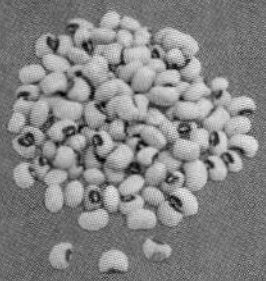	Medium-size, oval-shaped pea.	Dark beige with a black dot on the skin; smooth texture; savory flavor.
Cannelini (kan-eh-LEE-nee) Beans 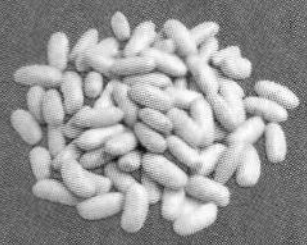	Larger than an American white bean.	Creamy white color; mild flavor; smooth texture.
Fava (FAH-vuh) Beans 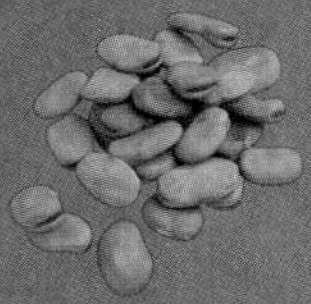	Large, flat, kidney-shaped bean.	Brown or white in color; fine texture, slightly firm.
Garbanzo (gahr-BAHN-zoh) Beans 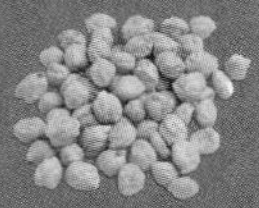	Medium-size, round bean; also called chick peas.	Beige color; firm texture; nutty flavor.
Great Northern Beans 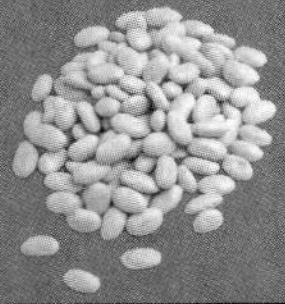	Medium-size, oval-shaped bean.	Creamy white color; powdery texture; mild flavor.
Green & Brown Lentils 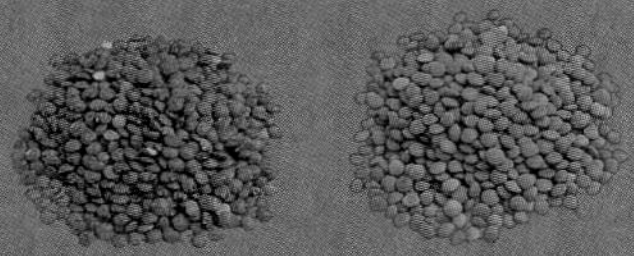	Disk-shaped, pea-size bean.	Green and brown in color.
Navy Beans 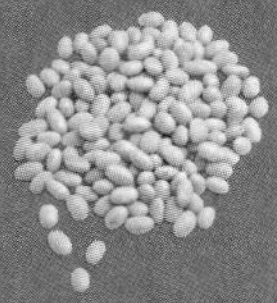	Small, oval-shaped bean.	White in color; powdery texture; mild flavor.
Peanuts 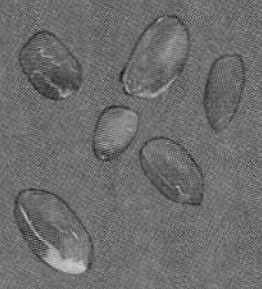	Oblong kernels.	Light brown in color; firm texture.

(Continued on next page)

Fig. 26-17 (Cont'd.).

LEGUME	DESCRIPTION CHARACTERISTICS	QUALITY
Pinto Beans	Medium-size, oval-shaped bean.	Beige and brown in color, typically mottled; powdery texture; earthy flavor.
Black Beans	Medium-size, oval-shaped bean. Also called turtle beans.	Creamy interior flesh with black shell or skin; sweet flavor.
Red Kidney Beans	Kidney-shaped bean.	Reddish-brown color; soft texture; robust flavor.
Soybeans	A round bean.	Black or yellow in color; bland flavor.
Yellow & Green Split Peas	Whole peas that have had the skin removed and are split in half.	Yellow and green color; soft, floury texture with a sweet taste.

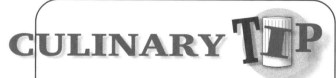

CULINARY TIP

NUTRIENTS IN LEGUMES—Legumes contain little fat and no cholesterol. Legumes are an excellent source of complex carbohydrates, protein, and soluble fiber. They provide iron, potassium, folate and other B vitamins, calcium, and zinc. Legumes are an essential protein source for people who follow a vegetarian diet.

QUALITY CHARACTERISTICS OF LEGUMES

When selecting legumes, consider the following quality standards. Legumes should be brightly colored and uniformly sized. They should not be marked, shriveled, damaged, or broken. Legumes are graded as:

• U.S. No. 1—The highest quality.
• U.S. No. 2—Above average quality.
• U.S. No. 3—Medium quality.

PURCHASING LEGUMES

When purchasing legumes, look for uniformly sized pieces, which ensure even cooking. The legumes should have smooth skin and should not look withered. Withering is a sign that the legumes are old. Legumes keep drying as they age, so purchase only enough to last one month. Older legumes require more cooking liquid and a longer cooking time.

Legumes can also be purchased in canned form. Although the canning process does destroy nutrients, some nutrients can be recovered by using the canning liquid.

Preprocessed legumes are also available. These legumes have already been soaked, which means they will take less time to cook. See Fig. 26-18.

STORING LEGUMES

As with other dry goods, legumes should be stored in a cool, dark, dry place with good ventilation. Keep opened packages of legumes in airtight, moisture-proof containers. Do not store bags of legumes on the floor. Pests may infest them. You should never store dry legumes in the refrigerator or in a humid area. They will begin to absorb moisture immediately and spoil. Legumes need to be protected from heat and light. Vitamin B_6 is found in beans and it is sensitive to light.

COOKING LEGUMES

All legumes must be cooked to be digestible. Cooking makes the nutrients, such as protein, more accessible to the body. The flavor of legumes varies with the product. Some are very flavorful by themselves while others are quite bland and require seasoning. Great Northern beans and Navy beans are examples that require seasoning.

Cooking legumes involves rehydration (ree-HI-dray-shun), the process of adding water back into the legume. Since the beans have been thoroughly dried, they need to become filled with water again. This usually is accomplished in two steps: soaking and simmering.

Fig. 26-18. Legumes can be purchased dried in bulk or canned. When would you use each form in food service?

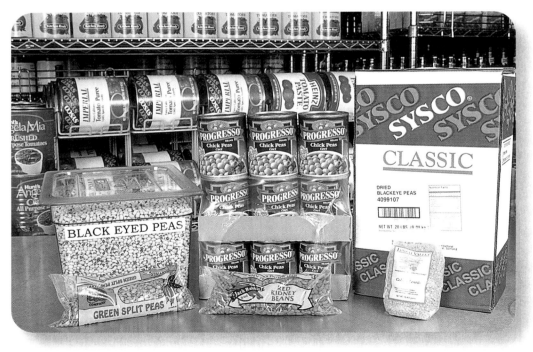

MOISTURE & MOLD IN LEGUMES

The USDA has procedures for detecting toxic, or mold-infected, legumes before food is sold. Once legumes are purchased, it is up to the foodservice operation to keep legumes safe from mold growth.

It is natural for the outside of legumes to host bacteria. However, this can become dangerous at high moisture levels when certain species grow and reproduce. The moisture content of a legume affects how long it remains nutritious and edible in storage. A moisture content of 10% or less is desirable.

Two types of fungi that cause the most concern are the various Aspergillus (as-puhr-JIH-luhs) and Fusarium (foo-sahr-EE-uhm) species of molds. Under certain conditions with some grains, legumes, and nuts, each type of mold can produce a toxic substance called aflatoxin (a-fluh-TAHK-suhn). Aflatoxin is a potent can-cer-causing agent. Once the food is infected, the aflatoxin can't be destroyed. There is no safe way to salvage legumes that have molded. If you discover mold growth, throw away the legumes immediately.

The easiest method to prevent mold growth in legumes is to keep them too dry for mold to grow. Aspergillus and Fusarium molds require moisture to reproduce.

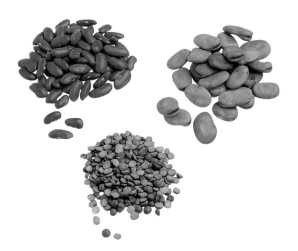

APPLY IT!

To estimate the moisture content in your legumes, try the following experiment.

1. Remove some legumes from the middle of the container in which they are stored.

2. Weigh 20 oz. of legumes and spread them in a large baking dish, not more than an inch deep.

3. Preheat the oven to 180°F. Place the dish in the oven for two hours, stirring occasionally.

4. After two hours, turn the oven off, but keep the dish in the oven until it has cooled.

5. Once cool, reweigh the legumes and compare them to the original weight of 20 oz. If the weight is 1 oz. less than the original weight, then the stored legumes have a moisture content of approximately 5%. If the weight is 2 oz. less, then they have a 10% moisture content.

Checking & Soaking Legumes

Before cooking legumes, you must get everything ready for preparation. Carefully sort through legumes before cooking. See Fig. 26-19. Remove any shriveled or discolored legumes. Also check for objects such as pebbles or stems that might have slipped into the package.

Next, rinse legumes in cold water repeatedly until the water is clear. Most legumes require soaking, but check the package to be sure. In general, the longer legumes soak, the less time they will take to cook. Remove any legumes that float. Insects may have eaten the insides of the legumes. The most efficient way to soak legumes is to leave them overnight in three times their volume of water in the refrigerator. An alternative method is to **quick soak** or soak for 1 hr. in 212°F water.

Simmering Legumes

After preparing the legumes, you will simmer them. Simmering legumes allows the hard, dry peas or beans to slowly reabsorb water. After soaking legumes, follow these general guidelines to cook legumes:

1. Bring the legumes and cooking liquid to a simmer. Simmering times can range from 30 minutes to 3 hours. When legumes are tender, but not too soft, they are ready to be used for food preparation.

2. Test for doneness by tasting a few beans.

☒ STORING COOKED LEGUMES

After legumes have been cooked, allow them to cool before using them. Keep the legumes in the cooking liquid while they cool. This will keep them moist. Use one of the following methods to cool legumes quickly:

- Divide the hot legumes into smaller quantities. Place them into pre-chilled shallow pans and refrigerate. See Fig. 26-20.
- Use an ice bath to bring down the temperature of the food. First divide the food into small, shallow pans. Place the pans in ice water in a sink.
- Use cold paddles, such as Rapid Kool™, that you fill with water and freeze. Stirring legumes with cold paddles will help cool them quickly. Sanitize the paddles every time you use them.

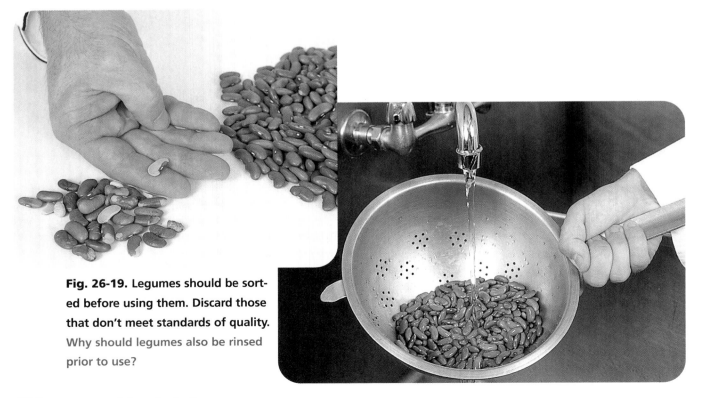

Fig. 26-19. Legumes should be sorted before using them. Discard those that don't meet standards of quality. Why should legumes also be rinsed prior to use?

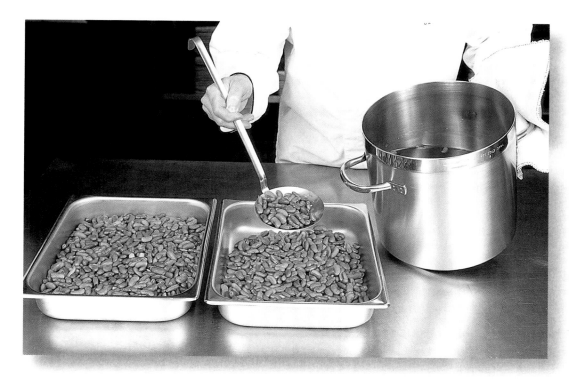

Fig. 26-20. Properly cool cooked legumes for storage. Identify three ways you can cool legumes.

Often, more legumes are prepared than will be used. In this case, cooked legumes can be stored in the refrigerator. You will need to use them within three days. Legumes that won't be used within the three-day period can be frozen. Package the cooked legumes in an airtight, moisture-proof container. To keep them moist, add just enough cooking liquid to cover them. Label the container with the date and contents. Frozen legumes can be stored for six months.

✖ PLATING & SERVING LEGUMES

Legumes can be used in salads, soups, stews, or casseroles. They also can be served alone or with rice. Legumes can also be used as a meat substitute in dishes such as lasagna or chili. For a change of pace, use legumes in place of common side dishes such as mashed potatoes.

SECTION 26-3 Knowledge Check

1. Name five types of legumes.
2. Identify the quality characteristics of legumes.
3. Describe mise en place for legumes.

MINI LAB

Working in teams, prepare and cook legumes. Share your finished product with the other teams. Discuss the results and what other dishes would use these legumes.

SECTION SUMMARIES

26-1 There are eight categories of fruit. Fruits have at least one seed.

26-1 The quality characteristics of each fruit vary with each type of fruit, its season, and its form.

26-1 Fruits are available fresh, canned, frozen, or dried, each requiring different purchasing and storing procedures.

26-1 Fruits can be cooked using either dry or moist cooking methods.

26-2 There are eight classifications of vegetables, or edible plants, including the squash family, roots and tubers, and leafy greens.

26-2 The quality characteristics of vegetables vary with each type. All vegetables are judged on their appearance and the condition they are in when they arrive on the market.

26-2 Vegetables are available fresh, canned, frozen, or dried, each requiring different purchasing and storing procedures.

26-2 By applying the appropriate cooking technique, tender vegetables that are packed with nutrition and taste can be served.

26-3 There are dozens of types of legumes used in a variety of dishes around the world. The most commonly used legumes in food service are navy beans, pinto beans, and lentils.

26-3 Legumes should be brightly colored and uniformly sized. They shouldn't be marked, discolored, shriveled, or broken.

26-3 Legumes can be purchased in bulk form, in cans, or preprocessed and ready to cook.

26-3 Before cooking legumes, they must be soaked in water.

CHECK YOUR KNOWLEDGE

1. Summarize the key quality characteristics for fruit from one of the eight categories.
2. List the nutrients found in fruits.
3. Explain how fresh fruit is graded.
4. How is fresh fruit purchased?
5. What is ethylene gas? How does it affect fruit?
6. What vegetables are also classified as fruits?
7. Name three quality characteristics of potatoes.
8. Describe the USDA grading system for vegetables.
9. How should you store dry legumes? How should you store cooked legumes?
10. What is rehydration?

CRITICAL-THINKING ACTIVITIES

1. You are in charge of selecting and purchasing fruit for your foodservice operation. How do you determine which fruits to buy? How do you know if the fruits meet the standards of quality?
2. Imagine that you've just made garlic mashed potatoes for 20 people, and the entrée is 30 minutes late. How will you keep the potatoes hot until they are served?

WORKPLACE KNOW-HOW

Decision making. Your manager has asked you to store the fruits and vegetables that have just been delivered. Explain how you will store the potatoes, bananas, oranges, tomatoes, leafy greens, frozen corn, and dried split peas.

LAB-BASED ACTIVITY: Cooking Fruits or Vegetables

STEP 1 Working in teams, you will be comparing the results of cooking fruits or vegetables for different lengths of time.

STEP 2 Choose a fruit or vegetable to use for this lab. Some choices might be:

Fruits
- Apples
- Pears
- Blueberries
- Peaches
- Plums
- Cranberries
- Apricots
- Bananas
- Mangos
- Pineapple
- Plantains

Vegetables
- Broccoli
- Green beans
- Spinach
- Carrots
- Cauliflower
- Squash
- Turnip greens
- Green cabbage
- Red cabbage
- Brussels sprouts
- Onions

STEP 3 Create a chart like the one shown below.

STEP 4 Prepare your fruit or vegetable for cooking. Simmer the fruit or vegetable for 10 minutes.

STEP 5 After 10 minutes, remove one serving of the fruit or vegetable to a plate. Allow the remaining fruit or vegetable to continue cooking for another 10 minutes.

STEP 6 Examine this serving of your fruit or vegetable. Record your responses on the chart. Taste the fruit or vegetable and record the flavor changes.

STEP 7 Repeat Step 5 and fill in the chart with your observations.

STEP 8 Repeat Step 6.

STEP 9 Repeat Steps 5 and 6 again.

STEP 10 Answer the following questions:
- What conclusions can you draw as you review your chart?
- Which stage of cooking do you prefer for the doneness of this fruit or vegetable?
- How can length of cooking time and cooking method impact a foodservice operation?

Cooked Fruit or Vegetable Evaluation

Cooking Time	Texture of Fruit or Vegetable	Color of Fruit or Vegetable	Color of Cooking Liquid	Flavor of Fruit or Vegetable
10 minutes				
20 minutes				
30 minutes				

Chefs & Cooks

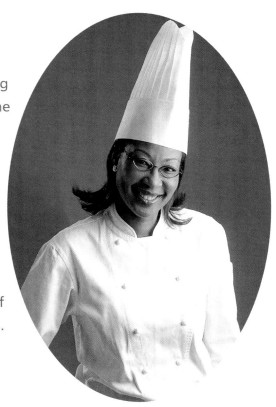

Whether a restaurant prides itself on home-style cooking or international dishes, its chefs and cooks can determine the reputation it will have. Chefs and cooks prepare and cook the food. Depending upon the type and size of the establishment they work for, chefs usually supervise the work of cooks.

Regardless of specialty, chefs and cooks must rely on their judgment and experience as they constantly taste, smell, and season the foods being cooked. They must be able to work independently and as members of a team, under extreme pressure, and in crowded spaces. Chefs and cooks make sure the food tastes good and is visually appealing, always keeping in mind the goal of pleasing the customer.

Executive chefs are highly skilled chefs with years of experience. They have many duties, including hiring and supervising the cooking staff, planning menus, and ordering food.

Sous chefs, also known as area chefs, are in charge of running the kitchen. They assist the executive chef and make sure that the staff is cooking, portioning, and garnishing food properly.

Sauce chefs prepare fish, stews, sautéed dishes, braised or roasted entrées, and sauces.

Garde mangers are cold-food chefs who prepare appetizers, salads, ice carvings, buffets, and cold meat preparations.

Roast cooks specialize in oven-roasted, baked, fried, and grilled items.

Vegetable cooks make pastas, vegetables, and soups.

Pastry chefs are trained in the art of making hot, cold, and frozen desserts and pastries.

Restaurant chefs, also known as line cooks, are responsible for à la carte dishes.

Tournants are cooks who take the place of absent staff members.

In a very large foodservice operation, the following cooks would also be present:

Soup cook, legume cook, fish cook, hors d'oeuvre cook, buffet cook, butcher, preserver cook, grill cook, fry cook, and staff cook.

Working in the Real World...

CAREER PROFILE

KEY SKILLS: In-depth knowledge of the foodservice industry; good eye-hand coordination; team player with good interpersonal and leadership skills; planning and organizational skills.

AVERAGE SALARY: $27,000–$74,000+

EDUCATION/TRAINING: Culinary degree; restaurant experience.

RECOMMENDED SUBJECTS: Food service, nutrition, accounting, and business management.

EMPLOYMENT OPPORTUNITIES:

- Openings will be plentiful through 2012 as the foodservice industry expands.
- Advancement depends on skill, training, and work experience.
- Chefs with supervisory experience may advance to executive chef.

CAREER RESEARCH ACTIVITY

1. Research the working conditions often faced by chefs and cooks. What classes and work experiences would help prepare you to face those working conditions? Present your findings in an oral report.

2. Find a résumé for a garde manger or a sous chef on the Internet. Describe that person's career path to the class.

EXECUTIVE CHEF

I am Kevin Milonzi, former executive chef of the Atomic Grill in Providence, Rhode Island. My pathway toward executive chef started at Johnson & Wales University where I earned a culinary arts degree. After graduation I joined the Atomic Grill staff as a sous chef. I worked hard and was eventually promoted to chef.

At the Atomic Grill, I was responsible for the daily kitchen operation. Scheduling, ordering, and training were just part of my duties. I helped create the restaurant's new **fusion** (FYOO-zhuhn) menu, which uses foods from a variety of cultures. I constantly adapted new ingredients and styles in my kitchen, while communicating these new concepts to the staff.

Running a successful kitchen requires having confidence in your abilities and the ability to build a strong team. Without a kitchen staff that is willing to work toward a common goal, your skills as a chef are meaningless—unless you plan on cooking 300 meals a night by yourself. The keys to team building are training, follow-up, and effective communication.

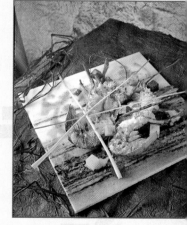

The rewards for being an executive chef are good, but the job requires long hours and working weekends and holidays. However, being an executive chef is a perfect way for me to express creativity, since food makes a perfect palette (pah-luht) for displaying my art.

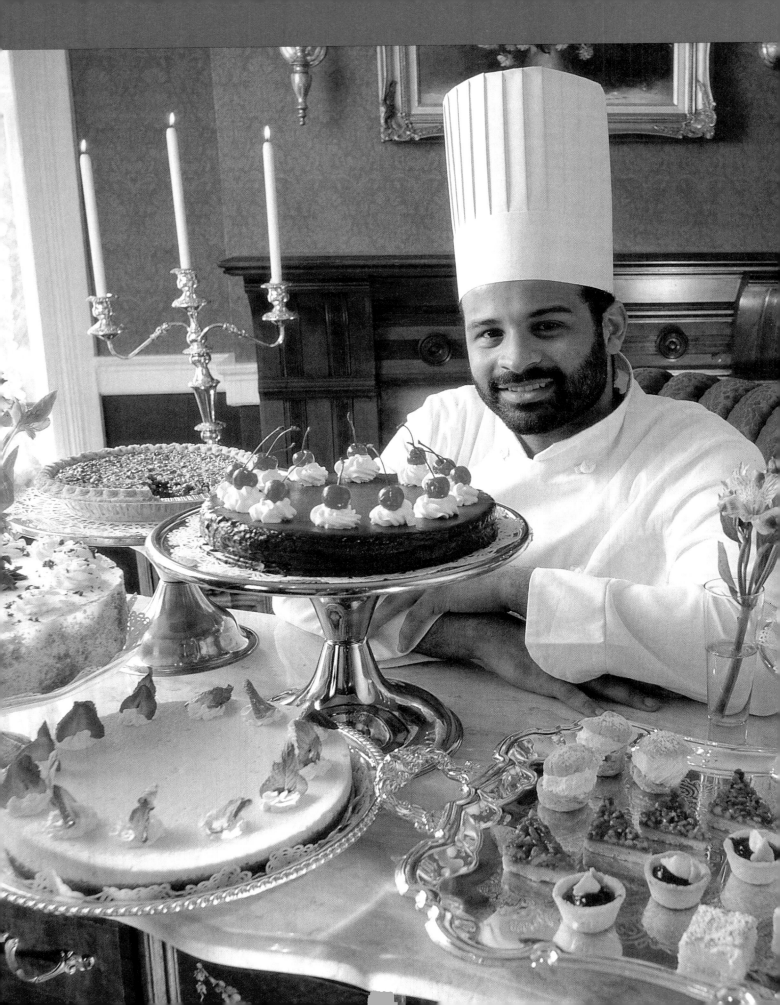

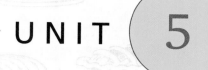

Baking &
Pastry
Applications

Baking Techniques

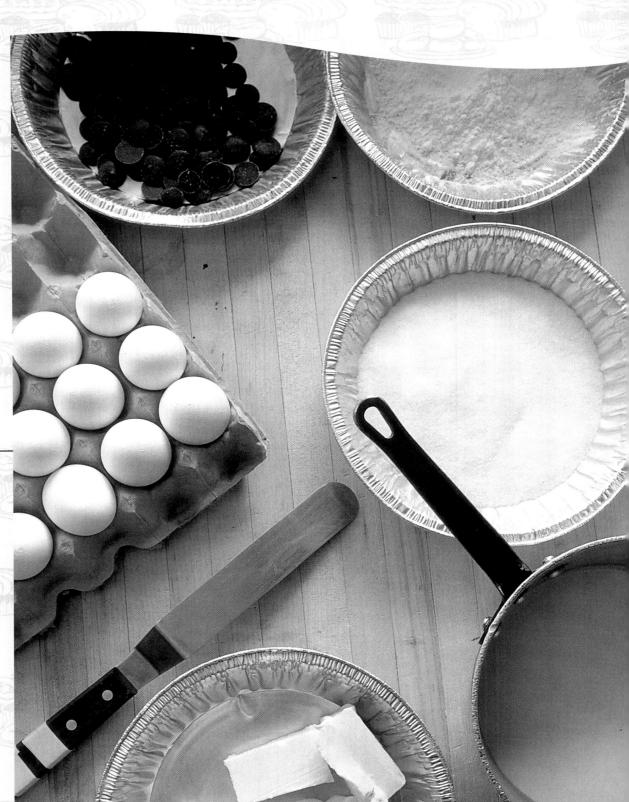

Bakeshop Formulas & Equipment

KEY TERMS

OBJECTIVES

After reading this section, you will be able to:

- Explain baking formulas.
- Contrast volume and weight measurements.
- Use a baker's balance scale.
- Convert a baking formula to a new yield.
- Explain the function of various bakeshop equipment and tools.

KEY TERMS

- formula
- scaling
- baker's percentage
- sheeter
- proofing cabinet
- stack oven
- convection oven
- reel oven
- molds
- rings

BAKING is an exact science that requires precise measuring and accuracy. Baking also requires the use of special baking equipment and smallwares to produce professional products. The type of equipment found in a bakeshop is customized for that particular operation. The size of the operation and how many goods it produces determine the need for specific equipment and tools.

BAKESHOP FORMULAS

Although you may add a dash of this and a pinch of that when you're making a pot of chili, you'll never use such imprecise measurements in a commercial bakeshop. A baker uses a **formula**—a recipe that includes the precise amount of each ingredient. These amounts are often listed as percentages of the total formula. The success of a formula is determined in large part on accurate ingredient measurement and following instructions carefully.

Accuracy is crucial in baking because most baked products are made from the same basic ingredients—flour, water, egg, fat, and a leavening agent. You'll learn more about these ingredients in Section 2 of this chapter. The difference between two baked products often lies in the proportion of each ingredient in the formula. If the proportions are off, you will end up with a different product or an unacceptable product. That's why it's important to read through a formula several times to make certain you understand it. Adding ingredients in the exact order specified in

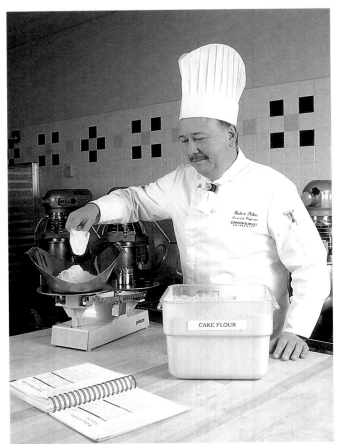

Fig. 27-1. Baking ingredients must be measured accurately and consistently. How can you ensure that your measurements meet these standards?

dients on a balance scale. Bakers refer to weighing as **scaling**. Many of the dry ingredients used in baking, such as flour, are easily and accurately weighed. Liquid ingredients, such as eggs and milk, can also be weighed, but are sometimes measured. Corn syrup, honey, and molasses are always weighed. Measuring ingredients by weight gives consistent, reliable results.

Using a Balance Scale

Professional bakers use a balance scale or a digital electronic scale for measuring. See Fig. 27-2. When you use a balance scale, it must balance before and again after you use it. To use a balance scale, follow these steps:

1. Place the scale scoop or container on the left side of the scale. You can also use waxed paper if the ingredient amount is small.

2. It is important to compensate for the weight of the scoop or container. Do this by placing pound weights on the right side of the scale and adjusting the ounce weights on the horizontal bar until the left and right sides balance.

3. To obtain a specific amount of an ingredient, add weights to the right side of the scale that equal the desired weight of the ingredient. You may have to make adjustments using the scale and the ounce weights on the horizontal bar.

4. Add the ingredient to the scoop, container, or waxed paper on the left side of the scale until the scale is balanced.

the formula is also important for success with baked products. Remember, you can't make adjustments once an item goes into the oven. A baked product's ingredients must be measured accurately from the start. See Fig. 27-1.

✖ BAKESHOP MEASUREMENTS

Bakeshop ingredients are measured by weight or volume. Volume is the space an ingredient occupies. Weight measures the mass or heaviness of something. These two methods of measurement often produce very different results. For example, if a formula calls for 8 oz. of flour, you cannot substitute 1 c. of flour. Assuming that 8 oz. = 1 c. can ruin the final product.

Because accurate and consistent measurement is so important, bakers tend to weigh most ingre-

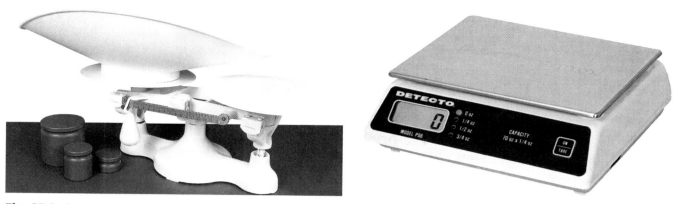

Fig. 27-2. Commercial bakeshops use a balance scale or a digital electronic scale to weigh, or scale, ingredients.

Using Math Skills

Bakers often convert an entire formula to make the desired number of servings. That's why it's important to have good basic math skills. For example, what if a cake formula makes five 8-in. cakes, but your bakery needs to make ten cakes?

Original Formula (Five 8" cakes)		New Formula (Ten 8" Cakes)
2 lbs.	egg whites	4 lbs.
12 oz.	cake flour	1 lb., 8 oz.
12 oz.	confectioners' sugar	1 lb., 8 oz.
¼ oz.	cream of tartar	½ oz.
1 lb., 4 oz.	granulated sugar	2 lbs., 8 oz.
⅛ oz.	salt	¼ oz.
¼ oz.	vanilla extract	½ oz.
⅛ oz.	almond extract	¼ oz.

Notice that the new formula simply doubles each ingredient. That's because you're making ten 8-in. cakes instead of five.

Many professional bakers use formulas that contain percentages. A percentage is a rate or proportion of 100. In other words, if 5% of the eggs are cracked, this means that 5 out of 100 eggs are cracked. Formulas are often expressed in baker's percentages. A **baker's percentage** means that each ingredient is a certain percentage of the weight of the total flour in the formula. The weight of flour is significant because it is the core ingredient of baked goods.

For example, if one kind of flour is used, its weight is 100%. If two kinds of flour are used in a formula, their total weight is 100%. To determine the percentage of each ingredient used in a formula, all ingredients must be expressed in the same unit, such as pounds. Once all the units are the same, the following calculation is used:

$$\frac{\text{weight of ingredient}}{\text{weight of flour}} \times 100\% = \% \text{ of ingredient}$$

For example, you're trying to find the percentage of water used in a formula for bread dough. The formula calls for 15 lbs. of bread flour and 9 lbs. of water. Calculate the percentage as follows:

$$\frac{9 \text{ lb. (weight of water)}}{15 \text{ lb. (weight of flour)}} \times 100\% = 60\% \text{ water}$$

So, the baker's percentage of water is 60%.

Baker's percentages allow you to compare the weight of each ingredient. What is especially convenient about baker's percentages is that one ingredient can be changed without recalculating the percentage for each ingredient. Keep in mind that the total percentages of all the ingredients will always add up to more than 100%.

THE BAKER'S PERCENTAGE

The Baker's percentage allows you to change the yield of a formula without changing the quality of the final product. For example, a formula for Quick Coffee Cake yields 6 lbs. However, you want to prepare 10 lbs. of Quick Coffee Cake. You must first determine the weight of flour for the new yield. You can then use the baker's percentage to calculate the rest of the ingredient amounts.

To determine the weight of flour, follow these steps:

1. Take the total percentage of the original formula. Change it to a decimal by moving the decimal two places to the left.

$$368\% = 3.68$$

2. Convert the new yield to ounces by multiplying by 16 (16 oz. in a pound).

$$10 \text{ lbs. (new yield)} \times 16 \text{ (oz.)} = 160 \text{ oz.}$$

3. Divide the new yield by the decimal figure from Step 1 to determine the weight of the flour. If needed, round the result to the next highest number.

$$160 \text{ (oz.)} \div 3.68 = 43.4 \text{ oz.}$$

So, 43 oz. is the weight of the flour for the new yield. Using this number and the baker's percentages of the original formula, you can determine the weight of the other ingredients. Simply multiply the new flour yield by the baker's percentages to determine the new ingredient amounts.

Quick Coffee Cake

INGREDIENT	AMOUNT	BAKER'S PERCENTAGE
Whole eggs	10 oz.	36%
Vegetable oil	12 oz.	43%
Water	1 lb. 8 oz.	86%
Pastry flour	1 lb. 12 oz.	100%
Baking powder	1 ¼ oz.	4%
Dried milk solids	3 oz.	11%
Salt	½ oz.	2%
Granulated sugar	1 lb. 8 oz.	86%
TOTAL	6 lbs. 6 ¾ oz.	368%

TRY IT!

1. Determine the weight of the remaining ingredients to yield 10 lbs. of Quick Coffee Cake.
2. Convert the formula to yield 15 lbs. of Quick Coffee Cake. First determine the weight of flour; then calculate the other ingredients.

LARGE BAKESHOP EQUIPMENT

Bakeshop equipment is exposed to wet, sticky ingredients and extreme changes in temperature. It's important for bakeshop equipment to be durable and of good quality. It must also be able to withstand the demanding workload and changing temperatures in commercial kitchens.

Mixers

Mixers are essential to every bakeshop and perform a variety of functions. They're used to mix, knead, or whip batters and doughs. The most common mixer in the bakeshop is the bench mixer. See Fig. 27-3. It comes with three basic attachments:

- Spiral dough hook.
- Flat beater or paddle.
- Whip.

There are tabletop, or bench, mixers for small volumes and floor mixers for larger volumes. Mixer capacity ranges from 5–140 quarts. Commercial bakeshops typically use floor models with at least a 30-qt. capacity. These mixers have adapter rings that allow you to use several different-sized bowls on one machine.

Fig. 27-3. A mixer and three attachments.

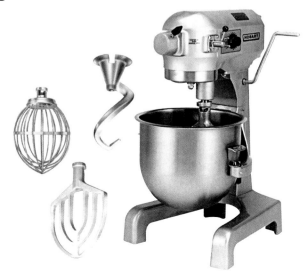

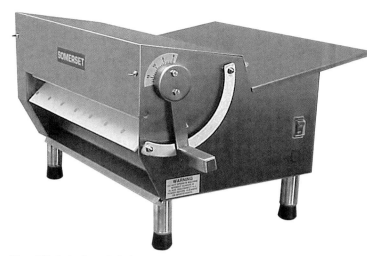

Fig. 27-4. Industrial sheeters are used to roll and fold doughs. What else can a sheeter do?

Sheeter

A **sheeter** is a piece of equipment that rolls out large pieces of dough to a desired thickness. It's used mostly for rolling and folding doughs, such as puff pastries, croissants, and Danish pastries. It also can be used to flatten pie or pizza dough. See Fig. 27-4.

Proofing Cabinets

A **proofing cabinet**, also called a proofer, is a freestanding metal box on wheels that is temperature- and humidity-controlled. It can be used to keep baked products warm or to proof yeast doughs. A proofing cabinet allows dough to rise slowly in a humidity controlled, low-heat environment before baking. See Fig. 27-5.

Bakery Ovens

Commercial ovens are invaluable pieces of equipment in the bakeshop. These ovens are used to produce a large variety of baked products. Both electric and gas models can be equipped with convection fans that circulate the oven's heated air. Some ovens even come with steam injection for proper volume and crust development in bread baking. Certain specialty bread bakers use old-world types of ovens that are brick-lined and fueled by wood.

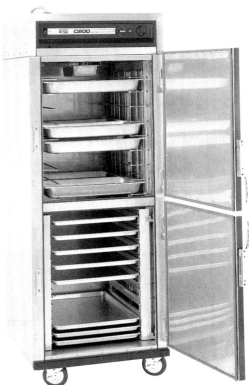

- **Convection oven.** A **convection oven** has a fan that circulates the oven's heated air. This fan allows you to cook foods in about 30% less time and at temperatures approximately 25°–35°F lower than temperatures in a conventional oven. Convection ovens range in size.

- **Reel oven.** With shelves that move or rotate like a Ferris wheel, a **reel oven** is used when all items need the same baking conditions. In other words, a reel oven bakes a quantity of similar items evenly. All items are exposed to the same temperature and humidity.

A reel oven is also called a rotating or revolving oven because its shelves rotate within the oven chamber. Furthermore, the movement of the baked goods creates convection currents similar to those made by a convection fan. Reel ovens are easier to load and unload than deck ovens because you don't have to bend down or reach up.

- **Deck oven.** This freestanding rectangular oven, also known as a **stack oven**, has a series of well-insulated shelves stacked on top of one another. Because each of these shelves has a separate door and temperature control, you can bake a variety of items at once. Deck ovens are used to bake a variety of items. You'll find the deck oven in most bakeries and pizza kitchens. See Fig. 27-6.

Deck ovens offer bakers a great deal of flexibility. Bakers who use such ovens can produce large or small amounts of baked goods because each deck has a separate control. Different products can be baked in each deck due to the separate controls.

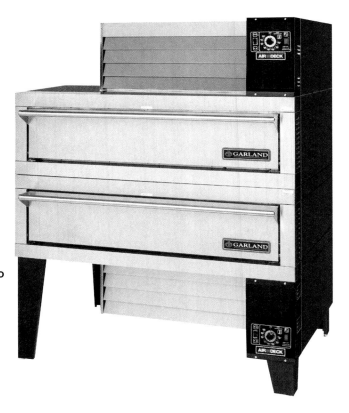

Fig. 27-6. Deck ovens are used in high-volume baking to cook a variety of products at once.

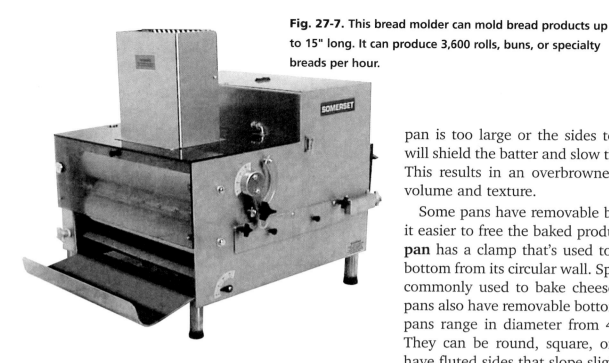

Fig. 27-7. This bread molder can mold bread products up to 15" long. It can produce 3,600 rolls, buns, or specialty breads per hour.

❎ BAKESHOP SMALLWARES

A commercial bakeshop needs various hand tools for cutting, molding, scooping, dividing, and finishing. Many tools are used to form, cut, glaze, and decorate various baked products. Depending on the function of a particular bakeshop, however, the equipment used may vary greatly. See Fig. 27-8 on page 612 (**Baking & Pastry Tools**).

Pans

Bakeshop pans are available in many types, sizes, shapes, and thicknesses. Choosing the correct pan for the job is important because it can affect the final outcome of the product. The surface of a pan will affect the outcome of the product, too. A pan with a shiny surface will reflect some heat away during the baking process so there is less surface browning. A pan with a darker surface tends to retain the heat.

The correct size and shape of baking pan is important in obtaining good texture, height, and appearance. If you put too much batter in a cake pan, the cake will rise and spill over the top. The cake may also collapse. On the other hand, if the pan is too large or the sides too high, the sides will shield the batter and slow the baking process. This results in an overbrowned cake with poor volume and texture.

Some pans have removable bottoms that make it easier to free the baked product. A **springform pan** has a clamp that's used to release the pan's bottom from its circular wall. Springform pans are commonly used to bake cheesecakes. Some tart pans also have removable bottoms. These shallow pans range in diameter from 4½ to 12½ inches. They can be round, square, or rectangular and have fluted sides that slope slightly.

Sheet pans are another common bakeshop pan. These shallow, rectangular pans come in full, half, and quarter sizes and are used to make a variety of baked goods, including rolls, biscuits, cookies, and sheet cakes.

Molds & Rings

Bakeshop molds and rings are also available in a wide variety of types, shapes, sizes, and thicknesses. As with pans, it's important to choose the correct ring or mold for the job. **Molds** are pans with a distinctive shape. They range from small, round, ceramic pans to long, narrow molds used for breads. A soufflé (soo-FLAY) mold, for example, is a round, porcelain mold with a ridged exterior and a smooth interior. It comes in 2- to 3-qt. sizes and as individual, small dishes called ramekins (RAM-uh-kihns). These molds are used to bake soufflés.

Rings are a type of container that have no bottom. They come in various heights and are usually round, but they can also be square. Rings are used to produce round or square breads or baked dessert items.

Fig. 27-9 shows a variety of pans and molds used in the bakeshop. The type of pan, mold, or ring used will depend on the product being prepared in the individual bakeshop.

Baking & Pastry Tools

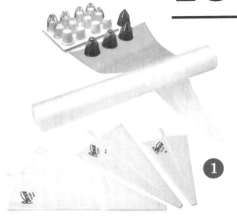

1. Pastry bags

Pastry bags can be made of nylon, plastic-lined cotton, canvas, polyester, or plastic. They are cone-shaped with two open ends. The smaller end is pointed and can be fitted with decorator tips of different sizes and shapes. The larger end can be filled with doughs, fillings, icing, or whipped cream. When the bag is squeezed, the contents are forced through the decorator tip.

2. Pastry brushes

These flat-edged brushes are used to brush liquids such as butter on dough before, during, or after cooking.

3. Pastry pattern cutters

Pastry pattern cutters are used to cut dough into specific shapes.

4. Bench scraper

Also called a dough cutter, this handheld rectangular tool has a stainless steel blade and a handle made of slip-resistant plastic or wood. The bench scraper can be used to clean and scrape surfaces and to cut and portion dough.

5. Rolling pins

This long, cylindrical tool is used to roll out bread and pastry doughs and shape cookies. The bakers' rolling pin is made from hardwood and has handles on each side. The French rolling pin is also made from hardwood, but does not have handles. Rolling pins should not be submerged in water for cleaning.

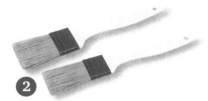

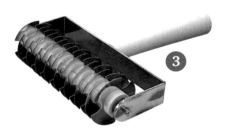

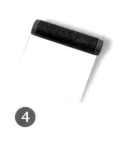

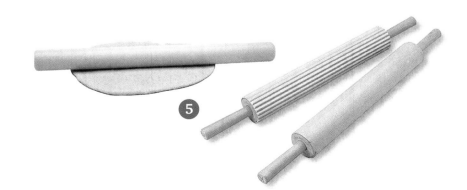

Fig. 27-9.

Pans & Molds

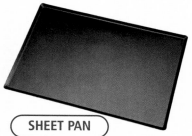
SHEET PAN

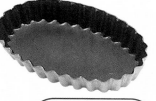
SOUFFLÉ MOLD

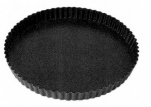
FLUTED, OBLONG TART PAN

TART PAN

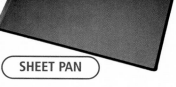

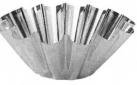
BRIOCHE PAN

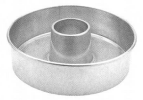
TUBE PAN

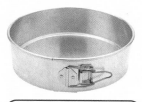
SPRINGFORM PAN

RAMEKIN

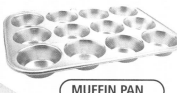
MUFFIN PAN

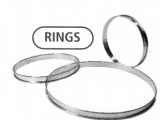
RINGS

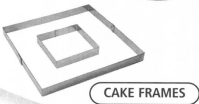
CAKE FRAMES

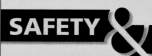

SAFETY & SANITATION

SANITIZING PASTRY BAGS—If you're using a non-disposable pastry bag, wash the bag in warm, soapy water after each use. To do this, remove the decorator tip, and turn the bag inside out. Wash both the bag and tip thoroughly. Then rinse and sanitize them. Stretch and hang the bag to let it air dry.

SECTION 27-1 Knowledge Check

1. Explain why accurate measurement is so important in baking.
2. Describe how a sheeter is used.
3. Explain how a pan's surface affects the outcome of the baked product.

MINI LAB

Weigh 2 lbs. of flour, 16 oz. of sugar, and 2 oz. of yeast using a balance scale. Then measure 32 oz. of water using a volume measure.

SECTION 27-2

Bakeshop Ingredients

KEY TERMS

- gluten
- crumb
- staling
- shortening
- hydrogenation
- leavening agent
- fermentation
- extracts
- batter
- dough

OBJECTIVES

After reading this section, you will be able to:

- Explain the importance of using exact ingredients.
- Identify the different categories of ingredients and their roles in the baking process.
- Explain the role of flavorings, chocolate and cocoa, additives, and nuts in baking.
- List techniques used to mix batters and doughs.
- Describe the impact of carryover baking.

FLOUR, fat, sugar, milk, eggs, flavorings—from this simple list of ingredients, you can make an endless variety of baked products. Ingredients are more than just parts of a baking formula. They add flavor, texture, and visual appeal to all types of baked products. In this section, you will learn about basic baking ingredients and mixing techniques.

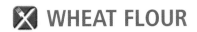

✖ USING EXACT INGREDIENTS

Baking, unlike cooking, leaves little margin for error. You can't just substitute the same amount of cake flour for bread flour and expect to come up with the same end result. To become a successful baker, you must understand how key ingredients work together. Baking formulas have been developed using exact types of ingredients. If the formula is not followed precisely, the product's texture and taste will be affected.

✖ WHEAT FLOUR

Wheat flour is the main ingredient in many baked goods. The proteins and starch in flour give these products structure. The classification of flour is based on the type of wheat it comes from—soft or hard. Hard wheat flour comes from kernels that are firm, tough, and difficult to cut. Bread flour is one type of hard wheat flour.

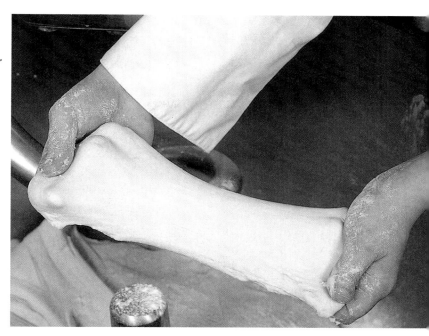

Fig. 27-10. Gluten gives dough its stretchiness, allowing it to be pulled and shaped. What other benefits does gluten give to dough?

Hard wheat has a high protein content. When wheat flour is mixed with water, certain proteins form **gluten**, a firm, elastic substance that affects the texture of baked products. The higher a flour's protein content, the more potential it has to form gluten. See Fig. 27-10.

Gluten is the substance that makes bread dough strong and elastic. Without gluten, you couldn't stretch the dough and hold in the gases that make it rise. The dough would collapse, resulting in poor volume and a coarse crumb. **Crumb** is the internal texture of a baked product.

Soft wheat flour, such as cake flour and pastry flour, comes from a soft wheat kernel. This type of flour has a low protein content, making it ideal for tender baked products such as cookies and pastries. Bread flour, cake flour, and pastry flour are all types of wheat flour.

- **Bread flour.** Bread flour is used for breadmaking. It has a high gluten-forming protein content. These proteins allow the bread to rise fully and develop a fine crumb. They also give the bread a chewier, firmer texture. Bread flour is used to make yeast breads, pizza, and bagels.

- **Cake flour.** Cake flour is lower in protein than bread flour and pastry flour. Cake flour produces a softer and more tender product than bread flour. Cake flour is bleached with chlorine (KLOR-EEN) to help produce a fine, white crumb in cakes.

- **Pastry flour.** The protein content of pastry flour is between that of bread flour and cake flour. It is used in pie dough, cookies, muffins, and quick breads. It is used for cakes only if cake flour is unavailable.

Other types of flours used in the bakeshop are listed in Fig. 27-11 on page 616.

LIQUIDS

Liquids are an essential part of baking. The most common liquids used in baking are water, milk, and cream. Liquids can also be found in eggs, sugar syrups, and butter, which contains about 15% water.

Accurate measurement of liquids is important because too much or too little can affect the outcome of the baked product. For example, adding too much water in pie dough will cause excess gluten formation, which may result in a tough texture.

- **Water.** Water is the most common liquid ingredient used in baking, especially for breads. It has many uses besides moistening dry ingredients. Water is necessary for gluten structure to form in flour. Also, water temperature is used to adjust temperatures. This applies to bread dough in particular, where dough temperature is important. Because water is tasteless, odorless, and colorless, it doesn't affect the flavor or color of baked products. It also adds no fat or calories.

- **Milk and cream.** Milk is another important liquid ingredient. Its protein, fat, and sugar content make it a valuable addition to baked products, ice creams, and custards. Milk also improves the flavor and texture of bread and other baked goods.

Fig. 27-11.

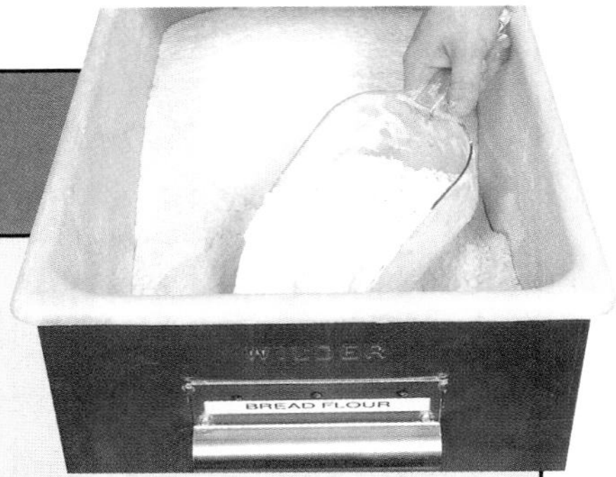

OTHER TYPES OF FLOUR	CHARACTERISTICS
Whole wheat flour	• Dark flour made from whole wheat grains. Only the outer hull is removed. • Fine or coarse ground. • May be combined with bread flour or all-purpose flour for better volume and milder flavor. • High protein, but moderate gluten content. • Often combined with bread flour for better gluten structure in breads.
Cracked wheat flour	• Dark flour made from cut, not ground, whole wheat grains. • Usually soaked or partially cooked before adding to dough in order to soften the flour. • Must be mixed with bread flour or whole wheat flour when used in baked goods.
Non-wheat flours	• Whole or milled flours made from corn, rye, barley, buckwheat, oat, and other grains as well as from potatoes and soybeans. • Varying colors, textures, and gluten levels. • Usually mixed with bread flour to provide a better gluten structure.

Some of these improvements include:
- Yielding a soft, rather than crispy, crust on items such as cream puffs or éclairs (ay-KLARES).
- Adding more color or flavor to crusts when applied to the surface of the baked product.
- Extending shelf life by delaying staling. **Staling** is the process by which moisture is lost, causing a change in the texture and aroma of food. Staling causes the crumb to be dry and the crust to become soft and moist.

Dried milk solids are also used in baked goods. Since milkfat can reduce milk's shelf life, dried milk solids are usually purchased as nonfat dry milk. Nonfat dry milk can be reconstituted with water or used dry. If kept dry, it is easier to use and can be stored without refrigeration. You can sift it with dry ingredients or mix it with shortening, before adding the water separately.

Dairy products such as buttermilk, yogurt, and sour cream are also used in the bakeshop. These products contain live bacteria that convert milk sugar into acid. The acid in buttermilk, for example, provides a whiter, more tender crumb in biscuits. See Fig. 27-12.

Another common dairy product, heavy cream, has a high fat content. This fat content allows it to tenderize baked goods. Cream is often whipped for toppings, chilled desserts, and fillings such as pastry cream. It's used as a liquid ingredient in custards, sauces, and ice creams. You will learn more about desserts in Chapter 30.

FATS

During the baking process, fats surround the flour particles and prevent long strands of gluten from forming. This tenderizes the baked good. Fats also add to the flavor, moistness, browning, flakiness, and leavening, depending on the type of fat. In baking, solid fats are referred to as **shortening**. Purified oils are made solid by a process called hydrogenation. **Hydrogenation**

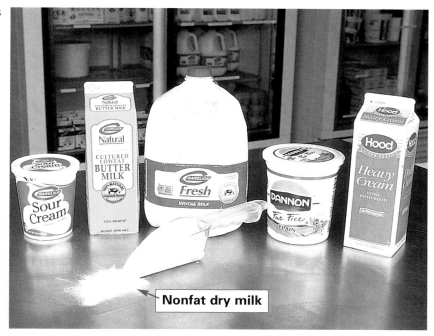

Fig. 27-12. Milk and other dairy products help tenderize baked goods.

Nonfat dry milk

(hy-drah-juh-NAY-shuhn) involves making oils solid by the addition of hydrogen to the oil. The most common types of fat used in the bakeshop include all-purpose shortening, emulsified shortening, oil, butter, and margarine. See Fig. 27-13.

■ **Vegetable shortening.** When most people hear the word "shortening," they think of a solid, white, flavorless fat used for baking. This type of shortening, known as vegetable shortening, is made from purified oils that have been hydrogenated to make them solid and less likely to become rancid. Vegetable shortening has a fairly high melting point, which makes it ideal for forming flaky pie doughs. It is also a good choice for frying and for making cookies and cakes.

■ **Emulsified shortening.** Some shortenings contain emulsifiers. Emulsified shortenings are also called high-ratio shortenings because they allow the baker to add a high ratio of water—and sugar—to a cake or icing. Some high-ratio shortenings look like all-purpose shortenings.

High-ratio liquid shortenings look like creamy oils. Some cake formulas are designed to use high-ratio liquid shortenings. These cakes will be extra moist, airy, and tender and will have a longer shelf life than cakes made with other fats. Other fats cannot replace high-ratio liquid shortenings because of their unique characteristics.

■ **Oil.** Oils are fats extracted from plants such as soybeans, corn, peanuts, and cottonseed. They are liquid at room temperature and neutral in flavor and color because they are highly refined. Because oil blends more easily throughout a mixture, it can coat more strands of gluten. Therefore, oil causes baked products to be more tender. Oil is used in quick breads, some pie crusts, deep-fried products like doughnuts, and rich sponge cakes like chiffon (shi-FAWN).

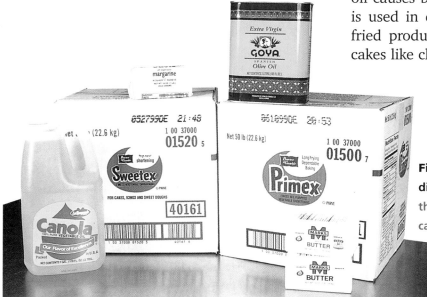

Fig. 27-13. Commercial bakeshops use many different types of fats in baking. Which of these fats might be used to make moist, airy cakes with a long shelf life?

■ **Butter.** Have you ever tasted a frosting that seemed to melt in your mouth? That frosting was probably made with butter. Butter can be purchased with or without salt. Unsalted butter is used in baking because of its pleasant flavor. Because butter is soft at room temperature, however, doughs made with butter are sometimes hard to handle. Butter is only 80% fat, so it produces a less tender baked product than shortening.

■ **Margarine.** Margarine is typically a hydrogenated vegetable oil with color, flavor, and water added. Margarines have improved over the years. While they cannot match butter's superior flavor, they are less likely to spoil and are usually lower in saturated fat. Margarines can be purchased either salted or unsalted.

⊠ SUGARS & SWEETENERS

Sugars and sweeteners add a sweet, pleasant flavor to baked products. Flavor, however, is not their only contribution to baking. The other functions of sugars and sweeteners include:

- Creating a golden-brown color.
- Stabilizing mixtures such as beaten egg whites for meringue (muh-RANG).
- Providing food for yeast in yeast breads.
- Retaining moisture for a longer shelf life.
- Tenderizing baked products by weakening the gluten strands and delaying the action of other structure builders such as egg protein.
- Serving as a base for making icings.

Refined Sugars & Sweeteners

Sugar is produced from sugarcane or sugar beets. The cane or beet is crushed to extract the juice. The juice is then filtered and gently heated to evaporate the water. Through a series of heat-induced steps, the sugar is crystallized (KRIST-uh-lized), or turned into crystals, and separated from the dark, thick molasses that forms. It must be refined to produce sugar grains of various sizes. Various sugars and sweeteners are used in the bakeshop. See Fig. 27-14.

■ **Molasses.** Molasses is the thick, sweet, dark liquid made from sugarcane juice. There are many grades of molasses available. Premium grades have a golden-brown color and a mild, sweet flavor. Lower grades are typically darker in color with a less sweet, stronger flavor. This stronger color and flavor is often desirable in baked products.

■ **Brown sugar.** Brown sugar is a soft-textured mixture of white sugar and molasses. It can be light or dark in color. Store brown sugar in airtight containers to prevent moisture absorption.

■ **Turbinado sugar.** Turbinado sugar is raw sugar that has been steam-cleaned. Its coarse crystals are blond colored and have a delicate molasses flavor. Turbinado sugar is used in some baked products and beverages.

Fig. 27-14. Many different types of sugars are used in baking. Try to identify each type of sugar shown here.

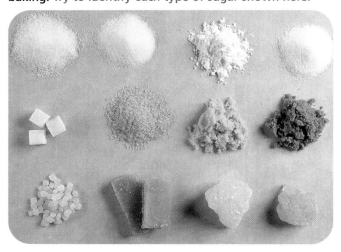

- **Coarse sugar.** Coarse sugar, also known as sanding sugar, consists of large, coarse crystals that don't dissolve easily. It's used to decorate items such as doughnuts or cakes.
- **Granulated sugar.** Regular granulated sugar is often referred to as extrafine white sugar or table sugar. It is the most common sugar used in the bakeshop. Granulated sugar is used in cooked icings, candies, and other baked products.
- **Confectioners' sugar.** Confectioners' sugar, also known as powdered sugar, is granulated sugar that has been crushed into a fine powder. Confectioners' sugar also contains about 3% cornstarch, which helps keep the sugar from clumping. It is often used in uncooked icings and glazes and as a decorative "dusting" on baked products.
- **Superfine sugar.** Superfine sugar is more finely granulated than regular white sugar. As a result, it dissolves almost instantly. Superfine sugar is perfect for making sweetened cold liquids and egg white meringues less gritty. Meringues can be used for such items as toppings on pies.
- **Corn syrup.** Corn syrup is produced from the starch found in corn. The starch granules are removed from corn kernels and treated with acids or enzymes to create a thick, sweet syrup. Light corn syrup has no color, while dark corn syrup has a molasses-like flavor. Corn syrup does not crystallize easily, so it is a popular ingredient in frostings, candies, jams, and jellies.
- **Maple syrup.** Maple syrup adds a unique flavor to baked products. It is made from the sap of a maple tree. Syrups are graded according to their color and flavor. The lighter and milder the syrup, the higher grade it will receive.
- **Honey.** Honey is a thick, sweet liquid made by bees from flower nectar (NECK-tur). The type of flower affects the final flavor and color of the honey. Honey is widely used to give baked products a distinct, sweet flavor. It should be stored in a cool, dry place. Refrigerated honey will crystallize and form a gooey mass. If this happens, the honey can be heated in the microwave in small amounts or in a pan of hot water over low heat.

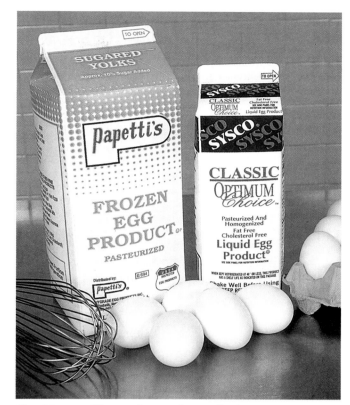

Fig. 27-15. Different forms of eggs fit the varying needs of commercial bakeshops.

✖ EGGS

Eggs are the second most important ingredient in baked products. Eggs come in a variety of sizes. Formulas listing the amount of eggs by number instead of weight have based the formula on large eggs, which weigh about 2 oz. each.

Commercial bakeshops use egg yolks instead of whole eggs when a richer, more tender product is desired. They also use egg whites in place of whole eggs when baking low-fat products.

Forms of Eggs

Shell eggs and egg products, such as liquid frozen eggs, dried eggs, and liquid refrigerated eggs, are used in baking. Egg products can be purchased as whole eggs, egg whites, or egg yolks. See Fig. 27-15.

■ **Shell eggs.** Shell eggs are eggs sold in their shells. They are often called fresh eggs. If stored properly at 41°F or below, they will last up to four weeks beyond the packing date. Shell eggs are purchased in flats, each of which holds 2½ dozen, or 30 eggs. There are twelve flats in a case, meaning that one case contains 30 dozen or 360 eggs.

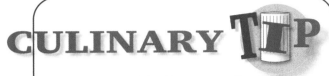

EGG FRESHNESS—You can tell whether an egg is fresh by putting the whole egg in a glass of water. If it floats, the egg is old.

■ **Egg products.** Egg products are eggs that have been broken, removed from the shell, and pasteurized. The whites can be separated from the yolks, and additives included if necessary. For example, frozen egg yolks have 10% sugar added to prevent them from gelling. The egg products are then packaged and refrigerated, frozen, or dried and packed in pouches.

Egg products are popular because of their convenience. They can be substituted for shell eggs in many baked products. Frozen egg products must be thawed in the refrigerator, so plan ahead when using them. Do not let them sit at room temperature, as egg products are highly perishable. Dried eggs are often used in prepared mixes such as for cakes. High-quality, dried egg whites are often preferred for making meringues over liquid egg whites because they are more stable.

Functions of Eggs

Eggs serve a variety of functions during the baking process. These functions include:

- **Structure.** Because of their protein content, eggs give structure to baked products such as cakes. They also help thicken some products such as custard sauces.
- **Emulsification** (i-MUHL-suh-fuh-KAY-shun). Egg yolks have natural emulsifiers that help blend ingredients smoothly.

- **Aeration** (AR-AY-shun). Beaten or whipped eggs assist in leavening because they trap air that expands when heated, causing baked products to rise.
- **Flavor.** Eggs add a distinct flavor to baked goods.
- **Color.** Egg yolks add a rich, yellow color to baked products. Eggs also add color to crusts during the browning process.

❌ LEAVENING AGENTS

A **leavening agent** is a substance that causes a baked good to rise by introducing carbon dioxide (CO_2) or other gases into the mixture. The gases expand from the heat of the oven, stretching the cell walls in the baked product. The end result is a light, tender texture and good volume. The main leavening agents are air, steam, baking soda, baking powder, and yeast.

Air

Air is an important leavening agent in all baked products since air is added during the mixing process. Angel food cake is a good example of a baked product that relies on air as a leavening agent. You can add air to a mixture by whipping egg whites. See Fig. 27-16.

Steam

Steam is another important leavening agent. It is created during the baking process when water evaporates to steam and expands. Because water in one form or another is in all baked products, steam is an important leavening gas. It is especially important to items such as puff pastries and croissants.

Baking Soda

Baking soda, or sodium bicarbonate (SO-dee-um by-CAR-buh-nate), is a chemical leavening agent that must be used with acid to give off CO_2 gas. There are many sources of acid used in bak-

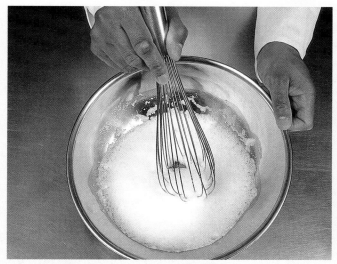
When whisking light mixtures, hold the whisk like a pencil, with the balloon end pointing away from you.

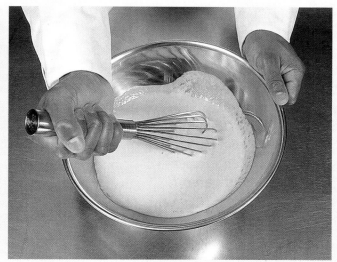
When whisking heavier mixtures, it is less tiring if you hold the whisk with the balloon end facing you, slightly bending the wrist.

Fig. 27-16. Air is incorporated into a mixture through physical means. How does air affect the item's texture and volume?

ing, such as buttermilk, sour cream, and yogurt; fruits and fruit juices; most syrups, including honey and molasses; and chocolate. The CO_2 gas is what causes the baked products to rise. Mix baking soda thoroughly, or it will leave an unpleasant aftertaste.

Baking Powder

Baking powder is made up of baking soda, an acid such as cream of tartar, and a moisture-absorber such as corn starch. When mixed with a liquid, baking powder releases CO_2. The type used in the bakeshop is double-acting. This means that when it first comes in contact with moisture, it gives off CO_2. When it comes into contact with heat, it gives off more CO_2. Double-acting baking powder can be fast- or slow-acting. Fast-acting varieties react more quickly when mixed with liquids. The slow-acting varieties require more heat to release CO_2. Baking powder is used as a leavening agent in cakes, cookies, muffins, and quick breads.

Yeast

Yeast is a living organism. During a process called **fermentation** (FUR-mun-TAY-shun), yeast breaks down sugars into carbon dioxide gas and alcohol, which are necessary for the rising process in products such as bread. Yeast products get their distinctive aroma and flavor from this process. The types of yeast most commonly used in bakeshops are compressed yeast, dry active yeast, and quick-rise dry yeast. See Fig. 27-17.

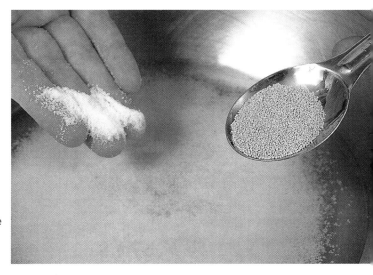

Fig. 27-17. Commercial bakeshops use different types of yeast to cause baked goods to rise. Describe how to activate the following types of yeast: compressed, dry active, quick-rise dry.

- **Compressed yeast.** Sometimes called fresh or wet compressed yeast, this type of yeast is moist and must be refrigerated. Compressed yeast is available in 0.6-oz. cubes or 2-lb. blocks. It should be creamy white, have a crumbly texture, and smell like freshly baked bread. To use compressed fresh yeast, crumble it into warm water. Don't use compressed yeast that looks brown, feels slimy, or smells sour. Compressed yeast rapidly deteriorates at room temperature.

- **Dry active yeast.** Dry yeast has had most of its moisture removed by hot air, which leaves granules of dormant yeast that are "asleep." Dry yeast must be reactivated in liquid that is between 100°F and 110°F before being added to other ingredients. Dry active yeast is available in ¼-oz. packets, 4-oz. jars, or 1- to 2-lb. vacuum-sealed bags. Unopened packages can be stored in a cool, dry place for several months. Once opened, containers of dry active yeast should be kept frozen. When substituting active dry yeast for compressed yeast, use 50% less than called for in the formula.

- **Quick-rise dry yeast.** Also called instant yeast, quick-rise dry yeast is similar in appearance to dry active yeast. However, its leavening action is much quicker, speeding the rising of dough. Quick-rise dry yeast provides closer results to compressed yeast. To use quick-rise dry yeast, blend it with the dry ingredients. Then add water that is between 100°F and 110°F to activate the yeast. Quick-rise dry yeast lasts at least one year in unopened packages or when stored frozen.

Fig. 27-18.

SPICES	USES IN THE BAKESHOP
Allspice	Used in cakes and puddings; allspice is the dried, unripe berry of a tropical tree; available whole or ground; combines flavors of cinnamon, nutmeg, and cloves.
Anise	Used in cakes, cookies, and candies; anise is the dried seed of a plant; available whole or ground; licoricelike flavor.
Cardamom	Used in pastries and baked goods; cardamom is the seed of a native Indian herb; available whole or ground; sweet, peppery flavor.
Cinnamon	Used in cakes, cookies, pies, breads, and desserts; cinnamon is the thin, dried inner bark of an evergreen tree; available ground or in sticks; warm, spicy flavor.
Cloves	Used in baked goods such as breads and pies; cloves are the dried flower buds of an evergreen tree; available whole or ground; warm, spicy flavor.
Ginger	Used in baked goods such as cookies and cakes; ginger is the root of a tropical plant; available dried or fresh; sweet, peppery flavor.
Nutmeg	Used in custards, pies, breads, and other baked goods; nutmeg is the kernel or seed of the fruit of an evergreen tree; available whole or ground; sweet, warm, spicy flavor.
Poppy Seed	Used in breads, rolls, and other baked goods; poppy seed is the dried, ripened seed of a Middle-Eastern plant; nutty flavor.

Salt

Salt also has an important role in baking. It enhances the product through its own flavor as well as bringing out the flavor of other ingredients. Salt also acts on gluten and results in an acceptable texture. A certain amount of salt is also necessary to slow down or control fermentation in yeast products. However, salt can negatively react in baked goods if it is not measured accurately or if it is added at the wrong point in the mixing process.

✖ FLAVORINGS

Flavorings include extracts and spices. Although flavorings don't usually influence the baking process, they do enhance the flavor of the final baked product.

- **Extracts. Extracts** are liquid flavorings that contain alcohol. They are mostly concentrated, volatile oils or essences diluted with alcohol. Vanilla extract is the exception. It is made by passing alcohol through the vanilla bean, with little or no heat, to extract flavor.
- **Spices.** Spices add to the enhancement of food and baked goods by adding flavor, color, or aroma. Most spices come from the bark, roots, flower buds, berries, or seeds of aromatic plants or trees. While not commonly thought of as spices, coffee beans and vanilla pods also fall into this category. Citrus zest, or the outer skin of oranges, lemons, and limes, is considered a spice, too.

Ground spices release their flavor quickly and are often purchased in quantities that can be used within three months. The flavor of whole spices comes out over long cooking periods such as those used in baking. Spices should be used carefully so they don't overpower the food. The spices used frequently in the bakeshop are listed in Fig. 27-18. For more information on spices, see Chapter 16.

✖ CHOCOLATE & COCOA

Chocolate and cocoa add body, bulk, and a unique color and flavor to a wide variety of baked products. Both items are made from the cacao (cuh-CAY-oh) bean. The "meat" of the cacao bean is roasted and ground into a thick substance called chocolate liquor. Cocoa butter is a by-product of cocoa powder production. More steps are then taken to create a variety of chocolate or cocoa products. The most common varieties in the bakeshop are unsweetened chocolate, semisweet chocolate, liquid chocolate, cocoa powder, and Dutch-process cocoa powder. See Fig. 27-19.

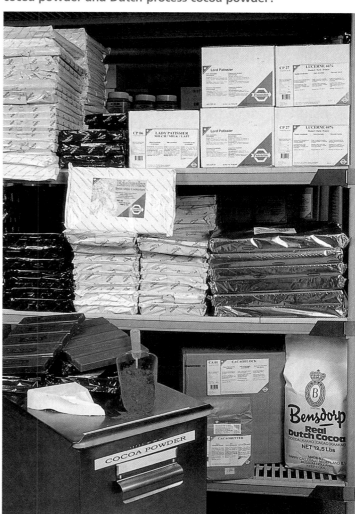

Fig. 27-19. All varieties of chocolate and cocoa come from the cacao bean. What is the difference between cocoa powder and Dutch-process cocoa powder?

■ **Unsweetened chocolate.** This form of chocolate is also known as bitter or baking chocolate. It is the pure, hardened substance that results from roasted and ground cacao beans. Unsweetened chocolate has no added sugar or milk solids. It is bitter because it contains no sugar. Unsweetened chocolate gives baked products an especially rich taste because it still contains all of the cocoa butter from the bean.

■ **Semisweet chocolate.** Sugar, lecithin (LEH-suh-thun), and vanilla are added to create semisweet or bittersweet chocolate. Semisweet chocolate is often used in chocolate chip cookies and glazes.

■ **White chocolate.** White chocolate is made from cocoa butter, sugar, vanilla, lecithin, and dried or condensed milk. There is no chocolate liquor in white chocolate.

■ **Cocoa powder.** This is the dry, brown powder that remains once the cocoa butter is removed from the chocolate liquor. It is used mostly in baking and has no added sweeteners or flavorings. Cocoa powder absorbs moisture and provides structure, as does flour.

■ **Dutch-process cocoa powder.** This type of cocoa has a darker color and milder flavor than regular cocoa. It is less likely to lump and produces a milder, smoother chocolate flavor. Dutch-process cocoa can be substituted for unsweetened chocolate when adjustments are made to the amount of cocoa and shortening used.

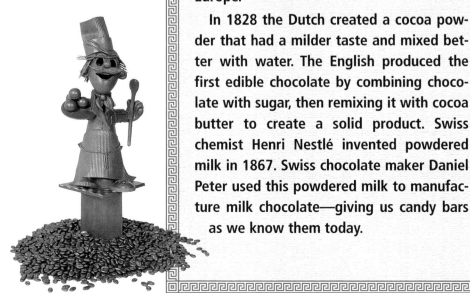

a LINK to the Past

CHOCOLATE

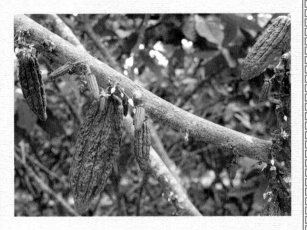

Whether it appears in cookies, candy, or drinks, chocolate is one of the world's favorite foods. It probably comes as no surprise to you that America leads the world in chocolate consumption.

Chocolate and cocoa come from the fruit of the cacao tree. For many years cocoa was used to make hot chocolate—but only by those who could afford it. As domestic cultivation of the cacao tree grew, prices fell and hot chocolate was enjoyed throughout Europe.

In 1828 the Dutch created a cocoa powder that had a milder taste and mixed better with water. The English produced the first edible chocolate by combining chocolate with sugar, then remixing it with cocoa butter to create a solid product. Swiss chemist Henri Nestlé invented powdered milk in 1867. Swiss chocolate maker Daniel Peter used this powdered milk to manufacture milk chocolate—giving us candy bars as we know them today.

Fig. 27-20.

ADDITIVE	FOOD ITEMS	PURPOSE
Thiamin Niacin Riboflavin Iron	• Flours, breads	• Nutrients
Beta carotene Red No. 3 Green No. 3 Yellow No. 6	• Margarine • Candies • Various baked products	• Coloring agents
Lecithin	• Chocolate, baked products, margarine	• Emulsifier
Carrageenan Pectin Modified starches	• Ice cream, cream cheese, sherbets, fruit fillings, puddings, pie fillings	• Thickeners and stabilizers
Glycerine	• Cake icings	• Humectant (used to retain moisture and keep foods soft)
Chlorine Potassium bromate Benzoyl peroxide Ascorbic acid	• Cake flour • Bread flour • All flour • Bread flour	• Bleaching and maturing agents
Sodium bicarbonate Potassium carbonate	• Baking powder • Dutch-processed cocoa powder	• Acids, alkalis, and buffers (used to adjust and control acidity or alkalinity)
Gum and starch derivatives	• Frozen desserts	• Fat replacers
Polydextrose	• Baked products, puddings	• Bulking agent (used to provide texture and body in reduced-fat goods)

ADDITIVES

Additives are used in the bakeshop to color, thicken, provide texture in, and replace fat in baked products. See Fig. 27-20 for a list of common additives used in the bakeshop.

NUTS

Nuts are often used to provide flavor, texture, and color in baked products. Fig. 27-21 shows the nuts most commonly used in commercial bakeshops. For more information on nuts, see Chapter 16.

Fig. 27-21.

NUTS	USES IN BAKING
Almonds	Used in breads, cakes, pastries, marzipan, and as decorations; sweet almonds are eaten, bitter almonds are used as a source of flavorings and extracts; available whole, slivered, ground, sliced, and in flour or meal form.
Chestnuts	Used to flavor buttercreams and fillings, and as a decoration for cakes and cookies; sweet flavor; available dried, chopped, and canned as a paste.
Coconuts	Used in cakes, cookies, pies, and desserts; available grated or flaked and may be sweetened or unsweetened; desiccated (de-si-KATE-ed) coconut is dried, unsweetened coconut that has been ground to a fine meal.
Hazelnuts	Also known as filberts; used in candies, baked goods, and desserts; can be made into a paste for flavoring buttercreams and fillings; available whole in the shell, whole shelled, or chopped.
Macadamia Nuts	Used in cakes, cookies, and ice creams; smooth, buttery flavor; available roasted and salted; very expensive.
Peanuts	Used in pastries and candies, such as peanut brittle; often combined with chocolate creations; available raw, dry roasted, in granules.
Pecans	Used in pies, breads, and desserts; mild and sweet flavor; available shelled in halves or pieces; expensive, but other nuts can easily be substituted.
Pine Nuts	Used in breads, cookies, and pastry; available raw or toasted; resemble almonds in flavor.
Pistachios	Used in cakes, pastries, and to flavor buttercreams and ice creams; mild flavor and fine texture; available shelled, roasted, and salted.
Walnuts	Used in cookies, brownies, cakes, muffins, and ice creams; available in halves, which are mostly used for decoration, and pieces.

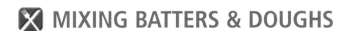 MIXING BATTERS & DOUGHS

Batters and doughs are formed when the dry and liquid ingredients are combined to create baked products. **Batters** contain almost equal parts of dry and liquid ingredients. Batters are usually easy to pour. Cakes and muffins are examples of baked products made from batters.

Doughs contain less liquid than batters, making it easy to work doughs with your hands. Doughs may even be stiff enough to be cut into shapes. Many types of breads are made from dough. There are a variety of ways to mix batters and doughs. Nine ways are described here.

1. **Beating.** Agitating (A-juh-TATE-ing) ingredients vigorously to add air or develop gluten is called beating. You may use a spoon or a bench mixer with a paddle attachment for beating.

2. **Blending.** Mixing or folding two or more ingredients together until they're evenly combined is called blending. Use a spoon, whisk, rubber spatula, or bench mixer with a paddle attachment for blending.

3. **Creaming.** Vigorously combining softened fat and sugar to add air is called creaming. Use a bench mixer on medium speed with a paddle attachment for creaming.

4. **Cut in.** To cut in, mix solid fat with dry ingredients until lumps of the desired size remain. Use a pastry cutter or a bench mixer with a paddle attachment to cut in fat.

5. **Folding.** Gently adding light, airy ingredients such as eggs to heavier ingredients by using a smooth circular movement is called folding.

6. **Kneading.** Working a dough by hand or in a bench mixer with a dough hook to develop gluten and evenly distribute ingredients is called kneading.

7. **Sifting.** Passing dry ingredients such as flour through a wire mesh to remove lumps, blend, and add air is called sifting. Use a rotary sifter or a mesh strainer for sifting.

8. **Stirring.** Gently blending ingredients until they're combined is called stirring. Use a spoon, rubber spatula, or whisk for stirring.

9. **Whipping.** Vigorously beating ingredients to add air is called whipping. Use a whisk or a bench mixer with a whip attachment for whipping.

CULINARY TIP

CARRYOVER BAKING—Baked products continue to bake for a short time after being removed from a hot oven. This process is called **carryover baking**. The chemical and physical changes that occur during the baking process do not stop immediately. The product continues to bake because of the heat contained in the product. If you don't take carryover baking into account, you will end up with overbaked products.

SECTION 27-2 Knowledge Check

1. Why is gluten so important in the baking process?
2. Describe what leavening agents do for baked products.
3. Contrast batters and doughs.

MINI LAB

Choose a bakeshop ingredient to research. Use print and Internet resources to create a poster that explains where the ingredient comes from and how it is used to create baked products.

SECTION SUMMARIES

27-1 Commercial bakers use formulas because accuracy ensures a consistent final food product.

27-1 Commercial bakers prefer to use weight measurements for accuracy.

27-1 A baker's balance scale is an accurate measuring tool.

27-1 Bakers rely on several commercial ovens that enable them to produce a variety of baked goods.

27-1 Proofing cabinets offer a controlled environment that allows dough to rise properly and consistently.

27-1 Commercial bakeshops rely on a variety of small tools to help with preparation and baking.

27-2 Wheat flour, liquids, fats, sugars and sweeteners, eggs, and leavening agents are the ingredients that play central roles in the baking process.

27-2 A wide range of flavorings can be used to enhance the flavor of baked goods.

27-2 Different varieties of chocolate, cocoa, and nuts add unique flavors and colors to baked goods.

27-2 Additives are used to color, thicken, provide texture in, and replace fat in baked products.

27-2 There are many ways to mix batters and doughs, including beating and folding.

27-2 Carryover baking can have a great impact on the end product.

CHECK YOUR KNOWLEDGE

1. Why is measuring ingredients accurately so important in baking?
2. What makes the deck oven so flexible?
3. Why is it important to sanitize pastry bags?
4. Contrast bread, cake, and pastry flour.
5. Name one advantage and one disadvantage of baking with margarine instead of butter.
6. What are three functions of eggs in the baking process?
7. Describe two ways that you can mix doughs and batters.
8. How does carryover baking impact baked products?

CRITICAL-THINKING ACTIVITIES

1. What might happen if a baker measured dry ingredients in measuring cups instead of weighing them on a scale? Explain your answer.
2. Suppose you are looking at different types of ovens to purchase for a new bakery. What factors would you consider in your decision-making process?
3. Why is it important for a baker to know the protein content of different types of flour? Give an example of when this knowledge would be needed.

WORKPLACE KNOW-HOW

Problem Solving. Ten cherry pies were baked according to the formula. After cooling, their crusts are dry and too brown. Draw some conclusions about why this might have happened. How could it be prevented?

LAB-BASED ACTIVITY: Measuring Ingredient Yields

STEP ❶ Working in teams, review the ingredients for Chocolate Applesauce Cake shown below. The formula yields six 9-in. cakes, or 8 lbs. 9½ oz. You want to make ten 9-in. cakes, or 14 lbs., 5 oz.

STEP ❷ Create a chart similar to the one below and determine the amount of ingredients you would need to yield ten 9-in. cakes. Use the following steps:

- Add the baker's percentage. Change the total to a decimal by moving the decimal two places to the left.
- Convert the new yield (14 lbs., 5 oz.) to ounces by multiplying pounds by 16.
- Divide the new yield (in ounces) by the decimal figure to determine the weight of the flour. If needed, round the result to the next highest number.

- Change each ingredient's baker's percentage to a decimal by moving the decimal two places to the left.
- Multiply each of these numbers by the weight of the flour to determine the new ingredient amount. If needed, round the results to the next highest number.

STEP ❸ After filling out your chart, practice measuring each ingredient with the appropriate tool: baker's or electronic scale, measuring cups or spoons, or volume measures.

STEP ❹ Note which ingredients were hard to measure. Compare your results with the class.

Chocolate Applesauce Cake

Ingredient	Yield : Six 9-in. Cakes	Yield: Ten 9-in. Cakes	Baker's Percentage
Flour, cake, sifted	1 lb., 11 oz.	?	100%
Cocoa powder, sifted	1½ oz.	?	6%
Baking soda, sifted	¾ oz.	?	3%
Baking powder, sifted	¾ oz.	?	3%
Salt	¾ oz.	?	3%
Cinnamon, ground	¾ oz.	?	3%
Sugar, brown	2 lbs., 4 oz.	?	133%
Oil, vegetable	1 lb., 5 oz.	?	78%
Eggs, whole	13 oz.	?	48%
Applesauce	12 oz.	?	44%
Buttermilk	1 lb., 8 oz.	?	89%
TOTAL	8 lbs., 9½ oz.	?	510%

Yeast Breads & Rolls

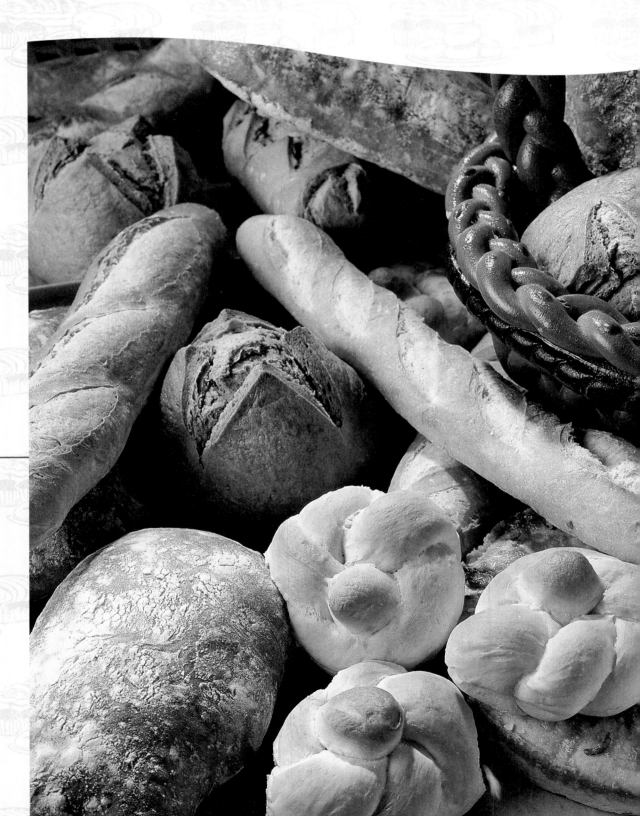

Yeast Dough Basics

KEY TERMS

- leavens
- peel
- starter
- hard lean dough
- soft medium dough
- sweet rich dough
- rolled-in fat yeast dough

OBJECTIVES

After reading this section, you will be able to:

- Describe the characteristics of quality yeast products.
- Identify types of yeast.
- Distinguish various types of yeast doughs.
- Identify products made from regular yeast doughs and rolled-in fat yeast doughs.

FROM bagels to flaky croissants, breads are usually a part of every meal. Yeast breads appeal to your eyes, nose, and taste buds. Learning about the characteristics of quality yeast products is important to foodservice professionals. It will help you plan a variety of nutritious and flavorful menu accompaniments that delight customers.

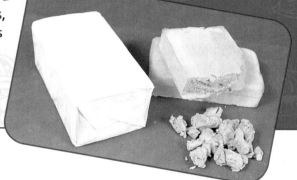

✖ LEAVENING

Yeast breads and rolls are made from dough. Dough is a mixture of flour, water, salt, and other ingredients to which yeast has been added. Yeast **leavens** (LEH-vuns), or causes dough to rise as it fills with CO_2 bubbles. This process is called fermentation. See Fig. 28-1.

Quality yeast products are the result of a careful balancing act. The leavening action of the yeast is balanced with the development of gluten. Gluten, along with wheat protein, gives bread texture. The formation of gluten is controlled by mixing water and wheat flour, and by the way dough is handled during preparation. Most yeast doughs are oven-baked in pans, on sheets, or pushed into the oven on peels. A **peel** is a wooden board that a baker uses to slide breads onto the oven floor or hearth (HARTH).

Yeast

As described in Chapter 27, the three most commonly used yeasts in baking are compressed yeast, active dry yeast, and quick-rise dry yeast. See Fig. 28-2.

Be sure to note which form of yeast is called for in a formula. Dry yeast is about twice as strong as compressed yeast, yet the two forms are similar in taste when the correct proportions are used.

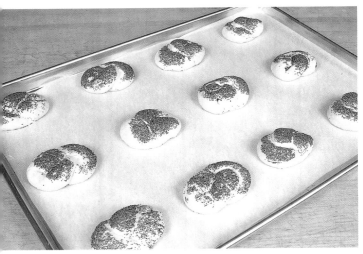

Fig. 28-1. The leavening action of yeast increases the volume of the dough. What kinds of products can be made from yeast dough?

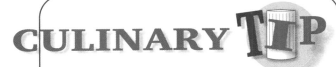
When substituting compressed yeast for dry yeast, use double the amount of dry yeast called for in the formula. When substituting dry yeast for compressed yeast, use half the amount. Too much or too little yeast will affect the yeast fermentation. Quick-rise dry yeast can be used in the same proportions as active dry yeast.

All yeast is sensitive to temperature. Yeast growth slows down at temperatures below 34°F. Temperatures above 138°F kill yeast cells. The ideal temperature range for yeast fermentation is 78°F–82°F.

Since yeast loses its potency as it ages, all yeast is labeled with an expiration date. Yeast must be used before this date to produce the best quality yeast products.

Starters

The unique flavor and texture of some breads, such as sourdough, come from the use of a starter. A **starter** is a mixture of flour, yeast, sugar, and a warm liquid that begins the leavening action. A portion of the starter is then used to leaven dough. Sourdough starters are also available as active dry cultures and are used much like dry yeast.

Other Yeast Dough Ingredients

The variety of yeast products you see in a bakery display case all begin with flour, water, and yeast. The type and amount of additional ingredients, along with factors such as shaping and baking methods, determine the end product. Each ingredient in a yeast dough carries out a special function with regard to the end product. See Fig. 28-3.

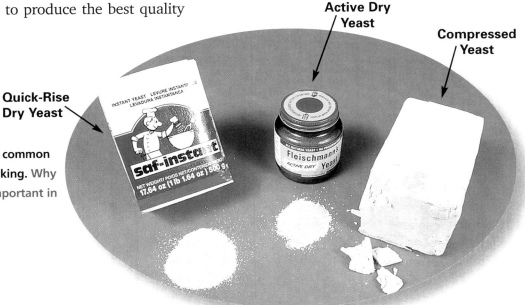

Quick-Rise Dry Yeast

Active Dry Yeast

Compressed Yeast

Fig. 28-2. Here are three common types of yeast used in baking. Why is temperature control important in preparing yeast doughs?

Fig. 28-3.

INGREDIENT FUNCTION	FLOUR	SALT	SUGAR	FAT	MILK SOLIDS	WATER	YEAST
Binds ingredients	✔	✔				✔	
Absorbs liquids	✔	✔	✔		✔		
Adds to shelf life	✔	✔	✔	✔	✔	✔	✔
Adds structure	✔	✔	✔	✔		✔	
Affects eating quality	✔	✔	✔	✔	✔	✔	✔
Adds nutritional value	✔		✔	✔	✔		✔
Affects flavor	✔	✔	✔	✔	✔		✔
Affects rising	✔	✔	✔			✔	✔
Affects gluten	✔	✔	✔	✔		✔	
Adds texture	✔	✔	✔	✔	✔		✔
Colors crust	✔	✔	✔	✔	✔		
Affects shape	✔		✔		✔		
Affects volume	✔	✔			✔		✔
Adds tenderness			✔	✔	✔		

Choosing the appropriate flour is critical to the preparation of quality yeast breads and rolls. Different types of flour give the product different qualities. For more information on flour, see Chapter 27.

☒ REGULAR YEAST DOUGHS

Yeast products are generally classified according to the type of dough used to produce them. Regular yeast doughs are prepared by combining yeast with the other ingredients into one mixture. The three most common regular yeast doughs used in foodservice operations are:

- Hard lean doughs.
- Soft medium doughs.
- Sweet rich doughs.

Hard Lean Doughs

A **hard lean dough** consists of 0–1% fat and sugar. Hard lean doughs are the most basic yeast doughs. They are often made solely from flour, water, salt, and yeast. Hard lean doughs yield products with a relatively dry, chewy crumb and a hard crust. The crumb is the internal texture of a bread or roll. The crust is the outer surface of a bread or roll. See Fig. 28-4.

Fats make a hard lean dough easier to handle, but they also soften the crumb. In commercial baking operations, chemical dough conditioners such as chlorine dioxide (KLOR-een die-AHK-side) are sometimes used. These conditioners may be added to strengthen the glutens that give hard lean-dough products their dense structure.

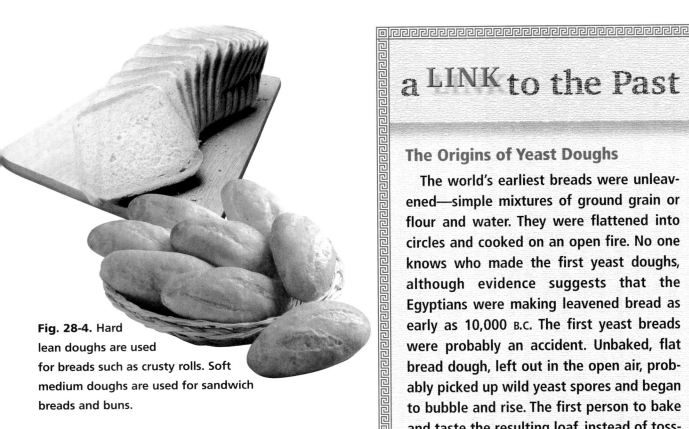

Fig. 28-4. Hard lean doughs are used for breads such as crusty rolls. Soft medium doughs are used for sandwich breads and buns.

Similar to traditional hard lean doughs are whole-grain breads, rye breads, and sourdoughs. Their textures are much more dense because of the coarser, heavier flours and hotter baking methods used. The crumb is chewier and the crust is usually darker and crisper.

CULINARY TIP

ENRICHING HARD LEAN DOUGHS—Hard lean doughs are stiff, dry, and more difficult to work with than soft medium doughs. Therefore, some bakers add oil. You can add eggs or oil to hard lean doughs to make them richer. Whole eggs may be added for color, fat, or additional moisture.

a LINK to the Past

The Origins of Yeast Doughs

The world's earliest breads were unleavened—simple mixtures of ground grain or flour and water. They were flattened into circles and cooked on an open fire. No one knows who made the first yeast doughs, although evidence suggests that the Egyptians were making leavened bread as early as 10,000 B.C. The first yeast breads were probably an accident. Unbaked, flat bread dough, left out in the open air, probably picked up wild yeast spores and began to bubble and rise. The first person to bake and taste the resulting loaf, instead of tossing it out as spoiled, opened up the world of yeast breads and rolls.

Today, yeast is a part of every yeast bread formula. Yeast provides the leavening action in many of the baked goods produced in food service. Foodservice professionals know how to expertly use yeast to produce the breads and rolls desired. From sourdough to Kaiser rolls and Pullman loaves, yeast is the ingredient that gave rise to this portion of the foodservice industry.

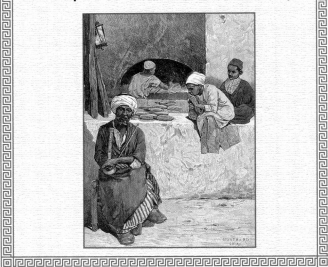

Soft Medium Doughs

Soft medium doughs produce items with a soft crumb and crust. The percentage of fat and sugar in these doughs is 6–9%. Soft medium dough is elastic and tears easily.

Yeast products made from soft medium dough include Pullman bread. Pullman bread is white or wheat sandwich bread that is made into squared-off loaves. These loaves get their shape from baking in a 2-lb. loaf pan that's enclosed on all sides. Other soft medium dough products include dinner rolls, such as cloverleaf and Parker House rolls.

Sweet Rich Doughs

At the other extreme of regular yeast doughs, are sweet rich doughs. A **sweet rich dough** incorporates up to 25% of both fat and sugar. Because sweet rich doughs use such large amounts of fat and sugar, their structure is soft and heavy. The high gluten content of bread flour helps sweet rich doughs support the additional fat and sugar.

Most sweet rich doughs are moist and soft. In working with a sweet rich dough, you may be tempted to add more flour to make the dough easier to handle. However, adding flour will toughen the final product. Use only a light dusting of flour on your hands and work surfaces when working with sweet rich doughs.

Many sweet rich dough products are famous for their golden yellow crumb and brown crust. The traditional means of achieving this golden color is to add numerous eggs to the dough. However, the egg can break down the gluten and make the dough too heavy. Many commercial kitchens use yellow food coloring to enhance the color of dough. You can also add shortening to increase the dough's richness. Some examples of sweet rich dough products are yeast-raised coffee cakes, cinnamon buns, and doughnuts. See Fig. 28-5A.

Fig. 28-5A. Sweet rich doughs can be used to create a vast array of taste-tempting bread products.

ROLLED-IN FAT YEAST DOUGHS

In addition to regular yeast doughs, bakers use rolled-in fat yeast doughs to make rolls and pastries. Rolled-in doughs differ from regular yeast doughs in their preparation.

When making a **rolled-in fat yeast dough**, combine the fat into the dough through a rolling and folding action. This process yields a dough made of many thin, alternating layers of fat and dough. As the dough bakes, the heated fat layers release moisture in the form of steam. The steam becomes trapped between the layers of dough, pushing them apart and lifting them. The finished products of rolled-in fat yeast doughs are notable for their rich, flaky texture. Two popular kinds of rolled-in fat yeast dough products are croissants and Danish pastries.

Rolled-in fat yeast doughs traditionally use butter for the fat layers. Butter adds a rich flavor and aroma, but it is difficult to handle while rolling and folding. Warm butter is too soft to roll, and cold butter cracks when folded. Instead, you may want to use other high-moisture fats, such as margarine or shortening. They may be substituted partially or completely for the butter. This will improve handling ability and lower costs.

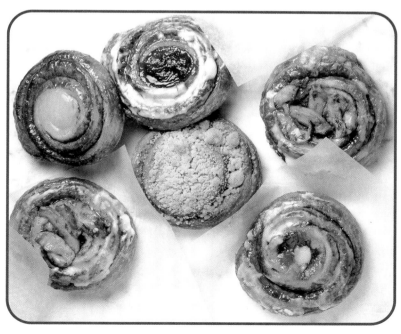

Rolled-in fat yeast doughs also differ from regular yeast doughs in gluten development. Gluten develops during folding and rolling, so little kneading is required with rolled-in fat yeast doughs. Overdeveloping the gluten in a rolled-in fat yeast dough will make the finished product tough and chewy. Larger foodservice operations often use sheeters to ensure consistent rolled-in fat yeast dough production.

Croissants

Croissants (kwah-SAHNTS) are crescent-shaped, flaky rolls. Croissant dough is a soft, wet mixture of bread flour, yeast, cold milk, salt, butter, and a little sugar. You can add dry milk solids and cold water instead of milk. The cold water or milk slows the leavening action of the yeast. Eggs are not part of the traditional formula, but can be added for additional richness. Butter or another high-moisture fat equal to 25–50% of the weight of the dough is rolled in.

A freshly baked croissant should be light golden brown. It should have a flaky, layered texture and an open grain or crumb. Croissant dough can be shaped into traditional crescents or the tighter half circles that Swiss and German bakers call gipfels (gayp-fels).

Danish Pastry

Danish pastry dough is sweeter and richer than croissant dough. Danish pastry is usually eaten as a breakfast or dessert item. Unlike croissant dough, Danish pastry dough is rich in eggs. It can also include milk.

Danish pastry is also softer, flakier, and more tender than croissants. These characteristics, along with a more intense flavor, are due to the Danish pastry's higher percentage of rolled-in fat. This percentage can range from 10–50%. See Fig. 28-5B.

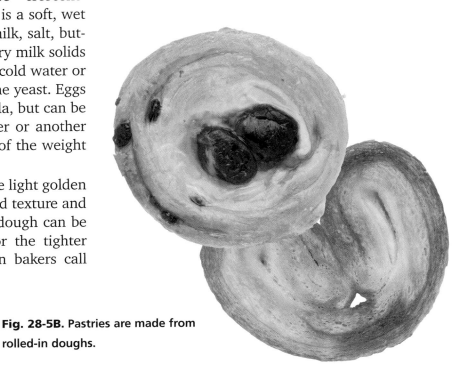

Fig. 28-5B. Pastries are made from rolled-in doughs.

SECTION 28-1   Knowledge Check

1. Describe the characteristics of quality yeast products.
2. What is a "starter" and how is it used?
3. Name the three types of regular yeast doughs. Give examples of products made from each type.

MINI LAB

Imagine that you work in a small bakery. The bakery's croissants keep turning out heavy and chewy. What three factors might be responsible for this? Offer a solution for each factor.

Yeast Dough Production

KEY TERMS

- preferment
- kneading
- let down
- punching
- bench rest
- shaping
- panning
- proofing
- slashing
- docking
- oven spring

OBJECTIVES

After reading this section, you will be able to:

- Explain proper methods of preparing yeast breads and rolls.
- Describe the process of fermentation in yeast doughs.
- Identify common causes of failure in yeast bread production.
- Prepare quality yeast breads.

THE production of quality yeast breads and rolls requires good technique, patience, and creativity. To produce a good yeast product, you will need to learn different dough mixing methods. The process of making yeast breads and rolls is a fascinating one. This section will help you understand that process. Practice will help you produce quality yeast dough products.

YEAST DOUGH PREPARATION

Yeast breads and rolls can be prepared by traditional "hand" methods. However, larger quantities and faster turnover times are often required. Yeast breads and rolls can also be prepared through an automated process known as continuous bread making.

The steps involved in making yeast breads vary depending on the type of dough used and the item being produced. However, the same general stages apply to all yeast dough products.

1. Scaling ingredients.
2. Mixing and kneading.
3. Fermentation.
4. Dividing dough.
5. Rounding dough.
6. Bench rest.
7. Shaping dough.
8. Panning dough.
9. Final proofing.
10. Baking dough.
11. Cooling dough.
12. Packaging dough.

Keep the following quality guidelines in mind when producing yeast breads and rolls:

- Maintain personal cleanliness at all times.
- Keep utensils, materials, and machinery clean and in good working order.
- Use the best quality ingredients.
- Read all formulas carefully and measure ingredients properly.
- Maintain the appropriate environmental temperatures.
- Regulate dough temperatures.
- Serve only freshly baked and properly stored yeast products.

✖ MIXING METHODS

There are three basic methods of mixing yeast dough ingredients: the straight-dough method, the modified straight-dough method, and the sponge method. Each of these methods gives its own characteristics to the finished product. Each method also affects the activity of the yeast and the formation of the gluten.

Fig. 28-6. A bench mixer is used to mix the ingredients of yeast breads and rolls.

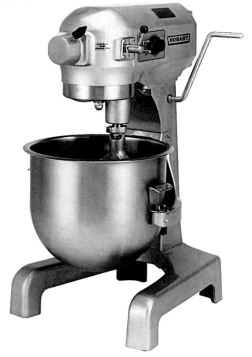

Straight-Dough Method

You will use the straight-dough method to mix the ingredients for most basic breads. The straight-dough method calls for mixing all the ingredients together in a single step. Ingredients may be mixed by hand or with a bench mixer. See Fig. 28-6.

In doughs mixed by the straight-dough method, the yeast begins acting on all the ingredients immediately. As you continue mixing or working the dough, the gluten develops.

Modified Straight-Dough Method

The modified straight-dough method breaks the straight-dough method into steps. These steps allow for a more even distribution of sugars and fats throughout the dough. This modification is commonly used when preparing rich doughs.

1. Dissolve the yeast in part of the water.
2. Combine the fat, sugar, salt, milk solids, and flavorings.
3. Mix well, but do not whip.
4. Add eggs one at a time, as they are absorbed into the mixture.
5. Add the rest of the liquids and mix briefly.
6. Add the flour and the dissolved yeast last.
7. Mix until a smooth dough forms.

Sponge Method

Some yeast products, such as crusty hearth breads or sweeter doughs, benefit from the sponge method. The sponge method allows the yeast to develop separately before it is mixed with the other ingredients. This method results in a more intense flavor and a lighter, airy texture. The sponge method makes a very soft, moist, and absorbent dough. Here are the basic steps:

- Combine 50% water with 50% flour.
- Add the yeast. Sugar or malt may also be added to this mixture to promote faster yeast growth.

USING THE "240 FACTOR"

Because the desired dough temperature for yeast doughs is 80°F, and $80 \times 3 = 240$, the correct water temperature is often called the "240 factor." You can control water temperature by adding ice to cool the water until the sum of the temperatures involved reaches 240°F. Several factors affect dough temperature, including:

• Flour temperature.

• Room temperature.

• Friction temperature of the mixer speed. This is 10–20°F for first speed, 20–30°F for second speed, and 30–40°F for third speed. In most cases, the friction temperature used is 30°F.

• Water temperature.

Of these, only the water temperature can be easily modified by the baker. Commercial bakers have developed a formula for calculating the correct water temperature to achieve the desired dough temperature, no matter what the other temperatures may be.

The following example shows how the desired dough temperature is used to calculate the ideal water temperature:

Step 1. Check the desired dough temperature in the formula.

Step 2. Multiply the desired dough temperature by 3.

Step 3. Add together the flour, room, and friction temperatures.

Step 4. Subtract the result of Step 3 from 240°F in Step 2.

Step 5. The result of Step 4 is the correct water temperature for achieving the desired dough temperature.

For example:

1. Desired dough temperature $= 80°F$
   Flour temperature $= 66°F$
   Room temperature $= 70°F$
   Friction temperature $= 30°F$
2. $80°F \times 3 = 240°F$
3. $66°F + 70°F + 30°F = 166°F$
4. $240°F - 166°F = 74°F$
5. The ideal water temperature is 74°F.

TRY IT!

Find the ideal water temperature for yeast rolls considering the following factors: the desired dough temperature $= 80°F$; the flour temperature $= 62°F$; the room temperature $= 78°F$; and the friction temperature $= 30°F$.

• Cover the sponge. Let it rise in a warm place for two to three hours or until it doubles in bulk.

• Combine the sponge with the remaining ingredients either by hand or in a mixer.

One modification of the sponge method is sometimes called the preferment method. **Preferment** is the process of removing a portion of the dough. It is kept dormant for 8–24 hours and then added to the next day's bread products. This method enhances the fermentation, color, and taste of the final baked products.

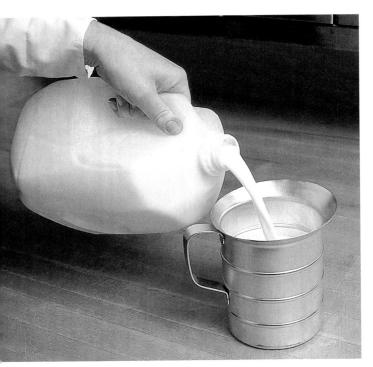

Fig. 28-7. Accurate measuring of ingredients contributes to successful yeast dough products.

SCALING INGREDIENTS

Accurate measurement, or scaling, of all ingredients is critical in the preparation of yeast doughs. Successful formulas are based on proportional mixtures of ingredients. Too much or too little of an ingredient will affect yeast activity, gluten formation, and product quality.

Use a baker's scale to weigh all ingredients that are denser than milk or water. This includes flour, yeast, shortening, eggs, honey, molasses, malt, and oil. Milk and water may be measured with volume measures. See Fig. 28-7.

Scale each ingredient separately. Make sure the weight of each ingredient corresponds to the weights called for in the formula. In some formulas, ingredients are given as a percentage of the total weight of the flour. Foodservice operations usually post procedures for converting percentages to weights and weights to percentages.

MIXING & KNEADING

When you mix dough ingredients thoroughly, it ensures even yeast distribution, gluten development, and a uniform mixture. Once the ingredients are mixed, the dough must be kneaded to further develop the gluten. **Kneading** means to work the dough until it is smooth and elastic.

1. Grasp the dough and bring it toward you. See Fig. 28-8A below.

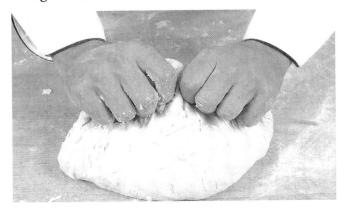

2. Form a fist and push the dough away with your knuckles. See Fig. 28-8B below.

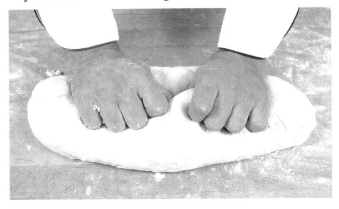

3. Repeat the process until the dough is smooth and elastic. See Fig. 28-8C below.

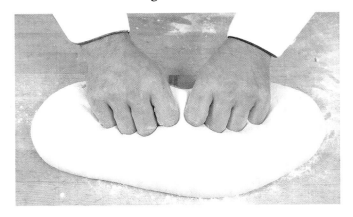

In continuous bread making or commercial baking, mixing and kneading are done in a spiral mixer. There are four stages to this process.

■ **Pickup.** Use a low speed to mix the water and yeast. If oil is used, add it immediately after the liquid ingredients. Then incorporate the dry ingredients, and add solid fats or shortenings last. Once all ingredients have been added to the mixer, turn the speed to medium.

■ **Cleanup.** During this stage the ingredients come together into a ball around the dough hook. The bottom of the mixing bowl can be clearly seen. At this stage all liquid is absorbed into the flour.

■ **Development.** During this longest stage of mixing and kneading, oxygen is incorporated into the dough and gluten is developed. The dough will be uneven in color and will tear easily.

■ **Final clear.** This stage is reached when proper gluten has developed. To verify gluten formation, cut off a small piece of dough and stretch it apart with your fingers. It should stretch to such a thinness that light can be seen through the dough. You should also be able to stretch the dough several times without it breaking. At this point, remove the dough from the mixer.

CULINARY TIP

OVERMIXING—If you overmix or overknead a regular yeast dough, you will cause the ingredients in the dough to "let down." A **let down** is a condition in which the ingredients in a dough completely break down. Overmixed dough is warm and sticky and falls apart easily. Adding flour can help offset overmixing to a certain extent.

✖ FERMENTATION

Once a regular yeast dough has been kneaded thoroughly by hand or has reached the final clear stage in a mixer, the dough is ready for fermentation. Fermentation (fuhr-muhn-TAY-shuhn) is the process by which yeast converts the sugars in dough into alcohol and carbon dioxide. Gases that are trapped in the gluten cause the dough to rise.

For fermentation to take place in dough, do the following:

• Shape the kneaded dough into a ball.

• Coat it with a thin film of oil.

• Cover the dough to keep it from drying out. Avoid popping any bubbles that may appear beneath the dough surface.

• Place the dough in a proofing cabinet, or proofer, which shields the dough from drafts and temperature changes.

Use a probe thermometer to measure the dough temperature before placing it in the proofer. See Fig. 28-9. If you're not using a proofer, regularly measure dough temperature throughout fermentation. Remember that allowing dough to become too cool will slow yeast action, while heat over 90°F will cause fermentation to accelerate.

Fermentation is complete when the dough has approximately doubled in size. You can test whether fermentation is complete by inserting two fingers into the dough up to the knuckles and then removing them. If the finger pressure leaves a slight impression around which the dough closes very slowly, fermentation is complete. The dough is then ready to be punched.

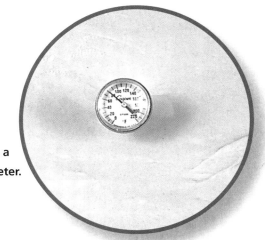

Fig. 28-9. This is a dough thermometer.

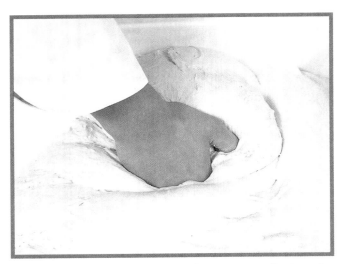

Fig. 28-10. To punch down dough, press your fist into the middle of the dough. Then fold the outer edges to the middle.

Punching

The action of turning the sides of the dough into the middle and turning the dough over is called **punching**. See Fig. 28-10. This is done by pressing gently and firmly, not by hitting or kneading the dough. Punching accomplishes four important actions.

■ **Maintaining the dough temperature.** By effectively turning the dough inside out, punching moves the cooler exterior surfaces to the middle. This evens the dough temperature.

■ **Releasing carbon dioxide.** If too much of the gas developed during this first stage of fermentation remains within the dough, it will become concentrated and slow the later stages of fermentation.

■ **Introducing oxygen.** Punching the dough incorporates oxygen from the air.

■ **Developing gluten.** Any handling of the dough strengthens the gluten.

Dividing Dough

Once the dough has been punched, it must be divided for baking. Commercial bread formulas give portions by weight. To divide dough, use a bench scraper to cut the dough into uniform pieces. See Fig. 28-11. Weigh the pieces on a baker's scale, as when scaling ingredients.

You will need to work quickly when portioning dough. Fermentation continues during this process. The last pieces portioned may become overfermented if there is any delay. Keep the large mass of dough covered as you work so its surface does not dry out. If any small pieces of dough are left, divide them evenly and add them to the larger pieces. Tuck them under each portion so they will be well incorporated. Otherwise the smaller pieces will ferment too fast.

Rounding Dough

Divided dough must be rounded, or shaped, into smooth balls. To do this, put the dough on the bench. With the palm of your hand, cup the dough with a circular motion, working the dough with your fingertips. This will cause the dough to form into a smooth, firm, round ball.

Rounding dough provides it with a skin to prevent the loss of too much carbon dioxide. Some formulas call for the dough to be folded over during rounding. This provides a kind of secondary punching after dividing. If the dough is not rounded, it will rise and bake unevenly, with a lumpy or rough surface.

Fig. 28-11. Use a bench scraper to divide dough.

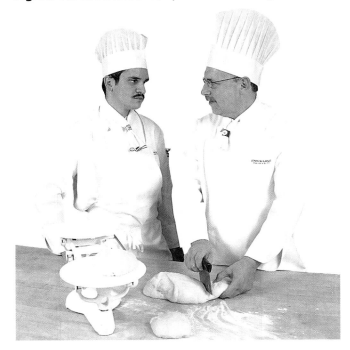

When rounding, perform each of the subsequent actions, such as shaping and panning, in the same order, so the dough ferments consistently. The first portion rounded should also be the first piece to be shaped, and so on.

Bench Rest

Depending on the formula, at this time the rounded portions may need to be placed in bench boxes or left covered on the work bench. A bench box is a covered container in which dough can be placed before shaping. This short, intermediate proofing stage, called a **bench rest**, allows the gluten to relax. The dough becomes lighter, softer, and easier to shape.

Shaping Dough

Once the portions have been properly rounded and, if necessary, rested, they must be shaped. **Shaping** forms the dough into the distinctive shapes associated with yeast products. Some general principles apply to the shaping process.

- **Work quickly.** Fermentation continues during shaping. Cover the portions you are not working with to prevent them from drying out.
- **Shape pieces in order.** Start with the first piece you rounded. Maintain the same order to ensure consistency.
- **Use very little flour.** A dusting of flour on your hands and the work surface will keep the dough from sticking. Too much will dry it out.
- **Place any seam at the bottom.** Seams, or the places where edges of the dough meet, should be straight and tight. The seam is the weakest part of the piece. Seams can open during baking and ruin the product's shape.
- **Shaping loaves.** Although bread loaves come in a wide variety of textures and tastes, there are essentially two ways to shape dough into loaves. Pan loaves are rolled and placed, seam down, into prepared loaf pans. In baking, loaves receive their characteristic shape from the support offered by the high sides of the loaf pans. Free-form loaves, such as braided loaves, are shaped by hand. They

are baked, seam side down, on flat pans or paddles, or directly on a hearth. Use the following steps to make braided loaves:

1. Divide dough into three parts. Roll into three equal strips. See Fig. 28-12A below.

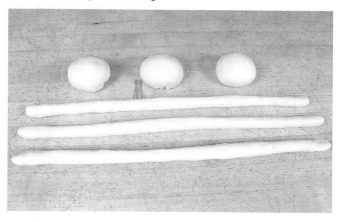

2. Cross strip 2 over strip 3. Cross strip 1 over strip 2. Cross strip 2 over strip 1. Repeat until half the bread is braided. See Fig. 28-12B below.

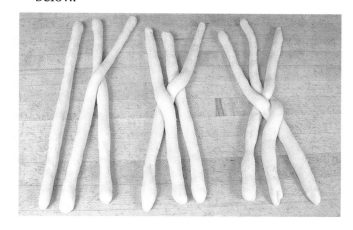

3. Flip the bread over so the three unbraided strips are facing you. Repeat step 2 until the whole loaf is braided. See Fig. 28-12C below.

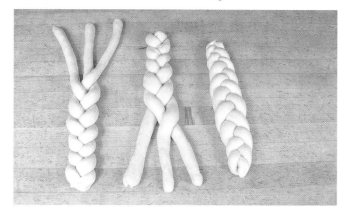

Soft Rolls

PASTRY TECHNIQUE:
See the Method of Preparation.

NUTRITION:
Calories: 141
Fat: 4.35 g
Protein: 2.62 g

Variations:
1. Rolls
2. Pecan rolls
3. Cinnamon rolls
4. Coffee cakes

YIELD: 26 LBS., 15 OZ. (18 DOZEN)   SERVING SIZE: ONE, 2-OZ. ROLL

INGREDIENTS

9 lbs.	Water
1 lb.	Dry milk solids
1 lb.	Sugar, granulated
8 oz.	Yeast, compressed
14 lbs.	Flour, bread
4½ oz.	Salt
1 lb.	Shortening, vegetable

METHOD OF PREPARATION

1. Gather the equipment and ingredients.

2. Scale the ingredients.

3. Soften the compressed yeast in part of the water. The water temperature should be 78°–82°F.

4. Use the straight-dough method for mixing the dough. Combine all of the ingredients in the bench mixing bowl.

5. Mix until proper gluten development occurs. To test the gluten development, cut a small piece of dough from the mass in the bowl. Stretch the dough to a thinness that allows light to clearly shine through. If the dough can be stretched a few times without tearing, it is ready for fermentation.

6. Lightly coat the dough with oil before putting it into the proof box.

7. Ferment the dough.

8. Punch the dough down when it is almost double in bulk. To test the dough for punching readiness, insert two fingers into the dough. If the indentation remains, the dough is ready for punching.

9. Divide the dough using a bench scraper.

10. Round the dough.

11. Allow the dough to rest for a short time to relax the gluten.

12. Shape the rolls.

13. Place the rolls in parchment-lined or lightly-greased pans.

14. Put the panned rolls into the proofing cabinet to ferment prior to baking. The rolls are properly proofed when almost double in bulk, or when the dough closes around a finger indentation without collapsing.

15. Bake the rolls at 375°F for 20 minutes or until evenly browned.

■ **Shaping rolls.** Yeast rolls are like individually portioned loaves. Shape rolls with the same care used to shape loaves. This will produce items with an attractive, even surface and uniform size.

Depending on the formula, rolls may be shaped and baked on flat sheets, like free-form loaves. They may also be placed in special pans that offer additional structure during baking. Cloverleaf and butterflake rolls, for example, are baked in greased muffin pans. Brioche (bree-OSH) rolls, like brioche loaves, are baked in special fluted tins. Pan rolls, Parker House rolls, and knots are baked on flat sheets or in shallow baking pans.

When panning rolls, allow enough room between the rolls to ensure even browning. Avoid crowding. Most formulas indicate how many rolls will fit on a sheet and how they should be placed. See Fig. 28-13.

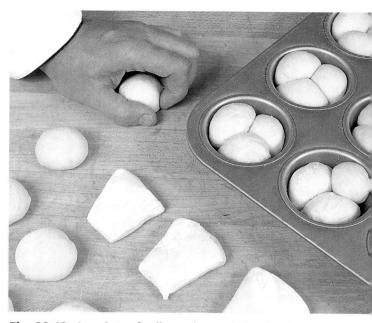

Fig. 28-13. A variety of rolls can be made by shaping dough, ranging from simple pan rolls to more elaborate Brioche, Parker house, clover leafs, and knots.

Panning Dough

Shaped dough is ready for **panning,** or placing in the correct type of pan. Some items should be shaped directly on the pan such as baguettes and hearth-style breads. Each formula specifies the size and type of pan to be used and indicates how the pan should be prepared. In general, perforated pans dusted with cornmeal are used for baking lean doughs. Sheet pans lined with parchment or lightly greased are used for soft medium doughs.

☒ FINAL PROOFING

The final fermentation stage for regular yeast dough items is called final proofing. **Proofing** allows the leavening action of yeast to achieve its final strength before yeast cells are killed by hot oven temperatures. Yeast dough items are proofed once they have been shaped and panned.

Final proofing requires higher temperatures and humidity levels than fermentation—temperatures of 85°F–95°F and humidity levels of 80–90%. The use of a proofer is essential to maintain these conditions.

The length of the final proofing time depends on the type of dough. Most doughs are fully proofed when finger pressure leaves an indentation that closes slowly around the center but does not collapse. Fully proofed items are slightly less than double in size.

Proofing time is shortened for rich and sweet doughs. This is done to keep the weight of the heavier dough from collapsing during baking. Some other items, such as rye breads, are also deliberately underproofed. Underproofed dough is known as young dough. Overproofed dough—dough that has more than doubled in size during final proofing—is called old dough.

☒ WASHING, SLASHING & DOCKING

Many yeast dough products require special additional preparations before baking. These preparations, called washing, slashing, and docking, affect the baking quality and eye appeal of the finished items.

■ **Washing.** Applying a thin glaze of liquid to the dough's surface before baking is called adding a wash. Depending on the type of item and the wash used, washing can lighten or darken the crust's color, and make the surface shiny and glossy. See Fig. 28-14.

Apply the wash with a pastry brush, either before or after proofing. Check the formula for timing. If you apply the wash after proofing, be careful not to puncture the surface and deflate the dough. Use a small amount of wash for each item. Avoid puddling or dripping egg washes, which cause uneven browning. Excess washing can burn or cause items to stick to the pan.

Fig. 28-14.

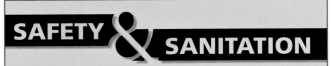

DESIRED EFFECT	TYPE OF WASH
A crisp crust	Water
A glossy, firm crust	Egg white & water
A deep-colored, glossy crust	Whole egg & water
A deep-colored, soft, glossy crust	Whole egg & milk
A deep-colored, soft crust	Milk

SAFETY & SANITATION

AVOIDING CONTAMINATION—Never apply an egg wash to a product that has already been baked. The egg will remain uncooked, presenting the risk of salmonella bacteria.

■ **Slashing.** Making shallow cuts in the surface of the item, done just before baking, is called **slashing**. Slashing, also called stippling, helps gases escape from hard-crusted breads during baking. This allows for higher rising and the development of a more tender crumb. Improperly slashed breads will burst or break along the sides during baking. The patterns made by slashing, which leave a scarred or cross-hatched impression in the baked crust, also add visual appeal. See Fig. 28-15. To slash dough, follow these guidelines:

• Use both hands, steadying the item with one hand while you cut with the other.

• Use a utility blade; a sharp, unserrated knife; or a clean, sharp razor. Blunt or serrated edges bruise or tear the surface of the dough.

• Make shallow, slightly angled cuts, just under the surface of the dough.

• Make all cuts of equal length, overlapping cuts by one-third of their length.

• Make the slashes on the full surface of the dough in a symmetrical pattern.

■ **Docking.** The process of making small holes in the surface of an item before baking is called **docking**. Used primarily with rich doughs or rolled-in doughs, docking allows steam to escape and promotes even baking. Docking also keeps rich doughs from rising too much during baking. Follow the formula's directions for docking. Use a sharp-tined fork or a skewer to dock the dough.

⊠ BAKING YEAST DOUGH

Baking is the process that changes dough into breads or rolls through the application of heat. Oven temperature and baking time are determined by five factors.

■ **Dough type.** Young, underfermented doughs require cooler oven temperatures, higher humidity, and longer baking times than fully proofed doughs. Old, overfermented doughs require higher oven temperatures, less humidity, and shorter baking times.

■ **Dough richness.** Lean doughs require higher oven temperatures and shorter baking times. Rich doughs require lower oven temperatures and longer baking times.

■ **Portion size.** Smaller items, such as rolls, require shorter baking times than larger items, such as loaves.

■ **Desired color.** The desired color of the crust often depends on the tastes of the customer. Higher oven temperatures and longer baking

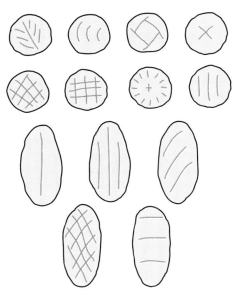

Fig. 28-15. Use a utility blade or sharp knife to make slashes. Why are many breads slashed before baking?

Baking with Steam

Breads with thin, crispy crusts, such as French and Italian loaves, benefit from the addition of steam to the oven during baking. The steam keeps the crumb soft while adding a glossy shine to the surface. As the sugars in the crust caramelize, a thin, crispy crust is formed. See Fig. 28-16.

Some bakery ovens are equipped to inject a desired amount of steam into the oven for several seconds depending on the type of bread and the formula. In ovens without steam injectors, a pan can be added with just enough water so the water evaporates during the early stages of baking.

Stages of Baking

As yeast dough products bake, their internal temperatures rise. Each of the four stages of the baking process contributes to the final product:

1. **Oven spring.** During the first five minutes of baking, the dough suddenly rises and expands as the yeast reacts to the heat of the oven. This final leavening effort, occurring before internal temperatures become hot enough to kill the yeast cells, is called **oven spring**. Steam injection helps achieve oven spring. Oven spring will not occur if there is too much salt or not enough yeast in the dough or if the dough was overproofed. At this early stage, the dough is very soft and will collapse if touched.

times generally yield a darker crust color than lower temperatures and shorter baking times. An egg wash can add color to a crust that must be baked at a low temperature or for a short time.

- **Weather.** Oven temperatures may need to be adjusted to compensate for less-than-ideal temperature and humidity conditions during dough preparation. Altitude (AL-tuh-tood), or the location of the baking site above sea level, affects baking, too. The moisture in dough evaporates more slowly at higher altitudes, such as those found in mountainous areas. Oven temperatures may be increased slightly to prevent the dough from expanding too much and breaking down the cell structure in the bread.

Formulas will list the ideal oven temperature and baking time. Slight adjustments may be necessary. Appropriate placement of pans in the oven is also important. Air and heat must be allowed to circulate freely around the pans. This can be accomplished by placing pans at the appropriate distance from the heating element. Crowding the oven slows baking time and results in unevenly baked items.

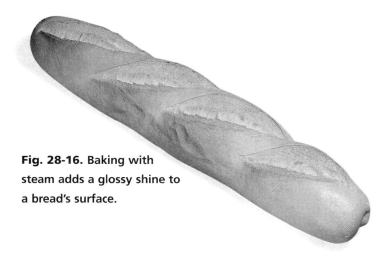

Fig. 28-16. Baking with steam adds a glossy shine to a bread's surface.

2. **Structure develops.** As the internal temperature rises from 130°F, starch granules in the dough begin to absorb moisture and swell up. At 150°F, the starches gel and become the final structure of the bread. At 165°F, the gluten begins to dry out and coagulate as the starch gel replaces it. The crumb is formed during this stage.

3. **Crust forms.** At 165°F, the crust begins to form as the starches and sugar on the surface of the dough brown and thicken. The product will appear done at this stage, but additional baking time is needed to evaporate the alcohol given off by the yeast. Yeast products removed from the oven too early will not taste right.

4. **Finished product.** By the time the internal temperature has reached 176°F, the alcohol will have evaporated. Finished products have an internal temperature of approximately 220°F.

Testing for Doneness

Appearance is not the best test for doneness. A better gauge of whether a product is done is the thump test. Tap the top of the loaf. If the loaf gives off a hollow sound, indicating that it is filled with air and not moisture, it's done. If the bottom of the loaf is damp or heavy, it probably requires additional baking. Watch rolls and small loaves carefully, as their bottom surfaces may burn before the crust color develops fully.

Another way to test for doneness is to look at the crust. If it is evenly brown on top and bottom, it's done. With practice, you will come to recognize the appropriate degree of browning and crust formation. Fig. 28-17 explains some causes of problems with yeast dough.

Fig. 28-17.

PRODUCT FAILURE	POSSIBLE CAUSE
Poor shape	• Too much liquid in dough. • Improper shaping of dough. • Incorrect proofing. • Too much steam in oven.
Blisters on crust	• Too much liquid in dough. • Improper fermentation.
Top crust separates from the loaf	• Loaf poorly shaped. • Top not slashed. • Dough dried out during proofing. • Lack of moisture in oven.
Large holes in crumb	• Too much yeast. • Overkneaded dough. • Inadequate punching of dough.
Poor flavor	• Improper fermentation. • Inferior, spoiled, or rancid ingredients.

COOLING & STORING YEAST PRODUCTS

Once a yeast dough product is removed from the oven, it must be cooled and stored properly to maintain the highest possible quality.

• Remove yeast products from their pans immediately.

• Place them on cooling racks or screens at room temperature. One exception is rolls baked on sheets. These may be left on the sheets to cool, if they are well spaced.

• Cool yeast products completely before slicing or wrapping.

■ **Glazing.** In some cases, you will brush melted butter or shortening or a glaze onto a hot yeast dough product immediately after removing it from the oven. Sweet dough products such as coffee cake and Danish pastry may be glazed with a mixture of water and sugar or corn syrup while they are still warm.

■ **Staling prevention.** Yeast dough products begin the process of staling as soon as they are baked. Staling causes yeast dough products to lose their freshness. During staling, the crust becomes moist and tough, while the interior crumb of the bread becomes dry and crumbly. Staling also causes breads to lose flavor. There are several procedures for slowing the staling process.

1. **Additions to dough.** Depending on the formula, ingredients such as malt syrup may be added to the dough at the mixing process to help slow staling. Commercial bakeries may also add chemicals such as monoglycerides (MAH-noh-glih-suh-ryds) and calcium propionate (PRO-pee-uh-nate) to lengthen shelf life.

2. **Adequate proofing.** Underproofed items stale more quickly than those that have received proper proofing.

3. **Avoid refrigeration.** Refrigeration speeds up the staling process of yeast breads.

■ **Proper packaging and storage.** Do not wrap products while they are still warm. Most breads should not be kept for more than one day in a foodservice operation. If you're keeping them longer than one day, wrap them tightly in moisture-proof wrapping and store them in a freezer to prevent staling. Wrap items with thin, crisp crusts, such as French baguettes, in paper. They will lose their characteristic crunchiness and become soggy if wrapped in plastic. Soft dough products can be packaged in paper or plastic. Sweet dough products can be packaged in a pastry box or wrapped in plastic. See Fig. 28-18.

SERVING BREADS & ROLLS

Yeast breads and rolls can be served at breakfast, lunch, or dinner. They can be part of or served with every course of a meal, from appetizers to salads to desserts.

A variety of spreads can be used with yeast breads and rolls. In addition to butter, other common spreads include cream cheese, flavored butter, jellies and jams, and olive oil.

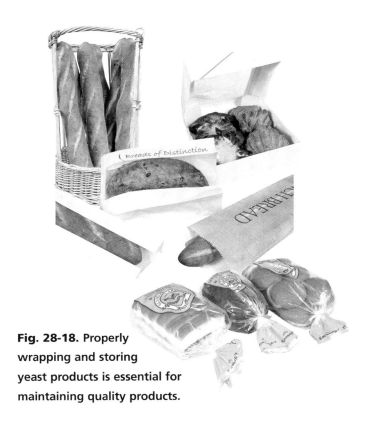

Fig. 28-18. Properly wrapping and storing yeast products is essential for maintaining quality products.

SECTION 28-2 Knowledge Check

1. List, in order, the stages involved in making regular yeast dough products.
2. Define fermentation and explain when it takes place.
3. Explain how to prevent staling in yeast doughs.

MINI LAB

Prepare the Soft Rolls formula on page 644. Follow the formula directions carefully. Serve and evaluate the rolls.

SECTION SUMMARIES

28-1 One characteristic of a quality yeast product is a texture that is full of tiny air holes.

28-1 Active dry yeast is one of three common types of yeast.

28-1 Yeast breads are made from dough, a mixture of flour, water, salt, yeast, and other ingredients.

28-1 Yeast dough products are generally classified according to the type of dough used to produce them.

25-1 Bagels, brioches, and croissants are examples of hard lean regular dough, sweet rich regular dough, and rolled-in fat yeast dough.

28-2 The straight-dough method is one of three proper methods used to produce yeast products.

28-2 The fermentation stage is reached after regular yeast dough has been kneaded thoroughly, either by hand or machine.

28-2 The common cause of failure in yeast bread production is often the lack of interaction between ingredients.

CHECK YOUR KNOWLEDGE

1. How are most yeast breads baked?
2. Describe the state of yeast at temperatures below 34°F and above 138°F.
3. Name the types of doughs that produce a hamburger bun, a Kaiser roll, and cinnamon raisin bread.
4. Explain the sponge method and its use.
5. What are the benefits of thoroughly mixing the yeast dough?
6. Explain what occurs in each stage of kneading dough with a commercial mixer.
7. Describe the let down stage. When does it occur?
8. Name two ingredients used as washes. What purpose do they serve?

CRITICAL-THINKING ACTIVITIES

1. Suppose that one of your bakery customers is following a low-fat diet. He is deciding between Italian bread, Parker House rolls, and croissants. Which of these do you think best matches his dietary needs? Explain your answer.
2. You have a basic formula for white yeast bread. What could you do to make the final product more flavorful?

WORKPLACE KNOW-HOW

Communication. Your catering team is preparing Danish pastries for a corporate breakfast meeting. You want each Danish pastry to be tender, flaky, and delicious. How will you communicate this to your team? What techniques will you emphasize to achieve these results?

LAB-BASED ACTIVITY:

Baking Brioche

STEP 1 In teams, review the formula for Brioche. Note the necessary ingredients and equipment that will be used.

STEP 2 Assign each team member a task and produce the baked product.

STEP 3 As you prepare the dough, note your team's observations to the following:

- What type of yeast was used? What is the optimal temperature for the yeast?
- What was the texture of the dough? How did it feel?
- Which mixing method was used?
- What bread-making stages were followed? What were your observations at each stage?
- How did you test for doneness?
- What are the characteristics of the end product?

STEP 4 Have a contest to determine which team produced the best Brioche. Evaluate each team's bread using the following categories:

- Shape.
- Volume.
- Crumb.
- Crust.
- Color.
- Tenderness.
- Taste.

Rate each category using the following scale:

1 = Poor; 2 = Fair; 3 = Good; 4 = Great

Brioche

YIELD: 10 LBS., 5 OZ.   SERVING SIZE: 2 OZ.

INGREDIENTS

3 oz.	Yeast, compressed
1 lb.	Milk, whole
2 lbs.	Eggs, whole
1 lb., 2 oz.	Flour, pastry
3 lbs., 6 oz.	Flour, bread
5 oz.	Sugar, granulated
1 oz.	Salt
2 lbs., 4 oz.	Butter, unsalted, soft

METHOD OF PREPARATION

1. Gather equipment and scale the ingredients.
2. Dissolve the yeast in the milk and eggs in a 5-qt. mixing bowl.
3. Add all of the dry ingredients to the yeast, milk, and egg mixture; mix on medium speed for 5 minutes.
4. Slice the butter into ½-in. pieces; incorporate into dough on medium speed for 2 minutes.
5. Refrigerate overnight on a floured surface. Cover with a damp cloth, and seal in a plastic bag.
6. On the next day, remove the dough from the refrigerator.
7. Scale into 2-oz. portions.
8. Mold the dough and place in lightly-greased brioche pans.
9. Proof the dough.
10. Brush the dough with an egg wash just before baking.
11. Bake at 375°F for approximately 20 minutes, or until brown on all sides.

Quick Breads

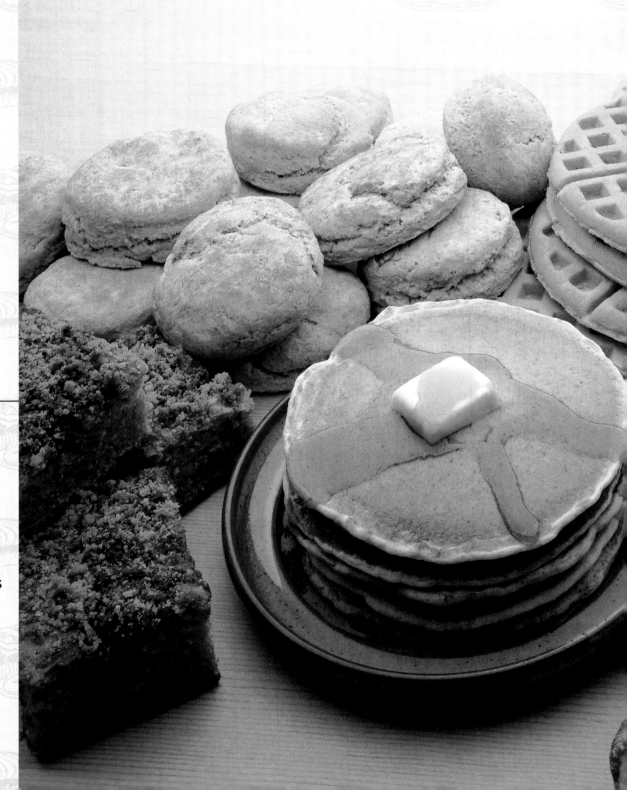

Quick Bread Basics

OBJECTIVES

After reading this section, you will be able to:

• Identify the characteristics of quick breads.

• Explain the functions of quick bread ingredients.

• Compare quick bread doughs and batters.

• Prepare quick breads.

QUICK breads are baked goods that can be served at breakfast, at lunch, or with dinner. Some examples of quick breads are pancakes, biscuits, muffins, scones, waffles, and loaf breads. These tender and flavorful baked goods don't require a lot of time or equipment to produce. As the name implies, quick breads can be made quickly.

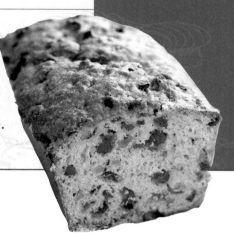

⊠ TYPES OF QUICK BREADS

Quick breads are those products that have a bread- or cake-like texture, but don't contain yeast. Therefore, quick breads don't need to rise or proof before baking. Instead of using yeast, quick breads use chemical leavening agents such as double-acting baking powder and baking soda.

Quick breads are typically baked on sheet pans or in loaf and muffin pans. Quick breads can be plain, lightly glazed, sprinkled with confectioner's sugar, or frosted. They can be served warm or cold. Quick breads include biscuits, scones, soda breads, muffins, pancakes, and waffles.

Typical ingredients in a quick bread product are flour, eggs, fat, sugar, salt, a chemical leavening agent, and a liquid.

■ **Flour.** Flour is the foundation of quick breads. A combination of hard and soft wheat flours produces the best quick bread products.

■ **Eggs.** Eggs provide added volume and structure. They are a natural leavening agent.

■ **Fat.** Fat is used to keep the baked product moist and tender. It also aids in creaming, or mixing.

■ **Sugar.** Sugar and other sweeteners, such as brown sugar or molasses, improve the flavor and color of quick breads. Sugar also aids in creaming.

■ **Salt.** Salt strengthens gluten and adds flavor.

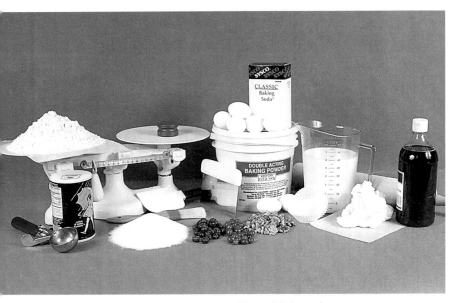

Fig. 29-1. These ingredients are used in quick breads.

Quick breads are produced by one of three methods: the biscuit method, the blending method, or the creaming method.

- The biscuit method requires cutting the fat into the dry ingredients. This is done until the fat and dry ingredients resemble corn meal. Then the liquid ingredients are added. This process produces flaky items such as biscuits.
- The blending method combines the liquid, sugar, liquid fat, and eggs at the same time. Then the dry ingredients are added to the mixture. The liquid fat and sugar act as a tenderizer. The blending method is most commonly used to make muffins and fruit breads.

• The creaming method involves using solid shortening instead of liquid fat. In this method, the sugar and pre-softened shortening are creamed together with a mixer on low speed until the mixture is light and fluffy. The eggs are then added one at a time. After the eggs are added, the dry and liquid ingredients are alternately added. Muffins made by the creaming method are more cake-like in texture.

The type of quick bread and the consistency of its dough or batter determine which method you should use.

■ **Doughs.** Quick breads can be made from soft doughs or batters. See Fig. 29-2. Soft doughs are thicker in consistency than batters. They can be

■ **Leavening agents.** Leavening agents, such as double-acting baking powder or baking soda, allow quick breads to leaven, or rise.

■ **Liquid.** The liquid, typically milk, adds moisture. It allows the dry ingredients to be blended into a batter or dough. Liquid also helps produce gluten.

The same ingredients are used in most quick breads. See Fig. 29-1. However, the proportion of these ingredients varies. The proportion of ingredients is determined by the product being made.

The flour used in quick breads ranges from wheat to oatmeal. Grains such as bran and cornmeal are often added for flavor and texture. Spices, nuts, fruits, and other ingredients may be added to alter the flavor of the product.

Fig. 29-2.

QUICK BREAD PRODUCTS	AMOUNT OF FLOUR	AMOUNT OF LIQUID	CONSISTENCY
Biscuits (soft doughs)	Three parts	One part	Sticky, pliable
Pancakes (pour batters)	One part	One part	Thin, pours
Muffins & Fritters (drop batters)	Two parts	One part	Thick, forms in drops

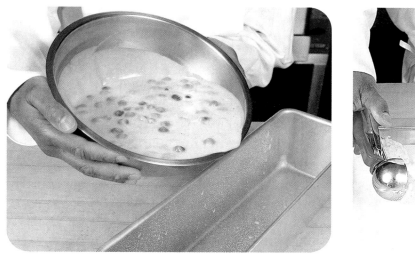
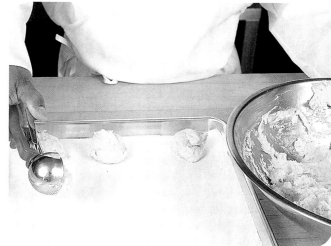

Fig. 29-3. Pour batters and drop batters have different consistencies.

rolled and cut into shapes prior to baking while batters cannot. Baking powder biscuits and scones are examples of soft dough quick breads.

■ **Batters.** Quick bread products, such as pancakes and muffins, are made from either a pour batter or drop batter. **Pour batters** vary in consistency. Some are so thin they can be poured from the mixing bowl to the cookware just like water. Others are almost as thick as drop batters. **Drop batters** are so thick they need to be scraped or dropped from a portion or ice cream scoop to the cookware. See Fig. 29-3.

LOAF BREADS

Loaf breads are similar in preparation to muffins. Like other quick bread products, loaf breads are made from flour, leavening agents, eggs, fat, sugar, salt, and a liquid. Baking powder is the chemical leavening agent used in loaf breads.

Loaf breads are made from a drop batter or a very thick pour batter. The baked product should have a uniform texture. The crust should be lightly browned, but not thick. The crumb should be tender and moist, not tough or dry. Loaf breads also should have rounded tops with a split down the center. See Fig. 29-4.

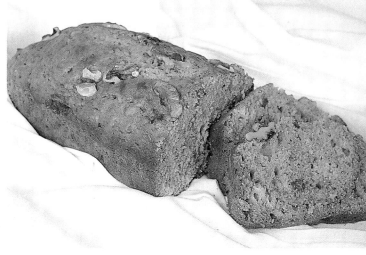

Fig. 29-4. The interior of a loaf bread should be moist and tender. What other characteristics indicate quality?

BAKING SODA VERSUS BAKING POWDER

Baking soda is sodium bicarbonate, or $NaHCO_3$. Since baking soda is a base, it can be mixed with an acid to produce carbon dioxide or CO_2. The CO_2 is what actually leavens the baked good. If you look through formulas that call for baking soda, there also should be an ingredient that's acidic, such as vinegar, fruit juice, or buttermilk. This acid is needed for the CO_2 to be produced.

If a formula calls for baking powder, an acidic ingredient probably isn't used. This is because baking powder is a combination of baking soda, cornstarch, and a powdered acid such as cream of tartar. As the baked good mixture is heated, the acid within the baking powder mixes with the baking soda and produces the CO_2 necessary to leaven the baked good.

APPLY IT!

Try this experiment to see how carbon dioxide is produced with baking soda and baking powder:

1. Add one teaspoon of baking powder to one bowl and one teaspoon of baking soda to another bowl. Add a tablespoon of water to each bowl. Record your observations.

2. Repeat the experiment, but this time pour a tablespoon of vinegar in each bowl instead of water. Record your observations.

■ **Mixing.** The time spent mixing loaf bread batter is crucial. Undermixing will result in a lumpy batter with dry pockets of flour. Overmixing will overdevelop the gluten. The batter will be stringy or elastic. The end product will be tough and will have **tunnels**, or large, irregular holes, in the crumb. When mixing loaf bread batter, you should mix the batter lightly. Mix it only long enough to blend all the ingredients.

■ **Flavor.** You can alter the flavor of loaf breads by substituting or adding ingredients. For instance, add walnuts, cranberries, or zucchini to make walnut bread, cranberry bread, or zucchini bread. You can also use bananas or pumpkin to make banana bread or pumpkin bread.

⊠ PREPARING LOAF BREADS

Once the mixture is ready, allow it to relax for 3–5 minutes. Then you can bake it. To produce loaf breads, follow these guidelines:

1. Gather and assemble all ingredients, utensils, and smallwares.

2. Grease the bottom of deep pans, such as loaf pans.

3. Prepare the loaf bread batter using either the creaming or blending method. The choice will depend on the formula.

4. Heat a conventional oven to 400°F.

5. Scale the appropriate amount of loaf bread batter into the greased pans. Allow the batter to rest. Place the loaf pans in the oven.

6. Place a shallow trough of oil down the center of the top of the loaf bread batter. This will prevent uneven splits.

7. Bake at 400°F for the length of time specified in the formula. Check for doneness. If the loaf is firm to the touch and springs back, it is done.

8. Remove the loaf breads from the oven. See Fig. 29-5.

QUICK BREADS & GLUTEN

Unlike yeast breads, very little gluten is developed in quick breads. This is a desired result. Quick breads should be tender, not chewy. Too much gluten will result in a less tender product.

Quick breads use leavening agents, such as baking soda or baking powder instead of yeast and fermentation to rise. They won't work if there is too much gluten in the mixture. Too much gluten will make the mixture heavy instead of light.

LEAVENING QUICK BREADS

Leavening agents allow quick breads to rise quickly without proofing. A leavening agent is a substance that causes dough or batter to rise. The two most common leavening agents are double-acting baking powder and baking soda.

■ **Purchasing leavening agents.** Purchase leavening agents, such as baking powder, in the smallest unit possible. It's true that you may receive better prices when buying in larger quantities. However, if the leavening agents are not used within a short time, they will deteriorate. This will result in low-quality baked products. The money saved buying bulk quantities is then wasted. Leavening agents must maintain their freshness in order to be effective.

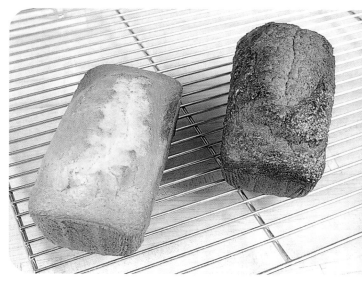

Fig. 29-5. Loaf breads are done when they are firm to the touch and spring back.

■ **Storing leavening agents.** Store leavening agents in air-tight containers. Keep the containers in a cool, dry place. Always keep the lids on the containers, even if you use the leavening agents frequently throughout the day. This will prevent contamination, moisture absorption, and spillage.

If cared for properly, baking soda and baking powder can have a shelf life of 2–4 months. They can lose approximately 10% of their potency each month.

SECTION 29-1 Knowledge Check

1. Name three characteristics of quick breads.
2. Explain how quick bread doughs differ from batters.
3. How are quick breads leavened?

MINI LAB

Evaluate one formula for biscuits, one for muffins, and one for a loaf bread. Determine what equipment would be needed to prepare the batters and doughs. Compare results with your classmates.

Making Biscuits

OBJECTIVES

After reading this section, you will be able to:

• Explain the biscuit method of mixing.

• Identify quality characteristics of biscuits.

• Prepare quality biscuits.

BISCUITS are a popular baked item in many foodservice operations. They are typically served at breakfast. Biscuits vary greatly in shape, size, and filling, and are simple to make. Proper mixing is the key to producing quality biscuits. Overmixing will produce tough biscuits.

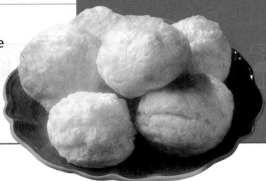

☒ THE BISCUIT METHOD

The basic ingredients in biscuits are flour, a leavening agent, shortening, sugar, salt, and milk. Sometimes eggs and butter are used to improve quality and flavor.

Eggs also build structure. They increase the volume of biscuits, acting as a natural leavening agent. If you decide to add eggs to your biscuit mixture, you will need to adjust the amount of other leavening agents in the formula.

The biscuit method is used most often when making dough products such as biscuits and scones. As you have read, the **biscuit method** involves cutting in the fat with the dry ingredients. This method typically is performed by using a mixer on low speed. Be careful not to overmix.

To make biscuits using the biscuit method, use the following procedure:

1. Gather and assemble all ingredients, utensils, and smallwares.

2. Prepare the sheet pan. Grease the sheet pan with a commercial pan grease or line the pan with parchment paper.

3. Scale, or measure, the ingredients. The measurements must be exact if the biscuits are to maintain quality.

4. Sift all the dry ingredients into the mixing bowl.

5. Cut the shortening into the dry ingredients. This will result in a mixture containing small pieces of fat. This step can be performed using the mixer with either the paddle or pastry knife attachments.

6. Whisk the eggs and milk together in a separate stainless steel bowl.

7. Add the combined liquid ingredients to the flour mixture. Mix lightly. Be careful not to overmix. Overmixing will make the biscuits tough.

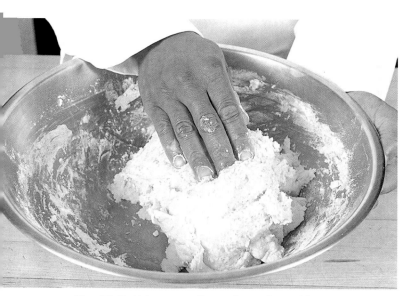

Fig. 29-6. Using your fingertips to knead biscuit dough keeps the dough from becoming tough.

8. Take the mixed dough to a pre-floured bench and set it down. Flour the top of the dough by dusting it with bread flour.

9. Knead the dough lightly using your fingertips only. Then fold it in half and rotate it 90°. Continue this process about 5–10 times. Do not overknead. Overkneading will make the biscuits tough. The dough should be soft and elastic, but not sticky. See Fig. 29-6.

10. Allow the dough to rest 15 minutes before rolling.

CULINARY TIP

CUTTING BISCUITS—When cutting biscuits into shapes, make your cuts as close together as possible. The goal is to eliminate scrap. Scraps will need to be reworked, rerolled, and cut, and reworked dough is tougher. For this reason, a pastry cutter or knife often is the best tool to use when cutting biscuit dough into shapes.

Cutting & Forming Biscuits

After the dough is prepared, you are ready to shape your biscuits. Biscuits can be rolled and cut into a variety of shapes.

1. Roll the prepared dough onto a pre-floured surface. The dough should be rolled out to about ½-inch in thickness.

2. Check the dough's depth. Make sure the dough is uniform in thickness. Biscuits double in height during baking.

3. Cut the dough into shapes using a round hand cutter or pastry knife. When using a hand cutter, be sure to cut straight into the dough. Do not twist the cutters. Twisting can prevent the dough from rising correctly. See Fig. 29-7A below.

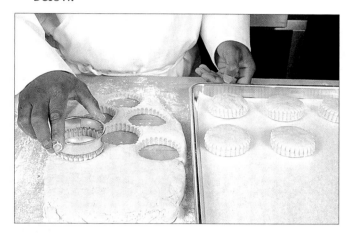

4. Place the raw biscuits on a sheet pan lightly greased with commercial pan grease or lined with parchment paper. The sides of the dough should not be touching. Brush the tops of the raw biscuits with egg wash prior to baking. This will make the crust golden in color. See Fig. 29-7B below.

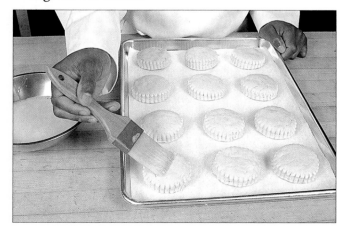

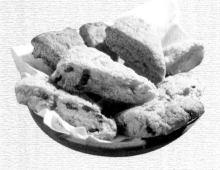
Baking Biscuits

As soon as the biscuits are shaped and placed on the sheet pan, allow them to relax for 10 minutes before baking. This will allow the gluten to react and help the chemical reaction of the baking powder or baking soda. Place the sheet pans in a hot conventional oven. Oven temperature should be between 400°F and 425°F. Bake the biscuits for approximately 8–10 minutes. The tops of the biscuits should be lightly browned.

Remove the sheet pans from the oven and allow the biscuits to cool on wire racks. Serve the biscuits immediately. Butter, jam, preserves, and honey can accompany the biscuits.

⊠ QUALITY BISCUITS

When checking the quality standards for biscuits, you should first make sure the mixture is thoroughly blended. This must be achieved without overmixing. If the mixture is overmixed, the baked product will lack quality.

Rolled and cut biscuits should be light, tender, and flaky. Properly kneading and cutting the dough determines this quality. Overkneading or twisting the hand cutters can **deflate**, or cause the dough to lose volume. Biscuits should have high volume.

The following quality standards should be achieved when baking biscuits.

■ **Appearance.** Rolled and cut biscuits should all be the same size. They should have flat tops and straight sides.

■ **Color.** Biscuits should have a golden brown crust. The crumb should be creamy or flaky, depending on the type of biscuit.

■ **Texture.** Rolled and cut biscuits should be light, tender, and flaky. Flaky biscuits should easily separate into layers when broken apart. This separation is due to the fat that melts between the layers during baking. The fat separates the layers. See Fig. 29-8.

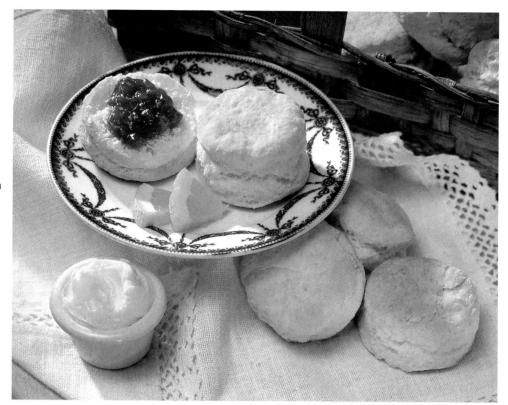

Fig. 29-8. Quality biscuits are a favorite accompaniment to many meals.

■ **Flavor.** Biscuits should have a pleasing, delicate flavor. A bitter flavor may indicate too much baking powder or baking soda. You may want to add different flavor ingredients to the mixture to increase quality. Such ingredients include herbs, chives, cheese, and bacon.

COOLING & SERVING BISCUITS

Biscuits can be cooled on wire racks after baking. However, they are best served when hot. You can serve biscuits throughout the day. Most food-service operations offer them at all meals. Honey, jam, preserves, and butter can be spread on biscuits to add more flavor.

SECTION 29-2 Knowledge Check

1. Summarize the biscuit method of mixing.

2. Explain how biscuits are cut and formed.

3. Name three quality standards or characteristics of biscuits.

MINI LAB

Working in teams, prepare biscuit dough. Practice rolling and cutting the biscuit dough. Bake the dough and serve the biscuits to the class. Evaluate each team's product for tenderness, flakiness, and flavor.

Making Muffins

OBJECTIVES

After reading this section, you will be able to:

• Explain the blending method of mixing.

• Explain the creaming method of mixing.

• Identify quality characteristics of muffins.

• Prepare quality muffins.

MUFFINS can be bread- or cake-like in texture depending on the method used to mix the ingredients. Muffins can be different shapes and sizes. Muffins usually have fruit or nuts added to the mixture to add flavor and texture to the baked product.

THE BLENDING METHOD

The blending method is used to produce muffins, loaf breads, pancakes, and waffles. The **blending method** involves using oil or liquid fat to blend the ingredients. Batters for these baked goods are sometimes interchangeable. For example, bran muffin batter can be poured into a loaf pan instead of a muffin pan. The end result is bran loaf bread instead of bran muffins. You only would need to adjust the baking time.

The basic ingredients in muffins are flour, leavening agent, eggs, oil, sugar, salt, and a liquid. Flour blends may be used to increase the nutritional value of the product.

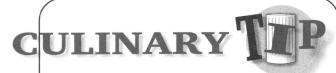
CULINARY TIP

USING LINERS—To bake muffins that have a moist, tender exterior, line the muffin pans with paper cups. If you want muffins with a crust, omit the liners. Instead, grease the bottoms and sides of the muffin pans.

Muffins are made from a drop batter. They are leavened by a leavening agent, such as baking powder. The structure of the muffin is achieved when the flour, starches, gluten, and egg proteins coagulate during heating. To blend muffins:

1. Sift the dry ingredients into a separate mixing bowl. Add sifted, dry ingredients to the liquid and sugar mixture. See Fig. 29-9A below.

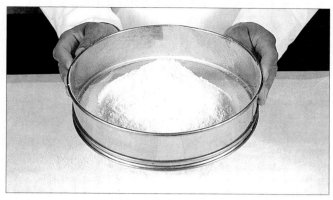

2. Combine and blend the liquid ingredients with the sugar until smooth. See Fig. 29-9B below.

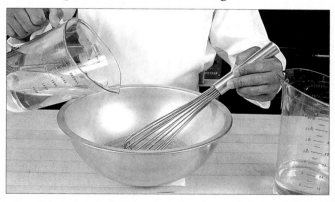

3. Mix together until the dry ingredients are just moistened. Do not overmix. This will make the batter tough. The batter should look lumpy. See Fig. 29-9C below.

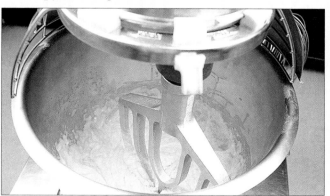

THE CREAMING METHOD

When preparing cake-like muffins made with solid shortening, you will need to use the **creaming method** of mixing. The creaming method involves combining the sugar and fat first until light and fluffy. Use the following steps for the creaming method.

1. Gather and assemble all ingredients, utensils, and smallwares.

2. Scale the ingredients.

3. Sift the dry ingredients into a separate mixing bowl and set aside.

4. Combine the solid fat and the sugar in the mixing bowl until smooth, fluffy, and creamy. Use the paddle attachment on the mixer.

5. Add the eggs one at a time. Blend well after each addition.

6. Add the flour and liquid ingredients alternately in approximately three parts. Continue to mix until the batter is smooth.

DIVIDING MUFFIN BATTER

Dividing the muffin batter involves transferring the batter from the bench mixing bowl into individual muffin pans. To avoid overmixing the batter, scrape downward from the outer edge of the mixing bowl.

It's also important to divide the batter evenly. This will ensure that the muffins are uniform in size. Using a portion scoop can help achieve this. You also can drop the batter into the pan by hand. To do this well requires practice. When filling the muffin pans, only fill them half full. Leave enough space for rising.

BAKING MUFFINS

When baking muffins, dry and liquid ingredients can be mixed ahead of time. Once they are combined, however, you will need to bake the muffins immediately. Otherwise, your muffins could lose volume. To bake muffins, follow these procedures.

1. Set the conventional oven temperature at 385°F–400°F and grease the muffin pan with commercial pan grease.

2. Using a portion scoop, lift the batter from the mixing bowl and drop or pour it into the prepared muffin pan. A portion scoop will provide equal-size muffins. Do not mix the batter when scooping it out. See Fig. 29-10.

3. Garnish the muffin batter with sugar, nuts, or streusel (STROO-suhl) toppings.

4. Place the muffin pans in the oven. Bake for the time listed on the formula. Test for doneness by pressing on the top of the muffin. If it springs back, it's done. The tops also should be a golden brown color.

5. Remove the muffin pans from the oven and let the pans cool on wire racks until the muffins are warm.

6. Turn the muffins out of the pan onto the cooling rack. If muffins stick, tap the bottom of the pan to loosen them.

QUALITY MUFFINS

Quality standards for muffins are similar to those for other quick breads. See Fig. 29-11. The tops should be golden brown, and the walls shouldn't be too thick. Muffins should be tender and moist. The crumb should break apart without crumbling. When producing muffins, ensure that the following quality characteristics are present.

- **Appearance.** Muffins should be round in shape with dome-shaped tops. They should be uniform in size.
- **Color.** Muffins should have a golden brown surface.
- **Texture.** The grain should be even. The muffin should be tender and moist, not dry or brittle. Muffins should not be filled with tunnels. Tunnels are a sign of overmixing.
- **Flavor.** The flavor should be sweet and pleasant with no bitter aftertaste from too much leavening.

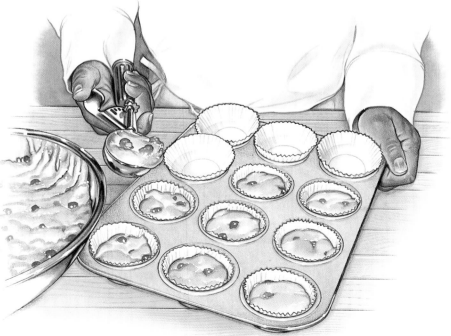

Fig. 29-10. A portion scoop will help you maintain consistent size muffins.

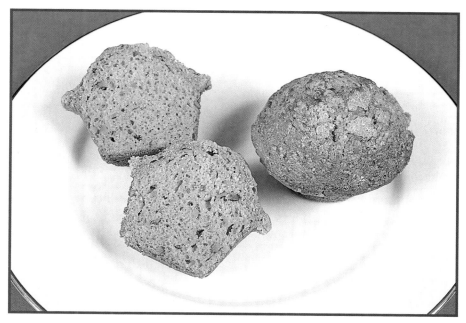

Fig. 29-11. Muffins should have a uniform shape and size, golden crust, and an even interior crumb.

⊠ COOLING & SERVING MUFFINS

Muffins are cooled in the pans until they are warm. The muffin pans should be placed on wire racks to allow air to circulate around the pans.

Muffins are better if made daily and served immediately. Muffin batter can be premade and refrigerated for three days prior to baking. It also can be frozen for two weeks. You can freeze muffin batter either before or after portioning.

To thaw the frozen batter, place it in the refrigerator. Allow it to thaw overnight. The batter will be ready to bake in the morning.

Muffins are served at breakfast, lunch, and sometimes dinner. They may be accompanied by jams and jellies.

SECTION 29-3   Knowledge Check

1. Contrast the blending and creaming methods.
2. Describe how to portion muffin batter.
3. Name three quality standards for muffins.

MINI LAB

Working in teams, make a variety of muffins. Evaluate the quality characteristics of each team's finished product. Compare the results.

SECTION SUMMARIES

29-1 Quick bread characteristics include a bread- or cake-like texture.

29-1 There are basic ingredients in all quick breads; the proportion of ingredients to each other determines the product being made.

29-1 Quick bread dough is thick and can be shaped, while quick bread batters vary in consistency.

29-1 Quick breads can be prepared using one of three methods.

29-2 The biscuit method is used in making dough products such as biscuits or scones.

29-2 Biscuits can be rolled and cut into various shapes using a round hand cutter or pastry knife.

29-2 To meet the standards of quality, biscuits should be golden brown, flaky, and have good flavor.

29-3 The blending method involves using oil or liquid fat to blend ingredients.

29-3 The creaming method involves combining solid fat and sugar before adding the remaining ingredients.

29-3 Muffins are made from drop batter and portioning is controlled by a portion scoop.

CHECK YOUR KNOWLEDGE

1. Name the basic ingredients of quick breads and describe their functions.
2. What are the three methods used to prepare quick bread mixture?
3. Compare pour batters with drop batters.
4. What are the two most common leavening agents used in quick bread?
5. Why might eggs and butter be added ingredients to biscuit dough?
6. What is the baking procedure for biscuits?
7. Contrast the basic ingredients of muffins and biscuits.
8. What is the leavening agent in muffins?
9. Explain the procedure for portioning muffins and preparing them for baking.
10. Describe the characteristics of a quality muffin.

CRITICAL-THINKING ACTIVITIES

1. When baking biscuits, a coworker adds yeast to the formula in addition to baking powder. What should you do? Explain your answer.
2. You have just mixed a batch of muffin batter and are ready to portion it. However, you can't locate the portion or ice cream scoop. How can you evenly portion the batter without overmixing it?

WORKPLACE KNOW-HOW

Problem solving. You have a quick-bread formula, but it is not labeled as to what type of quick bread it will produce. How can you determine what the end product will be?

LAB-BASED ACTIVITY: Making Banana Nut Bread

STEP ❶ Divide into four teams. Each team will prepare a batch of banana nut bread using a variation of the Banana Nut Bread formula.

- **Team A** will prepare the Banana Nut Bread using canned bananas without the nuts.
- **Team B** will prepare the Banana Nut Bread using canned bananas with the nuts added.
- **Team C** will prepare the Banana Nut Bread using fresh bananas without the nuts.
- **Team D** will prepare the Banana Nut Bread using fresh bananas with the nuts added.

STEP ❷ Prepare your team's Banana Nut Bread.

STEP ❸ Evaluate each team's Banana Nut Bread using the following checklist of quality characteristics:

✔ Uniform texture with thick walls.

✔ Rounded top with an even split down the center.

✔ Lightly browned crust, but not too thick.

✔ Tender, moist crumb—not tough or dry.

STEP ❹ Answer the following questions on a separate sheet of paper:

- How does the flavor and texture differ for each variation of Banana Nut Bread?
- What factors contributed to any differences in flavor and texture?
- How did the pre-preparation steps differ for your team's version of Banana Nut Bread from the other teams' pre-preparation steps?
- How did this impact the total preparation time?
- How did the total preparation time vary for each team's Banana Nut Bread?

Banana Nut Bread

YIELD: 6 LBS., 3 ⅝ OZ.   SERVING SIZE: 3 OZ.

INGREDIENTS

1 lb., 4 oz.	Sugar, granulated
6 oz.	High-ratio shortening
½ oz.	Baking soda, sifted
½ oz.	Lemon powder
⅛ oz.	Salt
8 oz.	Bananas, fresh or canned, mashed
2 oz.	Eggs, whole
1 lb., 8 oz.	Water, cold
1 lb.	Bread flour, sifted
1 lb.	Cake flour, sifted
½ oz.	Baking powder, sifted
4 oz.	Nuts, finely chopped
2 oz.	Banana compound

METHOD OF PREPARATION

1. Gather the equipment and ingredients.
2. Place granulated sugar, shortening, baking soda, lemon powder, and salt in a mixing bowl with paddle attachment; cream for 2 min.
3. Add the bananas and eggs to the mixture in the bowl; cream for an additional 1 min.
4. Add ⅓ of the water and mix at low speed.
5. Sift together the flours and baking powder.
6. Add the sifted ingredients to the mixture in two stages. Mix at low speed.
7. Add ⅓ of the water, and mix only until all ingredients are incorporated. Don't overmix.
8. Scrape the bowl well.
9. Add the nuts and banana compound.
10. Add the remaining water; mix well.
11. Scale evenly into 5 loaf pans, 19 oz. per pan.
12. Bake at 375°F until the loaves are light brown overall and firm in the center.
13. Cool. Then remove from the pans.

Desserts

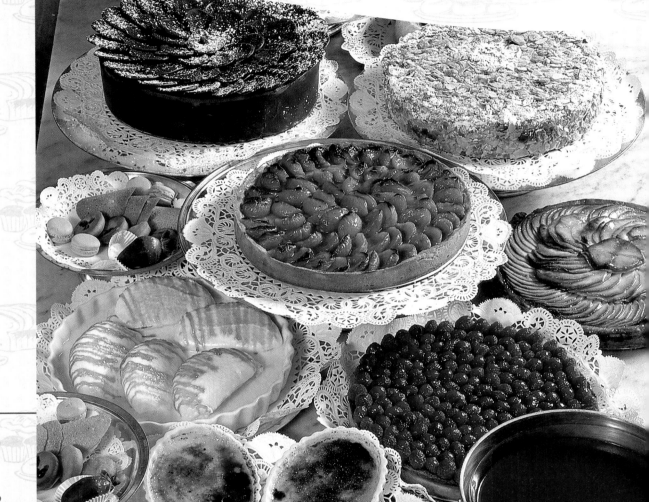

Cookies

KEY TERMS

- crisp cookies
- spread
- soft cookies
- chewy cookies
- double pan

OBJECTIVES

After reading this section, you will be able to:

- Identify characteristics and types of cookies.
- Mix, pan, and bake cookies.
- Cool, serve, and store cookies properly.

IT is nearly impossible to imagine a world without cookies. They are served in quick-service and family-style restaurants as well as in cafés where they may be served beside a dish of ice cream. It seems that almost any crunchy or flavorful ingredient—from candy to nuts to fruit—can turn basic cookie dough into a special dessert.

✖ COOKIE CHARACTERISTICS

Cookies are classified according to texture. They can be crisp, soft, or chewy. For example, biscotti (bee-SKAWT-tee) are hard and crispy, while a macaroon (ma-kuh-ROON) is chewy and soft. Sometimes the texture of a cookie, such as a chocolate chip cookie, is a matter of personal taste—some people prefer them soft and chewy, while others prefer them crispy. It is important to know the various types of cookies so that you get the desired shape.

Crisp Cookies

Crisp cookies have very little moisture in the batter. Most are made from stiff dough, without much liquid in the mix. They also have a high ratio of sugar.

During the baking process, crisp cookies **spread**, or expand, more than other cookies because of the greater amount of sugar they contain. Crisp cookies dry fast during baking because of their thinness and must be stored in air-tight containers without refrigeration. If they absorb moisture, they will turn soft.

Soft Cookies

Soft cookies have a much different ratio of ingredients than crisp cookies do. A **soft cookie** has low amounts of fat and sugar in the batter, and a high proportion of liquid, such as eggs. Corn syrup, molasses, or honey is often used along with granulated sugar. Syrups retain moisture after the baking process, providing a soft texture.

Soft cookies, as with most cookies, are finished baking when their bottoms and edges turn a light golden brown. Soft cookies, like crispy cookies, must be stored in air-tight containers and not refrigerated. When refrigerated, they absorb moisture and become soggy.

Chewy Cookies

All chewy cookies are soft, but not all soft cookies are chewy. **Chewy cookies** need a high ratio of eggs, sugar, and liquid, but a low amount of fat.

For chewy cookies, the gluten in the flour must develop during the mixing stage. The amount of gluten in a particular kind of flour determines how much the cookie will expand. Gluten provides both stretch and flexibility to the cookie, which gives it the chewy characteristic. Pastry flour is ideal for cookie production. However, a combination of cake flour and bread flour may be used for a chewier texture. See Fig. 30-1.

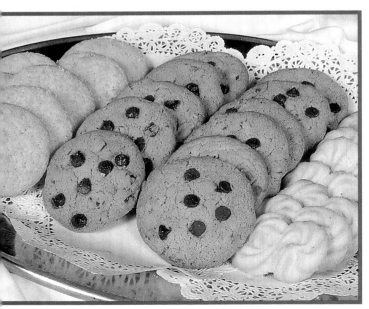

◪ COOKIE SPREAD

Some cookies require hand-labor to produce a particular molded shape. Although some cookies hold their shape while baking, most cookies will spread. The spread of a cookie is determined by six factors:

1. **Flour type.** Pastry flour is used for its medium gluten content, allowing for the proper spread.

2. **Sugar type.** Granulated sugar provides the proper amount of spread. If a finer grain of sugar, such as confectioners' sugar, is used, the cookie will spread less.

3. **Amount of Liquid.** A cookie batter with a high amount of liquid, such as eggs, will have an increased spread. For reduced spread, decrease the amount of eggs in the recipe.

4. **Baking soda.** In a cookie batter, the baking soda promotes the proper spread by relaxing the gluten. Baking soda is used as a leavening agent when it is combined with liquid and an acid.

5. **Fat Type.** The type of fat used in cookie dough also affects the spread of the cookie. When butter or margarine is used, more spread is created. When all-purpose shortening is used, less spread is created.

6. **Baking temperature.** Oven temperatures that are too low cause excessive spread. Oven temperatures that are too high give little or no spread.

◪ MIXING COOKIES

Most cookie doughs contain the same ingredients. Sugar, fat, eggs, flour, baking soda, and leavening agents, such as baking powder, are mixed together in varying amounts. Additional ingredients such as chocolate, nuts, or fruits may also be added. Either of the two methods that follow can be used to mix cookie doughs.

Fig. 30-1. Different cookie textures appeal to a variety of customers.

One-Stage Method

A few cookies, such as biscotti, are made using the one-stage method. Melted butter or oil is mixed in a single stage. All ingredients should be at room temperature and accurately measured. To make cookies using the one-stage method, follow these steps:

1. Put all the ingredients in a mixer.

2. Blend at low speed using the paddle attachment. It will usually take 2–3 minutes to blend the batter or dough.

3. Scrape down the sides of the bowl with a spatula as necessary to be sure all the ingredients are well blended.

Creaming Method

The creaming method is the most common procedure for mixing cookie dough. Creaming together sugar and fat, such as butter or shortening, makes a smooth mixture. It is smooth because air has been beaten into the fat and sugar cells. The air cells expand, lightening the cookies while they bake. A smooth mixture such as this will easily combine with other ingredients.

1. With all the ingredients accurately measured and at room temperature (70°F), use the paddle attachment on the bench mixer to cream sugar, fat, flavorings, and salt together. The mixture will become lighter in volume, texture, and color. Cream only slightly for a chewy cookie. Careful consideration should be given to the lightness of a cookie batter. Excessive lightness will cause a cookie to spread too much while it bakes. See Fig. 30-2A below.

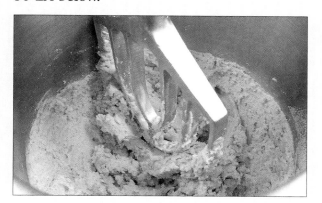

CULINARY TIP

ADDING EGGS—If eggs are added all at once, the mixture may curdle because the fat cannot absorb all the liquid immediately. Lecithin, which is found in egg yolks, is an emulsifier and helps in the creaming process. See Fig. 30-3 on page 672.

2. After creaming, add eggs in stages to allow for their proper absorption into the mixture. Blend them in at low speed. See Fig. 30-2B below.

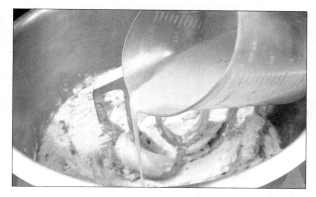

3. In a separate bowl, sift flour and other dry ingredients together.

4. Then add dry ingredients to the creamed mixture and continue to mix on low speed until the dry ingredients are incorporated. Be careful not to overmix the batter. Overmixing develops the gluten, preventing the cookie from spreading properly as it bakes. See Fig. 30-2C below.

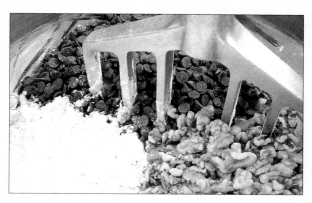

Fig. 30-3.

COOKIE DOUGH ERRORS	SPREADING	CRUMBLY	HARD	DRY	LACK OF SPREAD
Poorly mixed	✔	✔			✔
Too little sugar					✔
Too much sugar	✔	✔			
Too little flour			✔	✔	✔
Too much flour				✔	
Too much leavening		✔			
Too much baking soda	✔				
Not enough eggs		✔			
Too much shortening		✔			

☒ COOKIE TYPES

Cookies may be classified not only by texture and mixing methods, but also by type. The five basic types of cookies are drop, rolled, icebox, molded, and bar cookies.

It is easier to classify cookies by their type than by their mixing method. Mixing methods are relatively simple, but cookie types can vary a great deal. Regardless of the method used to make the cookie, it is important that all the cookies in a batch be of the same thickness and size.

Drop Cookies

Chocolate chip, peanut butter, and oatmeal are examples of drop cookies. The soft batter or dough for drop cookies uses the creaming process. Follow these steps to make drop cookies:

1. Choose a scoop for the size of cookie that is desired.

2. Drop the cookies onto parchment-lined baking sheets; if the recipe calls for greased baking sheets, be sure to follow directions.

3. Leave enough space between the cookies on the baking sheet to allow for even baking and spreading. Keep in mind how much a particular type of cookie will spread. Sometimes a recipe will recommend using a weight dipped in sugar to flatten each cookie. Most drop cookies will spread without being flattened. See Fig. 30-4.

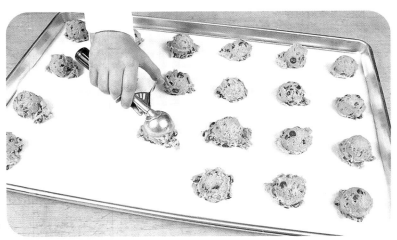

Fig. 30-4. Be sure to leave enough space between cookies to allow for even spread.

Rolled Cookies

Sugar cookies are examples of rolled cookies. To make rolled cookies, simply follow these steps:

1. Chill the dough for rolled cookies after mixing. Using as little flour as possible, roll out the dough to ⅛-in. thickness.

2. Use cookie cutters to cut out the cookies. To minimize the amount of wasted dough, cut the cookies as close together as possible. The dough can be rolled and cut twice. The scrap left over after the second cutting should be discarded because it will make tough cookies.

3. Place cookies on a parchment-lined baking sheet and bake.

Icebox Cookies

Icebox cookies are perfect for making sure that freshly baked cookies are always on hand. Drop cookie dough and sugar cookie dough work well for icebox cookies. The dough can be made ahead of time and stored in the refrigerator. Once the rolls of mixed dough have been placed in the refrigerator, the cookies can be sliced and baked as needed.

Molded Cookies

Crescents, almond lace, and tuile (TWEEL) are examples of molded cookies. Crescents are hand shaped before they are baked. Almond lace and tuile cookies are shaped after baking.

CULINARY TIP

USING BASIC COOKIE MIXES—It can be more cost-effective to use a basic cookie mix as the foundation for several types of cookies. Basic cookie mixes generally include flour, leavening, sugar, fat, and dehydrated eggs. Some mixes require the addition of liquid only. Others may require liquid, fat, and eggs.

Bar Cookies

These cookies are made from dough that has been shaped into long bars, baked, and then cut. Popular bar cookies are hermits, coconut bars, and fruit bars. Follow these steps to make bar cookies:

1. Weigh the dough into 1¾ lb. units.

2. Mold the dough into cylinders that are as long as the sheet pan.

3. On each parchment-lined sheet pan, place three strips spaced a fair distance apart. Use your fingers to flatten the dough to ¾-in. wide and ¼-in. thick.

4. Brush the dough with an egg wash if the recipe calls for it, and then bake. Egg wash is a mixture of egg yolk or white with water or milk.

5. After the cookies have baked and cooled, cut the strips into bars about 1¾-in. wide. See Fig. 30-5 below.

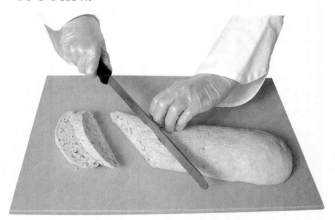

✖ BAKING & COOLING COOKIES

Always use clean, unwarped pans for baking cookies. Lining the pans with parchment paper keeps cookies from sticking to the pan. It also allows for even browning.

Because of their small size and high sugar content, cookies can burn quickly. The heat from the pan that continues to bake the cookies once they are removed from the oven is called carry over baking. For this reason, it is better to slightly underbake cookies. To prevent burning the bottoms or edges of cookies before they are done, **double pan** them by placing the sheet pan inside a second pan of the same size. This double-pan technique is especially good for rich dough. When baking two sheets at one time on separate oven racks, reverse them halfway through the baking process. This ensures even baking.

Cookies are done when the bottoms and edges turn light golden brown. Be sure not to remove cookies from the pans until they are firm enough to handle. Some cookie varieties, such as drop cookies or macaroons, will crack if they are cooled in a draft or too quickly.

✖ STORING COOKIES

Be sure that cookies are completely cooled before storing them. Cookies are best kept in airtight containers away from moisture. They should not be refrigerated. Cookies have the best flavor and texture for only a few days. It is important to properly wrap cookies to ensure their freshness. See Fig. 30-6.

Most types of cookies can be frozen for up to three months. They should be carefully wrapped to keep the freezer's dry air from pulling out moisture. Use heavy-duty freezer bags, aluminum foil, or plastic freezer containers.

Often cookies are served as part of a dessert buffet, with sorbet (sor-BEY) or ice cream, or at a reception. Whether they are simple or elaborate concoctions with fillings and frostings, cookies appeal to nearly everyone.

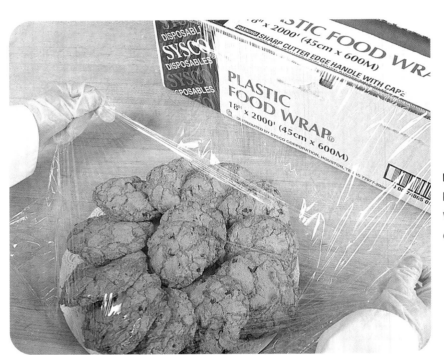

Fig. 30-6. Properly wrapping cookies will help ensure their freshness when served. Why do you think that cookies dry out easily if not wrapped properly?

SECTION 30-1 Knowledge Check

1. Identify the factors that influence the spread of a cookie.

2. Identify the five different types of cookies.

3. Choose one type of cookie and explain how to make it.

MINI LAB

In teams, produce a batch of one of the types of cookies introduced in this section. Sample each team's cookies. Evaluate each team's cookies for spread, consistency, and texture.

Cakes

OBJECTIVES

After reading this section, you will be able to:

- Describe five types of cakes and their mixing methods.
- Demonstrate how to scale and pan cakes.
- Bake, cool, and serve cakes.

CUSTOMERS often look forward to something sweet, such as cake, for a conclusion to a good meal. Cakes are made of eggs, flour, sugar, fat, leavening, and flavorings. They can be as simple as a pound cake or as elaborate as a wedding cake. This section introduces different types of cakes and how to make them.

✖ TYPES OF LAYER CAKES

There is an almost limitless variety of cake formulas. Different textures and tastes result from the type of fat and the different ingredients used. The five basic varieties of cakes are:

- Pound cakes.
- Sponge or foam cakes.
- Angel food cakes.
- Chiffon cakes.
- High-ratio layer cakes.

Cake ingredients either weaken or strengthen a cake's structure and determine its texture, moisture, and sweetness. For example, sugar and fat, used in proper amounts, help weaken cake structure and give the cake tenderness. On the other hand, eggs and flour both have proteins that, when baked, join together to give the cake support. See Fig. 30-7.

The starch in flour also helps stabilize the cake by absorbing liquid when it is mixed. Liquid, such as milk or water, forms gluten when it combines with flour. When mixed, gluten gives structural support to the cake.

■ **High-fat cakes.** These cakes generally use baking powder as the leavening agent. High-fat cakes, such as pound cake, also require that air cells be creamed into the center of the fat cell. The air cells then pick up the leavening gases that the heat of the oven releases.

■ **Low-fat cakes.** Low-fat cakes, such as sponge cakes, are leavened from air that is whipped into the egg batter. These cakes have a light and springy texture. This makes them a good choice for desserts such as a torte that has many layers with cream and fruit between them.

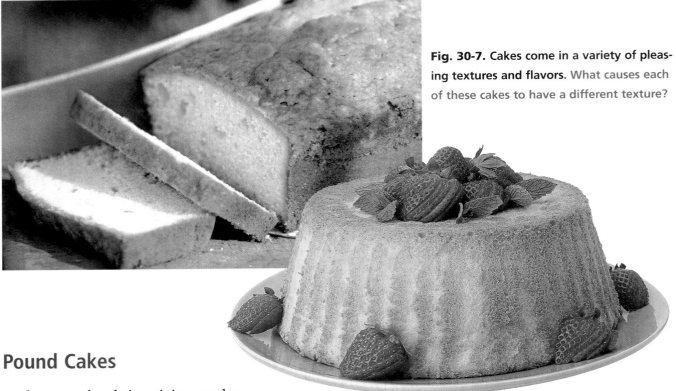

Pound Cakes

The pound cake's origin can be traced back to England. **Pound cakes** contain a pound each of butter, flour, sugar, and eggs. They are flavored to taste using vanilla, almond, or lemon. The butter pound cake is a familiar example, and is considered to be the basis for all layer cakes.

A pound cake can be frozen for up to two months, or kept refrigerated for a week. Many other variations on the basic pound cake have been developed, such as lemon poppy seed or chocolate pound cake.

Sponge or Foam Cakes

Sponge cakes, which are also called foam cakes, have an airy, light texture because of large amounts of air whipped into the eggs. This type of cake does not rely on butter or modern types of fat such as all-purpose shortening or **emulsified shortening**—a type of fat that helps create a smooth consistency throughout the mixture. Instead, sponge or foam cakes have a base of whipped, whole eggs.

European sponge cake, which is called **genoise** (zhen-WAHZ), is the most common example. Genoise can be the basis for special desserts with layers of jam, chocolate, or fruit filling. Because whole eggs are used in the batter, sponge cakes are richer than angel food cakes.

Angel Food Cakes

Angel food cakes are a type of foam cake that is made with egg whites—not egg yolks. The air whipped into the egg whites leavens the cake. Once the egg whites have been whipped, the cake batter must be finished quickly, or it will collapse when the air beaten into the egg whites escapes.

Usually angel food cakes are baked in tube pans. The pans are left ungreased so that as the batter rises it can attach to the sides of the pan. To prevent the cake from collapsing as it cools, the pan is turned upside down, and the cake left to cool inside the pan. Angel food cake may be served plain, frosted, topped with a chocolate or fruit-flavored glaze, or served with whipped cream or fresh fruit. Because angel food cakes contain no egg yolks or other fat, they are a healthier alternative to other cakes.

Vanilla Chiffon Genoise

YIELD: 10 LBS., 6 OZ. (SEVEN 9-IN. CAKES)   SERVINGS: 70

PASTRY TECHNIQUES:
Whipping, Combining

Whipping:
1. Hold the whip at a 45° angle.
2. Create circles, using a circular motion.
3. The circular motion needs to be perpendicular to the bowl.

Combining:
Bringing together two or more components.
1. Prepare the components to be combined.
2. Add one to the other, using the appropriate mixing method (if needed).

HAZARDOUS FOODS:
Egg yolks
Egg whites

NUTRITION:
Calories: 225
Protein: 4.74 g
Fat: 8.99 g

INGREDIENTS

2 lbs.	Egg yolks
3 lbs.	Sugar, granulated
12 oz.	Oil, vegetable
2 lbs.	Egg whites
2 lbs., 4 oz.	Flour, cake, sifted
1 oz.	Baking powder
5 oz.	Water, room temperature
To taste	Extract, vanilla

METHOD OF PREPARATION

1. Gather the equipment and scale the ingredients.
2. Properly grease the cake pans.
3. Place the egg yolks and half of the granulated sugar in a 5-qt. mixing bowl; whip to full volume.
4. Continue mixing on medium speed, and slowly incorporate the oil.
5. In another 5-qt. mixing bowl, whip the egg whites to a medium peak; slowly add the remaining granulated sugar to make a meringue.
6. Sift together the cake flour and baking powder.
7. Combine the water and vanilla extract.
8. Alternately add the flour and water mixtures into the yolk mixture by hand.
9. Fold the meringue into the batter.
10. Scale 1 lb., 8 oz. batter into each greased, paper-lined, 9-in. cake pan.
11. Bake at 360°F until spongy in the center.

Chiffon Cakes

Chiffon (shef-FON) **cakes** are a variation of genoise cakes. They are made by using whipped egg whites, or meringue (muh-RANG), to lighten a mixture. The egg yolks and part of the sugar are whipped to full volume and then the flour is added to the yolk and sugar mixture. Finally, the egg whites and the remaining sugar are whipped to form the meringue, and then folded in.

Chiffon cakes have less saturated fat and cholesterol than any cake except angel food, and about half the fat of a pound cake. Like angel food cakes, chiffon cakes are cooled upside down. Chiffon cakes can be stored in the freezer for up to two months or refrigerated for up to three days.

High-Ratio Layer Cakes

High-ratio layer cakes contain a high ratio of both liquids and sugar, giving the cake a very moist and tender texture. It is necessary to use a high-ratio shortening or emulsified shortening to help absorb the quantity of liquids. These cakes have a tight and firm grain due to the mixing method. The paddle attachment is used on the bench mixer to limit the amount of air that is mixed into the batter. Wedding cake is an example of a high-ratio layer cake.

✖ CAKE MIXING METHODS

Mixing cake batter is an important step when making a cake. A properly mixed cake has the desired texture and grain. Air is blended into the batter and all ingredients are mixed completely. Each mixing method produces a certain kind of cake. Bakers use the following five standard methods. See Fig. 30-8.

Creaming Method

The creaming method was once the standard method for mixing a cake. To begin with, all ingredients should be at room temperature and accurately scaled. Then use the following steps:

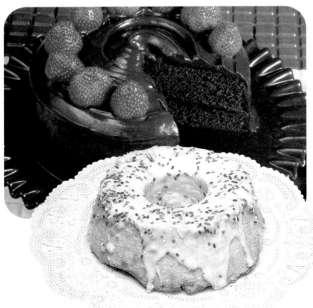

1. Cream the butter or all-purpose shortening, sugar, and salt. Cream the mixture on medium speed for about 4–6 minutes, until it is lighter in volume, texture, and color.

2. Add the eggs and other liquids gradually in small amounts. Beat the mixture on low speed after each addition to fully incorporate the eggs without curdling.

3. Add the sifted, dry ingredients and mix on low speed to incorporate the dry ingredients with the wet ingredients.

Blending Method

The blending method is often called the two-stage method, because the liquids are added in two stages. This method produces a smooth batter that makes a moist, tight, and firm-grained cake. The blending method is used for making

Fig. 30-8.

TYPE OF CAKE	MIXING METHODS
High-fat or Shortened Cakes	• Creaming method. • Two-stage or blending method.
Low-fat or Foam-type Cakes	• Foaming or sponge method. • Angel food method. • Chiffon method.

high-ratio cakes, which means using large amounts of liquids and sugar as well as emulsified shortenings to absorb the liquids and sugar.

- Blend the sifted flour, sugar, chemical leaveners, and other dry ingredients for 30 seconds on medium speed.
- Add the emulsified shortening and half of the liquids.
- Mix on low speed until the ingredients are moistened.
- Increase the speed to medium and mix for 5 minutes.
- Scrape the sides of the bowl and add the remaining liquid.
- Blend on low speed for 3 minutes.

Sponge or Foam Method

In the sponge method, leavening is formed from air that is trapped in the beaten eggs. When the ingredients are warmed to room temperature, the foam has a greater volume, creating a sponge-like texture. Follow these steps to prepare sponge cakes:

1. Once all ingredients are at room temperature, melt the butter and set it aside.
2. Heat sugar and eggs in a double boiler, stirring constantly, to about 110°F.
3. Beat the eggs at high speed for 10–15 minutes, until they are thick and light. When properly beaten, the foam will fall in a ribbon-like shape when you lift the beater.
4. Sift all of the dry ingredients; then carefully fold them into the foam. Because the foam can easily be deflated, most bakers do this step by hand.
5. Fold in the melted butter, but do not overmix.
6. Pan and bake the batter at once so that it doesn't lose volume.

Angel Food Method

Angel food cakes have no fat and are based on egg-white foam. They do, however, contain a large amount of sugar. To properly whip the egg whites, do not add all of the sugar to them at once. Gradually add the sugar as you whip the egg whites to create high-volume foam. Follow these steps to make angel food cake:

1. Whip the egg whites with half the sugar, salt, and cream of tartar to full volume.
2. Sift the remaining half of the sugar with the flour. Fold the sugar and flour mixture into the egg-white foam just until it is absorbed.

Chiffon Method

The chiffon method is closely related to the angel food method. Follow these steps to make chiffon cakes:

1. Whip the egg yolks and half of the sugar to full volume. They will be a light pale yellow.
2. Fold in sifted flour and other dry ingredients.
3. Whip the egg whites and the remaining half of the sugar until a meringue with medium to stiff peaks forms.
4. Gently fold the meringue into the yolk mixture a small amount at a time. See Fig. 30-9.

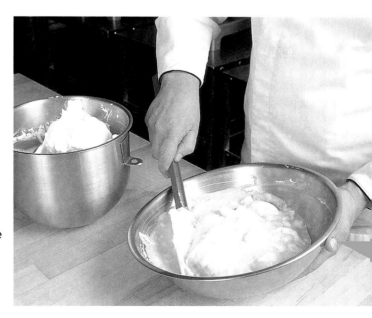

Fig. 30-9. Carefully folding meringue into the chiffon cake mixture incorporates air and makes the final product fluffy.

ADJUSTING FOR ALTITUDE

According to where you live, you may need to make adjustments to your cake recipes. The higher the altitude, the lower the air pressure or atmospheric (at-mohs-SFEAR-ik) pressure. This means that a higher percentage of liquid evaporates at high altitudes than it does at low altitudes. Because liquid evaporates from cakes as they bake, they may end up tasteless and tough.

For high altitude areas, use the following for recipes that include a leavening ingredient:

- For altitudes of about 2,000 ft., decrease the amount of baking powder or other leavening agent called for in the recipe by 15%.
- For altitudes of about 5,000 ft., decrease the level of baking powder or other leavening agent called for in the recipe by 40%.
- For altitudes at about 8,000 ft., decrease the amount of leavening agent by 60%.

Above 3,000 ft., the baking temperature for cakes should be increased by 25°F. This temperature will help prevent liquid evaporation.

$$\frac{\text{wt. of ingredient}}{\text{wt. of flour}} \times 100\% = \% \text{ of ingredient}$$

APPLY IT!

You are catering a family reunion in Denver. You plan to make a large sheet cake for the party. The sheet cake formula calls for 5 oz. of baking powder.

1. Denver is 5,280 ft. above sea level. How should the formula be adjusted?
2. If you alter the amount of leavening, how will other ingredients such as flour and eggs need to be altered?

⊠ PANNING & SCALING CAKES

To keep cakes from sticking, baking pans are usually coated with fat and flour or lined with parchment paper. This allows the cake to release easily from the pan. Commercial pan preparations are also available, such as spray pan release, which is a type of grease.

Pans should be filled one-half to two-thirds full, so that the batter does not spill over the sides of the pan as it rises. Spread the batter evenly using an offset spatula. Don't work the batter too much, or air cells will collapse and the cake will not rise properly. When making multiple cakes or when making a multi-tiered cake, always fill pans to the same level. If one pan has more batter, it will be larger and require longer to bake than the other cakes. For all but foam cakes, tap the filled pans firmly on a bench or counter to let large air bubbles escape before baking.

Pan Preparation

It is important to have the pans prepared before the batter is mixed. Pans should be filled as soon as possible after mixing is complete so that air cells in the batter do not collapse.

Most pans are either sprayed with an oil and flour mixture or greased and dusted with a bit of flour. See Fig. 30-10. Extra flour should always be tapped out of the pan so that the bottom of the cake does not get doughy. Some baked items can be placed on pans lined with parchment paper.

Scaling Cake Batters

Because it is important that cakes be consistently the same size, the batter is scaled before it is panned. How a batter is scaled is based on the amount of liquid in the batter and the amount of handling a batter can withstand.

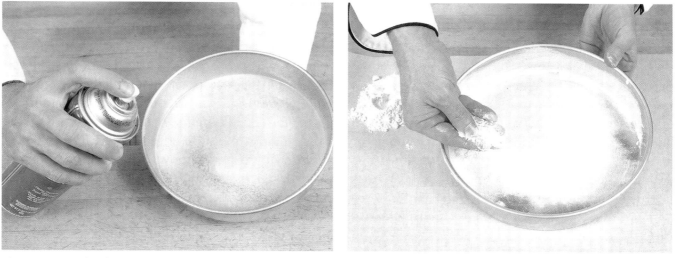

Fig. 30-10. Both of these pan preparation methods help a properly baked cake release easily from the pan after baking.

■ **Creaming method.** These thick batters do not pour easily. To scale cakes made by the creaming method:

1. Place a prepared cake pan on the left side of the scale.
2. Balance the scale to zero.
3. Set the scale for the desired weight.
4. Add batter to the prepared pan until the scale balances. See Fig. 30-11.

■ **Blending method.** These batters can be scaled the same way. However, because they have more liquid, they can also be measured by volume:

1. Place an empty volume measure on the left side of the scale.
2. Balance the scale to zero.
3. Set the desired weight and pour the batter into the volume measure until the scale balances.
4. Pour the batter into the prepared pan, being careful to scrape out all of the batter from the volume measure.

■ **Sponge or foam method.** To keep beaten eggs from collapsing in these batters, handle the batter as little as possible.

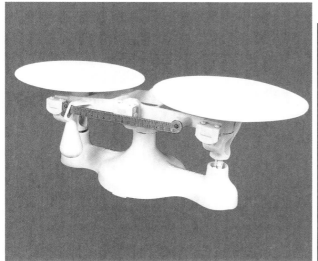

Fig. 30-11.

PAN TYPE & SIZE	SCALING WT.
High-fat Cakes	
• Round 8 in.	• 14–18 oz.
• Square 9 in. × 9 in.	• 24 oz.
• Loaf 2¼ in. × 3½ in. × 8 in.	• 16–18 oz.
Low-fat Cakes	
• Round 8 in.	• 10 oz.
• Sheet 18 in. × 26 in., ½-in. thick (for jelly roll or sponge roll).	• 2½ lb.
• Tube (angel food and chiffon) 10 in.	• 24–32 oz.

BAKING CAKES

Baking the cake completes the chemical reactions begun when the batter was mixed. Preheat the oven to the correct temperature. If the oven is too hot, the cake may set before it has risen fully, or it may set unevenly, causing the crusts to be too dark. A temperature that is too low creates poor texture and volume, since the cake won't set fast enough. Cakes also may collapse when oven temperatures are too low.

Ovens and the shelves in them should be level. When pans are placed in the oven, they should not touch each other. The air needs to flow between the pans for the cakes to bake evenly.

It is important to keep the oven door closed in order not to disturb cakes while they bake. Cakes may fall if they are disturbed before they finish rising or become partially browned.

■ **Determining doneness.** Three tests for doneness may be used with cakes. A cake is done if:

• A pick or cake tester comes out clean when inserted into the center of the cake.

• The center of the cake's top springs back when lightly pressed.

• It pulls slightly away from the sides of the pan.

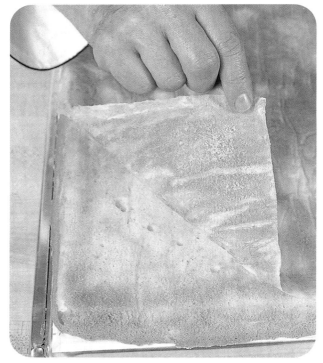

COOLING CAKES

Cakes may break if turned out of the pan too early. Always cool cakes at least 15 minutes before removing them from the pan. When turning out sheet cakes, lightly sprinkle the top with granulated sugar. Place an empty sheet pan with the bottom side down on top of the cake. Turn both pans upside down and remove the top pan from the cake. If parchment paper has been used to line the pan, peel it off the cake. See Fig. 30-12.

To remove a chiffon or angel food cake from the pan, loosen the cooled cake using a spatula or knife. Put a cooling rack or tray on top of the cake pan. Turn the cake pan and rack over carefully holding on to both. Carefully remove the pan from the cake.

ICING & BUTTERCREAMS

Icing improves a cake by forming a protective layer around the cake that seals in moisture. Icing also adds richness and flavor. Fudge-type icings hold up well on cakes and last longer in storage. To use after storage, simply heat the icing in a double boiler until the icing can be spread.

Buttercream is usually used to make cakes, tortes, and desserts taste better and look more attractive. Here are five types of buttercreams:

1. Simple buttercream is made by combining butter, shortening, confectioners' sugar, egg whites, and vanilla.

2. French buttercream is made with beaten egg yolks and butter.

3. Italian buttercream is made with Italian meringue and butter.

4. German buttercream is made with butter, emulsified shortening, and fondant—a sugar syrup.

5. Swiss buttercream is made with Swiss meringue and butter.

Fig. 30-12. Slowly remove parchment paper from the baked cake.

Icing Cakes

When deciding what type of icing to use, be sure that the icing is not too heavy for the cake. Dense cakes pair well with fudge-type icings and simple or German buttercreams. However, lighter buttercreams such as Swiss and Italian, whipped cream, and fruit fillings go well with sponge cakes. Simple syrups can also be used.

Before spreading the icing, tap off any loose crumbs from the cake that would interfere with a smooth appearance. When spreading the icing on a layer cake, do not spread too much on the first layer. The iced cake should have a uniform appearance with an even amount of icing all over it. Icing should not ooze out the side after the layers have been placed.

To ice the top layer, start from the center and work out to the edges. Then spread the icing down the sides of the cake. Be sure to smooth the surface before adding decorations. See Fig. 30-13.

✕ STORING & SERVING CAKES

Cakes should be wrapped in air-tight containers or plastic wrap and stored in the refrigerator until needed. If cakes have not been decorated and have been properly wrapped, they can be kept frozen for up to one month.

Frosted cakes should be stored in the refrigerator until they are served. Because frosting easily absorbs refrigerator odors, decorated cakes should be boxed or covered before they are placed in the refrigerator. Always bring cakes to room temperature before serving them.

Sheet cakes keep fresh and moist longer than layer cakes. Sheet cakes can be stored after they are baked, then cut into various shapes, such as bars or squares, prior to being served.

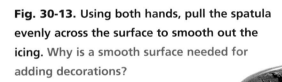

Fig. 30-13. Using both hands, pull the spatula evenly across the surface to smooth out the icing. Why is a smooth surface needed for adding decorations?

S E C T I O N 30-2   Knowledge Check

1. Contrast chiffon cakes and pound cakes.
2. Explain one of the five methods for mixing cakes.
3. Describe the process for icing a cake.

(MINI LAB)

In teams, produce a cake. Be sure to add icing or a topping. Evaluate each team's cake on appearance, texture, and flavor.

Pies

OBJECTIVES

After reading this section, you will be able to:

- Prepare mealy or flaky pie dough.
- Describe the different types of pie fillings.
- Prepare pie crusts and pie fillings.
- Demonstrate proper pie storage.

A few ripe peaches sweetened and baked in a crust with a lattice-work top make an appetizing pie. Fruit pies, cream pies, and custard pies have long been considered favorite American desserts. This section presents the basics of pie dough and pie fillings.

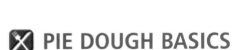 PIE DOUGH BASICS

Basic pie dough is sometimes called 3-2-1 dough. This ratio refers to the weight of three parts flour, two parts fat, and one part water. Successful pie crusts are based on gluten development in the flour and the mixture of flour and fat.

Using proper technique is an important factor in making pie dough. It also helps to understand how the ingredients work together.

■ **Pastry flour.** Pie dough is made from pastry flour because the high gluten content in bread flour absorbs most of the liquid. This makes the dough tough and rubbery. However, pastry flour has enough gluten to keep the dough together so it can be rolled out.

■ **Vegetable shortening.** Butter or vegetable shortening is used to make dough. With a high melting point of 90°F–100°F and consistent qual-

ity, vegetable shortening is the best fat for a pie dough. The shortening should be cut into the flour. The size of the fat particles in the dough determines its flakiness.

■ **Water.** Water or milk at 40°F or colder is added to the dough to form gluten when mixed with flour. It is important not to overmix pie dough or it will become tough. The cold temperature of the water is also important so that the fat in the dough firms up. The crust will fall apart if not enough liquid is added. In contrast, the crust becomes tough if too much liquid is used, because too much gluten develops.

■ **Salt.** Salt tenderizes the gluten and enhances flavor. To be sure it is distributed evenly, either dissolve salt in the liquid before adding it to the dough or sift it with the flour.

Fig. 30-14.

DOUGH	USES
Flaky Dough	• Pie top crusts; prebaked pie shells.
Mealy Dough	• Fruit pies, custard pies, cream pies; bottom crust.

Types of Pie Dough

Two-crust pies have both a bottom and a top crust. The top crust may be partially open in a lattice-work pattern or decorated with dough cutouts. Single-crust pies are often filled with cream or custard mixtures.

A pie is frequently judged by its flaky and tender crust. The two types of pie dough are flaky and mealy. See Fig. 30-14.

■ **Flaky pie dough.** Flour is not completely blended with the fat for flaky dough. Flaky pie dough is either long-flake or short-flake. In long-flake, the fat is about the size of walnuts, which creates a very flaky crust. This is used for the top crust of pies. In short-flake, the fat is in pieces about the size of peas. The gluten develops after the water is added and the dough is mixed. Then the moistened flour and fat form flaky layers when the dough is rolled out. This dough is often used for two-crust pies.

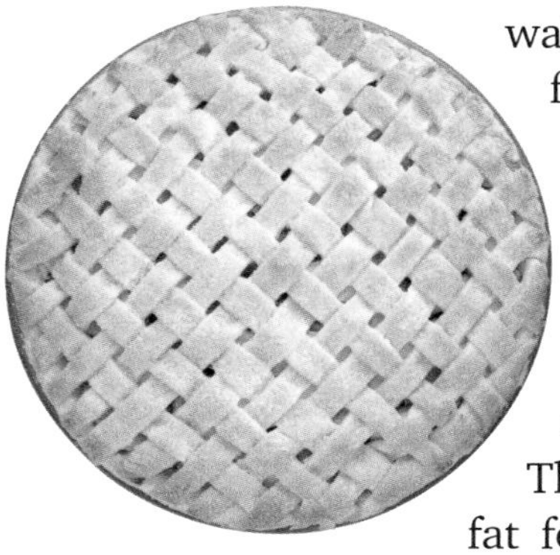

■ **Mealy pie dough.** The texture of mealy pie dough resembles coarse cornmeal. The fat is blended into the flour more completely than it is for flaky dough. Mealy dough also requires less water or milk. The flour particles in mealy dough are more highly coated with fat and will not absorb as much liquid. Because the baked dough is less likely to absorb moisture from the filling, the crust won't be soggy. For this reason, mealy dough is used for the crust in custard and fruit pies.

✖ MIXING PIE DOUGH

It is important not to overmix pie dough. To keep the dough flaky, pie dough should normally be mixed by hand. Pastry flour should be sifted together with the salt before mixing to lessen clumping. Next, the fat is cut into the flour until the fat is the size of peas. The cold liquid is then added and all ingredients are mixed until the dough holds together.

Dough should be covered with plastic wrap and chilled before using. Some pastry chefs refrigerate the dough overnight so that the gluten can relax. This allows the dough and fat to firm for easy handling and rolling. Because pie dough should not be kept refrigerated longer than one week, the dough can also be frozen in 8- to 10-oz. portions. If freezing the dough, wrap it in air-tight packaging and defrost it overnight in the refrigerator before use.

The mixing method for both flaky and mealy dough varies only slightly. The fat is cut into the sifted flour for both kinds of dough. However, the fat in flaky dough is left in pieces the size of walnuts or peas, while the fat in mealy dough is blended to a cornmeal-like consistency. The larger pieces of fat determine the flakiness of the dough.

✖ SHAPING PIE DOUGH

After the dough has been chilled, it is ready to be shaped. If the dough is too cold, allow it to soften slightly before working it.

■ **Scaling the dough.** For a 9-in. top crust, use 7 oz. of dough. For a 9-in. bottom crust, use 8 oz. of dough. Add 1 oz. to the top crust and 2 oz. to the bottom crust for each additional inch of crust diameter.

■ **Dusting the bench and rolling pin with flour.** Do not use too much flour when dusting the bench and rolling pin. Since flour makes the dough tougher, use only what is needed to keep the dough from sticking when rolling it out. See Fig. 30-15.

Combining:
Bringing together two or more components.
1. Prepare the components to be combined.
2. Add one to the other, using the appropriate mixing method (if needed).

NUTRITION:
Calories: 135
Protein: 1.83 g
Fat: 9.69 g

CHEF NOTE:
1. The dry milk solids and the sugar can be sifted at the beginning with the pastry flour. The process would be continued in the same manner.
2. Basic pie dough can be used for many applications. The nutrition analysis is based on 1 oz. of dough.

Basic Pie Dough

YIELD: 1 LB., 8¼ OZ. (THREE, 8-OZ. CRUSTS)   SERVING SIZE: 1 OZ.

INGREDIENTS

12 oz.	Flour, pastry
8 oz.	Shortening, vegetable
¼ oz.	Salt
4 oz.	Water, ice-cold
0–1 oz.	Dried milk solids (optional)

METHOD OF PREPARATION

1. Gather the equipment and scale the ingredients.

2. Sift the flour to aerate it, removing lumps and impurities.

3. Cut the shortening, by hand, into the flour.

4. Dissolve the salt in the cold water.

5. Incorporate the water into the flour until it is sticky. Do not over-work the dough.

6. Allow the dough to rest and chill properly, preferably overnight.

7. Divide the dough into 3, 8-oz. portions.

8. Roll out the dough on a lightly floured pastry cloth. Roll the dough to about a ⅛-in. thickness in a circular form. The dough should be about 1 in. larger than the inverted pie pan.

9. Fold the rolled-out dough in half and carefully place the dough over half the pie pan. Unfold the dough to cover the entire rim of the pie pan. Gently pat the dough from the center of the pan out to work out any air bubbles under the crust.

■ **Rolling out the dough.** Roll the dough to a ⅛-in. thickness all over, after lightly flattening it. Roll the dough from the center to outer edges in all directions. Check the dough occasionally to be sure it isn't sticking. When you have finished rolling, the dough should be perfectly round.

■ **Panning the dough.** Roll the dough tightly around the rolling pin to lift it without breaking. Unroll the dough into the pan. Without stretching it, press the dough into the sides of the pie pan. Be sure there are no air bubbles between the pan and the dough.

Fig. 30-15. Use only enough flour to keep the dough from sticking to the rolling pin. Why is it important to flatten pie dough with a rolling pin?

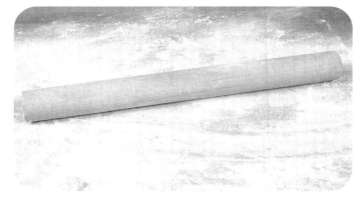

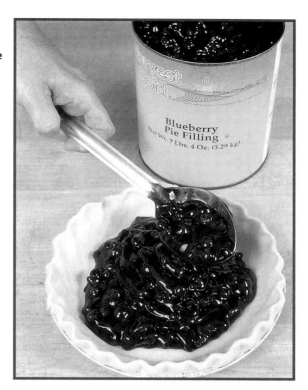

Fig. 30-16. Ready-prepared pie fillings make pie production quick and easy.

■ **Fluting single crust pies.** Fluting the edges of the crust gives a nice finish to the pie. **Fluting** is a manner of decorating the crust by making uniform folds around the edge of the pie. Fold under the extra dough extending beyond the edge of the pan and bring it above the pan's rim, even with the edge. Press thumbs together diagonally to make a ridge around the dough.

■ **Sealing and fluting two-crust pies.** Place the cold filling in the bottom crust and then place the top crust on top of the filling. Use a small amount of water or egg wash to moisten the edge of the bottom crust, and seal the two crusts together. Tuck the edge of the top crust under the bottom crust. Flute the crust and apply an egg wash or a glaze to the top crust if desired.

✖ BAKING PIE SHELLS

Sometimes bakers prepare pie shells in advance, which is known as **baking blind**. The dough is fitted into a pan and pierced with fork tines or a dough docker so that blisters will not form in the dough as it bakes. An empty pie pan is placed on top of the dough and turned upside down to bake. Another method is lining the shell with parchment paper and filling the shell with dried beans or pastry weights. These procedures keep the dough from both blistering and shrinking.

✖ PIE FILLINGS

A variety of fruit, custard, and cream pie fillings can be used. Some fillings are added before the crust is baked. However, some fresh fruit and cream fillings are placed in pre-baked crusts. Specialty pies may contain ice cream or cream cheese fillings, and their assembly may require a combination of the methods mentioned.

Cooked Fruit Fillings

Cooked fruit fillings can be purchased ahead of time, or made on the premises. Ready-made fillings are purchased in 10-lb. cans or 20- to 45-lb. pails for commercial use. See Fig. 30-16. There are two methods for preparing fruit fillings at your foodservice operation: the cooked juice method and the cooked fruit and juice method. In both methods, the fruit filling must cool before it is added to the unbaked shells. Fruit pies are baked between 400°F and 425°F until the crust has an even, golden brown color.

Types of Starches

Various starches are used to thicken pie fillings. Remember to always mix starches with sugar or a cold liquid before adding them to a hot liquid. This procedure helps avoid a lumpy filling.

• Cornstarch sets up a gel that allows the filling to hold its shape when sliced.

• Modified starch, also called waxy maize, is a type of corn product used for fruit pies that will be frozen. Modified starches make a clear, soft paste instead of a gel. These starches don't break down when frozen.

- Tapioca or flour starches are less often used because they cloud the pie filling.
- Pregelatinized starch is precooked. This starch is good to use if the fruit does not need to be cooked before filling the pie shell.

Cream Pie Fillings

Cream pies are filled with flavored pastry cream, which is a thickened egg custard. Cornstarch thickens cream filling and helps it to retain its shape. The filling is cooked on the range and then placed in a prebaked crust. Often cream pies are topped with a **meringue**, which is made of sugar and stiffly beaten egg whites. To lightly brown the meringue topping on a pie, bake the meringue at 400°F until the surface is lightly browned. Examples of cream pies include coconut, lemon, and chocolate. Whipped cream is also used as a topping on cream pies.

Custards

Custard pie fillings are made with eggs. When the pie bakes, the egg protein firms the pie. The secret to making a good custard pie is not to overcook the filling. One way to avoid overbaking is to begin the baking process in a hot oven (400°F–425°F) for the first 10 minutes to set the crust. Then cook the filling slowly by reducing the oven temperature to between 325°F and 350°F.

Soft Pies

Similar to custard pies, soft pies also have eggs in them that firm the pie when it bakes. Pecan is a type of soft pie. This type of pie is baked in the same manner as custard pies.

Chiffon Pies

Chiffon pies are based on either cooked fruit or cream filling. They are stabilized with gelatin that is added to the hot filling. When the filling is cool, a meringue is folded into the filling. The filling is then placed in a prebaked shell and chilled.

a LINK to the Past

Desserts Colonial Style

The word "dessert" comes from the French word desservir (day-zer-VEER), which means "to remove all dishes from the table." As early as 1640, pies, tarts, and cobblers were popular desserts in America. The saying, "as American as apple pie," is popular today, but the apple pie did not originate in America. Deep-dish fruit pies were common in Germany and France long before appearing in the colonies.

Wealthy colonists enjoyed rich desserts such as flummery (FLUHM-muh-ree). A carryover from an ancient British dessert, flummery was made by boiling oatmeal and the water it soaked in until it was smooth and gelatin-like. It was often topped with cream, nuts, raisins, and syrups. In the 18th century, flummery became a soft cream custard, thickened by gelatin and topped with nuts, syrups, and preserves.

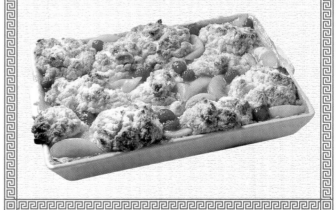

✕ BAKING PIES

For the first 10 minutes, pies should be baked at 400°F–425°F. High heat helps the bottom crust set so that it doesn't soak up extra moisture. Fruit pies, however, are baked in high heat for the entire baking period. To keep from overbaking custard pies, reduce the temperature to between 325°F and 350°F after the first 10 minutes of baking.

Determining Doneness

Gently shake custard or other soft pie to determine if it is done. It has finished baking if no liquid shakes. The pie continues to cook after it is removed from the oven, so a pie with a soft center will continue to firm up. Another way to test for doneness is to insert a knife in the pie's center. If the pie is done, the knife will come out clean.

The best way to judge if a fruit pie has finished baking is to follow the guidelines given in the formula. Baking times will vary, based on the type of fruit used, but crusts should be golden brown.

Fig. 30-17. Pie à la mode is a popular dessert with many customers.

✕ STORING & SERVING PIES

To keep bacteria from growing, custard pies and cream pies must be refrigerated. A baked fruit pie can be kept at room temperature for serving. Unbaked pie shells or unbaked fruit pies may be frozen for as long as two months. A baked fruit pie generally does not freeze well. Neither do meringue-topped, cream, or custard pies.

Pie à la mode, or pie with ice cream, is a familiar dessert item on many menus. The pie is heated, and a scoop of ice cream is placed on top of or beside the pie. See Fig. 30-17.

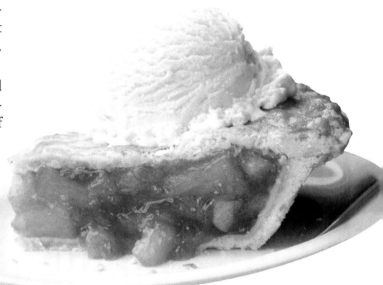

SECTION 30-3 Knowledge Check

1. Describe two types of pie dough.
2. Choose one method of preparing pie dough and explain it.
3. Name the three major types of pie fillings.

MINI LAB

Work in teams to make pies. Choose the best type of pie dough to accompany either a fruit, cream, or custard pie. Share your team's pie with the class. Evaluate each team's pie dough and filling.

Specialty Desserts

OBJECTIVES

After reading this section, you will be able to:

• Explain how ice cream desserts differ.

• Make custards and puddings.

• Store and serve desserts properly.

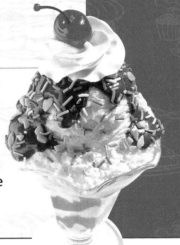

S O M E desserts may not be baked goods, or even cooked items. They may use a combination of preparation methods. These specialty desserts often accompany elegant meals. Frozen desserts, puddings, custards, mousse (moos), chiffons (shef-FONS), and Bavarians (bah-VERY-ahns) are included in this section.

✗ FROZEN DESSERTS

Dessert options include a variety of frozen dishes. A few of the frozen desserts are ice cream, frozen yogurt, sherbet, and sorbet.

■ **Ice cream.** Ice cream is one of the most versatile and popular frozen desserts. It may be served plain in a cone or dish, or as the basis of a rich dessert with fruit or chocolate shavings.

Custard-style ice cream is made with cooked vanilla custard that consists of cream, milk, eggs, sugar, and flavorings. American-style ice cream has no eggs. American style is uncooked and is made with milk, cream, sugar, and flavorings.

■ **Frozen yogurt.** Frozen yogurt includes the typical ingredients for American ice cream with the addition of yogurt. Starches or heavy creams are sometimes added to provide smoothness.

Fruits and other flavors, such as chocolate or vanilla, are the most common additions to yogurt. Nonfat, frozen yogurt is made from nonfat yogurt, which is a common addition to menus.

■ **Sherbet.** Sherbet combines fruit juices, sugar, water, and a small amount of cream or milk to increase smoothness and volume. If the milk or cream is omitted, the result is called **sorbet** (sor-BEY) in French. Sorbets are served as an intermezzo (inter-MET-zo) between courses at a formal meal to cleanse the palate for the next course. It is also served as a light dessert to finish a meal.

Ice cream and sherbet are both mixed constantly in a churn as they freeze. Otherwise, they would freeze in solid blocks. The circulation of air increases the volume and ice crystals remain small. See Fig. 30-18.

Fig. 30-18. Ice cream, frozen yogurt, sherbet, or sorbet adds a refreshing conclusion to a meal. When would you serve each?

✖ CUSTARDS & PUDDINGS

Custards are made of eggs, milk or cream, flavorings, and sweeteners. Custards are baked or cooked in a double boiler on the range. Custard can be served alone; as the base for fruit pies, tarts, or ice cream; or for a dessert sauce.

Pudding is a dessert made from milk, sugar, eggs, flavorings, and cornstarch or cream for thickening. Chocolate, butterscotch, and vanilla are the most common types of pudding.

Stirred & Baked Custards

Stirred custards are made on the range in a double boiler or saucepan. To keep the custard from overcooking, it must be stirred constantly. These custards, therefore, do not set as firmly as baked custards do. Stirred or baked custard is used as a dessert sauce, or can become part of a more complex dessert.

■ **Baked custard.** Baked custards work on the same principle as stirred custards: the eggs must coagulate and the custard must become thick, not runny. Thickening occurs during the baking process. If overbaked, the protein in the eggs coagulates too much. This leads to a curdled, broken, and watery custard. Custards should be taken from the oven when the center is still slightly fluid. To make a baked custard, follow these steps:

1. Mix eggs, sugar, salt, and vanilla in a bowl until blended.
2. **Scald** milk in double boiler by heating it to just below simmering. To scald means to heat just below the boiling point.
3. Slowly pour the milk into the egg mixture. Be sure to stir it constantly.
4. Pour the custard into cups that are arranged in a shallow hotel pan.
5. Skim off any bubbles that form on top of the custard.
6. Pour water into the hotel pan, making sure that the level of water is equal to the level of the custard in the cups.
7. Bake the custard at 325°F for the length of time indicated in the formula or until it is set, such as the consistency of firm gelatin.
8. Remove the custard from the oven, being careful not to spill the hot water. Cool and then store the custard covered in the refrigerator.

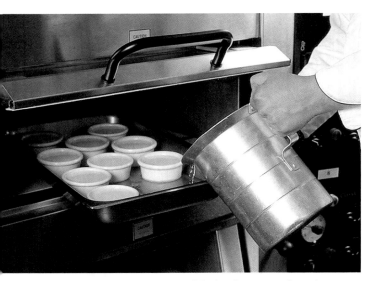

Fig. 30-19. A bain marie will help the custard cook properly. What other foods can you think of that require the use of a bain marie?

■ **Smooth custard.** When making a custard, it is important to add small amounts of hot liquid gradually while beating the egg and liquid mixture. This helps keep the custard from curdling. When custard curdles, the eggs separate from the solids, making it tough. Custards should be velvety and smooth. A bain marie, or a water bath, is used to insulate the custard pan so that the custard doesn't bake too quickly. When baking the custard, keep the oven at a low setting between 325°F and 350°F. If you are cooking custard on the range, the double boiler should be kept at between 165°F and 170°F. See Fig. 30-19.

Puddings

Puddings are popular, profitable, and economical. A good pudding results from careful preparation and a trusted recipe. The most common dessert puddings in foodservice operations are starch-thickened and baked.

■ **Starch-thickened puddings.** Starch-thickened puddings, also called boiled puddings, require starch as the thickening agent. To cook the starch, the pudding is boiled in a saucepan. Pastry cream is a good example of starch-thickened pudding. The resulting mixture can be poured into molds and chilled. To serve these puddings, unmold

them and garnish them with chocolate shavings, fresh mint, or fruit such as raspberries.

■ **Baked puddings.** Two popular styles of baked puddings are rice pudding and bread pudding. Both of these desserts are made by adding a large amount of either rice or bread to the custard. Baked puddings are often topped with rich sauces to enhance their appearance and make them more flavorful.

✖ BAVARIANS, CHIFFONS & MOUSSES

Bavarians, chiffons, and mousses are all based on ingredients and techniques discussed earlier. Custard, whipped cream, and fruit fillings thickened by starches can be combined to make these airy desserts.

A **Bavarian**, or Bavarian cream, is made of whipped cream, gelatin, and a flavored custard sauce. The gelatin is softened in cold water or another liquid. Then it is dissolved in a hot custard sauce and cooled until it is nearly set. Next, whipped cream is folded in, and the entire mixture is put in a mold to set.

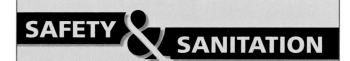

PREVENTING FOODBORNE ILLNESS—Cream desserts, such as custard, can carry foodborne bacteria. Follow these safety guidelines:
• Store cream desserts in food-grade plastic.
• Don't use leftover creams or sell day-old cream products, such as eclairs or cream puffs.
• Keep cream desserts covered when cooling to prevent a skin from forming.
• Cool cream quickly in a shallow pan to avoid contamination.
• Use pasteurized egg products when preparing Bavarians, chiffons, and mousses.

The amount of gelatin is key in a good Bavarian cream. While too much gelatin makes the Bavarian rubbery and overly firm, too little gelatin makes the dessert too soft to hold its shape. Be sure to measure accurately.

Chiffons can be served as chilled desserts, not only as pie fillings. The process of making a chiffon is similar to the one above for Bavarians except that meringue is substituted for the whipped cream. Other chiffon bases may be fruit fillings and pastry cream.

Mousse is a light and airy dessert made with both meringue and whipped cream to enhance the lightness. Fresh fruit or melted chocolate often serves as a base for mousse. Mousse is often served in eye-catching containers, such as hollowed fruits and special molds. See Fig. 30-20.

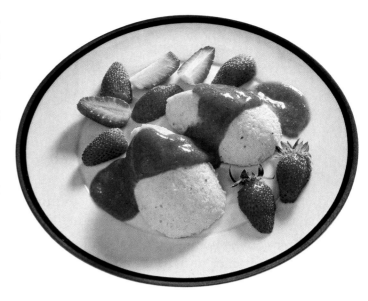

Fig. 30-20. Adding whipped ingredients, such as cream or meringue, make chilled desserts light and airy.

✖ STORING & SERVING DESSERTS

Any dessert with eggs or cream must be kept refrigerated or frozen until it is served. Ice cream and sherbet should be kept at 0°F or below to keep large ice crystals from forming. Before serving a frozen dessert, it should be held at 8°F–15°F for 24 hours, so that it will be soft enough to serve.

Parfaits (pahr-FAYS) and sundaes are two popular desserts. A parfait is a frozen dessert flavored with heavy cream. Sundaes contain one or more scoops of ice cream topped with garnishes, fruits, or syrups.

In general, the following guidelines can be used for serving special desserts:
- All elements of the dessert should work together to offer a pleasing flavor.
- Contrasting flavors, colors, and textures can be served together as long as the final effect is pleasing.
- The appearance, texture, and taste of each item must be of the highest quality.

SECTION 30-4 Knowledge Check

1. Explain how sherbet and sorbet differ.
2. Give two guidelines to follow when making a custard.
3. Identify the common ingredients in Bavarians, chiffons, and mousses.

MINI LAB

As a team, prepare a dessert and present it to the class as a plated dish. Evaluate each team's dessert and discuss what you learned from this experience.

SECTION SUMMARIES

30-1 Cookies offer more variety of form, texture, and type than any other bakery item.

30-1 The different types of cookies vary in mixing and panning methods and baking time.

30-1 After cooling cookies, store them in an airtight container until serving.

30-2 The five types of cakes have two basic categories of batter, each of which has a different mixing method.

30-2 Bakers often scale the batter in pans to ensure uniformity in baking.

30-2 Bake time and oven temperature must be carefully observed, as well as the proper procedure for cooling cakes.

30-3 Flaky and mealy pie doughs are chosen for different types of end products.

30-3 Fruit, custard, and cream are all varieties of pie fillings.

30-3 Baked pies can either be refrigerated or left at room temperature depending on type, while unbaked pies may be frozen until needed.

30-4 Frozen desserts offer a wide range of variety from ice cream to sherbet.

30-4 The most common dessert puddings in foodservice operations are starch-thickened and baked puddings.

30-4 Store egg and cream dessert ingredients in the refrigerator or freezer for safety.

CHECK YOUR KNOWLEDGE

1. How does the type of flour used change the formation of a cookie?

2. Compare rolled and drop cookies.

3. Describe a pound cake.

4. List distinctive characteristics of angel food cake.

5. Compare high-fat and low-fat cakes.

6. Describe three tests for cake doneness.

7. Explain how icing helps improve a cake.

8. Explain 3-2-1 pie dough.

9. Describe flaky dough and when it's used.

10. What ingredients are used in frozen desserts?

CRITICAL-THINKING ACTIVITIES

1. If you wanted to increase the spread of a cookie and you had used all your milk and eggs, what could you add?

2. Why do you think that high-ratio cakes require a high amount of emulsified shortening to absorb the liquids?

3. Would waxy maize be an adequate thickener for frozen yogurt? Why or why not?

WORKPLACE KNOW-HOW

Problem solving. Your foodservice operation has decided to serve a frozen dessert at a summer reception that will be held in a nearby park. What dessert would you recommend and how will you store it until you are ready to serve it?

LAB-BASED ACTIVITY: Making Cream Puffs

STEP ❶ In teams, prepare the Basic Cream Puffs.

STEP ❷ Prepare one of the following fillings:
- Custard filling
- Pudding
- Sweetened fruit, or ice cream

STEP ❸ Choose one or more of the following toppings:
- Confectioners' sugar
- Frosting
- Hot fudge sauce
- Whipped topping
- Fresh fruit
- Nuts
- Ice cream

STEP ❹ Split cream puffs almost all the way around, or cut in halves almost down to the bottom crust. Fill one half of the puff with the filling and put the halves together. Place on a dessert plate.

STEP ❺ Add the topping and plate your dessert.

STEP ❻ Explain why the filling and the topping go well together.

STEP ❼ Evaluate your dessert using the following rating scale.

Poor = 1; Fair = 2; Good = 3; Great = 4

Basic Cream Puffs
YIELD: 25 CREAM PUFFS   SERVING SIZE: 2 OZ.

INGREDIENTS:

8 oz.	Unsalted butter or shortening
¼ oz.	Salt
¼ oz.	Granulated sugar
1 lb.	Water or whole milk
10½ oz.	Sifted bread flour
1 lb.	Eggs

METHOD OF PREPARATION

1. Gather the equipment and ingredients.
2. Place the butter, salt, granulated sugar, and water or milk in a medium pot.
3. Bring to a boil.
4. Add all of the sifted flour at once.
5. Stir with a wooden spoon for approximately 5 min. or until the mixture forms a ball that does not stick to the inside of the pot.
6. Cook at this point for an additional 3 min.
7. Remove from the heat, and place the mixture in a mixing bowl.
8. Mix on low speed until cooled slightly.
9. Add the eggs gradually; mix at low speed; make sure the eggs are fully incorporated before the next addition.
10. When the eggs are fully incorporated, use a pastry bag and tip to pipe the mixture into the desired shapes on parchment-lined sheet pans. Makes about 25, 2-oz. cream puffs.
11. Bake at 400°F–425°F until brown and dry on the inside.

Baking & Pastry

Baking and pastry employees use a variety of doughs and batters to produce breads, cakes, muffins, pies, biscuits, pastries, and elegant desserts. Attention to detail, good eye-hand coordination, and an artistic flair are key skills for those interested in baking and pastry.

Baking and pastry workers must be skilled in basic bread and pastry techniques, and have an in-depth knowledge of how ingredients function together. These individuals find work in all types of settings, from small neighborhood bakeries to large hotel catering operations.

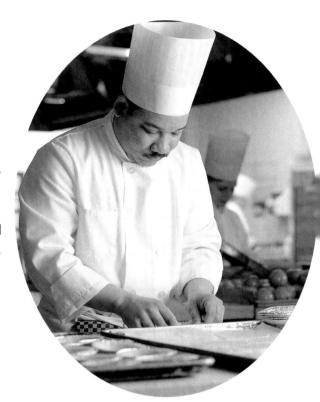

Baker's helpers assist bakers in preparing non-dessert baked items, such as breads and rolls.

Baker and pastry apprentices work closely with the baker or pastry chef in preparing baked products and fancy desserts.

Pastry cooks work under a pastry chef. They prepare items such as desserts and specialty cakes for all occasions.

Pastry chefs are responsible for the preparation of pastries and desserts. They supervise pastry cooks and bakers. Pastry chefs may also be responsible for creating new formulas.

Bakers generally prepare breads and rolls. In some operations, they also bake cakes and pies. In large operations, each baker may focus on a different type of baked product.

Production bakers must be familiar with large retail baking systems, product development, bakery management, and sales.

Confectionery food technologists work with developing bakery and confectionery products, and establish specifications for raw materials used in food products. Experience with making products is essential.

Chef instructors are experienced chefs who choose, after many years of experience, to become instructors at the high school or college level.

In large bakery and pastry operations, you may find the following work opportunities available:

District sales managers, cake decorators, production supervisors, bakery/food scientists, executive pastry chefs, and flavorists.

Working in the Real World...

EXECUTIVE PASTRY CHEF

My name is Casey Shiller and I am the executive pastry chef for the Boeing™ Leadership Center. As part of my job, I supervise the preparation of all cakes, pies, cookies, muffins, breakfast pastries, plated desserts, breads, and pastries. The foundation for my career started with my education at Johnson & Wales University. I graduated with honors with a Bachelor of Science in Pastry Arts and Baking.

Throughout my career, the work experiences I have had have allowed me to continually develop my technical skills in pastry arts and baking. Among the prestigious properties that I have worked are the Trump Plaza Hotel-Casino®, Trump Taj Mahal Hotel-Casino®, the Trump Worlds Fair Hotel-Casino® in Atlantic City, New Jersey; and The Ritz-Carlton® Amelia Island near Jacksonville, Florida.

I'm also a faculty member at St. Louis Community College. I teach classes in baking, pastry, chocolates, wedding cakes, and confectionary art. I'm an active member of the American Culinary Federation (ACF), the US Pastry Alliance, and the St. Louis Chefs de Cuisine Association. I also coach the Missouri State Junior Culinary Team.

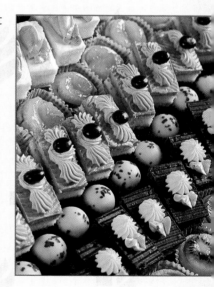

In the year 2000, I was named one of the "Top 10 Rising Star Pastry Chefs 2000," by Chocolates à la Carte®. I have also earned several gold and silver medals for my chocolate sculptures and plated desserts at the New York Food Show.

JOHNSON & WALES UNIVERSITY

National High School Recipe Contest

High School seniors compete for college scholarships!

Have you created your own recipes?
Are you considering a culinary arts career?

In the fall of each year since 1989, Johnson & Wales University, the world's largest food service educator, has invited high school seniors to submit their own original recipes into competition for thousands of dollars in Johnson & Wales tuition scholarships.

- Regional experts and celebrity judges from all areas of food service evaluate contest entries and bring excitement to the competition.

- Scholarships are awarded in amounts up to full tuition in the College of Culinary Arts at Johnson & Wales University. All scholarships apply to full-time, day-school study and are renewable for up to four years. Actual receipt of a scholarship is subject to the student being otherwise qualified and accepted for admission to Johnson & Wales University.

- A $500 J&W grant is awarded for all complete entries.

- The National Competition will be held at one of Johnson & Wales University's four campuses. The University arranges free transportation and accommodations for each student finalist whose entry is selected for national competition.

The Johnson & Wales National Recipe Contest is held in cooperation with the American Cancer Society and the American Heart Association. Because it is important to develop good dietary habits early in life to reduce cancer risks and heart disease, the American Cancer Society and the American Heart Association have published the following nutritional and dietary guidelines based on scientific research. You are encouraged to make healthful menu choices and take these guidelines into consideration when planning your entry to the Johnson & Wales University National High School Recipe Contest.

GENERAL JUDGING CRITERIA

CRITERIA	MAX POINTS
Overall quality, flavor, taste, texture, doneness	40
Presentation	20
Creativity	20
Nutritional Value	100
Kitchen Score: Mise en Place; Sanitation/Cooking Techniques	100
TOTAL SCORE	280

For the current year's contest details, entry form, deadlines, judging criteria, contest guidelines, and competition dates, log onto:
www.jwu.edu/admiss/recipecontest

American Heart Association®

■ Some vegetables and fruits, such as mushrooms, tomatoes, chili peppers, cherries, cranberries and currants, have a more intense flavor when dried than when fresh. Use them when you want a burst of flavor. Plus, there's an added bonus: when they're soaked in water and reconstituted, you can use the flavored water in cooking.

■ Shrimp, lobster, crab, crayfish and most other shellfish are very low in fat. But ounce for ounce, some varieties contain more sodium and cholesterol than do poultry, meat or other fish.

■ Some fish have omega-3 fatty acids, which may help lower the level of lipids (blood fats). Some fish high in omega-3 fatty acids are: Atlantic and Coho salmon, albacore tuna, mackerel, carp, lake whitefish, sweet smelt, and lake and brook trout.

■ Some wild game, such as venison, rabbit, squirrel and pheasant are very lean; duck and goose are not.

■ Oils that stay liquid at room temperature are high in unsaturated fats. They include corn, safflower, soybean, sunflower, olive and canola (rapeseed) oils. All are low in saturated fatty acids and can be used to help lower blood cholesterol in a diet low in saturated fatty acids.

■ Use egg whites in place of whole eggs. In most recipes one egg white and a little acceptable vegetable oil will substitute nicely for a whole egg.

American Cancer Society®

■ Add fresh or dried fruits like chopped apples, raisins, prunes, kiwi or orange sections to green leafy salads.

■ Substitute applesauce for oil in muffins, quick breads and cakes. Use puréed prunes or baby food prunes instead of oil in brownies or chocolate cake.

■ Substitute whole wheat flour for up to half of the white flour called for in a recipe.

■ Use evaporated skim milk instead of whole milk or cream in baked goods, sauces and soups.

■ Use low-fat or non-fat yogurt to replace all or part of the sour cream or mayonnaise in a recipe. Replace all or part of the ricotta cheese with low-fat cottage cheese. Use a purée of cooked potatoes, onions and celery as a creamy base for soups instead of dairy cream or half-and-half.

■ Use low-fat cooking methods like roasting, baking, broiling, steaming or poaching. Use either a cooking spray, broth, water or a well-seasoned cast iron pan to sauté meats. If you must use oil or margarine, cut the amount in half.

GENERAL CONTEST GUIDELINES

To enter the contest, submit your original recipes for one of the following categories:

- **Healthful Dinner**—a hot entrée as well as a vegetable and a starch.
- **Healthful Dessert**—a hot or cold plated dessert.

Contest judges look for innovative combinations and streamlined preparation. An interesting variation on a traditional recipe is more apt to score well than the use of exotic and difficult-to-obtain ingredients.

Contest Requirements

- Each student may submit only one contest entry.
- Participants entering the National High School Recipe Contest are ineligible to compete in any other national contest that Johnson & Wales University sponsors.

Portion Sizes

- The dinner or dessert must consist of four servings.
- The dinner or dessert dish will be presented on four 12" round, off-white plates supplied by Johnson & Wales University.

Preparation Time

- Preparation time must not exceed three hours. No prior preparation is allowed (i.e., no overnight processes or procedures).

Recipe

- Recipes must be typed on plain 8½" x 11" paper.
- List ingredients in order of preparation. The method of preparation and/or ingredients cannot be changed once the recipe has been submitted.
- List and describe the steps in the preparation process and itemize the quantities and types of ingredients required.
- Include a list of ingredients and equipment required.

Photographs

Two (2) copies of an original 4" x 6" color photo of your prepared entrée (one serving) must accompany your entry. These photos will be used for comparison purposes. (Quality and clarity of photographs are important.)

Signature

The entry form must be signed by your parent or guardian and your foods teacher or guidance counselor, attesting to the originality of your recipe.

Healthful Dinner Requirements

- Entrée must be a meat, fish, poultry, or vegetarian dish.
- Entrée must be accompanied by a side dish of a starch and a vegetable.
- Presentations must be enhanced by a garnish. The garnish must complement the entrée, be edible, and appear on the recipe and ingredient list.
- Recipes should be nutritionally balanced according to the American Heart Association (AHA) and American Cancer Society (ACS) guidelines.

Healthful Dessert Requirements

- Plated dessert may be either a hot or a cold plated item.
- Presentations must contain four (4) components of plated desserts:

  The Main Item is an individual serving of a dessert—usually between 3-5 oz.

  The Sauce(s) is usually between 1-2 oz. One sauce is all that is necessary, but multiple sauces are often used on a plated dessert.

  The Garnish can be a simple dusting of powdered sugar or a more complex use of sorbet or ice cream. The garnish must complement the dessert, be edible, and appear on the recipe and ingredient list.

  The Crunch Component is a decorative cookie that gives textural contrast to the main item. It is always used when the main item itself does not contain "crunch" *(flour)*, but it can be used for any dessert if desired.

- Recipes should be nutritionally balanced according to the American Heart Association (AHA) and American Cancer Society (ACS) guidelines.

Helpful Hints

- Be specific on sizes, amounts, and types of products needed. No convenience food items may be used. All recipes, including pasta, must be made "from scratch" (i.e., no pudding mixes, cake mixes, etc.).
- Regional seasonality should be taken into consideration (i.e., dessert should reflect the Western U.S. in late fall to early spring).
- Using ice cream as the main item of the dessert is discouraged due to time constraints.

HEALTHFUL DESSERT RECIPE

Fruit Passion: Berry, Kiwi, and Orange Cornucopia

YIELD: 4 SERVINGS

Cornucopia

INGREDIENTS

1 lb. shredded phyllo dough
spray grease release

METHOD OF PREPARATION

1. Pull shredded phyllo dough into long strands.
2. Spray metal cones with grease release.
3. Wrap phyllo dough around cone forms and spray again.
4. Bake in a 350°F oven until golden brown, about 7-10 minutes.

Filling

INGREDIENTS

4 oz. Neufchâtel cheese, softened
⅓ c. lemon-flavored low-fat yogurt
1 tbsp. confectioners' sugar

METHOD OF PREPARATION

1. Beat Neufchâtel cheese in a small bowl.
2. Stir in yogurt and confectioners' sugar.

Fruit Mixture

INGREDIENTS

1 pt. blackberries
1 pt. raspberries
1 pt. strawberries
2 each kiwi
½ c. Mandarin oranges

METHOD OF PREPARATION

1. Clean blackberries, raspberries, and strawberries.
2. Hull and cut strawberries so that they are the same size as the other berries. Cut some blackberries in half for size (if needed). Peel and cut kiwi.
3. In a bowl, gently mix all fruit and chill.

Kiwi Coulis

INGREDIENTS

4 each kiwi

METHOD OF PREPARATION

1. Peel and purée kiwi in a food processor.
2. Strain and pour into a squeeze bottle for use garnishing.

Strawberry Coulis

INGREDIENTS

1 pt. strawberries
½ oz. cornstarch
Water as needed

METHOD OF PREPARATION

1. Clean strawberries.
2. If needed, add cornstarch to enough water to form slurry and use to thicken.
3. Pour into a squeeze bottle for use garnishing.

Blackberry Coulis

INGREDIENTS

1 c. blackberries

METHOD OF PREPARATION

1. Clean blackberries.
2. Purée in a food processor and strain.
3. Pour into a squeeze bottle for use garnishing.

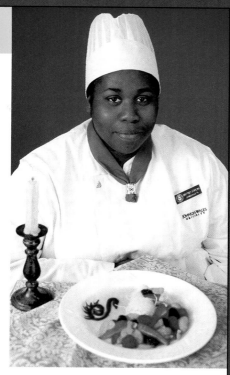

Brittney Starling
Eastside High School
Gainesville, Florida

PLATING INSTRUCTIONS

1. Gently pipe filling into cornucopia.
2. Arrange fruit mixture to appear as though spilling out of cornucopia.
3. Garnish with strawberry coulis, blackberry coulis, and kiwi coulis.

Baked Striped Bass with Mango Salsa, Roasted Red Bliss Potatoes and Zucchini Fans, and Curried Haricots Verts with Carrot

YIELD: 4 SERVINGS

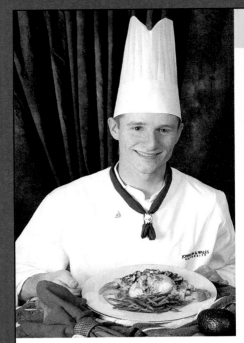

William Schibel, Jr.
Central Bucks East High School
Doylestown, Pennsylvania

Baked Striped Bass with Mango Salsa

INGREDIENTS

2 lbs. striped bass filet, bones removed
½ red onion
1 tsp. olive oil
1 red bell pepper
4 ripe mangos, peeled and diced
Juice of 4 limes; 1 tbsp. set aside
2 tbsp. finely chopped cilantro
½ tsp. ancho chili powder
Salt and pepper to taste
2 ripe avocados

METHOD OF PREPARATION

1. Preheat oven to 350°F.
2. Lay filets on a cutting board with the "good" side up. Using a boning knife, cut a slit down the center of the top of the filet lengthwise from the top to the bottom, being careful not to cut all the way through to the cutting board. Create a "pocket" by opening up the slit. Place in the refrigerator on a sheet pan lined with parchment paper.

3. Remove the skin from the onion and brush with ½ tsp. of the olive oil, grill and dice ¼ inch. Place in mixing bowl.
4. Cut the red pepper in half, remove the seeds, brush with the remaining ½ tsp. olive oil, grill and dice ¼ inch. Add to onion.
5. Add the mango, lime juice, cilantro, chili powder, salt and pepper to the onion and red pepper and mix well.
6. Stuff the pockets of the filets with the mango salsa, reserving ½ c. for garnish. Season each filet with salt and pepper. Cut each filet in half to create 4 portions.
7. Bake in preheated oven for approximately 20 minutes or until internal temperature of fish is 145°F.
8. Avocodo Fans: Peel avocados and remove pits. Quarter and brush with lime juice.
9. Place 1 portion in the center of each preheated dinner plate.
10. Place 1 avocado fan next to each filet and place a heaping tbsp. of salsa at the top of the fan.

Roasted Red Bliss Potatoes and Zucchini Fans

INGREDIENTS

8 each red bliss potatoes, washed and striped (peel a strip of skin off, going around lengthwise)
2 zucchini, washed and sliced in ⅛ in. rounds
3 tbsp. minced shallot
3 tbsp. chopped basil
1 tbsp. minced fresh ginger
Salt and black pepper to taste

METHOD OF PREPARATION

1. Blanch potatoes in boiling, salted water until almost done.
2. Strain carefully; set potatoes on paper towels and cool in the refrigerator.
3. Slice potatoes in ⅛ in. thick rounds and put them in a large stainless steel bowl.
4. Add the rest of the ingredients to the bowl and toss gently.
5. Line up 2 bamboo skewers for each serving on a sheet pan and place aluminum foil across the top of each pair to make a "crib." On each crib, alternate 6 pieces of potato and 6 pieces of zucchini.
6. Bake at 350°F for 25 minutes.
7. Transfer fans to one side of each dinner plate next to the Baked Striped Bass.

Curried Haricots Verts with Carrot

INGREDIENTS

1½ lbs. haricots verts
1 tbsp. extra virgin olive oil
¼ lb. carrots, julienned
1 tsp. curry powder
1 tbsp. freshly chopped basil
Salt and black pepper to taste

METHOD OF PREPARATION

1. Blanch haricots verts in boiling, salted water for 1 minute; shock and drain well.
2. Heat olive oil in a sauté pan over medium heat. Add the blanched beans, carrots, and the rest of the ingredients to the pan and sautée for approximately 3 minutes.
3. Stack moderately tall next to the fish on the remaining side of the dinner plate.

Reach for the Stars

YIELD: 4 SERVINGS

Creamy Lemon Custard

INGREDIENTS

1½ c. sugar
⅓ c. cornstarch
1½ c. water
2 tbsp. lemon peel, grated
½ c. lemon juice
8 oz. low-fat cream cheese, softened
5 drops yellow food coloring

METHOD OF PREPARATION

1. In medium saucepan, combine sugar and cornstarch.
2. Gradually stir in water; blend until smooth.
3. Cook over medium heat for 10-12 minutes, or until mixture boils and thickens, stirring constantly.
4. Remove from heat and stir in lemon peel and lemon juice.
5. In medium bowl, beat cream cheese until smooth.
6. Slowly stir in hot filling mixture and food coloring into cream cheese until well blended.
7. Cool for 30 minutes.

Angel Food Cake

INGREDIENTS

¾ c. flour
¾ c. sugar
12 large egg whites, room temperature
1½ tsp. cream of tartar
1¼ tsp. vanilla extract
½ tsp. almond extract
¾ c. sugar

METHOD OF PREPARATION

1. Preheat oven to 375°F.
2. In a small bowl, combine flour and ¾ c. of sugar.
3. In a separate large bowl, beat the egg whites with cream of tartar, vanilla and almond extracts until soft peaks form.
4. Gradually add ¾ c. of sugar and continue beating at high speed until stiff peaks form.
5. Gradually add flour mixture to egg whites, folding in gently until blended.
6. Pour batter into ungreased 10 in. tube pan.
7. Bake in pre-heated oven for 30-40 minutes. Continue baking until crust is golden brown.
8. Immediately invert cake and allow to cool completely.

Raspberry Sauce

INGREDIENTS

⅓ pt. fresh raspberries
2 tbsp. confectioners' sugar

METHOD OF PREPARATION

1. In a food processor, blend the raspberries until they become liquefied.
2. Add the confectioners' sugar and mix together until blended.
3. Pour into a squeeze bottle.

White Chocolate Sauce

INGREDIENTS

6 oz. white chocolate disks

METHOD OF PREPARATION

1. Melt chocolate over a double boiler until smooth.
2. Pour ⅔ of chocolate into a squeeze bottle.
3. Take the remaining chocolate and pour into a pastry bag with a plain tip.
4. On a sheet of wax paper, squeeze out designs of the white chocolate and freeze for about 10 minutes.

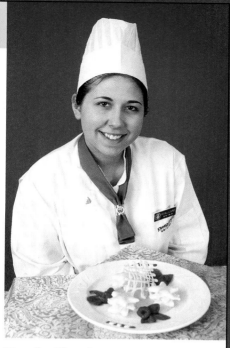

Rochelle Courey
North Royalton High School
North Royalton, Ohio

PLATING INSTRUCTIONS

1. Using a serrated knife, slice the cake horizontally to create four layers.
2. Use a star-shaped cookie cutter to cut out nine stacks of star-shaped cake pieces, 36 in total.
3. Create 12 stacks in this order: slice of cake, spoonful of custard, slice of cake, spoonful of custard, slice of cake.
4. Drizzle four plates with sauces and place four stacks on each plate. Garnish with white chocolate design.

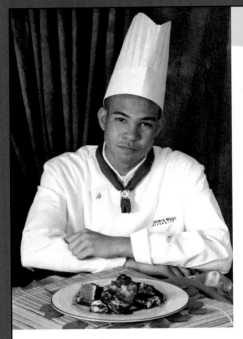

Jason Johnson
Silver Creek High School
San Jose, California

Sesame Seed Encrusted Tuna, Garlic-Flavored Mixed Vegetables, Nori Rolls, and Blood Orange Sauce

YIELD: 4 SERVINGS

Sesame Seed Encrusted Tuna

INGREDIENTS

4 each, 4 oz. tuna steaks cut 1 in. thick
Salt, black pepper, and cayenne pepper to taste
2 tsp. wasabi powder
Water as needed
½ c. white sesame seeds
1 tbsp. olive oil

METHOD OF PREPARATION

1. Season tuna steaks with salt, black pepper, and cayenne.
2. Prepare wasabi by blending wasabi powder with enough water to form a firm paste. Allow paste to sit for 5 minutes before using. Coat tuna steaks with wasabi paste and refrigerate until needed.
3. When ready for service, coat the tuna with sesame seeds. Heat a sauté pan to very hot and add olive oil. Sear tuna on all sides; tuna should be cooked medium-rare. Slice ¼ in. thick. Serve with Garlic-Flavored Mixed Vegetables, Nori Rolls, and Blood Orange Sauce.

Garlic-Flavored Mixed Vegetables

INGREDIENTS

1 tbsp. Canola oil
1 c. macedoine of carrots
1 c. macedoine of zucchini
1 c. macedoine of yellow squash
1 c. thinly sliced mushrooms
4 tbsp. granulated garlic
Pinch of salt

METHOD OF PREPARATION

1. Heat canola oil and sauté carrots until almost tender. Add the rest of the vegetables and sauté until tender.
2. Add the garlic and salt. Set aside.

Nori Rolls

INGREDIENTS

2 c. Calrose short grain rice
3 c. water
3 tbsp. black sesame seeds
1½ tbsp. light soy sauce
2 tbsp. rice wine vinegar
4 each Nori wrappers
1 red bell pepper, julienne

METHOD OF PREPARATION

1. Wash rice three times in cold water and drain well. Place rice into a medium saucepan and add water. Bring to a boil, cover, reduce heat, and cook on very low for 20 minutes. Let rest for 5 minutes.
2. Meanwhile, dry sauté sesame seeds to toast, then toss gently into the cooked rice along with the soy sauce and vinegar.
3. Place approximately ½ c. of rice on nori wrapper and spread evenly over entire wrapper. Place 3 to 4 strips of red pepper in the center of the wrapper and roll sushi style. Slice on the bias and set aside.

Blood Orange Sauce

INGREDIENTS

Juice of 6 blood oranges
4 oz. canned pineapple juice
2 tbsp. heavy cream
2 tbsp. light corn syrup
Pinch of sugar
2 tbsp. miso paste
¼ tsp. cornstarch slurry

METHOD OF PREPARATION

1. Combine all ingredients in a saucepan over medium heat.
2. Whisk until sauce is smooth and slightly thickened. Set aside.

Garnish

INGREDIENTS

3 blood oranges cut in segments
20 chives
½ c. chopped green onions

PLATING INSTRUCTIONS

1. Pack vegetables into a 3-in. ring mold and place on the center of the plate.
2. Fan tuna slices decoratively.
3. Place two nori rolls on plate.
4. Drizzle sauce over tuna.
5. Garnish with: blood orange segments, chives, and sprinkling of green onions.

Warm Bittersweet Chocolate Cakes with Raspberry Purée

YIELD: 4 SERVINGS

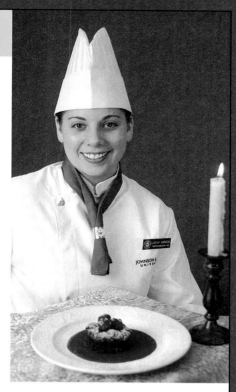

Lindsay Olivia Swinson
St. Margaret's High School
Tappahannock, Virginia

Warm Bittersweet Chocolate Cakes

INGREDIENTS

Nonstick cooking spray
1 tsp. cocoa powder for dusting
8 oz. bittersweet chocolate, finely chopped
¼ c. margarine
Dash of salt
⅓ c. cholesterol-free egg substitute

6 tbsp. sugar substitute (Splenda)
2 tbsp. cocoa powder
1 tbsp. fresh orange zest, finely grated
3 large egg whites
12 whole raspberries for garnish
3 tbsp. confectioners' sugar for dusting

METHOD OF PREPARATION

1. Preheat oven to 400°F. Lightly grease four (7-oz.) ramekins and dust with cocoa powder. Place ramekins on a small baking sheet.
2. Combine the chocolate and margarine in a double boiler until melted, then whisk until mixture is glossy with a smooth consistency.
3. Remove mixture from heat and stir in the salt, then allow to cool slightly.
4. Using a large bowl and mixer on high speed, beat the egg substitute, half of the sugar substitute, the 2 tbsp. of cocoa, and orange zest until consistency is thick.
5. Spoon the chocolate mixture into the egg substitute mixture and beat until well blended, resulting in a thick mixture.
6. In another bowl with clean beaters, beat the egg whites on medium-high speed until foamy and thick.
7. Sprinkle the remaining sugar and increase the speed to high until firm, glossy peaks form.
8. Spoon half of the beaten egg whites onto the chocolate mixture, whisking until blended. Then add the remaining whites and stir gently until just blended. Spoon into the prepared ramekins.
9. Bake the cakes until puffy with cracked tops, approximately 15 minutes.
10. Remove from oven. Run a small knife around the inside of each ramekin to loosen the cake and invert onto serving platters.

Raspberry Purée

INGREDIENTS

1½ c. frozen raspberries
⅛ c. water
⅓ c. powdered sugar
½ tsp. fresh lemon juice

METHOD OF PREPARATION

1. Using a blender, combine the raspberries, water, and confectioners' sugar, pulsing until a smooth purée forms.
2. Press purée through a sieve.
3. Stir in lemon juice.

PLATING INSTRUCTIONS

1. Cover the center of plate with 3 tbsp. of raspberry purée.
2. Center the cake in the middle of plate, garnish with 3 raspberries, and dust with powdered sugar.

Honey-Baked Pork Tenderloin, Green Beans, and Garlic Mashed Potatoes

YIELD: 4 SERVINGS

Honey-Baked Pork Tenderloin

INGREDIENTS

- 1½ lbs. pork tenderloin (Note: may be in two pieces)
- ½ c. sweet yellow pepper, trimmed, seeded, and diced
- ½ c. sweet red pepper, trimmed, seeded, and diced
- ¼ c. onion, finely chopped
- ¼ c. celery, finely chopped
- 1 clove garlic, crushed
- ½ c. whole-wheat breadcrumbs, toasted
- 1 egg substitute, beaten
- ⅛ c. chopped pecans, toasted
- ¼ tsp. pepper
- 3 tbsp. apple juice, unsweetened
- 2 tbsp. honey
- Vegetable spray

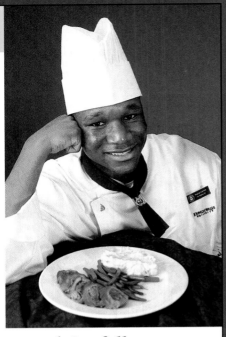

Marcel Canfell
Beaufort-Jasper Academy
for Career Excellence
St. Helena Island, South Carolina

METHOD OF PREPARATION

1. Preheat oven to 350°F.
2. Rinse pork roast under cold, running water and pat dry. Set aside.
3. Coat a medium nonstick skillet with cooking spray; place over medium-high heat until hot.
4. Add yellow pepper, red pepper, onion, celery, and garlic and sauté until tender-crisp. Drain.
5. Combine vegetable mixture, breadcrumbs, egg substitute, pecans, and pepper in a medium bowl; stir well.
6. Butterfly the pork by cutting down the center of the meat, about ¾ of the way through. Slice each side of the meat in the same manner, until the whole piece of meat opens flat.
7. Spread the stuffing mixture over the meat, leaving about 1 inch around the edges. Roll the meat up tightly, and secure by tying with kitchen twine.
8. Place meat in a small roasting pan that has been sprayed with vegetable spray.
9. Combine apple juice and honey, stirring well. Brush pork roast with half of apple juice-honey mixture. Bake at 350°F for 1½ to 2 hours or until the internal temperature reaches 155°F, basting occasionally with remaining apple juice-honey mixture.
10. Allow meat to set for about 20 minutes, then slice and plate.

Green Beans

INGREDIENTS

- 1 lb. fresh green beans, washed and trimmed
- 1 tsp. olive oil

METHOD OF PREPARATION

1. Blanche green beans by plunging into boiling water for 30 seconds, then immediately plunging into ice water until cool; drain.
2. When ready to serve, heat the olive oil in a nonstick sauté pan until hot. Add green beans and quickly stir fry until tender-crisp and hot.

Garlic Mashed Potatoes

INGREDIENTS

- 2 c. baking potatoes, peeled and cubed
- 2 cloves garlic, minced
- ½ c. skim milk
- 1 tsp. fresh chives, snipped
- Salt and pepper to taste

METHOD OF PREPARATION

1. Cook potato cubes in boiling water until tender. Drain potatoes well.
2. Mash potatoes, adding milk, garlic, and chives. Season to taste.

Raspberry & Kiwi Parfait Baskets

YIELD: 4 SERVINGS

Baskets

INGREDIENTS

3 tbsp. sweet butter, plus extra for greasing
3 tbsp. superfine sugar
4 tbsp. corn syrup
½ tsp. allspice
1 tsp. almond extract
¼ c. all-purpose flour
2 tbsp. whole wheat flour

METHOD OF PREPARATION

1. Preheat oven to 350°F.
2. Put butter, sugar, and corn syrup in a pan and stir over medium heat until melted. Simmer for 3 minutes; remove from the heat.
3. Stir in allspice, almond extract, and flour; mix until smooth. Set aside for 10 minutes.
4. Cut 2 sheets of parchment paper to measure approximately 8 in. square each. Place on cookie sheet. Drop enough of the mixture on the parchment paper to make two circles, each measuring 4 in. in diameter. Allow plenty of space between them as they will spread.
5. Bake for 15 minutes, then mold into basket shapes over 2 upturned cups or ramekins. Repeat three times to make a total of 6 baskets. Let set.
6. Break two of the baskets into pieces for use later.

Filling

INGREDIENTS

½ c. low-fat cottage cheese, strained through cheesecloth
¼ c. low-fat sour cream
4 tbsp. softened Neufchâtel cheese
1½ tbsp. Splenda
½ tsp. vanilla extract
¼ tsp. grated lemon peel
¼ tsp. lemon extract

METHOD OF PREPARATION

1. Blend all ingredients until smooth.
2. Keep chilled until ready to use.

Raspberry Sauce

INGREDIENTS

12 oz. frozen raspberries
5 tbsp. water
2 tbsp. Splenda
¾ tsp. Knox unflavored gelatin

METHOD OF PREPARATION

1. Heat raspberries with sugar and 3 tbsp. water.
2. Strain through cheesecloth or sieve.
3. Dissolve gelatin in 2 tbsp. boiling water.
4. Mix with raspberry juice and cool.

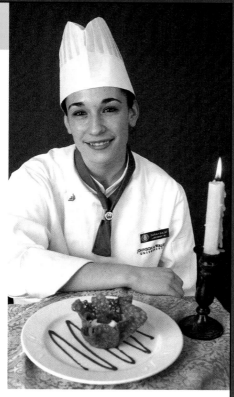

Sara Baum
Mamaroneck High School
Larchmont, New York

PLATING INSTRUCTIONS

1. Place one basket shape on each plate.
2. Layer each basket with sliced fresh kiwi and a spoonful of cheese mixture.
3. Garnish with kiwi slices, fresh raspberries, and crunchy basket pieces.
4. Place raspberry sauce in bottles and drizzle on each plate.

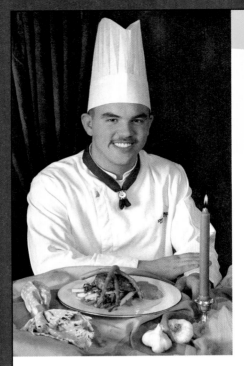

Chris McDonald
Plantation High School
Plantation, Florida

Mahi Mahi with Seasonal Vegetables, Sweet Potatoes, and Asparagus

YIELD: 4 SERVINGS

Mahi Mahi

INGREDIENTS

½ c. olive oil
2 tbsp. balsamic vinegar
1 tsp. honey
1 tsp. chopped garlic
¼ c. peeled, seeded, and chopped tomato
¼ tsp. salt
¼ tsp. black pepper
⅓ c. packed chopped herbs: basil, dill, tarragon, and parsley

. . . .

4 each Mahi Mahi fillets
Creole seasoning, as needed
1 tbsp. olive oil

METHOD OF PREPARATION

1. Vinaigrette: Combine olive oil, balsamic vinegar, honey, garlic, tomato, salt, pepper, and herbs; whisk well to blend. Hold in refrigerator.
2. Season the Mahi Mahi fillets with Creole seasoning.
3. Heat olive oil in a large skillet over medium heat. Add the fish fillets to hot oil and sear until they are lightly golden and flake easily with a fork, approximately 4 to 6 minutes per side.
4. Plate each Mahi Mahi fillet on top of seasoned vegetables and top with vinaigrette.

Seasonal Vegetables

INGREDIENTS

1 tbsp. olive oil
⅛ head white cabbage, cored and chiffonade
⅛ head red cabbage, cored and chiffonade
½ tsp. salt
¼ tsp. black pepper
2 c. thinly sliced red onion
4 medium sized carrots, julienne
1 medium sized zucchini, julienne
1 medium sized yellow squash, julienne
⅓ c. water

METHOD OF PREPARATION

1. Heat olive oil in large skillet over medium-high heat. Add the white cabbage, red cabbage, salt, and pepper, and cook for two minutes, stirring occasionally.
2. Add the onions and cook for two more minutes, stirring occasionally.
3. Add the carrots and cook for two more minutes, stirring occasionally.
4. Add the zucchini, yellow squash, and water, and cook for two more minutes or until crisp, stirring occasionally.

Sweet Potatoes

INGREDIENTS

2 large sweet potatoes, cut into thick slices
1 tbsp. nutmeg
2 tbsp. honey

METHOD OF PREPARATION

1. Boil potato slices in water until soft.
2. Drain and mash with nutmeg and honey.
3. Place a serving of sweet potatoes to one side of the Mahi Mahi.

Asparagus

INGREDIENTS

12 asparagus spears

METHOD OF PREPARATION

1. Boil asparagus until tender and drain.
2. Drape three asparagus spears across the top of each Mahi Mahi fillet.

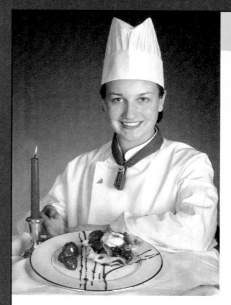

Michelle Moser
Downingtown High School
West Chester, Pennsylvania

Almond and Chocolate Tuile Nest

INGREDIENTS

2 oz. unsalted butter
3 large egg whites
¼ tsp. pure almond extract
2 oz. all-purpose flour
2 oz. confectioners' sugar
½ tsp. salt
2 tsp. cocoa powder (Dutch processed)

METHOD OF PREPARATION

1. Preheat oven to 350°F.
2. Melt butter. In small bowl combine butter, egg whites, and almond extract. Set aside.
3. Sift together flour, sugar, and salt.
4. In medium bowl combine flour mixture and butter mixture.
5. Remove ⅓ c. batter, place in custard cup and add to it the cocoa. Allow both batters to rest for 30-45 minutes at room temperature.
6. Using a parchment cone, drizzle some of the chocolate batter onto a non-stick baking mat in a circular pattern. Spread approximately 2 tbsp. almond batter on top of the chocolate so that it becomes a rough circle with a diameter of 6 in.

Almond and Chocolate Tuile Nest with Fresh Berry Mix and Hard-Crack Strawberries

YIELD: 4 SERVINGS

7. Bake the Tuile at 350°F for 4 to 6 minutes. The edges of the cookie will be golden brown.
8. Immediately remove cookie and drape over small ramekin, or shallow baking dish. Allow to cool in the shape of a nest. Set aside until ready to use.

Berry Mix with Lemon Simple Syrup

INGREDIENTS

4 oz. water
4 oz. sugar
½ lemon, zest
½ lemon, juice
1 lb. strawberries, fresh
4 oz. blueberries, fresh
4 oz. raspberries, fresh

METHOD OF PREPARATION

1. Combine water, sugar, lemon zest, and lemon juice in small saucepan.
2. Boil and continue to heat until 225°F. Set aside.
3. Wash fruit.
4. Quarter strawberries.
5. In medium bowl, combine fruit and syrup; set aside until ready to use.

Quick Crème Fraiche

INGREDIENTS

4 oz. heavy cream
1½ oz. sour cream (reduced fat)
2 tsp. granulated sugar

METHOD OF PREPARATION

1. In a medium bowl whisk together heavy cream, sour cream, and sugar until soft peaks form when whisk is lifted.
2. Cover and refrigerate until ready to use.

Chocolate Ganache

INGREDIENTS

2 oz. semi-sweet chocolate
2 oz. heavy cream

METHOD OF PREPARATION

1. Grate chocolate into small bowl.
2. Heat cream to boiling; pour over grated chocolate and stir until well combined.
3. Cover and set aside until ready to use.

Hard-Crack Strawberries

INGREDIENTS

16 oz. water
16 oz. granulated sugar
12 medium to small strawberries

METHOD OF PREPARATION

1. In large saucepan, heat sugar and water to 300°F.
2. Dip strawberries in sugar, place on non-stick baking mat to cool until ready to use.

Garnish

1 small bunch fresh mint
1½ lemon, zest

PLATING INSTRUCTIONS

1. Using a parchment cone, pipe ganache onto plate to resemble a tree with one branch on the right-hand side.
2. Fill Tuile with ¼ of berry mixture and place on plate "resting" on the tree branch.
3. Top the nest with a generous tbsp. of crème fraiche; garnish with lemon zest and sprig of mint.
4. Place three hard-crack strawberries on the left-hand side of the plate for balance.

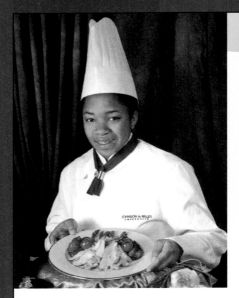

Colby Felix
DelMar High School
San Jose, California

Grilled Honey Dijon Rosemary Chicken Breast

INGREDIENTS

2 tbsp. Dijon mustard
1 tsp. honey
4 tsp. fresh rosemary, finely chopped
½ tsp. salt
¼ tsp. black pepper
4 each 3- to 4-oz. chicken breasts

METHOD OF PREPARATION

1. In a large bowl, combine all ingredients except chicken. Mix well to create a marinade.
2. Coat chicken with marinade.
3. Cook breasts on a broiler or grill over medium heat to an internal temperature of 165°F.
4. Turn breast ¼ turn on presentation side. Slice on the bias and fan on plates.

Herbed Cream Sauce

INGREDIENTS

2 tbsp. flour
2 c. skim milk
6 oz. crimini mushrooms, sliced
1 tsp. Dijon mustard
1 tsp. honey
2 tsp. granulated garlic
1 tsp. black pepper
2 tsp. fresh rosemary, minced
½ c. chicken stock

Grilled Honey Dijon Rosemary Chicken Breast with Herbed Cream Sauce, Sautéed Artichokes and Cherry Tomatoes with Garlic, Roasted Garlic Fettuccine, and Steamed Asparagus

YIELD: 4 SERVINGS

METHOD OF PREPARATION

1. In a sauté pan, dry sauté flour until lightly browned.
2. Pour flour and milk into a jar. Shake vigorously until completely blended, then strain.
3. Pour mixture into a saucepan and heat, stirring until mixture begins to thicken.
4. Add the remainder of the ingredients and continue stirring until the mushrooms are tender and the sauce is a medium consistency.

Sautéed Artichokes and Cherry Tomatoes with Garlic

INGREDIENTS

3 medium artichokes
2 tbsp. olive oil, divided
¼ tsp. salt
½ tsp. ground black pepper
Juice of 1 blood orange
1 tbsp. fresh oregano, minced
1 tbsp. freshly minced garlic
1 pt. cherry tomatoes

METHOD OF PREPARATION

1. Trim off stem of each artichoke flush with base. Pull back the leaves until you reach the center where the leaves are light in color. Trim the crown slightly and cut off the top third to half of the artichoke. Cut crowns into wedges and coat each with 1 tbsp. of the olive oil, salt, and black pepper.
2. Put remaining 1 tbsp. olive oil in a sauté pan over low heat. Add the artichokes and sauté on low until golden.

3. Cover and cook until they are just tender, stirring occasionally.
4. Add the blood orange juice, oregano, garlic, and cherry tomatoes. Sauté for another 1 to 2 minutes or until tomato skins start to wrinkle slightly.

Roasted Garlic Fettuccine

INGREDIENTS

1 lb. flour
¾ tsp. salt
3 egg whites
4 large bulbs roasted garlic
¼ to ½ c. water, as needed

METHOD OF PREPARATION

1. In a food processor, combine the flour, salt, egg whites, and roasted garlic. Pulse until ingredients form large crumbs.
2. Remove from processor and knead by hand to form a dough, adding water if needed. Cover with plastic wrap and allow dough to rest for 10 minutes.
3. Divide dough into 4 equal pieces. Roll dough into thin sheets. Cut into noodles.
4. Lightly dust noodles with flour and set aside.
5. Cook in boiling salted water until al dente. Drain.

Steamed Asparagus

INGREDIENTS

20 asparagus spears

METHOD OF PREPARATION

1. Steam asparagus until crisp-tender.
2. Shock in an ice bath, drain, and set aside until needed.
3. Reheat in boiling water for 1 minute to serve.

Chocolate Raspberry Bavarian

YIELD: 8 SERVINGS

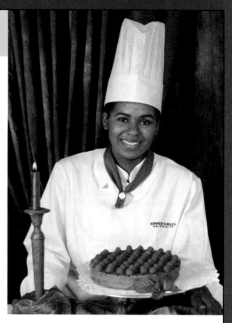

Tiffany Burnett
Martin Luther King, Jr. High School
Detroit, Michigan

Chocolate Angel Food Cake

INGREDIENTS

3 oz. sifted cake flour
3 oz. sugar, divided
1 oz. unsweetened cocoa
½ tsp. ground cinnamon
6 egg whites
½ tsp. cream of tartar
½ tsp. vanilla extract
1 pt. raspberries

METHOD OF PREPARATION

1. Preheat oven to 350°F.
2. Sift together the flour, half the sugar, cocoa, and cinnamon; set aside.
3. In a mixer, whip egg whites and cream of tartar in an extra-large bowl at high speed until foamy. Gradually add remaining sugar, whipping until soft peaks form.
4. Sift flour mixture into egg white mixture, folding in 2 tbsp. at a time.
5. Fold in vanilla.
6. Spoon batter into an ungreased 9-in. cake pan, spreading evenly with a spatula.
7. Bake for about 20 minutes, or until cake springs back when lightly touched. Remove cake from oven; cool.
8. Loosen cake from sides of pan. Put a parchment collar around the cake.
9. Top with Bavarian Cream and freeze until set.
10. Cover and chill until firm. Garnish with raspberries.

Bavarian Cream

INGREDIENTS

1 envelope unflavored gelatin
⅙ c. water
10½ oz. evaporated skim milk
1 egg, separated
1½ c. part-skim ricotta cheese
¼ c. plus 1 tbsp. sugar, divided
1 oz. unsweetened cocoa
¾ tsp. vanilla extract

METHOD OF PREPARATION

1. Sprinkle gelatin over water in medium pan. Let stand for 5 minutes.
2. Combine milk and egg yolk, stirring well. Add to gelatin mixture. Cook over low heat, stirring constantly until gelatin dissolves. Remove from heat.
3. Using paddle attachment on mixer, add cheese, ¼ c. sugar, cocoa, vanilla, and ⅓ c. of the gelatin mixture. Mix until smooth.
4. Combine remaining gelatin mixture and cheese mixture in large bowl and beat to consistency of unbeaten egg white. Beat at high speed for 1 minute.
5. Gradually add remaining 1 tbsp. sugar, beating until stiff peaks form and sugar dissolves. Chill for 10 minutes.
6. Whip the egg white and gently fold into chilled cheese mixture. Spoon on top of prepared cake and chill 3 hours, or until firm.

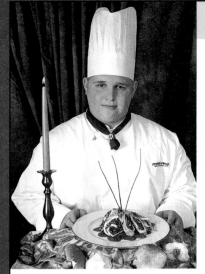

Matthew R. Betlach
Stoneman Douglas High School
Coral Springs, Florida

Spinach Portobello Roulades

INGREDIENTS

4 tbsp. olive oil, separated in half
1 small shallot, minced
2 garlic cloves, minced
3 large portobello mushrooms, diced
8 oz. fresh spinach, chiffonade
½ c. balsamic vinegar
¼ c. grated Parmesan cheese
Salt and pepper to taste

. . . .

2 each, 1-lb. whole skinless, boneless chicken breasts
Salt and pepper to taste
4 tbsp. olive oil

. . . .

24 baby spinach leaves
12 chives, 5 to 6 in. long

METHOD OF PREPARATION

1. Preheat oven to 375°F.
2. *Stuffing:* Heat 2 tbsp. olive oil in a sauté pan. Add the minced shallot and sweat until translucent. Add the minced garlic and cook until garlic starts to turn golden brown. Add the diced mushrooms and cook down for about 3 to 8 minutes. Add the remaining 2 tbsp. of olive oil and the spinach. When spinach starts to wilt, add the balsamic vinegar and cook for

Spinach Portobello Roulades, Roasted Garlic Sweet Potatoes, and Dijon String Beans

YIELD: 4 SERVINGS

1 to 2 more minutes on high heat. Remove pan from heat and strain any remaining liquid. Cool in refrigerator. When cooled, add the Parmesan cheese and season as needed with salt and pepper.

3. Place a chicken breast between two pieces of plastic wrap and pound with a meat mallet to flatten the breast to about ¼ in. thick. Repeat with other chicken breast.

4. Season the chicken with salt and pepper. Place a thin layer of the cooled stuffing on the flattened breast and roll breast up starting with the thinnest side and tuck sides in as you go; truss with butcher's twine.

5. Heat the 4 tbsp. olive oil and sear chicken roulades on all sides until browned.

6. Place in the oven and bake for 10 minutes or to an internal temperature of 165°F. Let rest for 5 minutes before slicing on the bias.

7. To plate: Place 6 baby spinach leaves on each warm dinner plate, stems facing inward. Place a mound of Roasted Garlic Sweet Potatoes in the center of the plate. Place 4 to 5 slices of the chicken roulade against the sweet potatoes, and arrange the Dijon Beans on the right side of the roulade. Place 3 chives on top.

Roasted Garlic Sweet Potatoes

INGREDIENTS

2 medium bulbs of garlic
1 tbsp. olive oil
1½ lbs. sweet potatoes
⅓ c. milk

METHOD OF PREPARATION

1. Preheat oven to 375°F.
2. Cut tops off the bulbs of garlic and place them in the middle of a sheet of aluminum foil. Drizzle olive oil over garlic; close foil and bake for 1 hour and 15 minutes. Remove from oven and let cool.
3. Pierce each sweet potato with a fork and place in oven for 1 hour, or until soft.
4. Remove roasted garlic from skins and place in a small bowl. Place milk in a small sauté pan and heat over low heat. When milk is simmering, whisk into the roasted garlic until mixture is smooth.
5. When sweet potatoes are soft, remove them from the oven and remove the skins. Place the sweet potatoes in a bowl and mash. Add the garlic-milk mixture and mix well. Do not overmix.

Dijon String Beans

INGREDIENTS

6 oz. fresh green beans
6 oz. fresh wax beans
1 tbsp. butter
¼ c. water
1 tbsp. Dijon mustard
3 tbsp. evaporated skim milk
2 tbsp. freshly chopped parsley

METHOD OF PREPARATION

1. Trim and clean the beans.
2. In a sauté pan, melt the butter and sauté the beans for 1 to 2 minutes. Add water and steam the beans for 8 minutes.
3. Mix the Dijon mustard and milk in a bowl.
4. When the beans are done, strain any leftover water. Add the beans to the mustard-milk mixture; add the parsley, and toss well.

Key Lime Chiffon Cake

YIELD: 16 SERVINGS

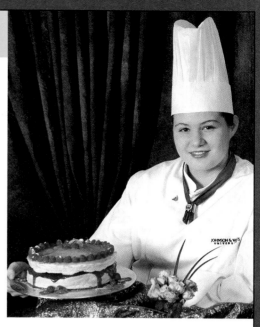

Courtney Hatch
Sun Valley High School
Indian Trail, North Carolina

Cake

INGREDIENTS

Non-fat, butter-flavored cooking spray
2 c. sifted cake flour
2 c. sugar
1 tbsp. baking powder
½ tsp. salt
½ c. applesauce, unsweetened
¾ c. egg substitute
½ c. water
1½ tsp. vanilla extract
Juice of 1 key lime
Grated zest of 4 key limes
8 egg whites at room temperature
½ tbsp. cream of tartar

METHOD OF PREPARATION

1. Preheat oven to 325°F.
2. Line two round 8-in. cake layer pans with parchment paper. Lightly spray the sides with cooking spray.
3. In a large mixing bowl, sift together cake flour, sugar, baking powder, and salt. Make a well in the middle.
4. In a separate bowl, beat together applesauce, egg substitute, water, vanilla, lime juice, and zest.
5. Pour wet mixture into flour mixture and blend well.
6. In a large mixing bowl, beat egg whites until frothy. Add cream of tartar and beat until egg whites form stiff peaks.
7. Take ½ c. of beaten egg whites and stir into flour and egg mixture to lighten it. Gently fold in the remaining egg whites. When blended, divide batter between the prepared pans.
8. Bake for 25 minutes or until cake is golden brown and begins to pull away slightly from sides. Do not open oven door until cake is almost done, or it may fall.
9. Run spatula around edges and turn out at once onto a wire rack. Cool completely.
10. To assemble, spread Raspberry Filling evenly on bottom layer of cake. Top with second layer and spread with Key Lime Topping. Decorate cake with key lime slices, raspberries, and mint sprigs on top of cake and around base. Dust with confectioners' sugar.

Raspberry Filling

INGREDIENTS

1 pt. fresh raspberries
1 tsp. lemon juice
¼ c. water
2 tbsp. cornstarch
¾ c. sugar

METHOD OF PREPARATION

1. In a blender, purée raspberries with lemon juice and half of the water (⅛ c.). Strain to remove seeds.
2. Mix remaining water with cornstarch to dissolve.
3. In a small saucepan, combine purée, cornstarch, and sugar. Cook over medium-low heat, stirring constantly, until mixture thickens.
4. Remove from heat and place in refrigerator to cool.

Key Lime Topping

INGREDIENTS

½ c. sugar
4 tbsp. cornstarch
⅔ c. water
5 tbsp. fresh key lime juice
1 tbsp. egg substitute

METHOD OF PREPARATION

1. In a small saucepan, combine all ingredients and cook over low heat, stirring constantly, until mixture thickens.
2. Remove from heat and let cool.

Glossary

A

à la carte (ah-lah-KART) **menu**—A menu that offers each food and beverage item priced and served separately. (12-1)

abrasion—A scrape that's considered to be a minor cut, such as a rug burn. (7-1)

accompaniments—Items that come with the meal, such as a choice of potato, rice, or pasta and a choice of vegetable. (12-1)

active listening—The skill of paying attention and interacting with the speaker. (2-1)

additives—Substances added to foods to improve them in some way. (11-1)

advertising—A paid form of promotion that persuades and informs the public about what a facility has to offer. (5-4)

al dente (al-DEHN-tay)—"To the bite"; to cook pasta so that it is not too soft or overdone. (25-1)

albumin—The clear white of an egg. (17-1)

amino acids—Small units of protein that have been broken down through digestion. (11-1)

angel food cakes—Foam cakes that are made with egg whites. (30-2)

antipasto—The Italian word for "before pasta"; a combination tray that typically includes cold meats, assorted cheeses, olives, marinated vegetables, and fruits. (18-4)

appetizers—Small portions of food meant to stimulate the appetite that are served as the first course of a meal. (3-2, 12-3, 21-2)

apprentice—A person who works under the guidance of a skilled worker in order to learn a particular trade or art. (1-3)

aroma—A distinctive pleasing smell. (16-2)

as-purchased (AP) price—The bulk price of an item. (14-1)

as-served (AS)—The actual weight of a food product that is served to customers. (14-1)

atmosphere—The "feeling" or "sense" that customers receive from the interior and exterior of a facility. (5-4)

au jus (oh-ZHOO)—To serve open-face sandwiches accompanied by the juices obtained from roasting meat. (19-2)

avulsion (auh-VUHL-shun)—A wound in which a portion of the skin is partially or completely torn off, such as a severed finger. (7-1)

B

bacteria (back-TEAR-ee-ah)—Tiny single-celled microorganisms that can make people very sick if they find their way into food. (7-2)

bain marie—A piece of equipment used to keep foods, such as sauces and soups, warm so they can be used in other dishes; also referred to as a water bath. (9-4)

baker's percentage—A type of measurement meaning that each ingredient is a certain percentage of the weight of the total flour in a formula. (13-1, 27-1)

baking blind—When bakers prepare pie shells in advance. (30-3)

balance—Dividing space to meet customer and preparation staff needs. (5-3)

banquette (bang-KEHT)—A type of seating arrangement in which customers are seated facing the server with their backs against the wall. (4-1)

barding—The process of wrapping a lean meat with fat, such as bacon, before roasting. (24-1)

base—A powdered or concentrated form of stock. (20-1)

baste—To spoon fat drippings that have collected in a pan over large birds, such as turkey, every 15–20 minutes. (23-2)

batch cooking—The process of preparing small amounts of food several times throughout a foodservice period. (11-3)

batonnet (bat-toh-nay)—¼-in.-thick matchstick-shaped cuts. (10-1)

batter—A semiliquid mixture that contains almost equal parts of dry and liquid ingredients, such as flour, eggs, and milk. (15-2, 27-2)

Bavarian (bah-VERY-ahn)—A dessert made of whipped cream, gelatin, and a flavored custard sauce; also called Bavarian cream. (30-4)

bench rest—A short, intermediate proofing stage for dough that allows the gluten to relax. (28-2)

biscuit method—A method of mixing that involves cutting in fat with dry ingredients. (29-2)

bisque—A specialty soup that is made from shellfish and contains cream. (21-1)

bivalve (BY-valv)—A mollusk that has two shells hinged together. (22-2)

blanching—Using the boiling method to partially cook food. (15-3)

blending method—A mixing method that involves using oil or liquid fat to blend ingredients. (29-3)

blends—Combinations of herbs, spices, and seeds that are used as flavorings. (16-1)

body language—Expressing your thoughts through physical action. (3-1)

boiling—A moist cooking technique in which you bring a liquid, such as water or stock, to the boiling point and keep it at that temperature while the food cooks. (15-3)

bolster—A shank or collar in the spot where the blade and handle of a knife come together. (10-1)

bouquet garni—A combination of fresh herbs and vegetables tied in a bundle with butcher's twine. (16-2)

bouquetière (boo-kuh-tyehr)—A bouquet of three or more vegetables arranged on a plate surrounded by other foods. (26-2)

braising—A long, slow combination cooking technique in which food is seared and then simmered in enough liquid to cover no more than ⅔ of the food. (15-3)

breading—Coating a food item with crumbs and egg. (15-2)

break even—What happens to an operation when projected cost equals projected income. (5-1)

brigade—A team of people in a foodservice operation in which each member specializes in a particular type of food preparation. (1-1, 18-1)

brochettes (broh-SHEHTS)—Combinations of meat, poultry, fish, and vegetables served on small skewers. (21-2)

broiling—A dry cooking method in which food is cooked directly under a primary heat source. (15-2)

brown rice—Rice that has had the hull, or outer covering, removed. (25-2)

brunoise (broon-WAZ)—⅛-in.-thick cubes cut from julienne slices. (10-1)

bulk—Large quantities of a single food product. (14-1)

business plan—A document that gives specific information about the future of a business. (1-4)

butler service—A type of meal service in which appetizers are carried on a serving plate at a standing event. (21-2)

butterflied—A fish that is dressed, then cut so the two sides lay open, yet are attached by skin. (22-1)

bypassing—When people or materials must walk or be moved past unrelated stations during the foodservice process. (5-3)

C

calamari (kah-lah-MAH-ree)—The Italian name for squid. (22-2)

calculate—The ability to work with numbers. (2-1)

calibrated (ka-luh-brate-ed)—Or adjusted; a food thermometer should be adjusted before each shift or each delivery, and if it is dropped. (8-2)

canapé (KAN-uh-pay)—A small, open-face sandwich that consists of two main parts, a platform, or base, and a cushion, or topping. (18-4)

candelabra (can-duh-LAH-brah)—A branched candlestick. (4-2)

cappuccino (kahp-uh-CHEE-noh)—A beverage made from espresso and steamed and foamed milk. (3-3)

caramelization (kar-muh-leye-ZAY-shuhn)—The process of cooking sugar to high temperatures. (15-1)

carbohydrates—The body's main source of energy, or fuel. (11-1)

cardiopulmonary resuscitation (CAR-dee-oh-PALL-mun-air-ee ree-CESS-ah-tay-shun)—Emergency care that is performed on people who are unresponsive, such as those who are unconscious because of choking, cardiac arrest, stroke, or heart attack. (7-1)

cardiovascular (CAR-dee-o-VAS-kyu-lur)—Heart-related. (11-1)

carryover cooking—The cooking that takes place after you remove something from the heat source. (15-2)

centerpieces—Decorative objects placed on tables to add beauty and interest. (4-2)

cephalopod (SEHF-uh-luh-pod)—A mollusk that has a thin internal shell. (22-2)

certification—Proof of expertise. (1-3)

chafing (CHAYFE-ing) **dish**—A device that holds a large pan of food over a canned heat source. (4-1)

chain—A restaurant operation that has two or more locations that sell the same products and are operated by the same company. (5-4)

chain restaurant—Many individual restaurants that all have the same atmosphere, service, menu, and quality of food. (1-4)

cheddaring—A process in which slabs of cheese are stacked and turned. (18-3)

chewy cookies—Cookies that have a high ratio of eggs, sugar, and liquid, but a low ratio of fat. (30-1)

chiffon (shef-FON) **cakes**—Cakes made by using whipped egg whites, or meringue, to lighten the mixture. (30-2)

chiffonade (shif-o-NOD)—To finely slice or shred leafy vegetables or herbs. (10-1)

cholesterol (kuh-LES-tuhr-ol)—A fatty substance found in all body cells and in all animal foods, such as meat, egg yolks, and dairy products. (11-1)

chowder—A specialty soup made from fish, seafood, or vegetables. (21-1)

chutney—A condiment made of fruit, vinegar, sugar, and spices. (26-1)

clarify—To remove particles in soup as they float to the top. (21-1)

clientele—The people who will be a business's main customers. (5-4)

clip-ons—A list of specials fastened to the menu. (12-3)

club sandwich—A triple-decker sandwich that features cold, sliced cooked turkey and ham (or bacon), cheese, tomato, and lettuce. The ingredients are layered between three slices of toasted bread and cut into four triangles. (19-2)

coagulate—To change from a liquid or semiliquid state to a drier, solid state. (15-1)

colander—A container with small holes in the bottom for rinsing and draining food. (25-1)

cold-pack cheese—A cheese product made from one or more varieties of cheese, especially Cheddar or Roquefort cheeses; also known as club cheese. (18-3)

collagen—Soft white tissue that breaks down into gelatin and water during slow moist cooking processes. (24-1)

combination cooking—Cooking techniques that use both moist and dry cooking techniques. (15-1)

commercial operations—Operations that earn more than enough to cover daily expenses, resulting in a profit. (1-2)

compensatory time—Extra pay or extra time off that employers must give to employees who work overtime. (2-3)

competitors—Businesses that offer similar products or services. (5-4)

competitors' pricing method—Method of determining menu selling prices in which a foodservice operation charges approximately what the competition is charging. (12-4)

compotes—Fresh or dried fruits that have been cooked in a sugar syrup. (26-1)

compotier (KAHM-pooht-tee-ay)—A deep stemmed dish used to serve compotes, candies, and nuts. (26-1)

condiments—Items such as mustard, pickle relish, and ketchup that are traditionally served as accompaniments to food. (4-2, 16-3)

connective tissue—The tissue that holds muscle fiber together. (23-1)

consommé—A concentrated, clear soup made from a rich broth. (21-1)

contaminated—Food that contains harmful microorganisms or substances that make food unfit to be eaten. (7-2)

continental menus—Table d'hôte breakfast menus that provide mostly a selection of juices, beverages, and baked goods. (12-1)

convection—The process during which the liquid closest to the bottom of a pan is heated and rises to the top, while the cooler liquid descends to the bottom of the pan. (15-3)

convection oven—An oven that has a fan that circulates the oven's heated air. This fan allows you to cook foods in about 30% less time and at temperatures approximately 25°-35°F lower than temperatures in a conventional oven. (27-1)

conversion factor—The number that results from dividing the desired yield by the existing yield in a recipe. (13-2)

cooking line—Arrangement of the kitchen equipment. (9-1)

cookware—Pots, pans, and baking dishes. (10-2)

corporation—A type of ownership created when the state grants an individual or a group of people a charter with legal rights. (1-4)

cost per portion—The cost of the amount of food you would serve to an individual customer. (14-1)

coulis (koo-LEE)—A sauce made from a fruit or vegetable purée. (20-2)

count—The number of individual items used in a recipe to indicate the size of each item. (13-2)

cover—An individual place setting that includes flatware, glassware, and dishes. (3-2)

creaming method—A mixing method in which ingredients like softened fat and sugar are combined first until light and fluffy. (29-3)

crêpes (krayps)—Small, thin pancakes made with egg batter. (19-1)

crisp cookies—Cookies that have very little moisture in the batter. (30-1)

critical control point—A step in the flow of food where contamination can be prevented or eliminated. (8-2)

cross-contamination—Contamination caused by the movement of chemicals or microorganisms from one place to another. (7-2)

cross-train—To provide work experience in a variety of tasks. (1-1)

croutons (KROO-tawnz)—Small pieces of bread that have been grilled, toasted, or fried and sometimes seasoned. (18-2)

crudité (kroo-dee-TAY)—The French word for "raw," or in this case, raw vegetables. (18-4)

crumb—The internal texture of a baked product. (27-2)

crust—The outer surface of a bread or roll. (27-2)

crustaceans—Shellfish that have a hard outer shell and jointed skeletons. (22-2)

cryovaced (cry-OH-vacked)—To shrink-wrap food items for purchasing and shipping. (26-1)

curdle—The separation of eggs and solids, resulting in a tough yet watery egg dish. (17-2)

curing—Preserving pork with salt, sugar, spices, flavoring, and nitrites. (24-2)

cycle menu—A menu that is used for a set period of time, such as a week, a month, or even longer. (12-1)

D

daily values—The amount of nutrients a person needs every day based on a 2,000-calorie diet. (11-2)

deductions—The money withheld from your gross pay for taxes, insurance, and other fees. (2-3)

deep-fried—A dry cooking method in which foods are completely submerged in heated fat or oil at temperatures between 350°F and 375°F. (15-2)

deflate—To lose volume in dough. (29-2)

deglaze—To remove any leftover scraps of food from a pan; then add a small amount of hot water or stock and cook on top of the range. (15-3)

dehydrated—An item from which the water has been removed. (17-1)

dehydration—Fluid imbalance. (11-2)

demi glace—A concentrated brown stock that has been reduced. (24-3)

demitasse (DEHM-ee-tahs)—A half-size cup in which espresso is traditionally served. (3-3)

devein (dee-VANE)—To remove the intestinal tract of a shrimp. (22-2)

diabetes—An illness that affects the body's ability to convert blood sugar into energy. (12-2)

direct contamination—Contamination that occurs when raw foods, or the plants or animals from which they come, are exposed to toxins. (7-2)

direct labor—Wages paid to employees. (5-1)

direct marketing—A form of advertising in which materials, such as letters and advertisements, are mailed directly to customers. (5-4)

disability—A physical or mental impairment that substantially limits one or more major life activities. (6-2)

discrimination (dis-kri-muh-NAY-shun)—The unfair treatment of people based on age, race, gender, ethnicity, religion, physical appearance, disability, or other factors. (2-3, 6-2)

distractions—Things that turn your attention to something else; disrupt active listening. (2-1)

docking—The process of making small holes in the surface of an item before baking. (28-2)

double pan—To place a sheet pan inside a second pan of the same size to prevent burning the bottom or edges of cookies before they are done. (30-1)

dough—A mixture that contains less liquid than batters, making it easy to work with your hands. (27-2)

drained weight—The weight of a food product without the packing medium. (26-2)

drawn—Fish that have had their gills and entrails removed. (22-1)

dredging—To coat foods with flour or finely ground crumbs. (15-2)

dressed—Drawn fish with the fins, scales, and possibly the head removed. (22-1)

dressing—The sauce that holds a salad together. (18-2)

drip loss—The loss of moisture that occurs as fish thaws. (22-1)

drop batter—Batters that are so thick they need to be scraped or dropped from a portion or ice cream scoop to the cookware. (29-1)

drupes—Fruits with stones, such as peaches. (26-1)

dry cooking techniques—Cooking techniques that use a metal and the radiation of hot air, oil, or fat to transfer heat. (15-1)

E

edible portion (EP)—The consumable food product that remains after preparation. (14-1)

elastin—A hard, yellow tissue that doesn't break down during cooking. (24-1)

empathy (EHM-pah-thee)—The skill of putting yourself in another's place. (2-3)

emulsified shortening—A type of fat that helps create a smooth consistency throughout a mixture. (30-2)

emulsifier—An additive, such as egg yolk, that allows unmixable liquids, such as oil and water, to combine uniformly. (18-3)

en papillote (ahn pah-pee-yoa)—A method of steaming that involves wrapping fish or shellfish in parchment paper with vegetables, herbs, and sauces or butters. (22-3)

enriched rice—Rice that has a vitamin and mineral coating added to the grain. (25-2)

entrée (AHN-tray)—A main dish. (12-1)

entrepreneur (ahn-truh-pruh-NYOOR)—A self-motivated person who creates and runs a business. (1-4)

entry level—Beginning jobs that require little or no experience. (1-2)

ergonomics (URH-guh-nah-mihks)—The science concerned with the efficient and safe interaction between people and the things in their environment. (6-2)

escargot (ess-kahr-go)—The French name for snails. (22-2)

espresso (ess-PRESS-oh)—A beverage made by forcing hot water and steam through finely ground, dark-roasted coffee beans. (3-3)

ethics—Your internal guidelines for distinguishing right from wrong. (2-3)

ethylene (eh-THUH-lean) **gas**—An odorless, colorless gas that is emitted by most fruits as they ripen. (26-1)

evaporates—When moisture escapes into the air. (15-1)

extenders—Items made from leftover low-cost ingredients. (12-3)

extracts—Concentrated liquid flavors that contain alcohol, such as lemon and vanilla, that are used as flavorings. (16-1, 27-2)

F

fabricated cuts—Smaller, menu-sized portions of meat. (24-1)

factor method—A common pricing method for restaurants with successful past performance records in which the food cost percent is divided into 100%. The resulting factor is multi-plied by the cost of the menu item, giving the menu selling price. (12-4)

fat cap—The fat that surrounds an animal's muscle tissue. (24-1)

fermentation (FUR-mun-TAY-shun)—The process in which yeast breaks down sugars into carbon dioxide gas and alcohol, which are necessary for the rising process in products, such as bread. (27-2)

fermented—Chemically changed, such as pickles made from certain vegetables that are fermented in flavored and seasoned brines or vinegars. (16-3)

fillets—The sides of fish. (22-1)

fine-dining—Restaurants that offer an upscale atmosphere, excellent food and service, and higher menu prices. (1-2)

finger foods—Hors d'oeuvres presented on platters from which each guest serves him- or herself. (18-4)

First In, First Out (FIFO)—The system of rotating stock in which items that are stored first are used first. (8-3, 14-2)

fixed menu—A menu that offers the same dishes every day for a long period of time. (12-1)

flambé (flahm-BAY)—To "flame" an item tableside as part of the preparation. (4-1)

flammable—Materials that are quick-to-burn. (7-1)

flatware—Dining utensils, such as spoons, forks, and knives. (4-2)

flavor enhancers—Seasonings that increase the way you perceive a food's flavor without changing the actual flavor. (16-1)

flavorings—Ingredients that change the natural flavor of the foods they are added to. (16-1)

flexibility—The ability to adapt willingly to changing circumstances. (2-1)

flow of food—The path food takes from receiving to disposal where hazards can be controlled and dangers minimized. (8-2)

fluting—A manner of decorating crust by making uniform folds around the edge of a pie. (30-3)

focaccia (foh-CAH-chee-ah)—An Italian bread flavored with olive oil and herbs. (19-1)

focal point—A single service point from which the server serves all customers. (4-1)

fondue—French word meaning "to melt." Refers to cooking or dipping foods into a central heated pot. (26-1)

food court—Several quick-service restaurants gathered into a single area, such as found in a mall or shopping center. (4-1)

foodhandler—A worker who is in direct contact with food. (8-1)

forecast—Anticipating future business needs, such as what things will cost, how much money will be needed, what staffing needs there will be, and what profits will be expected. (5-1)

formula—A special type of recipe used in the bakeshop that includes the precise amount of each ingredient. (13-1, 27-1)

franchise—A common form of ownership used by chain restaurants in which a franchise company sells the business owner the rights to its name, logo, concept, and products. (1-4, 5-4)

free enterprise—System in which businesses or individuals may buy, sell, and set prices with little government control. (1-4)

freezer burn—The discoloration and dehydration of frozen food caused by moisture loss as a food freezes. (9-2, 22-1)

full-service—Restaurants in which servers take customer orders and then bring the food to the table. (1-2)

fumet (fyoo-MAY)—A fish stock with lemon juice or other acids added to the water. (20-1)

fungi (fun-GUY)—Microorganisms found in soil, plants, animals, water, and in the air. (7-2)

G

garde manger (gahrd mohn-ZHAY)—The person responsible for the planning, preparation, and artistic presentation of cold foods; also called the pantry chef. (1-1, 18-1)

garnish—To use food as an attractive decoration. It is something that should add real value to the dish, by increasing its nutritional value and visual appeal. Garnish comes from the French word "garnir" which means "to decorate or furnish." (18-1)

gelatinization (juh-la-tuhn-uh-ZAY-shuhn)—The process in which starch granules absorb moisture when placed in a liquid. (20-2)

genetically engineered—Foods made by recombining genes. (6-1)

genoise (zhen-WAHZ)—European sponge cake that can be the basis for special desserts, with layers of jam, chocolate, or fruit filling. (30-2)

glaze—A stock that is reduced and concentrated. (20-1)

gluten—A firm, elastic substance that affects the texture of baked products. (27-2)

glycogen (GLY-kuh-juhn)—A storage form of glucose. (11-2)

grading—Applying specific standards of quality to food products. (6-1)

grain—The direction of muscle fibers, or treads, in meat. (24-3)

H

HACCP—Or Hazard Analysis Critical Control Points; the system used by foodservice establishments to help ensure food safety. (8-2)

hand sanitizers—Special liquids that kill bacteria on your skin, often without the use of water. (8-1)

hand tools—Handheld items used in a foodservice operation to cook, serve, and prepare food. (10-2)

hard lean dough—A type of dough that consists of 0–1% fat and sugar. (28-1)

hazard—A source of danger. (7-2)

heat transfer—How efficiently heat passes from one object to another. (10-2)

heat treated—Glass that is heated and then cooled rapidly. (4-2)

Heimlich maneuver—A maneuver used to remove an object blocking a choking victim's airway. (7-1)

herbs—The leaves and stems of plants that are used as flavor builders. (16-1)

high-heat cooking—Cooking at high temperatures, which can toughen proteins and dry out meat if used incorrectly. (24-3)

highlighting—A sales technique for emphasizing a particular menu item. (3-2)

holding—The process in which food is prepared ahead of time, then placed in an appropriate location and kept warm until someone orders it. (8-3)

hominy—Dried corn soaked in lye so that the kernels become swollen. As they swell, the outer layers loosen and are easily removed. (25-2)

hors d'oeuvre (ohr-DURV)—Very small portions of food served before a meal. (4-1)

hors d'oeuvre variés—A combination of plated items with enough hors d'oeuvres for one person. (18-4)

human resources—The staff of a foodservice operation. (5-1)

hydrogenation (hy-DRAH-juh-NAY-shun)—A process in which hydrogen is added to polyunsaturated fats, such as soybean oil, which changes it into a solid fat. (11-1, 27-2)

I

independent restaurant—A restaurant that has one or more owners and is not affiliated with a national name or brand. (1-4)

indirect labor—Operation's costs for such things as employee health insurance, taxes, and vacations. (5-1)

infuse—To extract the flavors of a substance by placing it in a hot liquid. (3-3)

irradiated food—Food that has been exposed to radiation to kill harmful bacteria. (6-1)

irradiation—A type of processing that eliminates potentially harmful microorganisms and enhances food safety. (24-2)

issuing—The process of delivering foods from storage to the kitchen as needed for use. (14-2)

J

job interview—A formal meeting between you and your potential employer. (2-2)

job lead—A possible employment opportunity. (2-2)

julienne (ju-lee-en)—⅛-in.-thick matchstick-shaped cuts. (10-1)

K

kale—A cabbage with curly green or multicolored leaves. (18-2)

keywords—Significant words that make it easier for employers to search an electronic résumé database for relevant information. (2-2)

kneading—To work dough until it is smooth and elastic. (28-2)

L

labor union—An organization of workers in a similar field. (2-3)

laceration (LASS-uh-ray-shun)—A deep cut or tear in the skin, such as a knife wound. (7-1)

lacto vegetarians—Vegetarians who eat or drink some dairy products, such as cheese and milk, but don't eat eggs. (11-2)

lacto-ovo vegetarians—Vegetarians who include dairy products and eggs in their diets. (11-2)

larding—The process of inserting long, thin strips of fat or vegetables into the center of a lean meat. (24-1)

laws—Established rules that protect various groups of people from discrimination and ensure that workers are treated fairly. (6-2)

leach—Dissolve. (11-3)

leadership—The ability to motivate others to cooperate in accomplishing a common task. (2-1)

leavening agent—A substance that causes a baked good to rise by introducing carbon dioxide or other gases into the mixture. (27-2)

leavens (LEH-vuns)—Causes dough to rise as it fills with carbon dioxide bubbles. (28-1)

legumes (lay-GOOMS)—A group of plants that have double-seamed pods containing a single row of seeds. (11-1, 26-3)

let down—A condition in which the ingredients in a dough completely break down. (28-2)

liner—An ingredient on a canapé that adds visual interest and texture, such as a small lettuce leaf. (18-4)

lockout/tagout—An OSHA procedure that requires all necessary switches on electrical equipment to be locked out and tagged when they are malfunctioning. (7-1)

lowboy—A half-size refrigerator unit that fits under the counter in each individual work station. (9-2)

low-heat cooking—Cooking at low temperatures, which is the best method for preparing large cuts of meat. (24-3)

lugs—Boxes, crates, or baskets in which produce is shipped to market. Lugs often hold 25–40 lbs. of produce. (26-1)

M

mandoline—A hand-operated machine used for slicing vegetables and fruits, such as potatoes and apples. (26-2)

marbling—Fat within an animal's muscle tissue. (24-1)

market form—The form poultry is in when purchased. (23-1)

marketing—The process of promoting and supplying goods and services to customers. (1-4)

marketplace—The physical location, the people, and the atmosphere of a particular geographic area. (5-4)

markup-on-cost method—Method of determining a food's selling price in which the food cost of an item is divided by the desired food cost percent. (12-4)

material safety data sheets (MSDS)—Records that OSHA requires employers to keep identifying hazardous chemicals and their components. (6-1)

mealy—A type of potato with thick skin and starchy flesh. (26-2)

mentors—Employees who have a solid understanding of their jobs and help tutor or train new employees. (5-2)

menu—A listing of the food choices a restaurant offers for each meal. (12-1)

menu board—A hand-written or printed menu on a board on a wall or easel. (12-3)

meringue (muh-RANG)—A mixture of sugar and stiffly beaten egg whites. (30-3)

mesclun (MEHS-kluhn)—A mix of baby leaves of lettuces and other more flavorful greens, such as arugula. (18-2)

microwaves—Invisible waves of energy that cause water molecules to rub against each other and produce the heat that cooks food. (9-3)

minimum internal temperature—The lowest temperature at which foods can be safely cooked or stored; below this temperature, microorganisms can't be destroyed. (8-2)

minimum wage—The lowest hourly amount a worker can earn. (2-3)

mirepoix (meer-PWA)—A mixture of coarsely chopped vegetables and herbs. (20-1)

mise en place (meez ahn plahs)—A French term that means "to put in place." (9-1)

moist cooking techniques—Cooking techniques that use liquid instead of oil to create the heat energy needed to cook the food. (15-1)

molds—Pans with a distinctive shape, ranging from small, round, ceramic pans to long, narrow molds used for breads. (27-1)

mollusks—Shellfish that have no internal skeletal structure and have shells covering their soft bodies. (22-2)

monounsaturated—Fats, such as olive and peanut oils, that are usually liquid at room temperature. (11-1)

mother sauces—The five basic sauces: sauce espagnole, tomato sauce, béchamel sauce, velouté, hollandaise sauce; also called leading sauces. (20-2)

musculoskeletal (muhs-kyoo-loh-skEH-luh-tahl) **disorders**—Conditions, such as carpal tunnel syndrome, lower back pain, and tendinitis, that are caused by repeated trauma to muscles or bones. (6-2)

N

networking—Making use of all your personal connections to achieve your career goals. (2-2)

noncommercial operations—Operations, such as government facilities, schools, and hospitals, that aim to cover daily expenses such as wages and food costs. (1-2)

nonedibles—Nonfood products, such as cleaning materials, paper goods, and smallwares. (14-2)

nonperishable—A product that will not spoil quickly when stored correctly. (4-2)

nutrient-dense—Foods that are low in calories but rich in important nutrients. (11-2)

nutrients—Chemical compounds that help the body carry out its functions. (11-1)

O

opaque—Cloudy. (16-4)

open-spit roast—To place a food, usually meat, on a metal rod or a long skewer and slowly turn it over a heat source. (15-2)

orientation—The process of making a new employee familiar with a foodservice organization, its policies and procedures, and specific job duties. (5-2)

oven spring—The sudden rise and expansion of dough as the yeast reacts to the heat of the oven. (28-2)

overhead costs—All costs outside food and labor. (1-4)

overstaffing—Scheduling too many people to work on a given shift. (5-1)

ovo vegetarians—Vegetarians who include eggs in addition to foods from plant sources in their diets. (11-2)

P

packing medium—A liquid used to protect the food product. (26-2)

paella (pi-AY-yuh)—A Spanish rice dish with meat or shellfish. (16-2)

pan-fry—A method of cooking in which a moderate amount of fat is heated in a pan before adding food. (15-2)

panning—The process of placing shaped dough in the correct type of pan. (28-2)

parasites (PAR-uh-sights)—Microorganisms, such as protozoa, roundworms, and flatworms, that live in or on a host to survive. (7-2)

parboiled rice—Converted rice that has been partially cooked with steam and then dried. (25-2)

parboiling—A moist cooking technique in which foods are put into boiling water and partially cooked. (15-3)

Parisienne scoop—A melon baller with a scoop at each end, one larger than the other. (10-2)

parstock—The amount of stock needed to cover a facility from one delivery to the next. (14-2)

partnership—A legal association of two or more people who share the ownership of the business. (1-4)

pasteurized—Heating products at very high temperatures to destroy harmful bacteria. (8-3, 17-1)

patronage (PAY-truh-nij)—The support of customers. (3-1)

peel—A wooden board that a baker uses to slide breads onto an oven floor or hearth. (28-1)

periodic-ordering—A method for determining how much goods to purchase by establishing how much product will be used in a given time period. (14-2)

perishable (PEHR-ih-shuh-bul)—Products that can spoil quickly, even when stored correctly. (4-2, 8-3)

perpetual inventory—A continuously updated record of what's on hand for each item. (14-2)

pesto (PEH-stoh)—An uncooked sauce made of olive oil, pine nuts or walnuts, a hard cheese such as parmesan, and fresh basil, garlic, salt, and pepper. (19-1)

phyllo—A type of pastry that can be used to create sandwich wraps. (19-1)

physical inventory—A list of everything that an operation has on hand at one time. (14-2)

phytochemicals—Natural chemicals found in fruits, vegetables, grains, and dry beans that seem to have anti-cancer properties. (11-2, 26-1)

pigments—The matter in cells and tissue that gives them their color. (15-1)

pilaf method—A method of cooking grains in which the grain is sautéed in oil or butter before adding the liquid; also called braising. (25-2)

pith—The white membrane of a lemon. (16-1)

poaching—Cooking food in a flavorful liquid between 150°F and 185°F. (15-3)

polenta (po-LEN-tah)—A food made from cornmeal that is gradually sprinkled into simmering water or stock and cooked until it becomes a thick paste. (25-2)

polyunsaturated—Fats such as corn, sunflower, and soybean oils that are usually liquid at room temperature. (11-1)

porous—The ability of an egg to absorb flavors and odors through the shell and lose moisture even when the shell is unbroken. (17-1)

portion size—The amount or size of an individual serving. (13-1)

positioning—The way a foodservice operation presents itself to the community. (5-4)

positive reinforcement—Praising an employee when a job or task is done correctly. (5-2)

pound cake—A type of cake that serves as the basis for all layer cakes; contains a pound each of butter, flour, sugar, and eggs. (30-2)

pour batter—A batter that varies in consistency; some are so thin they can be poured from the mixing bowl to the cookware just like water. (29-1)

preferment—The process of removing a portion of dough, keeping it dormant for 8 to 24 hours, and then adding it to the next day's bread products. (28-2)

preprocessed—Legumes that have already been soaked, which means they will take less time to cook. (26-3)

preset—To set items on the table before food is served. (3-2)

preset menu—A meal served to a group of customers who have decided in advance on the menu and the time of service. (4-2)

pressure-frying—A frying method in which foods are cooked more quickly and at lower temperatures than other frying methods; foods are extra crispy on the outside with their natural juices sealed on the inside. (23-2)

primal cuts—Large, primary pieces of meat separated from the animal; sometimes called wholesale cuts. (24-1)

printed menus—Menus that are handed to customers as soon as they sit down. (12-3)

prioritize—To put things in order of importance. (2-1)

prix fixe (pree-feks) **menus**—Menus that offer a complete meal for a set price and allow the customer to choose one selection from each course offered by the restaurant. (12-1)

probation (pro-BAY-shun)—The time period on a new job that gives your employer a chance to monitor your job performance closely to confirm you can do the job. (2-3)

processed cheese—A combination of ripened and unripened cheese. (18-3)

processing—The act of changing pork by artificial means, such as curing, aging, and smoking. (24-2)

product yield—The amount of food product left after purchasing or preparation. (14-1)

profit and loss statement—A statement that shows exactly how money flows in a business; sometimes called an income statement. (5-1)

proofing—The fermentation stage that allows the leavening action of yeast to achieve its final strength before yeast cells are killed by hot oven temperatures. (28-2)

proofing cabinet—An enclosed, air-tight metal container with wheels that holds sheet pans of food and in which the temperature and humidity are controlled; also called a proofer. (9-4, 27-1)

proportion—The ratio of one food to another and to the plate. (12-2)

psychological pricing method—A pricing method based on how a customer reacts to menu prices that is used once the selling price of a menu item is determined. (12-4)

public relations—Publicity and advertising that a foodservice operation uses to enhance its image. (5-4)

publicity—Free or low-cost efforts of a facility to improve its image. (5-4)

Pullman—Rectangular loaves of sandwich bread with flat tops and even texture. (19-1)

pulses—The dried seeds of a legume. (26-3)

punching—The action of turning the sides of a dough into the middle and turning the dough over. (28-2)

puncture—A deep hole in the skin, often caused by a pointed object, such as an ice pick. (7-1)

purée (pur-RAY)—Food in which one or more of the ingredients have been ground in a food processor, mashed, strained, or finely chopped into a smooth pulp; a soup thickened by grinding its main ingredient in a food processor. (11-3, 20-2)

Q

quality control—A system that ensures that everything meets the foodservice establishment's standards. (13-1)

quenelle (kuh-NEHL)—A purée of chopped food formed into shapes. (18-1)

quick breads—A type of bread made from quick-acting leavening agents, such as baking powder. (17-3)

quick soak—To soak legumes for 1 hour in 212°F water. (26-3)

quick-service—Establishments that quickly provide a limited selection of food at low prices. (1-2)

R

radiation—Energy waves that cook food by transferring energy from the cooking equipment to the food. (9-3)

radicchio (rah-DEE-kee-oh)—A cabbagelike plant with a slightly bitter, red leaf. (18-2)

raft—A floating mass that forms from the mixture of meat and eggs in a consommé. The raft traps the impurities that rise to the top of the broth. (21-1)

ramekins (RAM-uh-kins)—Small ceramic bowls. (17-1)

range of motion—Using the fewest body movements without unnecessary stress or strain. (9-1)

ready-made breads—Breads that are made in advance and delivered to foodservice establishments. (17-1)

receiving—Accepting deliveries. (8-3)

receptors—Groups of cells that detect stimuli. (16-4)

recipe—A precise set of directions for using ingredients, procedures, and cooking instructions for a certain dish. (13-1)

recipe conversion—Changing a recipe to produce a new amount or yield. (13-2)

recovery time—The time it takes for fat or oil to return to the preset temperature after food has been submerged. (15-2)

reduction—The process of evaporating part of a stock's water through simmering or boiling. (20-1)

reel oven—An oven with shelves that move or rotate like a Ferris wheel; bakes a quantity of similar items evenly. (27-1)

regulations—Rules by which government agencies enforce minimum standards of quality. (6-1)

rehydrate—To add water into. (26-1)

relishes—Coarsely chopped or ground pickled items. (16-3)

repetitive stress injuries—The potentially disabling ailments that develop among workers who must perform the same motions repeatedly. (2-3)

requisition—An internal invoice that allows management to track the physical movement of inventory. (14-2)

résumé (REH-zuh-may)—A summary of your career objectives, work experience, job qualifications, education, and training. (2-2)

rind—The outer surface of cheese. (18-3)

rings—A type of container that has no bottom and is used to produce round or square breads or baked dessert items. (27-1)

ripening—The process during which the bacteria and mold in an unripened cheese alter its flavor and texture. (18-3)

risotto—A rice dish in which the grain has been sautéed in butter, and then simmered in a cooking liquid, which has been added gradually to the rice until it is finished cooking. (25-2)

risotto method—A cooking method in which grain is first sautéed; then a small amount of hot liquid—often a soup stock—is added. The grain is stirred until all the liquid is absorbed. This process of adding liquid and stirring the grain is continued until the grain is completely cooked. (25-2)

risotto Milanese (rih-SAW-toh MIH-lah-neez)—An Italian dish which includes rice sautéed in butter before adding stock. (16-2)

rivets—Metal pieces that fasten the blade to the knife handle. (10-1)

rolled-in fat yeast dough—A type of dough in which the fat is combined into the dough through a rolling and folding action. (28-1)

rondelle—Disk-shaped slices made from cylindrical fruits or vegetables such as cucumbers or carrots; also called round. (10-1)

roux (roo)—A cooked mixture made from equal parts of fat and flour by weight. (20-2)

RTC—Or ready-to-cook; the term refers to poultry purchased in parts. (23-1)

rumaki—Appetizers that consist of blanched bacon wrapped around vegetables, seafood, chicken liver, meat, poultry, or fruits. (21-2)

S

sachet—A cheesecloth bag that holds herbs. It is tied with butcher's twine and then submerged in liquids. (16-3)

salsa—A condiment made of chiles, tomatoes, onions, and cilantro. (16-4)

sanitary—Clean. (7-2)

sanitation—Healthy or clean and whole; healthy and sanitary conditions and effective sanitary practices. (7-2)

sanitizing (SA-nuh-tyze)—A procedure that involves reducing the number of microorganisms on a surface. (7-2)

saturated fats—Fat that is solid at room temperature, including items such as lard, butter, whole-milk products, the visible fat on meat, and tropical (coconut, palm, and palm kernel) oils. (11-1)

sauces—Flavored, thickened liquids. (20-2)

sautéing (saw-TAY-ing)—A quick, dry cooking technique that uses a small amount of fat or oil in a shallow pan. (15-2)

savory (SAY-vuh-ree)—Stimulating and full of flavor. (16-4)

scald—To heat a liquid to just below the boiling point. (30-4)

scaling—Weighing bakeshop ingredients. (27-1)

scones—A type of quick bread that is often cut into triangle shapes. (17-3)

seared—Quickly browned. (15-2)

seasonings—Ingredients that enhance without changing the natural flavor of food. (16-1)

section—A group of tables a service staff member is responsible for serving; also called a station. (3-1)

semi-à la carte menu—A menu in which the appetizers and desserts are priced separately, and the entrée likely includes a salad or soup, potato or rice, vegetable, and possibly a beverage. (12-1)

semiperishable—Perishable items that contain an inhibitor that slows down the chemical breakdown of the food. These products include smoked fish, processed meats, and pickled vegetables. (14-2)

semolina (seh-muh-LEE-nuh) **flour**—A hard-grain wheat flour that is high in the proteins that form gluten. (25-1)

sensory evaluation—The systematic tasting of food by consumers and foodservice professionals. (16-4)

sensory perception—How our ears, eyes, nose, mouth, and skin detect and evaluate our environment. (16-4)

serrated—Knife blade that is toothed like a saw to slice coarse foods, such as bread and cake, without tearing them. (10-1)

serviette—A folded napkin placed on a dinner or service plate used for carrying flatware. (4-2)

sexual harassment—Any unwelcome behavior of a sexual nature, such as unwelcome advances, requests for sexual favors, and other verbal or physical conduct of a sexual nature. (2-3, 6-2)

shaping—The process of forming dough into the distinctive shapes associated with yeast products. (28-2)

sheeter—A piece of equipment that rolls out large pieces of dough to a desired thickness. (27-1)

shirred—Eggs that are covered with cream or milk and sometimes bread crumbs. They are prepared in ramekins lined with a variety of ingredients. (17-2)

shortening—What solid fats are referred to in baking. (27-2)

shrinkage—The percentage of food lost during its storage and preparation; the loss of water in meat as it cooks. (13-2, 24-1)

shucked—An oyster that has had the meat removed from the shell. (22-2)

side work—Clearly defined duties that every service member has to perform before opening the dining room to the public. (4-2)

simmering—A moist cooking technique in which food is cooked slowly and steadily in a slightly cooler liquid that's heated from 185°F–200°F. (15-3)

single-food hors d'oeuvre—An hors d'oeuvre consisting of one food item, such as jumbo shrimp. (18-4)

slashing—Making shallow cuts in the surface of an item, done just before baking; also called stippling. (28-2)

smallwares—Hand tools, pots, and pans used for cooking. (10-2)

soft cookies—Cookies that have low amounts of fat and sugar in the batter, and a high proportion of liquid, such as eggs. (30-1)

soft medium dough—A type of dough that is elastic, tears easily, and produces items with a soft crumb and crust. (28-1)

solanine (SOH-luh-neen)—A toxin that turns potatoes green and is not destroyed by heat and doesn't dissolve in water. (26-2)

sole proprietorship (proh-PRI-uh-tor-ship)—When a business has only one owner. (1-4)

solid waste—Waste that includes packaging material, containers, and recyclables. (6-1)

sorbet (sor-BEY)—A frozen desert made up of fruit juices, sugar, and water. (30-4)

soufflés—Puffed egg dishes. (17-1)

sous (soo) **chef**—The "under" chef who reports to the executive chef. (1-1)

specification—Or spec; a written description of the products a foodservice operation needs to purchase. (14-1)

spices—Flavorings that blend with the natural flavor of foods. (16-1)

spoken menu—A list of available foods and the prices of each that the server states to the customer after he or she is seated. (12-3)

sponge cakes—Cakes that have an airy, light texture because of large amounts of air whipped into the eggs; also called foam cakes. (30-2)

spread—Expand. (30-1)

springform pan—A pan with a clamp that's used to release the pan's bottom from its circular wall; commonly used to bake cheesecakes. (27-1)

stack oven—A freestanding rectangular oven that has a series of well-insulated shelves stacked on top of one another; also known as a deck oven. (27-1)

staling—The process by which moisture is lost, causing a change in the texture and aroma of food. (27-2)

standardized (STAN-duhr-dyzed) **recipe**—A set of written instructions used to consistently prepare a known quantity and quality of a certain food for a foodservice operation. (13-1)

standards—Established models or examples used to compare quality. (6-1)

starter—A mixture of flour, yeast, sugar, and a warm liquid that begins the leavening action. (28-1)

station—A group of tables a service staff member is responsible for serving; also called a section. (3-1)

steam table—A piece of equipment that keeps prepared foods warm in serving lines; also called a food warmer. (9-4)

steaming—Cooking vegetables or other foods in a closed environment filled with steam, such as in a pot with a tight-fitting lid. (15-3)

stewing—A combination cooking technique in which food is seared and then completely covered with liquid during cooking. (15-3)

stimuli—Things that cause an activity or response. (16-4)

stir-frying—A dry cooking technique similar to sautéing that uses a wok, a large pan with sloping sides. (15-2)

stocks—The liquids that form the foundation of sauces and soups. (20-1)

storing—Placing food in a location for later use. (8-3)

surimi (soo-REE-mee)—A combination of different kinds of white fish and flavoring, formed into different shapes. (22-2)

sushi (SOO-shee)—A Japanese dish of raw, fresh fish or seafood wrapped in cooked and cooled rice, often with a layer of seaweed to hold it together. (22-3)

sweating—The process of cooking vegetables in fat over low heat to allow them to release moisture. (21-1)

sweet rich dough—A type of dough that incorporates up to 25% of both fat and sugar. (28-1)

T

table d'hôte (tah-buhl DOHT) **menu**—A menu that lists complete meals—everything from appetizers to desserts and sometimes beverages—for one set price. (12-1)

table tents—Daily specials written on folded cards that stand on the table. (12-3)

tableside—At the table. (4-1)

tang—The part of the blade that continues into the knife's handle. (10-1)

thickening agent—An ingredient, such as cornstarch, that adds body to a sauce. (20-2)

tournéed (toor-NAYD)—A type of cut that results in vegetables with an oblong shape, seven equal sides, and blunt ends; also called turned. (18-1)

toxins—Harmful organisms or substances. (7-2)

trade publications—Professional magazines and newsletters that are produced by and for members of the foodservice industry. (2-2)

translucent—Clear. (16-4)

trends—General developments or movements in a certain direction within an industry. (1-2)

trim loss—The by-product material trimmed from the purchased product. (14-1)

trueing—The process of using a steel to keep a knife blade straight and to smooth out any irregularities; after the knife has been sharpened. (10-1)

trussing—Tying the legs and wings against a bird's body to allow for even cooking and to create an attractive final product when served. (23-1)

tuber—The short, fleshy underground stems of plants. (26-2)

tunnels—Large, irregular holes. (29-1)

turnover rate—The average number of times a seat will be occupied during a given block of time. (5-3)

U

underliner—A dish placed under another dish to protect the table from spills. (3-2)

unit cost—The cost of each individual item. (14-1)

univalve (YOO-nih-valv)—A mollusk that has a single shell. (22-2)

upselling—A sales technique for suggesting a larger size or better quality than the customer's original order. (3-2)

V

vacuum packed—Food that has been placed in an airtight container from which the air has been removed to prevent the growth of bacteria. (22-1)

vegans (VEE-guns)—People who do not eat any meat or animal products. (11-2)

vegetarians—People who do not eat meat or other animal foods. (11-2)

vendor—A company that sells products to the foodservice industry. (1-1)

vichyssoise (vi-shee-SWAZ)—A cold version of potato-leek soup. (21-1)

volume—The amount of space that a substance occupies. (13-2)

volume measures—Devices used to measure liquids in food service. (13-2)

W

waxy—A type of potato with thin skin and less starch than a mealy potato. (26-2)

weight—A measurement that tells how heavy something is. (13-2)

whetstone—A sharpening stone used to keep knives sharp. (10-1)

whey—The liquid portion of coagulated milk. (18-3)

work ethic—A personal commitment to doing your very best as part of the workplace team. (2-1)

work flow—The orderly movement of food and staff through the kitchen. (9-1)

work sections—Larger work areas that contain groups of similar work stations. (9-1)

work simplification—Performing a task in the most efficient way possible. (9-1)

work station—A work area that contains the necessary tools and equipment to prepare certain types of foods. (9-1)

workers' compensation—The legal responsibility of your employer to provide financial help to cover medical expenses and lost wages if you're injured on the job and can't work. (2-3)

Y

yield—The number of servings, or portions, that a recipe produces. (13-1)

yield percentage—The ratio of the edible portion of food to the amount of food purchased. (14-1)

Z

zest—The rind of a lemon that can be used as a flavoring. (16-1)

zoning—The process of dividing land into sections used for different purposes, such as residential, business, and manufacturing. (1-4)

Credits

Cover and Interior Design:
Squarecrow Creative Group

Cover Photography:
Kevin May

Aero, 221
Amana, 217
Amerex, 161
Archive Photos, 443
Art MacDillo's, Gary Skillestad, 40, 42, 53, 61, 71, 73, 95, 96, 104, 105, 162, 170, 175, 197, 204, 205, 389, 456, 486, 488, 530, 587, 647
Articulate Graphics, 257
Artville, Burke/Triolo, 248, 256, 270, 309, 317, 321, 333, 342, 407, 472
The Broaster Company, 520
Bunn-O-Matic, 85, 87, 225, 226
Cambro Manufacturing Company, 211, 225, 226, 247, 249
Candle Corporation of America, 225
Cleveland Range/A Welbilt Company, 218
Ken Clubb, 102, 103, 106, 158, 165, 380, 664
Corbis, 143, 186, 404
  James L. Amos, 220, 493
  AFP, 137
  Bettman/Corbis, 269
  Owen Franken, 281, 521, 624
  Hulton-Deutsch, 28, 169, 368
  Gianni Dagli Orti, 237
  Premium Stock, 424
  Rob & Sas, 23
  Underwood & Underwood, 92
  Michael Yamashita, 18
Dairy Management Inc., 691
Daydots, 166, 171, 172, 188, 192, 456
The Delfield Co., 209
Detecto Scale, 247, 607
The Edlund Co., 214, 239
Envision
  Mark Ferri, 263
  Peter Johansky, 286

Lisa Koenig, 268
Rita Maas, 268
Madeline Polss, 23, 268
FCCLA, 45
Foodpix, 72
  Susan Marie Anderson, 393
  Batista Moon, 99, 337-338, 459
  Bill Boch, 365, 487, 573
  Susan Bourgoin, 365, 366, 367, 443, 497
  Matt Bowman, 8, 254, 487, 689
  Burke/Triolo Productions, 107, 255, 364, 365, 366, 369, 370, 388, 400, 429, 470, 492, 573, 580
  John Burwell, 410, 423, 497, 573
  Steve Cohen, 402, 431, 442, 480
  Carol Conway, 270, 365, 618
  Ross Durant, 573
  Eisenhut & Mayer, 9, 358, 573, 580
  Thomas Firak, 436
  Thomas Francisco, 499
  Eric Futran, 10, 668
  Brian Hagiwara, 364, 436, 480, 660
  Gentl & Hyers, 371
  Martin Jacobs, 503
  John Kelly, 357
  Susan Kinast, 589
  Katherine Kleinman, 361, 367, 370, 571
  Alan Krosnick, 10, 652
  Scott Lanza, 383, 588
  Brian Leatart, 414
  Randy Mayor, 475
  Maximilian Stock, 365, 366, 370, 371, 423, 485, 487
  Alison Miksch, 397, 573
  Jan Oswald, 369, 422, 423, 438
  Scott Payne, 14-15
  Joe Pellegrini, 363
  Penina, 423, 438
  Christina Peters, 422, 487, 497, 676
  Judd Pilossof, 404
  Michael Pohuski, 9, 387, 468

Paul Poplis, 388, 422, 436, 457, 501, 573, 658
Kathryn Russell, 426, 430
Jeremy Samuelson, 200-201
Doug Schneider, 265
Laszlo Selly, 421
Scott Sims, 392, 470, 479
Rick Souders, 401
Eric Stampfli, 409
Ann Stratton, 436, 469, 653
Mark Thomas, 423
Sally Ullman, 422, 438, 475, 573
Jackson Vereen, 388, 455
Fountain Products, Inc., 566
FPG
  Ron Chapple, 86
  Spencer Jones, 7, 66
  Carlos Spaventa, 90
  Jonelle Weaver, 8, 278
David R. Frazier Photolibrary
  David R. Frazier, 25, 93, 131, 134, 136, 289, 290
  David Spaulding, 7, 140
Friedr Dick Corporation, 231, 233, 239, 241, 242, 243, 412, 413, 535
Tim Fuller, 266
Eric Futran, 7, 9, 10, 30, 31, 44, 49, 62, 67, 73, 79, 90, 92, 100, 101, 114, 121, 126, 148, 172, 212, 322, 334, 335, 338, 408, 495, 502, 600, 601, 602-603, 604, 630, 696, 697
Garland/A Welbilt Company, 206, 219, 610
Ann Garvin, 8, 9, 20, 21, 24, 27, 29, 35, 41, 46, 47, 58, 59, 68, 69, 71, 74, 76, 77, 78, 81, 84, 94, 98, 115, 116, 117, 118, 121, 122, 124, 125, 130, 132, 144, 145, 150, 151, 154, 156, 158, 161, 162, 164, 173, 176, 177, 178, 179, 180, 181, 182, 189, 193, 202, 203, 208, 215, 216, 220, 223, 230, 242, 243, 244, 245, 247, 249, 250, 271, 272, 273, 275, 279, 298, 299,

Index